Principles of
RHEUMATIC DISEASES

Principles of
RHEUMATIC DISEASES

Edited by

Richard S. Panush

University of Florida College of Medicine
Veterans Administration Medical Center
Gainesville, Florida

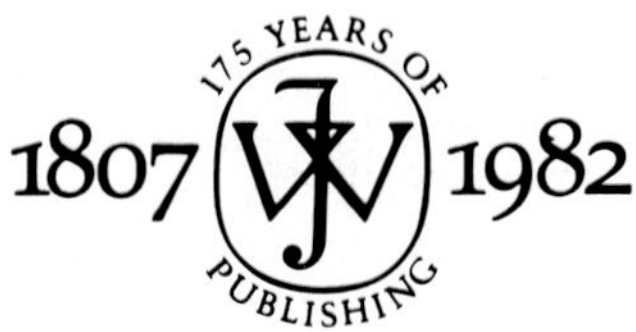

A WILEY MEDICAL PUBLICATION
JOHN WILEY & SONS / **New York • Chichester • Brisbane • Toronto**

Library of Congress Cataloging in Publication Data:

Main entry under title:

Principles of rheumatic diseases.

  (A Wiley medical publication)
  Includes index.
  1. Rheumatism—Immunological aspects.
I. Panush, Richard S. II. Series: Wiley medical
publication. [DNLM: 1. Rheumatism. 2. Arthritis.

WE 544 P957]
RC927.P68 616.7′23 81-1951
ISBN 0-471-05198-5 AACR2

Contributors

Roy D. Altman, M.D.
Professor
College of Medicine, University of Miami
Chief, Arthritis Division
Veterans Administration Medical Center
Miami, Florida

Merrill D. Benson, M.D.
Professor
Indiana University School of Medicine
Chief, Rheumatology Section
Veterans Administration Medical Center
Indianapolis, Indiana

Eric P. Brestel, M.D.
Assistant Professor
Section of Allergy and Clinical Immunology
College of Medicine, West Virginia University
Morgantown, West Virginia

Jacques R. Caldwell, M.D.
Clinical Associate Professor
Division of Clinical Immunology
College of Medicine, University of Florida
Gainesville, Florida

Andrei Calin, M.D., M.R.C.P.
Assistant Professor
Stanford University Medical Center
Director, Rheumatology Division
Veterans Administration Medical Center
Palo Alto, California

Lourdes C. Corman, M.D.
Assistant Professor
Divisions of Clinical Immunology and General Medicine
College of Medicine, University of Florida
Gainesville, Florida

Norman A. Cummings, M.D.
Professor
Chief, Division of Clinical Immunology and Connective
    Tissue Disease
Director, Arthritis Center
College of Medicine, University of Louisville
Louisville, Kentucky

Jeffrey C. Delafuente, M.S.
Assistant Professor
Department of Clinical Pharmacy
St. Louis College of Pharmacy, and
    Division of Allergy and Immunology
St. Louis University School of Medicine
St. Louis, Missouri

Andrea Dlesk, M.D.
Postdoctoral Fellow
Division of Clinical Immunology
College of Medicine, University of Florida
Gainesville, Florida

Bernard F. Germain, M.D.
Associate Professor
Director, Division of Rheumatology
College of Medicine, University of South Florida
Tampa, Florida

Norman L. Gottlieb, M.D.
Professor
Division of Rheumatology
College of Medicine, University of Miami
Miami, Florida

Robert G. Gray, M.D.
Clinical Assistant Professor
Division of Rheumatology
College of Medicine, Tufts University
Bay State Medical Center
Springfield, Massachusetts

Terry M. Hudson, M.D.
Associate Professor
Department of Radiology
College of Medicine, University of Florida
Gainesville, Florida

Jean M. Jackson, M.D.
Instructor
School of Medicine, Harvard University
Brigham and Women's Hospital
Boston, Massachusetts

J. Douglas Lee, M.D.
Section of Infectious Diseases
Department of Medicine
Marshfield Clinic
Marshfield, Wisconsin

Martha K. Lee, M.D.
Section of Rheumatology
Department of Medicine
Marshfield Clinic
Marshfield, Wisconsin

Selden Longley, M.D.
Associate Professor
Division of Clinical Immunology
College of Medicine, University of Florida
Assistant Chief, Medical Service
Veterans Administration Medical Center
Gainesville, Florida

Thomas A. Medsger, Jr., M.D.
Associate Professor
Division of Rheumatology and Clinical Immunology
College of Medicine, University of Pittsburgh
Pittsburgh, Pennsylvania

Arthur Mendelow, M.D.
Former Assistant Professor
Department of Orthopedic Surgery
College of Medicine, University of Florida
Veterans Administration Medical Center
Gainesville, Florida

Richard S. Panush, M.D.
Associate Professor
Chief, Division of Clinical Immunology
College of Medicine, University of Florida
Chief, Clinical Immunology Section
Veterans Administration Medical Center
Gainesville, Florida

Robert J. Quinet, M.D.
Section of Rheumatology
Ochsner Clinic
New Orleans, Louisiana

John S. Sergent, M.D.
Clinical Associate Professor
Division of Rheumatology
College of Medicine, Vanderbilt University
Nashville, Tennessee

Stanford T. Shulman, M.D.
Professor of Pediatrics
Northwestern University Medical School
Chief, Division of Infectious Disease
The Children's Memorial Hospital
Chicago, Illinois

Gerald H. Stein, M.D.
Assistant Professor
Division of Clinical Immunology
College of Medicine, University of Florida
Gainesville, Florida

John B. Winfield, M.D.
Professor
Chief, Division of Rheumatology and Immunology
School of Medicine, University of North Carolina
Chapel Hill, North Carolina

Michael Yaron, M.D.
Senior Lecturer
School of Medicine, Tel Aviv University
Head, Arthritis Research Unit and
    Department of Rheumatology and Physical Medicine
Ichilov Medical Center
Tel Aviv, Israel

Preface

Rheumatic diseases afflict large numbers of people and cause enormous suffering and disability. They constitute a fascinating group of nearly 200 diverse conditions that present stimulating challenges to the practicing clinician and the medical researcher. Rheumatic diseases range from the mundane, such as bursitis or osteoarthritis, to the esoteric, such as systemic lupus erythematosus, and reflect a complex array of biochemical and immunologic disturbances. Indeed, unraveling the pathogenesis of certain rheumatic disease has advanced our understanding of many basic biochemical and immunologic events—such as purine metabolism, immunoregulation, and the inflammatory response.

It is hoped that this book will communicate to readers some of the excitement of studying the rheumatic diseases. We have attempted to present basic concepts in clinical rheumatology, emphasizing pathogenetic and immunologic aspects of disease. The text is logically organized into sections relating to "Study of Rheumatic Diseases," "Immunology and Inflammation," "Rheumatoid Arthritis and Related Conditions," "Systemic Rheumatic Diseases," "Degenerative and Metabolic Diseases," and "Nonarticular Rheumatism." We hope this book will be of interest to practicing physicians and house staff, as well as medical and postgraduate students.

Richard S. Panush

Acknowledgments

I am grateful to many persons who helped in the preparation of this book. I learned much from the contributors, all of whom generously gave of their time and knowledge. My colleagues, Drs. Andrea Dlesk, Lourdes C. Corman, Paul Katz, Gerald H. Stein, and Selden Longley, helped substantially in compiling this volume. Preparation of the text would not have been possible without the efforts of many people in the office, particularly the superb assistance of Mrs. Alice W. Cullu. And finally, I am indebted to my parents and family, who have always supported my studies in medicine.

Financial support from the Veterans Administration and the Florida Chapter, Arthritis Foundation, helped sustain many of the activities of our unit, including preparation of this book.

Richard S. Panush

Contents

Part 5   DEGENERATIVE AND METABOLIC DISEASES

Part 6   NONARTICULAR RHEUMATISM

Principles of
RHEUMATIC DISEASES

Part 1

STUDY OF RHEUMATIC DISEASES

1

Structure and Function of Connective Tissue, Joints, and Synovial Fluid

Michael Yaron

Rheumatic diseases are among the great enemies of humanity. The ultimate goal of conquering these afflictions will depend on a better understanding of their etiology. Progress has been made during the past two decades in understanding the pathogenesis of rheumatic diseases, but much remains to be done. The pathologic processes of the rheumatic diseases occur in the connective tissue (joints and synovial fluid are specialized components of connective tissue). A basic understanding of connective tissue structure and function is necessary for dealing with the alterations that occur when a rheumatic disease intervenes.

CONNECTIVE TISSUE

Connective tissue is a diffuse organ system that provides support and protective covering of the body and its internal organs. It originates in the differentiation of embryonic mesoderm. Seventy percent of the wet weight of the body is of mesenchymal derivation. Connective tissue consists of cartilage, bone, tendons and their sheaths, ligaments, and fascia and forms the major substance of joints, dermis, bursae, and blood vessels. Nutrition to organs and their metabolic wastes must traverse the connective tissue. Inflammatory reactions in response to foreign materials, immunologic processes, or trauma occur in connective tissue.

Classification

Connective tissue may be of a fibrous type, cartilage, or bone. Fibrous connective tissue may be subdivided into loose and dense types. Connective tissue is composed of cells, ground substance, and fibrillar material. The principal cellular components of connective tissue are the fibroblast, chondrocyte, and osteocyte. These cells are responsible for the production of glycosaminoglycans (acid mucopolysaccharides), which are a major component of connective tissue ground substance. They also produce collagen, elastin, and reticulin, which are the fibrillar components of connective tissue. Specificity of connective tissue is determined by the type of parent cell (fibroblast, chondrocyte, osteocyte), the type of glycosaminoglycans in the ground substance, and the type, structure, and relative amount of fibrillar material. Lymphocytes, plasma cells, neutrophilic and eosinophilic leukocytes, histiocytes, and mast cells are additional cells found in connective tissue.

Cellular Elements

Fibroblasts are elongated cells with an ovoid nucleus. Their abundant cytoplasm contains ribosomes, polyribosomes, and rough endoplasmic reticulum, which take a basophilic stain with hematoxylin and eosin dye. Tropocollagen and proteoglycans accumulate before secretion in the smooth endoplasmic reticulum related to the Golgi apparatus. Pathologic accumulation of metachromatic glycosaminoglycans in cultured fibroblasts may be a diagnostic tool for the recognition of some inherited disorders of connective tissue. Mitochondria and, less frequently, lysosomes are also present in the fibroblast. Chondrocytes and osteocytes are specialized variants of fibroblasts that are responsible for the formation and maintenance of cartilage and bone, respectively.

Fibrillar Elements

Collagen

Collagen is the main fibrillar component of connective tissue. It represents about one-third of the total body protein. Collagen is widely distributed in the body and is the major component of tendons, fascia, ligaments, and dermis. It is a fibrous protein with a high tensile strength and is easily denatured by acid, alkali, or heat. The individual molecule of collagen (the collagen monomer) is called *tropocollagen*. The molecular weight of tropocollagen is about 300,000. The molecule is composed of three long polypeptide chains (α chains) consisting of approximately 1,000 amino acids each. They are wound together in the form of a triple helix stabilized by intramolecular hydrogen bonds as well as covalent cross links. The presence of three amino acids is characteristic of the collagen molecule; glycine, proline, and hydroxyproline constitute more than one-half of the collagen residues. Every third amino acid in the collagen polypeptide chain is glycine. The tropocollagen triple helix molecule contains three of the following chain types: $\alpha_1(I)$, $\alpha_1(II)$, $\alpha_1(III)$, $\alpha_1(IV)$, and α_2. The composition of different types of tropocollagen in different types of connective tissue is shown in Table 1.1.

The biosynthesis of collagen involves polypeptide synthesis, hydroxylation of proline and lysine residues, carbohydrate addition, extracellular aggregation into fibrils, and development of cross links. Polypeptide synthesis occurs on polyribosome aggregates of the endoplasmic reticulum in connective tissue cells. Ascorbic acid, molecular oxygen, and ferrous iron are needed for postribosomal hydroxylation of proline and lysine residues. The precursor transport form of collagen across the connective tissue cell membrane is a triple helix named *procollagen*. Extracellular removal of peptide extensions on the NH_2 terminal end of procollagen by a specific peptidase permits fiber formation. The cross linking of

Table 1.1. Composition of Tropocollagen in Different Types of Connective Tissue

Type	Chain Composition	Organ
I	$[\alpha 1\ (I)]_2\ \alpha 2$ (The only vertebrate collagen containing a mixture of two different α-chains)	Synovium Tendon Bone Adult skin Annulus fibrosus of intervertebral disc (periphery)
II	$[\alpha 1\ (II)]_3$	Articular cartilage Osteoid Epiphyseal growth plate Annulus fibrosus of intervertebral disc (center)
III	$[\alpha 1\ (III)]_3$	Synovium Fetal skin Vascular tissue
IV	$[\alpha 1\ (IV)]_3$	Basement membranes of renal glomerulus and lens capsule

collagen fibers depends upon the formation of aldehyde groups resulting from the deamination of lysine and hydroxylysine.

Reticulin Fibers

Reticulin fibers are closely associated with the deeper parts of basement membranes. They are also found around blood vessels and muscle fibers and in the parenchyma of solid organs, such as the kidney, spleen, and liver. Reticulin fibers are considered a form of collagen. They contain glycoprotein, retain silver after impregnation (argyrophilia), and react positively with the periodic acid-Schiff staining technique.

Elastic Fibers

Elastic material in the form of fibers and lamellae is found in arteries, ligaments, cartilage, lungs, and bronchi. It is formed from two morphologically distinct components: a central "amorphous" material made of protein elastin and a microfibrillar component made of a glycoprotein rich in cysteine. As in collagen, glycine occupies every third site on the polypeptide chain of elastin. In contrast to collagen, elastin contains only 1% hydroxyproline and no hydroxylysine. Some of the physical properties of elastin may be related to the presence of the unusual amino acids desmosine and isodesmosine. Elastic material synthesis may be impaired by copper deficiency or chelating agents since desmosine and isodesmosine synthesis requires a copper-dependent amine oxidase. In inflammatory disorders such as polyarteritis nodosa, elastic material located in the vascular wall may be destroyed by granulocyte elastase.

Ground Substance

The space between cells and fibers of connective tissue is occupied by an amorphous material, the ground substance. Proteoglycans are the principal compo-

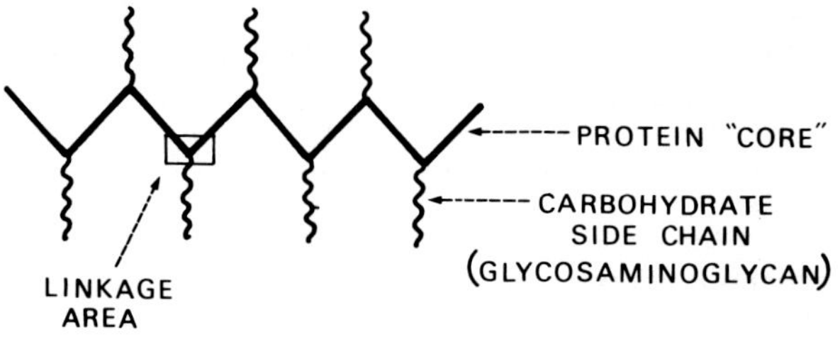

PROTEIN "CORE"

CARBOHYDRATE
SIDE CHAIN
(GLYCOSAMINOGLYCAN)

LINKAGE
AREA

Figure 1.1. Schematic representation of a proteoglycan.

nent of connective tissue ground substance, but they may also occur in certain cell granules, such as heparin in mast cells and chondroitin-4 sulfate in granulocytes. They are macromolecules consisting of a protein core to which glycosaminoglycan side chains are attached (Fig. 1.1). Many of the physical and chemical properties of connective tissue ground substances are due to their proteoglycan component(s). The proteoglycans may differ in their core protein as well as in their glycosaminoglycan side chains. Different glycosaminoglycans are found in different types of connective tissue. Synovial fluid and vitreous humor contain hyaluronic acid as virtually the sole glycosaminoglycan. Cartilage ground substance possesses chondroitin sulfate A and C and keratan sulfate, while chondroitin sulfate A is the major glycosaminoglycan constituent of adult bone.

Glycosaminoglycans are polymers of repeating groups of a hexosamine linked to a hexuronic acid. Keratosulfate is an exception, being a polymer of a hexosamine linked to a hexose (D-galactose) and not to a hexuronic acid. The glycosaminoglycan side chains are attached to the protein core by a glycosidic bond to the hydroxyl group of serine in the protein chain. The presence of a large number of polyanionic groups on the glycosaminoglycan molecule is responsible for several properties: Glycosaminoglycans may be precipitated from solution with polyvalent cations with which they form insoluble complexes (counterion binding); they react with polycationic dyes, such as toluidine blue or alcian blue, to display metachromasia; they behave as gels avidly binding water; and the anionic groups exclude other molecules from their "domain" (excluded volume properties). The glycosaminoglycans are highly viscous in solution, possibly explaining the soft tissue lubricant action of hyaluronate in synovial fluid.

In addition to proteoglycans, the ground substance of connective tissue also contains proteins derived mainly from the plasma. As much as 50% or more of the plasma albumin can be found in the ground substance of connective tissue.

CONNECTIVE TISSUE METABOLISM AND PHYSIOLOGY

We are just beginning to understand the physiology of connective tissue. Important contributions have been made in this field in the past few years, and a number of regulators of connective tissue metabolism are already known (Table 1.2). Further progress in this area may eventually lead to the control of pathologic processes occurring in connective tissue.

Regulators of connective tissue metabolism may affect connective tissue cell growth, synthesis, and degradation of ground substance and fibrillar components

Table 1.2. Some Regulators of Connective Tissue Metabolism

Hormones: Growth hormone, thyroxine, androgens, estrogens, adrenal corticosteroids
Drugs: Steroidal and nonsteroidal anti-inflammatory drugs, penicillamine
Osteoclast activating factor (OAF)
Connective tissue activating peptides (CTAP I, II, III)
Prostaglandins
Mononuclear cell factors
Ascorbic acid
Copper

of connective tissue. Castor has described and defined factors capable of stimulating connective tissue cell growth as well as the production of glycosaminoglycans and sulfate incorporation into glycosaminoglycans. These factors are termed *connective tissue-activating peptides (CTAP)*. Polypeptides capable of inducing connective tissue activation were found in lymphocytes, platelets, fibroblasts, and other cells. Prostaglandins, which have emerged as one of the principal mediators of the inflammatory process, may also play a major role in the regulation of connective tissue metabolism. Prostaglandins stimulate glycosaminoglycan synthesis in cultured human connective tissue cells. Connective tissue-activating peptides stimulate prostaglandin E_2 secretion by human fibroblasts. Factors derived from human mononuclear cells stimulate prostaglandin E_2 and collagenase production by cultured fibroblasts and have an inhibitory effect on their growth and collagen synthesis. Prostaglandin $F_{2\alpha}$-stimulated mouse fibroblast growth and its effect were potentiated by insulin. On the other hand, prostaglandin E_2 was found to have an inhibitory effect on dermal and synovial fibroblast growth in culture. An interferon inducer, polyinosinic-polycytidylic acid, or interferon itself stimulates both glycosaminoglycan and prostaglandin E_2 by human fibroblasts. It was therefore suggested that inflammation induced by viruses may be mediated by interferon and prostaglandins. Anti-inflammatory drugs inhibit prostaglandin E synthesis by human connective tissue cells. Stimulation of prostaglandin E and glycosaminoglycan synthesis induced in fibroblast cultures by connective tissue-activating peptides, human mononuclear cell factor(s), polyinosinic-polycytidylic acid, and interferon are also inhibited by steroidal and nonsteroidal anti-inflammatory drugs. Prostaglandins were found to stimulate bone resorption by rheumatoid synovia and may therefore play an important role in the bone destruction in rheumatoid arthritis. A stimulator of osteoclastic resorption of bone was found in supernates of stimulated human peripheral leukocytes and was named *osteoclast-activating factor (OAF)*. Collagenase is another important factor that may participate in joint destruction, alone or together with other proteinases present in different types of connective tissue, as shown in Table 1.3. Elevation of temperature may significantly affect the connective tissue activation process as well as collagenase activity; therefore it may be inadvisable to use deep heat on an inflamed joint.

Growth hormone, thyroxine, androgens, estrogens, and adrenal corticosteroids have all been implicated in the regulation of connective tissue metabolism. Cor-

Table 1.3. Articular Proteinases

	Matrix Compound Degraded			Enzyme Localization		
	Proteoglycan	Collagen	Elastin	Subcellular	Cellular[a]	Tissue
Cathepsin B	++	+	−	Lysosomes	C, F, M	Cartilage, synovium
Cathepsin D	++	−	−	Lysosomes	C, F, M	Cartilage, synovium
Cathepsin F	++	−	−	Membrane?	C	Cartilage
Cathepsin G	++	−	−	Azurophil granules	P	Synovial fluid
Elastase	++	++	++	Azurophil granules	P	Synovial fluid
Collagenase	−	++	−	?	F?, M	Synovium, synovial fluid
Metalloproteinase	++	−	−	?	F?, M	Synovium

[a] P, polymorphonuclear leukocytes; C, chondrocytes; F, fibroblasts; M, macrophages.

ticosteroids inhibit prostaglandin, hyaluronic acid, and collagen synthesis by connective tissue cells. They also may affect the connective tissue cell proliferation rate; their effect in this respect may differ substantially when different concentrations are used. Ascorbic acid may stimulate both hyaluronic acid and collagen synthesis in culture and, being a co-factor in the enzymatic hydroxylation of proline and lysine, it may be the cause of the damaged connective tissue in scurvy. Copper deficiency may cause the production of defective elastin, and penicillamine may inhibit and damage the cross linking of collagen and elastin molecules.

JOINTS

The connection area between rigid parts of the skeleton, either bones or cartilages, is termed a *joint*. Joints are made up of connective tissue. The composition of the joint connective tissue depends on the joint type. There are two main joint types: (1) joints with a cavity in which movement takes place, called *diarthroses* or *synovial joints* (e.g., the knee), and (2) joints without a cavity, with little or no movement, called *synarthroses*. Synarthroses may be subdivided into (a) fibrous joints (*syndesmoses*), such as the tibiofibular articulation, where bones are united by interosseous ligaments, (b) cartilaginous joints (*synchondroses*), such as the joint between the epiphyses and bodies of long bones, where the connecting medium is cartilage that eventually is converted into bone before adult life, (c) fibrocartilaginous joints (*symphyses*), such as the joints between the pubic bones and the vertebral bodies, where hyaline cartilage, fibrocartilage, and fibrous tissue contribute to the connection, and (d) bony joints (*synostoses*), such as in the adult skull sutures, where only a thin layer of fibrous tissue separates the indentating bony articulation.

Synovial (Diarthrodial) Joints

Joint Cavity and Membrane

Joint cavity formation begins at approximately 8 weeks of gestation. Synovial tissue arises from the primordial skeletal blastema. Flattened superficial cells facing the primitive joint cavity represent the early synovial intimal cells. Synovial joints (Fig. 1.2) permit different degrees of movement of the articulating bones. The extent of movement depends on the type of synovial joint (plane, hinge, condylar, ball and socket, ellipsoidal, pivot, or saddle joints). The articular surfaces of bone are covered with cartilage, usually of the hyaline type. A joint capsule and ligaments unite the articulating bones.

The synovial membrane is a vascular connective tissue that lines the inner surface of the joint capsule and ends at the margin of the articular cartilage. The synovial membrane produces the main components of synovial fluid and regulates its composition. The adult synovial membrane is not a continuous structure and lacks a basement membrane. It consists of an intimal layer of specialized connective tissue cells (synoviocytes) forming a loose layer, one to four cells in depth. Synovial cells are usually elongated and frequently exhibit long processes extending into the joint cavity. Electron microscopic studies of the intimal cell layer suggest that two primary cell types are present: a type A cell rich in phagocytic vacuoles, lysosomes, mitochondria, and filopodia, which appears to be involved in phagocytic activity, and a type B cell with an abundant endoplasmic reticulum, fewer vacuoles and vesicles, and smaller mitochondria, which appears to be involved in the synthesis of hyaluronate-protein of synovial fluid. Intermediate types of cells have also been described. The intimal synovial cells are embedded in a reticulin network. The subintimal layer of synovial tissue may be loose, fatty, or fibrofatty and contains types I and III collagen fibers. Mast cells, endothelial cells, macrophages, mesenchymal cells in the vascular adventitia, and unclassified connective tissue cells with a fibroblastic appearance are found in the subintimal layer of the synovial membrane.

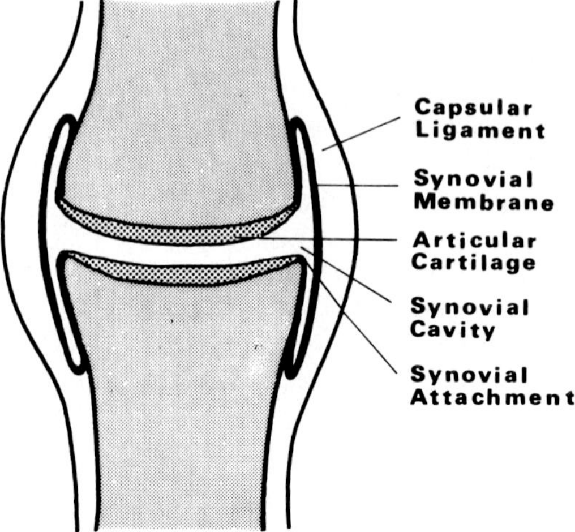

Figure 1.2. Schematic representation of a typical diarthrodial joint.

The synovial membrane is supplied by a rich network of blood and lymphatic vessels. Arteriovenous anastomoses are present, and shunting of blood circulation via these anastomoses is possible. Blood and lymph vessels are close to the joint cavity; substances from the blood diffuse into the synovial cavity, and vice versa.

Nerve endings found in the synovial tissue are usually the ones that accompany blood vessels and are part of the autonomic nervous system. The synovial membrane usually does not transmit stimuli of pain.

Cartilage

Normal articular cartilage is usually avascular and derives most of its nutrition from the synovial fluid. Some of its nutrition may come by diffusion from blood vessels in the underlying bony end plate and from the capillaries in the arterial circle at the periphery of the joint. The surface of normal articular cartilage is by no means smooth and consists of different sizes of undulations (primary, secondary, tertiary, and quaternary ridges) that play an important role in "squeezing" the synovial fluid and its nutrition into the cartilage. Articular cartilage is a connective tissue characterized by sparsity of connective tissue cells (chondrocytes) and by abundant ground substance.

Chondrocytes replicate until full growth has been attained, and then their replication rate slows down. There is evidence that replacement of articular cartilage may occur and that cartilage growth is involved in remodeling of adult joints after injury. Chondrocytes possess glycolytic, oxidative phosphorylation, cytochrome oxygenation, alkaline phosphatase, and lipase activity and are responsible for the production of ground substance and fibrillar components of cartilage. The abundant ground substance of normal cartilage is composed of water (about 70% of weight), electrolytes, protein, and glycosaminoglycans.

The hard and at the same time elastic properties of articular cartilage are due to the composition of its ground substance, especially to the glycosaminoglycan constituent. Chondroitin-4 sulfate (chondroitin sulfate A), chondroitin-6 sulfate (chondroitin sulfate C), keratan sulfate, and smaller amounts of chondroitin and hyaluronic acid are the glycosaminoglycan components of articular cartilage. With aging, the degree of polymerization of cartilage glycosaminoglycan decreases and the sulfate content increases. The relative amount of keratan sulfate increases with age, and at the same time the concentration of chondroitin sulfate A and water decreases. Articular cartilage stiffness and strength depend upon the structure and orientation of its collagen fibers. Collagen fibers constitute about one-half of the dry cartilage weight and are of type II $[\alpha 1 \ (II]_3$ (Table 1.1). Recent electron microscopic studies have shown dense interlacing bundles of collagen fibers lying parallel to the surface of the articular cartilage. This large amount of interlacing collagen fibers provides a strong and elastic surface mat and contains little proteoglycan. On the other hand, the articular matrix has a much larger relative proportion of proteoglycan in which collagen fibers are arranged at random. The cartilage area close to the bone end may be calcified to varying degrees.

Capsule and Ligaments

Joint capsule and ligaments are usually composed of irregularly arranged bundles of collagen fibers. Only in a few joints (e.g., those of the middle ear) are the joint capsule and ligaments composed almost entirely of elastic fibers. The capsule and ligaments possess proprioceptive nerve endings sensitive to position and movement and contain sensory fibers sensitive to twisting and stretching. The capsule and ligaments, unlike the synovial membrane, are highly sensitive to pain stimuli.

Lubrication

Joint lubrication plays an important role in reducing friction and thus joint wear. The structure and physical properties of opposing cartilage surfaces, the load applied on the joint, and the properties of the lubricant (synovial fluid) are the major factors in joint lubrication. Recent studies have shown that a glycoprotein fraction and not the hyaluronate protein complex may play a major role in joint lubrication. According to these studies, a glycoprotein is the major lubricant in fluid between opposing cartilage surfaces, while hyaluronate lubricates only the nonweight-bearing surfaces of the marginal synovial tissue. It is reasonable to believe that different forms of lubrication are important in different circumstances. For example, at high loads, boundary lubrication may play a key role, while when loading is sudden, squeeze-film lubrication is important. The special structure of cartilage and synovial fluid allows for synovial fluid to be squeezed into the cartilage when trapped by a load and by the undulations on the articulating cartilage surfaces. When pressure subsides, the fluid returns from the cartilage to the joint cavity. This type of lubrication is named *weeping lubrication,* and it probably also plays an important role in certain circumstances. The lubricating mechanisms of human joints are so effective that they bring the coefficient of friction during movement to values lower than that of ice sliding on ice. Improper lubricating mechanisms are related to joint pathology (see Chap. 24).

Synovial Fluid

In the sixteenth century, Paracelsus described the presence of a viscous, pale yellow, clear fluid in diarthrodial joints. Since it resembled egg white, he named it *synovia*. The synovial fluid is a dialysate of the blood plasma to which hyaluronate produced by synovial cells has been added. The ability of a blood plasma component to enter the synovial fluid usually depends on its molecular weight and size as well as on the permeability of the synovial blood vessels. It therefore appears that the synovial tissue acts as a semipermeable membrane, the properties of which may be altered by pathologic processes such as the ones resulting in inflammation. Synovial fluid may also be regarded as a specialized liquid ground substance of connective tissue in which the major glycosaminoglycan present is hyaluronic acid. Hyaluronate is a polymer with an estimated molecular weight range of 2 to 3×10^6, composed of equimolar proportions of glucosamine and glucuronic acid. The hyaluronate molecules are long linear interlacing chains that randomly coil and kink on themselves and are responsible for the viscosity of synovial fluid. The concentration of hyaluronate in normal joints is about 3.5 mg per g of fluid. During joint inflammation accompanied by a pathologic accumulation of synovial fluid, the hyaluronate molecular weight and concentration decrease. Because the amount of synovial fluid is much greater in an inflammatory effusion, the total amount of hyaluronic acid found in the joint space is significantly increased. When acetic acid is added to diluted synovial fluid, a precipitate composed of albumin and hyaluronate results. This precipitate is called a *mucin clot*. During inflammatory processes the mucin clot breaks easily. While the stable, unbreakable mucin clot in normal and noninflammatory synovial effusions is considered excellent or good, the one found in inflammatory fluids, which does not form a stable clot and breaks easily into smaller pieces, is regarded as poor. A poor mucin clot is one of the criteria for the diagnosis of rheumatoid arthritis (Table 10.1), although it may be found in other inflammatory joint diseases as well.

Normal synovial fluid does not contain fibrinogen and therefore does not clot in a test tube. Inflammatory synovial fluids do contain fibrinogen and will therefore clot in the test tube if an anticoagulant is not added. Normal synovial fluid is clear and contains only a small number of cells, most of them mononuclear (Table 1.4). During inflammatory or degenerative processes the amount of leuko-

Table 1.4. Normal Synovial Fluid

	Range	*Average*
Amount in knee, cc	0.13–3.5	1.1
pH	7.2–7.77	7.4
Leukocyte count, per cu mm	13–180	63
Polymorphonuclears, percent	0–25	6.5
Lymphocytes, percent	0–78	24.6
Monocytes, percent	0–71	47.9
Clasmocytes, percent	0–26	10.1
Unclassified phagocytes, percent	0–21	4.9
Synovial lining cells, percent	0–12	4.3
Total protein (g per 100 cc)	1.07–2.13	1.72
Albumin (g per 100 cc)		1.02
Globulin (g per 100 cc)		0.05
Immunoglobulins (mg per 100 cc)		
IgG	290–1200	490
IgA	30–290	110
IgM	6–110	43
a_2-Macroglobulin (mg per 100 cc)	22–175	81
Transferrin (mg per 100 cc)	44–202	107
Pyrophosphate (μm)	2.2–5	3.6
Cholesterol (mg per 100 cc)	21–23	22
Fibrinogen	0	0
Glucose	Approximately the same as in plasma	
Nonprotein nitrogen	Approximately the same as in plasma	
Electrolytes	Approximately the same as in plasma	
Uric acid	Approximately the same as in plasma	

Adapted from Jessar RA: The Study of Synovial Fluid, in JL Hollander and AJ McCarty, Jr, (ed): Arthritis and Allied Conditions. Lea & Febiger, 1972, Ch. 6.

cytes increases, and their number and polymorphonuclear percentage are proportional to the inflammatory activity. Inflamed joint fluid is cloudy. During inflammation there is also an increase in the protein and concentration of acute phase reactants. Glucose concentration is often decreased and can be very low in septic arthritis (Chap. 21). In normal synovial fluid most of the protein (60%–75%) is albumin. With the change of synovial membrane permeability during inflammation, there is an increase in the synovial fluid protein (mostly globulin) concentration that finds little access to normal synovial fluid because of its relatively high molecular weight. Electrolytes and other small molecules that pass easily through the synovial membrane are distributed in the normal synovial fluid in accordance with the Donnan theory of equilibrium across a semipermeable membrane. They will therefore be found in synovial fluid in concentrations similar to but slightly lower than those in serum. Cholesterol and pyrophosphate are also present in normal synovial fluid and may precipitate in certain pathologic processes. Concentrations of copper, iron, and aluminum have been reported to be increased in rheumatoid synovial effusions. The following enzymatic activities have been described in synovial fluid: beta glucuronidase, hyaluronidase, pepsin, trypsin, amylase, lipase, peroxidase, transaminase, alkaline, and acid phosphatase. These and other enzymes found in inflammatory synovial fluid, such as collagenase, may play an important role in the pathologic changes occurring in joint diseases. These enzymes may significantly change their level of activity with the changes in joint temperature occurring during inflammation. An important finding is the relatively low concentrations of complement in rheumatoid joint effusions. This finding and the occurrence of crystals in pathologic joint effusions will be dealt with in more detail in other chapters (Chaps. 3, 10, 25–27).

BIBLIOGRAPHY

Castor CW: Connective tissue activation: IV. Regulatory effects of antirheumatic drugs. *Arthritis Rheum* 15:504, 1972.

Castor CW: Connective tissue activation: VII. Evidence supporting a role for prostaglandins and cyclic nucleotides. *J Lab Clin Med* 85:392, 1975.

Castor CW: Synovial cell activation induced by a polypeptide mediator. *Ann NY Acad Sci* 256:304, 1975.

Castor CW: The physiology of the synovial cell and its contribution to disease processes, in Holt PJL (ed): *Current Topics in Connective Tissue Diseases*. Edinburgh, London, and New York, Churchill Livingstone, 1975, p 1.

Castor CW, Whitney SL: Connective tissue activation: XIII. Stimulation of sulfated glycosaminoglycan synthesis in human connective tissue cells by peptide mediators from lymphocytes and platelets. *J Lab Clin Med* 91:811, 1978.

Castor CW, Yaron M: Connective tissue activation: VIII. The effects of temperature studies in vitro. *Arch Phys Med Rehabil* 57:5, 1976.

Dayer JM, Krane SM: PGE_2 modulates collagenase production by cultured adherent rheumatoid synovial cells. *Arthritis Rheum* 21:552, 1978.

Dayer JM, Krane SM, Russel RGG, et al: Production of collagenase and prostaglandins by isolated adherent rheumatoid cells. *Proc Natl Acad Sci USA* 73:945, 1976.

Dayer JM, Robinson DR, Krane SM: Prostaglandin production by rheumatoid synovial cells: Stimulation by a factor from human mononuclear cells. *J Exp Med* 145:1399, 1977.

Dingle JT: Articular damage in arthritis and its control. *Ann Intern Med* 88:821, 1978.

Hamerman D, Rosenberg LC, Schubert M: Diarthrodial joints revisited. *J Bone Joint Surg* 52-A:725, 1970.

Harris ED Jr, Evanson JM, DiBona DR, et al: Collagenase and rheumatoid arthritis. *Arthritis Rheum* 13:83, 1970.

Harris ED Jr, McCroskey PA: Influence of temperature and fibril stability on degradation of cartilage collagen by rheumatoid synovial collagenase. *N Engl J Med* 290:1, 1974.

Holt PJL: Joint cartilage: Physiology and changes in arthritis, in Holt PJL (ed): *Current Topics in Connective Tissue Diseases.* Edinburgh, London, and New York, Churchill Livingstone, 1975, p 24.

Korn JH, Halushka PV, LeRoy EC: Suppression of growth and the phenotypic expression of fibroblasts by peripheral blood mononuclear cell supernatants: A role for prostaglandins. *Arthritis Rheum* 21:571, 1978.

Luben RA, Mundy GR, Trummel CL, et al: Partial purification of osteoclast-activating factor from phytohemagglutinin-stimulated human leukocytes. *J Clin Invest* 53:1473, 1974.

McDuffie FC: Synovial fluid components and characteristics, in Altman PL, Katz DD (eds): *Human Health and Diseases* (Biological Handbooks II). Bethesda, Md, Federation of American Societies for Experimental Biology, 1977, p 218.

Radin EL, Ehrlich MM, Weiss CA, et al: Osteoarthrosis as a state of altered physiology, in Buchanan WW, Dick WC (eds): *Recent Advances in Rheumatology,* Edinburgh, London, and New York, Churchill Livingstone, 1976, p 1.

Robinson DR, McGuire MB, Levine L: Prostaglandins in rheumatic diseases. *Ann NY Acad Sci* 256:318, 1975.

Robinson DR, Tashjian AH, Levine L: Prostaglandin stimulated bone resorption by rheumatoid synovia. *J Clin Invest* 56:1181, 1975.

Yaron M, Castor CW: Leukocyte connective tissue cell interaction. I. Stimulation of hyaluronate synthesis by live and dead leukocytes. *Arthritis Rheum* 12:365, 1969.

Yaron M, Yaron I, Allalouf D: Effect of some anti-inflammatory drugs on fibroblast-leukocyte interaction in vitro. *Ann Rheum Dis* 30:613, 1971.

Yaron M, Yaron I, Wiletzki Ch, et al: Interrelationship between stimulation of prostaglandin E and hyaluronate production by Poly (I) Poly (C) and interferon in synovial fibroblast culture. *Arthritis Rheum* 21:694, 1978.

2

Evaluation of Patients with Rheumatic Disease

Richard S. Panush

IMPORTANCE OF THE RHEUMATIC DISEASES

Rheumatic diseases have an enormous impact on the population of this nation. They cause the greatest disability of any group of diseases. More than 97% of all Americans over the age of 60 have radiologically detectable joint abnormalities. At least 50 million persons have some type of clinical arthritis, which is severe enough in 20 million to require medical care. Of these, an estimated 5 million have rheumatoid arthritis, 12 million have osteoarthritis, and the remainder have other rheumatic diseases. The cost to the country's economy, in terms of health care, disability, and lost work days, is staggering. Musculoskeletal diseases are the most prevalent cause of chronic disability and represent the second most frequent class of complaints made by patients to practicing physicians (Table 2.1).

Medical education and awareness of rheumatic diseases have been inadequate. Many medical schools have had no organized rheumatic disease unit. A recent survey showed that five states did not have a practicing rheumatologist. The American Rheumatism Association comprises approximately 3,200 physicians, of whom about 600 are board-certified rheumatologists, and many of these devote only a small portion of their time to clinical rheumatology. American Rheumatism Association members have an average of fewer than 400 patients each. Thus only about 3% of patients with rheumatic disease are cared for by rheumatologists (Table 2.1). The situation is unlikely to change significantly in the immediate future. Therefore, if patients with rheumatic disease are to receive adequate medical care, all physicians should have some familiarity with their problems.

It is perplexing that the rheumatologic history and physical examination have not excited greater interest among physicians, because problems presented by patients with rheumatic disease can be among the most challenging and satisfying in medicine. Studies of certain rheumatic diseases with immunologic features have been at the forefront of advances in clinical immunology. This work has significantly advanced our understanding of immunologic mechanisms of inflammation.

The musculoskeletal complaints presented by a patient can often be assessed immediately by the skilled physician through interview and examination. Be-

Table 2.1. Importance of Rheumatic Diseases in the U.S. Population

Prevalence
50 million with arthritis
20 million require care
12 million with osteoarthritis
5 million with rheumatoid arthritis
Human cost
Most prevalent cause of disability
Second leading complaint to physicians
$> \$4$ billion annual cost
Health care
$\sim$ 3,200 American Rheumatism Association members
$\sim$ 600 board-certified rheumatologists
$\sim$ 400 patients per rheumatologist's practice
$\sim$ Five states without rheumatologists

cause the musculoskeletal system is largely accessible and amenable to direct evaluation, in many instances additional and prolonged laboratory tests are unnecessary to establish a diagnosis. Thus many patients can be effectively managed in the office, which provides a satisfaction not always appreciated in other areas of medicine. Most patients with rheumatic diseases suffer chronic disability rather than acute, life-threatening problems. Therapeutic interventions that seem modest often translate into major functional benefits and greatly enhance the quality of the patient's life. Moreover, a proper diagnosis of rheumatic disease is necessary to preclude inappropriate use of therapeutic agents because many rheumatologic medications are potentially hazardous and should not be used unless clearly indicated.

RHEUMATOLOGIC HISTORY

History of the Present Illness

One of the first priorities when encountering patients with musculoskeletal complaints is to identify the organ system involved (Table 2.2). Indeed, not all pa-

Table 2.2. Rheumatologic History: Identification of the System Involved

Articular
Muscular
Neurologic
Vascular
Endocrinologic
Metabolic
Systemic
Nonarticular

Table 2.3. Rheumatologic History: Description of Articular Symptoms

---

Onset: gradual, insidious, abrupt
Character: progressive, remittent, exacerbating
Type of joint: large, small, axial, peripheral
Symmetry versus asymmetry
Type of symptom: pain, stiffness, swelling, erythema, warmth, loss of motion, additive, duration, relation to activity, intensity, time of day
External factors affecting symptoms
Functional abilities: activities of daily living

---

tients complaining of such symptoms have articular problems. In our practice we often see patients who appear with rheumatologic complaints yet have non-articular rheumatism, primary muscular disease, primary neurologic disease (peripheral neuropathies, compressive neuropathies, diabetic neuropathy, alcoholic neuropathy), vascular disease (thromboangiitis obliterans, arterial disease), endocrinologic or metabolic disease (diabetes mellitus, pernicious anemia with neuropathy, thyroid or parathyroid disease), or other systemic diseases (sarcoidosis, dysproteinemias, malignancy). The apparent complaint should be carefully delineated so that these possibilities are not overlooked.

Having determined that the patient's findings are articular, the physician should clarify whether the onset of illness was gradual, insidious, or abrupt (Table 2.3). It is also important to determine the duration and character of the illness—progressive, remittent, or exacerbating; frequency of remissions and exacerbations; and duration and intensity of remissions and exacerbations. Next, the specific symptoms need to be recognized. Which joints are involved—large, small, peripheral, or axial, and with or without symmetry? How are these symptoms manifested? Does the patient have difficulty walking, climbing, writing, eating, washing? The time of day of maximal symptoms is another important feature. Are symptoms most prominent in the morning and alleviated with activity, or do they tend to occur after activity and be most pronounced at the end of the day? Are they worse or better at night? With activity? With rest? Are there any discernible factors that ameliorate or aggravate symptoms, such as climate, temperature, environmental factors, heat, cold, or humidity? Are there any other factors relating to symptoms, such as intercurrent infection, occupation, environmental exposure, or drug use or abuse? Of course, the patient's age and sex will have been recorded. All of this information characterizes the nature of the patient's complaints adequately. Many of these factors are significant in the differential diagnosis of various types of rheumatic diseases, as will be stressed in the chapters dealing with individual diseases.

Review of Systems

A complete review of systems must be obtained, with particular attention to phenomena in other organ systems associated with rheumatic disease (Table 2.4). These phenomena include the headaches associated with temporal arteritis. Ocular symptoms of conjunctivitis, scleritis, and iritis may occur in certain systemic

Table 2.4. Rheumatologic History: Certain Associated Prenomena

---

Skin: photosensitivity, psoriasis, purpura, erythema nodosum, nodules, vasculitis, alopecia
Neuromuscular: neuropathies, headaches, myopathies
Ocular: conjunctivitis, scleritis, iritis, sicca complex
Gastrointestinal: xerostomia, ulcers, peptic ulcers, dysphagia, liver disease, colitis, diarrhea
Renal: stone, nephritis, urethritis
Pulmonary: pleuritis, infiltrates, nodules
Cardiovascular: pericarditis, hypertension, Raynaud's phenomenon, aortic insufficiency
Hematologic: adenopathy, splenomegaly
Constitutional: weight loss, fatigue, malaise, fever, chills

---

rheumatic diseases (rheumatoid arthritis and its variants), and keratoconjunctivitis sicca may occur in Sjögren's syndrome. Other visual changes may be noted in association with temporal arteritis. The cutaneous findings of psoriasis, purpura, erythema nodosum, vasculitis, and nodules should also be sought. Neurologic changes associated with the neuropathies of vasculitis, rheumatoid arthritis, and Sjögren's syndrome and the myopathies associated with systemic lupus erythematosus, scleroderma, and mixed connective tissue disease need also be appreciated. An array of gastrointestinal symptoms is found with certain rheumatic diseases: dry mouth with Sjögren's syndrome; ulcers with Behcet's syndrome, Reiter's disease, or lupus; dysphagia with inflammatory myositis; liver disease with systemic rheumatic disease; and colitis or diarrhea or both with Behcet's syndrome and Reiter's disease. Nephritis is usually associated with such systemic rheumatic diseases as lupus or vasculitis, urethritis with Reiter's disease, genital ulcers with Behcet's syndrome, and balanitis circinata with Reiter's disease. Pulmonary symptoms, such as interstitial fibrosis, pulmonary hypertension, pleurisy, infiltrates, and nodules, occur with certain systemic rheumatic diseases. Cardiovascular symptoms, such as pericarditis, hypertension, Raynaud's phenomenon, and aortic insufficiency, are seen with systemic rheumatic disease and rheumatoid arthritis and its variants. Adenopathy and splenomegaly frequently accompany the same disorders. Although this listing is, of necessity, brief, careful attention to all these possibilities is required for a complete history. Many of the specific associations will be covered in subsequent chapters.

Family History

A family history of any rheumatic disorder is an important consideration (Table 2.5). Many diseases, including gout, pseudogout, spondylarthritis, and osteoarthritis, as well as instances of rheumatoid arthritis, systemic lupus erythematosus, and scleroderma, occur in families.

Past Medical History

The therapeutic history of the patient is particularly important (Table 2.6). Drugs (birth control pills, antibiotics, diuretics, procainamide, hydralazine, anticonvulsants, amphetamines, or antihypertensives) can be identified that might have

Table 2.5. Rheumatologic History:
Other Features

Family history
Age, sex, race, ethnic background
Geographic history
Drug usage
Infectious exposure
Occupation, injuries, trauma
Socioeconomic status

---

precipitated or aggravated symptoms. All drugs that have been used to treat the patient's symptoms should be reviewed: aspirin, substituted salicylates, other non-steroidal anti-inflammatory agents (naproxen, ibuprofen, indomethacin, tolmetin, fenoprofen, sulindac), analgesics (acetaminophen, propoxyphene, ethoheptazine), oral or intra-articular corticosteroids, and other antirheumatic agents (gold salts, *d*-penicillamine, antimalarial or immunosuppressive agents). The duration, dose, effectiveness, and any adverse effects of drug therapy should be assessed. It is important to learn whether the patient has had any orthopedic procedures, physical therapy, or occupational therapy and whether any benefit was realized. It is useful to inquire about any pending litigation or compensation involved, to help assess if there is possible secondary gain from symptoms or disability.

Socioeconomic History

The physician should discern the functional capabilities of patients with musculoskeletal disease. Can they perform normal activities of daily living, including self-care (bathing, dressing, eating, toilet use), housework, and occupation (Table 2.5)? Does the patient have a hectic household to maintain? Does the economic standard of the patient's family depend on his or her ability to perform physical labor? What assistance does the patient receive in performing these various tasks?

Table 2.6. Rheumatologic History: Therapeutic History

Drugs that may precipitate or aggravate symptoms
    Birth control pills, antibiotics, diuretics, procainamide, hydralazine, methamphetamines, anticonvulsants, others
Drugs used for symptomatic relief
    Nonsteroidal anti-inflammatory drugs (aspirin, phenylbutazone, indomethacin, ibuprofen, fenoprofen tolmetin, naproxen, sulindac, meclofenamate)
    Analgesics (acetaminophen, propoxyphene)
    Steroids (oral and intra-articular)
    Antirheumatic (gold salts, antimalarials, *d*-penicillamine)
    Immunosuppressives
Duration, dosage, effectiveness, and toxicity of drugs
Surgical procedures
Physical and occupational therapy

Moreover, formulating a long-term therapeutic program usually necessitates questioning the patient about economic status and ability to sustain the family, as well as about health insurance and the cost of health care. If an occupation may have directly caused or exacerbated the symptoms, a change of job should be contemplated.

PHYSICAL EXAMINATION

The rheumatologic examination should be systematically incorporated into the general physical evaluation of patients (Table 2.7). Some have found it useful to begin by examining the patient's gait; evaluating the hands, wrists, elbows, and shoulders; then the head, eyes, ears, nose, throat, and neck; cardiopulmonary and abdominal examinations; evaluating the hips, knees, ankles, feet, and spine; and the neurologic examination. As in taking the history, it is important to search for extra-articular abnormalities that are often associated with rheumatic diseases.

It is not possible in this discussion to catalog all abnormalities and their clinical significance. However, certain abnormalities can be highlighted (Table 2.7). As the patient enters the room, the examiner should note the gait and ability to walk and carry out basic activities.

Examination of the hands includes observing the nails and joints, noting clubbing, rash, palmar erythema, tendons, and grip strength. Each joint, whenever possible, is assessed for the presence of erythema, warmth, tenderness at rest or during active or passive motion, range of active and passive motion, presence and quantitation of deformities, instability, swelling, crepitation, and palpable

Table 2.7. Rheumatologic Examination: Procedure

Gait: walking, activity
Hands: nails, clubbing, rash, palms, tendons, grip strength, individual joints
Wrists: carpal tunnel syndrome, neuropathy, tenosynovitis
Elbows: nodules, tophi, bursitis
Shoulders: glenohumeral joint, bursitis, tendinitis, capsulitis, acromioclavicular and sternoclavicular joints
Head: temporomandibular joint, hair, scalp, temporal artery, thyroid gland, tophi, cervical spine, head, eyes, ears, nose, throat
Pulmonary: pleuritis
Cardiac: pericarditis, aortic insufficiency
Abdominal: hepatomegaly, splenomegaly
Hips: bursitis, tendinitis, leg lengths
Knees: bursitis, stability, popliteal cysts, atrophy
Ankles: Achilles tendinitis, nodules, subtalar joint
Foot: tarsals, metatarsophalangeal joints, toes, nails
Spine: posture, motion, tenderness, measurements
Neurologic: neuropathy, myopathy

Table 2.8. Rheumatologic Examination: Joint
Assessment

Erythema
Warmth
Tenderness: rest, active and passive motion
Range of active and passive motion
Deformity
Instability
Swelling: synovial effusion, proliferation, or both
Crepitation
Rubs

or auscultatory rubs (Table 2.8). Distal and proximal interphalangeal joints are examined for range of motion, synovitis, cartilaginous or bony proliferation (Heberden's and Bouchard's nodes at the distal and proximal interphalangeal joints, respectively), and subluxation. Synovitis is usually felt by gentle ballottement of an effusion or synovial swelling. Cartilaginous or osteophytic proliferation is a hard, immobile swelling. With care and experience, one can readily identify subtle abnormalities. Motion, synovitis, and alignment of metacarpophalangeal joints are similarly evaluated.

At the wrists, one should look for tendinitis, dorsal or volar synovitis, carpal tunnel syndrome, or other neuropathies. The carpometacarpal and carpal, radiocarpal, and radioulnar joints of the wrist are examined as outlined (Table 2.8).

In the elbows, nodules, tophi, bursitis, and tendinitis should be sought. Synovitis of the elbow can be detected between the lateral epicondyle and olecranon process. This condition can be distinguished from tenderness at the medial or lateral epicondyles (epicondylitis) and olecranon bursitis, which occurs posterior to the olecranon process.

At the shoulder, the glenohumeral joint and periarticular structures should be examined for bursitis and tendinitis. The acromioclavicular and sternoclavicular joints are also evaluated at this time. Swelling of the shoulder is best perceived anteriorly. It is often difficult to differentiate between glenohumeral and periarticular abnormalities.

While examining the head, the physician should consider the temporomandibular joints, hair, scalp, temporal artery, thyroid gland, and auricle, the presence or absence of tophi, and the cervical spine. Particular attention should be given to motion and tenderness of the spine and tenderness or spasm of muscles.

During the cardiopulmonary examination, one listens particularly for rubs, effusions, or aortic insufficiency. The abdominal evaluation includes palpation for the presence of hepatomegaly or splenomegaly.

The examiner should determine the range of motion of the hip and look for bursitis or tendinitis in extra-articular areas. Flexion contractures are detected by holding one hip in complete flexion and then determining the extension of the other.

Similarly, one should not only manipulate the knee but also search for popliteal cysts and periarticular bursitis and tendinitis. Examination of the knee includes the evaluations listed in Table 2.8 as well as a determination of stability. Cruciate ligament stability is gauged by moving the tibia anteriorly and posteriorly with the femur fixed. Collateral ligaments are appraised by lateral and medial motion of the tibia. Swelling is usually felt in the suprapatellar area, medially or laterally.

At the ankle, both the talonavicular joint and the subtalar joint should be examined. True ankle synovitis is usually anterior and is reflected in the loss of flexion and extension. Subtalar disease limits inversion and eversion. Achilles tendinitis, tendon nodules, and periarticular abnormalities are perceived. Attention should be given to tarsals, metatarsophalangeal joints, toes, and nails of the feet. These joints and the small joints of the hand are examined in a similar fashion. Compressive or distal neuropathy is to be considered.

Posture, motion, tenderness, and quantitation of motion of the spine should be scrutinized. Measuring chest expansion may be useful. Lumbar motion is quantitated by the Shober test—measuring the distance between the fifth lumbar vertebra and a spot 10 cm superior to it (normal $\geq$ 4 cm). Paravertebral muscular tenderness and spasm should be assessed. Sacroiliac joint tenderness should also be determined. Neurologic examination should consider the presence of mononeuritis multiplex and distal and compressive neuropathies. The skin should be searched for nodules, dermatitis, purpura, alopecia, telangiectasia, muscosal lesions, or evidence of cutaneous vasculitis or vasospastic phenomena.

DIAGNOSTIC STUDIES

Diagnostic studies are discussed in detail in Chapters 3 and 4. In general, a careful history and physical examination of patients should provide the examiner with a fairly clear impression of the nature of the patient's illness. Depending on the clinical impression and differential diagnosis, certain other studies can be ordered (Table 2.9). In general, a complete blood count (including differential and platelet counts), erythrocyte sedimentation rate, urinalysis, and chest x-ray films are useful. In addition, x-ray films of the affected joints, tests for rheumatoid factors, antinuclear antibodies, "muscle enzymes" (creatine phosphokinase, glutamic oxalic transaminase, and lactic dehydrogenase), and serum uric acid, and analysis of synovial fluid are often helpful. A thorough rheumatologic his-

Table 2.9. Rheumatologic Evaluation: Generally
Useful Diagnostic Studies

Complete blood count and differential count
Erythrocyte sedimentation rate (Westergren method)
Urinalysis
Serum uric acid
Rheumatoid factors test
Antinuclear antibodies test
Synovial fluid analysis
Radiographs of selected affected joints

tory and physical examination will serve to reduce the number of expensive ancillary studies to those immediately pertinent.

ASSESSMENT

The interview, examination, and certain additional studies will usually confirm the rheumatologic diagnosis. This is a satisfying experience not only for the patient but also for the physician. Goethe's statement "Was Man weiss Man sieht" ("What one knows, one sees") is particularly applicable to the patient with rheumatic disease.

It is not enough, however, merely to establish a diagnosis. Since the patient usually has musculoskeletal disease and since the goal of therapy is to maintain the physical and financial independence of the patient, it is mandatory to reach a functional assessment. This is done, when appropriate, by determining the anatomic stage of disease, functional classification, and presence or absence of active disease as well as by carefully reviewing the patient's functional abilities and needs. Although developed for patients with rheumatoid arthritis, certain guidelines are useful for many other patients (see Chap. 10). Briefly, patients are classed I–IV depending on their functional abilities. Class I reflects complete functional ability; class II patients carry out normal activities adequately; class III patients are limited; and class IV patients are largely incapacitated. Patients can be "staged" depending on the progression of anatomic disease. By radiologic and clinical criteria, stage I patients have an early, mild form of the disease; stage II, moderate; stage III, severe; and stage IV, terminal. Patients are considered to have active disease when three of the four following criteria are met: Westergren erythrocyte sedimentation rate > 28 mm/hr, morning stiffness exceeding 45 minutes, six tender joints, or three swollen joints. All of these observations are considered in determining an optimal therapeutic program for each patient.

BIBLIOGRAPHY

Arthritis Foundation: *Arthritis. The Basic Facts.* Atlanta, 1976.

Arthritis Foundation: *Professional Manpower in Rheumatology.* New York/Atlanta, 1973.

Beetham WP, Polley HF, Slocumb CH, Weaver WF: *Physical Examination of Joints.* Philadelphia, WB Saunders Co, 1965.

Bilka PJ: Physical examination of the arthritic patient. *Bull Rheum Dis* 20:596, 1970.

Polley HF, Hunder GG: *Rheumatologic Interviewing and Physical Examination of the Joints,* ed 2. Philadelphia, WB Saunders Co, 1978.

Reynolds MD: Prevalence of rheumatic diseases as causes of disability and complaints by ambulatory patients. *Arthritis Rheum* 21:377, 1978.

Rodnan GP: Growth and development of rheumatology in the United States—A bicentennial report. *Arthritis Rheum* 20:1149, 1977.

3
Synovial Fluid Analysis

John S. Sergent

ASPIRATION OF SYNOVIAL FLUID

Indications and Contraindications

The possibility of infection in a joint is an absolute indication for synovial fluid aspiration. In addition, synovial fluid examination is necessary to establish a diagnosis of gout or pseudogout and is frequently helpful in establishing a diagnosis in chronic arthritis, including rheumatoid arthritis, osteoarthritis, and others. Finally, aspiration of synovial fluid is indicated for certain therapeutic considerations. In pyogenic arthritis, repeated aspirations (by needle or surgical drainage) are necessary as long as fluid is accumulating in order to minimize the risk of permanent cartilage damage. In addition, aspiration of tense, painful effusions of whatever etiology is frequently indicated for pain relief.

There are several relative contraindications to aspiration. The most important is a major bleeding diathesis, as in a patient with hemophilia and a circulating anticoagulant, or severe thrombocytopenia. Hemophilia itself is not an absolute contraindication, and tense, painful hemarthrosis should be aspirated if the factor VIII level can be corrected. Another relative contraindication is fear of introducing infection into the joint space, for example, in the setting of cellulitis associated with an effusion in the underlying joint.

Preparation of the Patient

The skin over the joint should be scrubbed, cleaned with disinfectant, and draped, just as for any other invasive procedure. Strict aseptic technique should prevail throughout the aspiration.

If the joint is distended with fluid, local anesthesia is unnecessary in most cases, since most of the pain comes not from the skin but from the synovium and trauma to the ligaments, periosteum, and other articular structures. In patients with gout and other arthritides accompanied by extensive cellulitis, the skin itself may be so tender that ethyl chloride and/or lidocaine will be required.

Knee

The knee is the easiest joint in the body to aspirate. In addition to being able to approach it easily with the needle, it is fairly simple to demonstrate even a small amount of fluid in the knee joint by use of techniques such as patellar ballottement, the "bulge" sign, and demonstration of a fluid wave.

The knee joint can be approached in several different ways. The easiest is from the medial aspect. A 20- or 22-gauge needle is inserted at approximately the midportion of the patella, beneath the patella, and is advanced laterally into the patellofemoral space. If only a small amount of fluid is present, an assistant can compress the knee from the lateral and superior aspects, forcing all of the fluid into the patellofemoral space. A common error has been to insert the needle too anteriorly, thus striking the patella or the patellar cartilage. This procedure induces pain, with reflex spasm of the quadriceps muscle, making entry into the patellofemoral space virtually impossible. It should be pointed out that relaxation of the quadriceps is essential for this approach, and for that reason sometimes the approach is not used, especially in children.

The lateral approach to the knee joint is also popular. Here the needle is usually oriented toward the superior aspect of the patella; again, it must be posterior to the undersurface of the patella. The patellofemoral space is entered, and fluid is aspirated without difficulty in most cases.

In the presence of extremely large effusions, the suprapatellar space is distended. This space can be easily entered, going either medially or laterally to the quadriceps tendon. Although this approach requires large effusions, it is simple and fast and is frequently the procedure of choice in children with acute arthritis.

Finally, if only a small amount of fluid is present, or if a patient is extremely obese, fluid can sometimes be aspirated from the tibiofemoral joint itself. Aspiration is usually done with the knee flexed at 90 degrees and the patient in a sitting position. This technique is not recommended for most situations.

Elbow

The elbow joint is approached with the patient holding the arm in approximately 90 degrees of flexion. The needle is inserted just proximal to the head of the radius, which can be identified by palpation over the elbow while the patient pronates and supinates the wrist. The needle is directed slightly posteriorly toward the olecranon and enters the joint space formed by the head of the radius and the lateral humeral epicondyle. The elbow can also be approached posteriorly, going over the lateral aspect of the olecranon. The medial aspect of the olecranon should be avoided, as the ulnar nerve passes over this area.

Ankle

The ankle joint can be approached anteriorly or laterally. The anterior approach, usually the simplest, involves placing the needle just medial to the tendon of the extensor hallicus longus muscle. This area can be identified by having the patient dorsiflex the great toe and palpating the area. A fossa is created just medial to the tendon, and the tibiotalar articulation can be identified in this fossa. The needle is directed horizontally into the joint. This process can be facilitated by having an assistant apply traction to the foot and heel to distend the joint space. The lateral approach to the ankle is about 1 cm above and anterior to the lateral malleolus.

Hip

The hip can be approached either anteriorly or laterally. The technique is difficult and should not be attempted by untrained persons. It is unusual to aspirate much fluid from the hip joint, and for that reason it is recommended that after aspiration, a small amount of radiopaque dye be injected and a radiograph obtained, to insure that the hip joint was in fact entered. Most hip joint aspirations are therefore performed in the radiology department under fluoroscopic control.

Shoulder

Before aspirating the shoulder joint, the examiner needs to be as certain as possible that he or she is dealing with true joint pathology, as opposed to the many periarticular complications that can arise in this area. The latter include subacromial bursitis, bicipital tendinitis, and rotator cuff tears. Many of these conditions can mimic true articular pathology, and the observer must become familiar with techniques of examination of this area.

The shoulder joint is best approached from the anterior aspect, inserting the needle about 1–2 cm below and slightly medial to the coracoid process.

Since the rotator cuff is usually torn in patients with longstanding rheumatoid arthritis, the subacromial bursa will communicate freely with the shoulder joint. In such patients, it may be sufficient to aspirate the bursa from a lateral approach. This technique is usually accomplished easily by placing the needle between the humoral head and the arch of the acromion.

Fingers and Toes

The metacarpophalangeal, metatarsophalangeal, and interphalangeal joints are all approached from the dorsal aspect, using a small (e.g., 25-gauge) needle. If the joint is distended with fluid, an adequate aspiration may be carried out by placing the needle tip just under the extensor tendon as it glides over the joint. In other situations, it will be necessary to insert the needle between the opposing cartilages, which can be painful. Gentle traction on the digit to pull the cartilages apart is helpful.

Wrist

The safest and most certain approach to the radiocarpal joint is from the dorsum, with the needle inserted just distal to the midportion of the radius. The intercarpal joints are usually difficult to aspirate unless they are bulging and tense, in which case they can be entered with a small needle while gentle traction is applied.

ANALYSIS OF SYNOVIAL FLUID

Once obtained, synovial fluid should be placed immediately into anticoagulated tubes, preferably with heparin. Before sending fluid to the laboratory, it is wise to consider the cost and relative benefit of each test ordered. For example, synovial fluid from a patient with gout can be examined for crystals by polarized light microscopy. If characteristic intracellular urate crystals are seen, most additional studies merely increase the expense for the patient, with no benefit.

Color and Turbidity

The synovial fluid should be examined immediately for color and turbidity. Normal synovial fluid is transparent, and it is possible to read a newspaper through a tube of it.

Although formal tests of viscosity are available, it is easy to place a drop of synovial fluid between one's fingers and test the viscosity grossly by rapidly separating the fingers. Normal synovial fluid will "string out" for several centimeters before snapping in two. In addition, the normal fluid has a distinctly oily consistency. A more watery consistency and the inability of the fluid to form a long string imply a reduced viscosity due to the depolymerization of hyaluronate. This condition is seen in most inflammatory states, either infectious or sterile.

Mucin Clot

The mucin clot test is performed by the dropwise addition of one part synovial fluid to four parts 10% acetic acid. Because of hyaluronate, normal synovial fluid will form a tight clot that does not fragment easily. A poor or friable mucin clot is seen in most inflammatory arthritides, including rheumatoid arthritis, septic arthritis, and gout. Patients with systemic lupus erythematosus and acute rheumatic fever usually have fair to good mucin clots, while those with osteoarthritis and arthritis following trauma usually have normal mucin clots. Like the synovial fluid viscosity test, the mucin clot test is essentially a test of the degree of polymerization of hyaluronate. The more highly polymerized this molecule is, the higher will be the viscosity and the tighter the clot formed with the addition of acetic acid.

Chemistries

Synovial fluid glucose is a useful chemistry examination in many conditions. Septic arthritis and tuberculous arthritis will reduce the synovial fluid glucose, and levels of less than 35 mg/dl are seen frequently. In addition, rheumatoid arthritis may show low synovial fluid glucose levels; occasionally the levels will be undetectable in very active rheumatoid arthritis. In borderline cases, fasting serum glucose should be compared to simultaneous synovial fluid glucose. A difference of 40 mg/dl or more is highly suggestive of infection.

Total protein of more than 3 g/dl indicates inflammation. Very high protein values, approaching those of serum, are seen in long-standing chronic inflammations such as rheumatoid arthritis and tuberculous arthritis.

Although not determined routinely, joint fluid pH correlates inversely with the amount of anaerobic metabolism taking place. It is a good index of neutrophil phagocytic activity. For example, a very low synovial fluid pH has been seen by some clinicians as an indication that a joint infection was not adequately controlled and suggests that either surgical debridement or the use of different anti-biotics should be attempted. This problem is especially true for aminoglycoside antibiotics, which are much less active at acid pH.

Lactic dehydrogenase, lysozyme, and other enzymes may be elevated if the white count is elevated and phagocytic activity is high. These studies are rarely of clinical usefulness. A variety of small molecules, such as electrolytes, may be ordered but provide no useful information. Occasionally, overzealous physicians and students order tests of synovial fluid uric acid levels to help diagnose gout. These tests also provide no useful or even interpretable information and add to the patient's expense.

White Cell Count and Differential

As noted in Table 3.1, normal synovial fluid usually contains approximately 100 white cells/cu mm, the majority of which are lymphocytes and other mononuclear cells. In osteoarthritis and similar conditions, synovial fluid cell counts of 2,000/ cu mm are occasionally seen, and it is not unusual to have as many as 30% neutrophilic cells. Active rheumatoid arthritis and gout will usually involve 5,000–25,000/cu mm white cells with almost 100% neutrophils. In any synovial fluid with a white blood cell count of greater than 25,000/cu mm, infection is highly suspect; a white count of greater than 50,000/cu mm presumes infection. However, it is recognized that occasional patients with rheumatoid arthritis will have extremely high white cell counts and, conversely, certain infectious conditions occasionally have low white cell counts. This latter condition applies especially to gonococcal arthritis, in which white cell counts in the range of 6,000–10,000/cu mm are fairly common.

Gram Stain and Culture

The Gram stain of a spun sediment of synovial fluid is occasionally very helpful in identifying quickly the likely causative organism in infectious states. For example, staphylococci, pneumococci, and other pathogens are usually visible on Gram stain if the particular organism is the cause of an active infection. With gonoccal arthritis, however, negative Gram stains are frequent, so that, as with many infections, negative data do not exclude the condition.

Synovial fluid can also be stained for tubercle bacilli, using acid-fast stains, and for fungi, using various silver stains.

Culture of synovial fluid should be done thoughtfully. If one suspects gonococcal arthritis, for example, culture of synovial fluid should be done immediately after the fluid is obtained on Thayer-Martin medium. Routine cultures for Gram-positive and Gram-negative organisms are done on the usual bacteriologic media, as are cultures for tubercle bacilli and fungi.

Examination for Crystals

The examination for crystals is performed by placing a drop of fresh synovial fluid (without anticoagulant) on a microscope slide. The slide is covered with a coverslip and examined immediately if possible. If this is not possible, the edge

Table 3.1. Characteristic Synovial Fluids in Various Diseases

Disease Category	Color and Consistency	WBC^b $(\times 10^3)/mm^3$	% $PMNs^c$	Protein (g/dl)	Glucose (% plasma)	Viscosity	Mucin Clot
Group II							
Osteoarthritis	Straw; clear	1–3	< 30	2–4	80–100	High	Good
Trauma	Straw; blood	1–3	< 30	2–4	80–100	High unless bloody	Good unless bloody
Systemic lupus erythematosus	Straw; may be cloudy	3–10	< 50	3–4	80–100	High	Fair–good
Group III							
RA	Straw; cloudy	10–30	> 90	5–8	5–75	Low	Poor
Reiter's syndrome	Straw; cloudy	10–30	> 90	5–8	80	Low	Fair–poor
Gout	Straw; clear	10–30	> 90	5–8	80	Low–mod.	Fair–poor
Rheumatic fever	Straw; clear	5–20	50–90	5–8	80	Low	Fair–poor
Group III							
Gonococcal arthritis	Straw; slightly cloudy	5–25	> 90	5–8	10–50	Low	Poor
Other bacterial infections	Creamy; thick	> 50	> 90	7–8	10	Low	Poor
Tuberculosis	Creamy; thick	10–20	60–80	7–8	10	Low	Poor

[a] Based on classification by Ropes and Bauer (1953).

[b] White blood cell count.

[c] Percentage of neutrophils.

of the coverslip should be covered with paraffin or nail polish to prevent drying. The slide should be examined as soon as possible, but up to 2 to 3 hours may elapse before reading becomes critical. If a longer time elapses, calcium pyrophosphate crystals may be digested by the phosphatases in the neutrophils and the possibility of in vitro crystallization of urate may obscure the picture.

When examined by simple light microscopy, most crystals cannot be clearly distinguished. Occasionally in acute gout enough crystals are present so that the diagnosis can be made with confidence by simple light microscopy. However, in most clinical situations, polarized light microscopy is necessary to identify the presence of crystals. In this technique, a polarizing lens is placed below the stage, often built into the light source itself. Above the stage is inserted a second polarizing lens, and the lens is rotated until the background is dark. In this setting, the axes of light transmission of the two lenses are at right angles to each other, and virtually all light is extinguished. If there is birefringent material, such as a crystal, between the two polarizing lenses, the crystal will further refract the light coming through the first polarizing lens, allowing some of it to get through the second lens. Thus, a crystal will appear as a bright object against a dark background. Further clarification of the type of crystal is obtained by placing a first-order color compensator between the two polarizing lenses. This compensator will refract the background light from the first polarizer, making the background appear red. Crystals are identified as positively and negatively birefringent based on their color when the color compensator is used. Thus, by convention, crystals such as urate that appear yellow when parallel to the long axis of the compensator and blue when perpendicular are declared negatively birefringent. Positively birefringent crystals are blue when parallel to the long axis and yellow when at right angles. Calcium pyrophosphate dihydrate crystals are positively birefringent.

The technique for identifying crystals, then, first involves focusing the microscope under ordinary light and high-dry magnification. The polarizing lenses are then placed at right angles to each other so that the background is virtually dark. The slide is then moved over the stage until a crystal is identified. Then the first-order color compensator is inserted and the stage rotated until the crystal is lying parallel to the long axis of the compensator. If the crystal is then yellow, it is identified as presumptively urate; if it is blue, it is presumed to be calcium pyrophosphate.

Uric acid crystals are usually long and needle shaped but may vary tremendously in length from 2 to 25 or 30 μm. The typical uric acid crystal is greater than 10 μm in length and often is seen both intracellularly and extracellularly. When intracellular, it is not uncommon to have three or four crystals within the same polymorphonuclear leukocyte, with some of the crystals apparently piercing the cell. Uric acid crystals are strongly birefringent, and if viewed with the polarizing lenses in place while the stage is rotated, the light transmission will be extinguished almost completely when the crystal is oriented 45 degrees from the long axis of the analyzer in either direction.

Calcium pyrophosphate dihydrate crystals are much more pleomorphic than urate. Thus, they may vary in size from 2 to 3 μm up to 10 to 12 μm. Their shape may be anything from squares or rhomboids to needles closely resembling urate crystals. The number of crystals seen also varies tremendously. Although cases of pseudogout have been observed in which the synovial fluid appeared purulent because of tremendous numbers of crystals, in the more usual situation only a few crystals are present, so that one must search the fluid carefully before ruling out pseudogout. In addition, calcium pyrophosphate crystals often are much less birefringent than urate crystals and therefore must be sought for more carefully. It is also common to find them both within cells and free in the fluid, and occasionally cells with two, three, or more pyrophosphate crystals are identified. Occasionally crystal identification is faster if a spun sediment is examined.

The inexperienced microscopist must remember that a number of other substances also have the ability to refract light and resemble crystals of various types. These include the following.

Fat Droplets

These droplets, known as *maltese crosses,* are common in a number of chronic effusions. Although they do not resemble urate or pyrophosphate crystals, the presence of a large number of fat droplets can make it difficult to see the smaller and frequently less birefringent crystals for which one is looking.

Bits of Collagen

Collagen fibers are often weakly birefringent and may be present in fairly large numbers, especially in osteoarthritis and posttraumatic arthritis. These fibers will be correctly identified if one uses high-power microscopy, because the characteristic curling of the collagen will be noted. Under low-power microscopy, however, these fibers may resemble small crystals.

Cell Interfaces

Often when two cells are in contact, the resultant interface will refract light and cause birefringence. For this reason, if a synovial fluid is grossly bloody, it is often impossible to rule in or out a crystal-induced synovitis. When one examines such a fluid using polarized light microscopy, one sees hundreds of refractile cell interfaces that can obscure any crystals present. For that reason, if synovial fluid becomes bloody while it is being aspirated, the aspiration should be discontinued immediately and an attempt made to get some of the fluid that has not been mixed with blood.

Steroids

A transient synovitis following intra-articular injection of microcrystalline corticosteroids has been attributed to an inflammatory reaction induced by these crystals. By polarized light microscopy they are strongly birefringent and needle shaped. They are usually positively birefringent, and there is considerable variation in size.

A special comment regarding aspiration of joints for the diagnosis of gout is in order. Although several milliliters of fluid are required for most of the analyses described, to establish the diagnosis of gout only one drop of fluid and a suitable microscope are needed. For this reason, it is reasonable to attempt to aspirate joints that may have only a small amount of fluid present. Thus, metatarsophalangeal joints and other small joints may be aspirated when acute gout is suspected. Because of the intense overlying cellulitis and edema, this aspiration needs to be done with some care; often the patient must be premedicated with a narcotic. In addition, it is sometimes useful to anesthetize the skin with ethyl chloride spray because of the intense tenderness of the overlying skin. The first metatarsophalangeal joint can be entered from above, approaching from either side of the extensor tendon of the great toe, using a tuberculin or insulin syringe with a 25- or 26-gauge needle. Frequently even the amount of fluid contained within the needle itself is adequate to identify crystals. The syringe can then be irrigated with sterile saline to obtain material for culture.

In persons suspected of having chronic polyarticular gout, it is frequently helpful to attempt to aspirate tophi. The most useful tophi for such purposes are in the ear, in the olecranon bursae, and around bony prominences such as the first metatarsophalangeal joint. If the tophus is very close to the skin surface, as it usually is in the ear, the skin should be pierced with a 20- to 22-gauge needle and a small amount of the chalky material scraped out on the tip of the needle. This material should then be examined by polarized light microscopy. If the tophus is in a deeper structure, such as the olecranon bursa, the tophus should be entered with a larger-bore needle, such as a 19-gauge needle, and a small amount of saline injected before aspiration is attempted. Chalky material is usually obtained and is then examined by polarized light microscopy.

Crystals from tophi will be densely packed, and no polymorphonuclear cells are usually seen.

Other Microscopic Studies

Tumor cells are occasionally identifiable on routine microscopy with Wright's stain, but if a tumor is suspected it is preferable to submit a sample of fluid for cytologic examination by the Papanicolaou technique.

Lupus erythematosus cells are easily identified in Wright's-stained preparations of synovial fluid from patients with antinuclear antibodies. Their demonstration in synovial fluid has no special significance.

Bits of cartilage may be seen in almost any synovial fluid, but persons with osteoarthritis occasionally have large numbers of collagen fibers in the fluid. As stated above, collagen may be birefringent.

Synovial Fluid Complement

Although much has been written in the last few years on the determination of synovial fluid complement levels in various diseases, these studies are usually of more help in understanding the pathogenesis of the inflammatory reaction than in establishing a diagnosis. However, it is generally true that synovial fluid (and other exudates) from patients with rheumatoid arthritis will usually have depressed complement levels. This finding is especially impressive when one considers the fact that the serum complement in rheumatoid arthritis is usually elevated. This dichotomy, low synovial fluid complement with high serum complement, is unique to rheumatoid factor-positive rheumatoid arthritis. However, in clinical situations, it is not always helpful to obtain this determination. It has been pointed out by some observers that synovial fluid complement levels in

Reiter's syndrome may be higher than in other inflammatory arthritides, but the overlap is large and this finding is not particularly helpful for diagnosis.

Rheumatoid Factor

The lymphocytes lining the synovial membrane in rheumatoid arthritis produce large amounts of immunoglobulin, a large portion of which are rheumatoid factors. In classic seropositive rheumatoid arthritis, both IgG and IgM rheumatoid factors are produced. In seronegative polyarthritis of various types, primarily IgG rheumatoid factor is found. As with synovial fluid complement, the identification of rheumatoid factor in joint fluid is of much help in understanding the pathogenesis of the inflammatory response in rheumatoid arthritis. However, as with the synovial fluid complement, testing for the presence or absence of synovial fluid rheumatoid factor is of little diagnostic value for the clinician. In fact, because of possible confusion resulting from such tests, routine evaluation of synovial fluid for rheumatoid factor is not recommended.

Antinuclear Antibody

As with rheumatoid factor, occasional patients will have antinuclear antibodies demonstrated in synovial fluids and other body cavities. The same problems of interpretation apply that exist for rheumatoid factor, and this test is also not recommended.

SYNOVIAL BIOPSY

Synovial biopsy, although infrequently necessary, is a highly useful test if one is considering a chronic infection, such as tuberculosis. Cultures in such cases are slow and often falsely negative, and rapid diagnosis often requires a biopsy. A number of biopsy needles are available for use in such situations, but surgical biopsy either by arthroscopy or by direct visualization is usually preferred.

Biopsy is also occasionally indicated to help establish the diagnosis in atypical cases of inflammatory joint diseases or if one suspects primary or metastatic synovial tumors.

BIBLIOGRAPHY

Cohen AS, Brandt KD, Krey PR: Synovial fluid. In Cohen AS (ed): *Laboratory Diagnostic Procedures in the Rheumatic Diseases,* ed 2. Boston, Little, Brown and Co, 1975.

Ropes MW, Bauer W: *Synovial Fluid Changes in Joint Diseases.* Washington, DC, Howard University Press, 1953.

Gatter RA: The compensated polarized light microscope in clinical rheumatology. *Arthritis Rheum* 17:253, 1974.

Ruddy S, Austen KF: The complement system in rheumatoid synovitis. I. An analysis of complement component activities in rheumatoid synovial fluids. *Arthritis Rheum* 13:713, 1970.

4

Diagnostic Studies
for the Rheumatic Diseases

Richard S. Panush

Eric P. Brestel

Jeffrey C. Delafuente

Selden Longley

A number of diagnostic studies have proved useful for evaluating patients with rheumatic diseases. It is important to understand the manner in which these tests are performed, their clinical significance, and their limitations, so that they can be meaningfully ordered and interpreted. As emphasized in Chapter 2, pertinent diagnostic studies should be selectively ordered after a careful history has been obtained and tentative impressions have been reviewed. Careless or excessive evaluation can be costly and confusing. This chapter will review (1) certain general laboratory studies, (2) studies relating to the neuromuscular system, (3) uric acid studies, (4) thermography, (5) humoral immune function, (6) cellular immune function, (7) tissue typing, and (8) tissue biopsy. Chapter 3 reviews the analysis of synovial fluid and biopsy of synovial membrane, and Chapter 5 contains a discussion of x-rays and scans of joints, arthrography, and arthroscopy.

GENERAL LABORATORY STUDIES

Baseline evaluation of most patients with rheumatic diseases will include a determination of hemoglobin, hematocrit, white blood count, differential count, examination of a blood smear, and urinalysis. Often chest x-ray and blood chemistry profiles are also needed.

Although most abnormalities encountered in these baseline studies are nonspecific, they help to assess the status of a patient. Many patients with chronic inflammatory arthritis have anemia. Coombs' test for hemolytic anemia is sometimes positive in persons with systemic lupus erythematosus (SLE) and infrequently in those with other rheumatic diseases. Leukopenia or thrombocytopenia should suggest SLE or Felty's syndrome. Leukocytosis occurs with steroid usage, crystal-induced synovitis, vasculitis, inflammatory arthritis, and particularly juvenile rheumatoid arthritis. Thrombocytosis is seen with inflammatory arthritis and in patients with active and extra-articular rheumatoid arthritis. Lymphopenia occurs with SLE and steroid usage. Neutropenia may be found in patients with Felty's syndrome, SLE, or as a complication of drug therapy. Eosinophilia has been reported with vasculitis, active and extra-articular rheumatoid arthritis, and toxic drug reactions and infrequently with SLE or progressive systemic sclerosis. Rouleau formation on the peripheral smear should suggest dysproteinemia and lead to additional appropriate immunologic studies (see below).

Proteinuria may be encountered with SLE, progressive systemic sclerosis, vasculitis, or amyloidosis. Similarly, sediment abnormalities can be due to nephropathy of SLE, scleroderma, or vasculitis. Many systemic diseases—rheumatoid arthritis, SLE, polydermatomyositis, progressive systemic sclerosis, vasculitis, sarcoidosis, or fungal infections—may be reflected by abnormalities, usually nonspecific, in the chest x-ray. Blood chemistry screens are appropriate for certain less common conditions with rheumatic manifestations—thyroid and parathyroid disease, diabetes mellitus, hepatic disorders, dysproteinemias, lipoproteinemias, hemochromatosis, Wilson's disease, and others (see Chap. 23).

NEUROMUSCULAR SYSTEM EVALUATION

Measuring serum muscle enzymes and performing electromyography, nerve conduction studies, and muscle biopsy are desirable in evaluating patients with myopathies. In patients with inflammatory myopathies (polydermatomyositis, vasculitis, mixed connective tissue disease, scleroderma, and Sjögren's syndrome), serum enzymes are often increased proportionally to the amount of muscle inflammation. Infrequently, enzymes may be increased in patients with muscular dystrophy, amyotrophic lateral sclerosis, or other neurogenic myopathies; endocrinopathic myopathies; toxic myopathies; after strenuous exercise or intramuscular injections; and in many nonmyopathic states.

Enzymes measured usually include serum glutamic oxaloacetic transaminase (SGOT), lactate dehydrogenase (LDH), creatine phosphokinase (CPK), and aldolase. Patterns of elevation vary in inflammatory myositis. Thus, in practice, all enzymes are usually measured in a given patient, and those values that best reflect the patient's disease course are sequentially followed.

The electromyogram (EMG) helps distinguish myopathies from neurogenic disorders. Inflammatory myositis, muscular dystrophy, and other myopathies are characterized by decreased muscle action potentials, increased polyphasic potentials, fibrillation, and monophasic potentials. In neurogenic disorders there are increased action potentials, polyphasic potentials, spontaneous fibrillation, and monophasic potentials. The EMG is not only a useful diagnostic adjunct but also helps select a site for muscle biopsy. A muscle contralateral to one with an abnormality documented by EMG is the recommended site because it is likely to be diseased yet would not be damaged by electrode insertion.

A muscle biopsy can often help establish a diagnosis in patients with muscular disorders. The site of the biopsy should be selected as one likely to contain diseased tissue. The specimen should be handled carefully, processed for histochemical studies and electron microscopic examination as well as light microscopy, and reviewed with an experienced pathologist whenever possible.

Nerve conduction studies help confirm entrapment neuropathies (carpal tunnel, tarsal tunnel, others) and differentiate mononeuritis multiplex from polyneuropathies.

URIC ACID STUDIES

Uric acid may be measured by several methods. Colorimetric assays use the ability of urate to reduce orthophosphotungstic acid to a blue product whose wavelength can be readily measured. Normal values for serum uric acid by this method are usually < 6 mg/100 ml. Colorimetric methods have been adapted for autoanalyzer use with often higher norms (< 8 mg/100 ml). A number of substances interfere with colorimetric determinations: ascorbic acid, acetaminophen, homogentisic acid, alpha-methyl-dopa, caffeine, theophylline, theobromine, and L-dopa in plasma and salicylate metabolites in urine. Another and more accurate uric acid assay is enzymatic, which spectrophotometrically determines uric acid concentrations in the ultraviolet range, where uric acid strongly absorbs, before and after uricase digestion. Normal levels by this method are generally < 7 mg/ 100 ml. A variation of the enzymatic method has been automated. Normal values for individual laboratories may vary and must be used in interpreting uric acid results. Since daily and seasonal variations of serum uric acid levels occur, values may need to be rechecked.

Serum hypouricemia may be found in certain diseases (xanthinuria, Fanconi syndrome, acute intermittent porphyria, hepatic disease, pernicious anemia, renal tubular transport defects, and neoplasms), with drug usage (allopurinol, aspirin, glyceryl guaiacolate, phenylbutazone, probenecid, sulfinpyrazone, coumarin derivatives, and x-ray contrast agents), and other conditions (alcoholism, toxic epidermal necrolysis, cirrhosis, hyperglycemia, myocardial ischemia, coronary artery obstruction, paraplegia and urinary tract infection, bleeding ulcer, fever of unknown origin, abdominal abscess, and Rocky Mountain spotted fever) (Table 4.1).

Hyperuricemia may be primary or secondary (Table 4.2). Primary hyperuri-

Table 4.1. Hypouricemia

Diseases
    Xanthinuria
    Fanconi syndrome
    Acute intermittent porphyria
    Liver disease
    Pernicious anemia
    Isolated tubular transport defect
    Neoplasia
Drugs
    Allopurinol
    Aspirin
    Glyceryl guaiacolate
    X-ray contrast agents
Miscellaneous disorders
    (See text)

Table 4.2. Hyperuricemia

Hematologic disorders (polycythemias, hemolytic anemias)

Neoplasia and lymphoproliferative disorders

Hypertension

Metabolic disorders (lipoproteinemias, acidosis, starvation, obesity)

Endocrinopathies (myxedema, hyperparathyroidism)

Renal insufficiency

Congenital disorders (glycogen storage disease, type I; Down's syndrome)

Psoriasis

Sarcoidosis

Drugs (diuretics, ethambutol, pyrazinamide, low-dose aspirin, lead)

---

cemia results from overproduction or underexcretion of uric acid or a combination of both. Deficiencies of hypoxanthine-guanine-phosphoribosyl-transferase and phosphoribosyl-pyrophosphate have been recognized in a small number of genetic hyperuricemias. Patients with glycogen storage disease (type I), with glucose 6-phosphatase deficiency, have excess available phosphoribosyl pyrophosphate with increased synthesis of uric acid and reduced tubular secretion as a result of their acidosis.

Secondary hyperuricemias similarly reflect problems with uric acid production or clearance or both in a variety of circumstances. Disease states associated with hyperuricemia include hematologic disorders (hemolytic anemias, polycythemias, myeloproliferative diseases), hypertension, metabolic disorders (lipoproteinemias, acidosis, starvation, obesity, hyperparathyroidism, myxedema), renal insufficiency, Down's syndrome, psoriasis, and sarcoidosis. Many drugs increase uric acid levels: diuretics (thiazides, triamterene, furosemide, clorthalidone, ethacrynic acid), ethambutol, pyrazinamide, low-dose aspirin, and chronic lead intoxication. The clinical significance and management of uric acid abnormalities will be further discussed in Chapter 26.

Measurements of urinary uric acid excretion also provide pertinent information about hyperuricemic patients and those with gout or renal calculi. Most normal persons eating a regular diet will excrete < 900 mg and, eating a purine-restricted diet, < 700 mg per 24 hr. Allopurinol is generally the drug of choice for patients with increased urinary uric acid; this drug reduces the risk of stone formation while lowering serum uric acid levels. Determining the ratio of urinary uric acid to creatinine has been recommended as a screening procedure for identifying patients with hypoxanthine-guanine-phosphoribosyl-transferase deficiency. Most normal populations had mean ratios of 0.30–0.50 and hyperuricemics 0.50–0.75. Patients with enzyme deficiencies had ratios exceeding 1.00.

THERMOGRAPHY

Thermography can be used to measure temperatures over joints. This procedure has documented and quantified joint inflammation. Methods require careful control of ambient temperature. Thermography is neither widely available nor widely used; its sensitivity and clinical value are not yet clear.

HUMORAL IMMUNE FUNCTION

Electrophoresis

Serum electrophoresis is a useful technique for evaluating serum proteins. Abnormalities of gammaglobulins (hypogammaglobulinemia, polyclonal or monoclonal increases) can be readily detected. Further studies of such patients to define the abnormalities more carefully would include radial immunodiffusion or immunoelectrophoresis. Unless the result of the serum protein electrophoresis is abnormal, additional laboratory studies (i.e., quantitative or qualitative Ig) are not usually informative.

Serum proteins may be separated on the basis of net charge by zone electrophoresis. The sample is applied to a supporting medium, usually cellulose acetate. An electropotential is placed across the medium, and serum proteins migrate toward the respective electrodes. The cellulose acetate strip is then stained, and the separated proteins appear visually as dense bands (Fig. 4.1). Five gross bands may be determined by this method and include albumin and the globulins alpha-1, alpha-2, beta, and gamma. Albumin migrates closest to the anode.

Scanning the strip permits quantitation of the amount of protein in each region. Some disease states give characteristic patterns. During acute illness, the alpha-1 and alpha-2 fractions may be elevated and the prealbumin, albumin, and transferrin proteins may be reduced. Occasionally, C-reactive protein increases in acute inflammatory states. This protein migrates in the gamma region and may be confused with monoclonal spikes of multiple myeloma. In chronic diseases, a diffuse increase of the gammaglobulins may be noted. These increases may be marked in chronic liver disease, SLE, rheumatoid arthritis, sarcoidosis, and Sjögren's syndrome. Hypogammaglobulinemia, multiple myeloma, Waldenström's macroglobulinemia, and alpha-1-antitrypsin deficiency may be suggested by abnormalities on serum electrophoresis. In patients suspected of having multiple myeloma, the urine may be concentrated and examined by immunoelectrophoresis for the presence of monoclonal light chains (see below).

Immunodiffusion in Gel

Simple gel diffusion is clinically advantageous in determining the qualitative presence of precipitating antibodies in hypersensitivity pneumonitis and in detecting the low-molecular-weight (7 S) IgM in some vasculitides and in lymphosarcoma-associated angioedemas.

The double-diffusion technique of Ouchterlony involves placing antigens and antibodies in wells cut into an inert supporting gel. A visible line of precipitation forms where the reagents are in equivalence. By this method antigens may be compared for identity, partial identity (cross-reactivity), or nonidentity against a given antibody (Fig. 4.2).

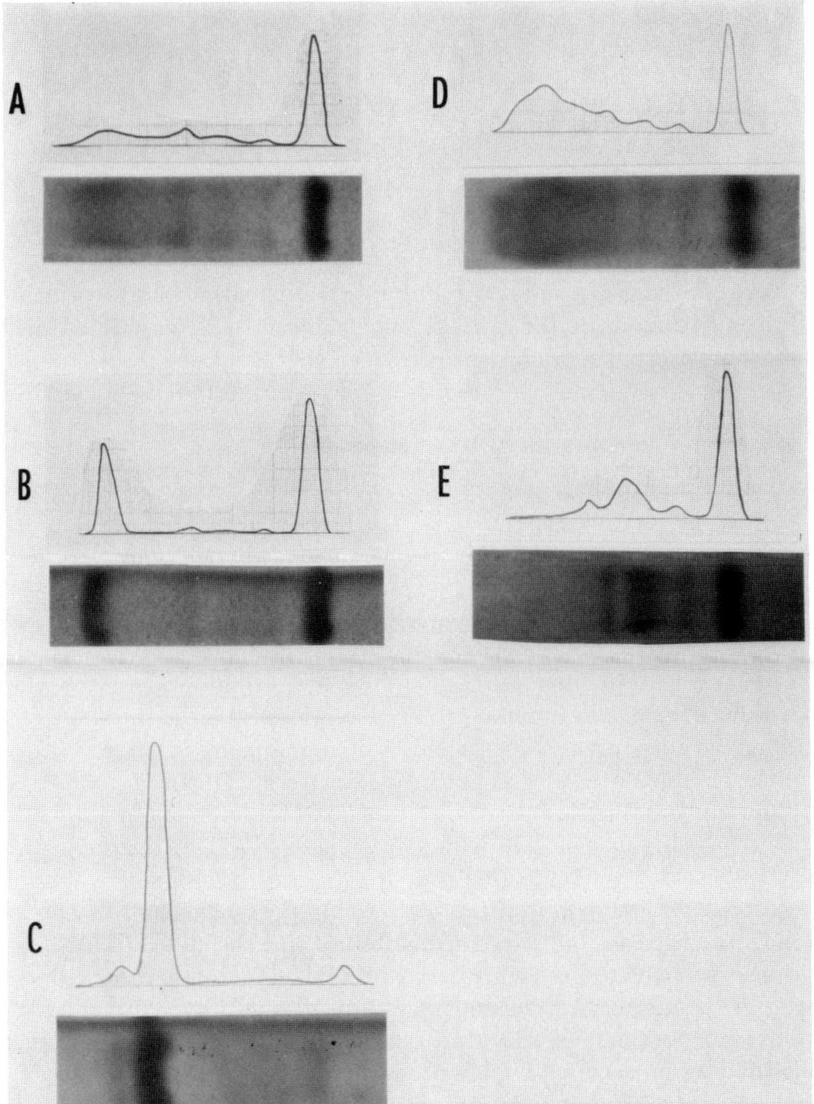

Figure 4.1. Zone electrophoresis of serum in cellulose acetate. Anode is toward right. (*a*) Normal human serum; (*b*) multiple myeloma serum; (*c*) urine with Bence Jones protein; (*d*) diffuse hypergammaglobulinemia; (*e*) hypogammaglobulinemia. (From Brestel EP, Delafuente JC, Longley S, Panush RS: Evaluation of patients with immunologic disease, in Waldman RH (ed): *Clinical Concepts of Immunology*. Baltimore, Williams & Wilkins Co, © 1979, p. 228. Reprinted by permission.)

Radial Immunodiffusion

Radial immunodiffusion is commonly used to quantitate IgG, IgA, IgM, C3, C4, the C1 esterase inhibitor, and other proteins. Antigens may be quantitated by being allowed to diffuse into gels containing dilute, specific antibody. Wells are cut into the gel, and the antigen samples or dilutions of a standard are applied to the wells. As the antigen diffuses into the gel, a visible precipitate forms, the area of which is proportional to the amount of antigen present (Fig. 4.3).

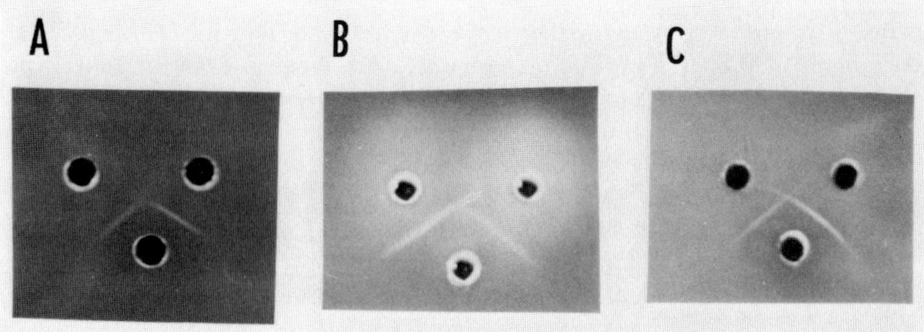

Figure 4.2. Ouchterlony immunodiffusion in gel. Illustration of (*a*) lines of identity; (*b*) lines of partial identity; (*c*) lines of nonidentity. (From Brestel EP, Delafuente JC, Longley S, Panush RS: Evaluation of patients with immunologic disease, in Waldman RH (ed): *Clinical Concepts of Immunology.* Baltimore, Williams & Wilkins Co, © 1979, p 229. Reprinted by permission.)

Quantitation of complement levels may be helpful in managing patients with SLE and glomerulonephritis and in certain others with complement-mediated diseases in whom disease and complement changes correlate. Immunoglobulin levels are altered in many diseases, with little specificity of patterns in individual patients. They are, therefore, usually quantitated in patients with hypogamma-globulinemia or monoclonal protein "spikes" on electrophoresis.

Immunoelectrophoresis

Immunoelectrophoresis is a qualitative tool and is at best semiquantitative. This method is commonly used for screening protein preparations for purity. It may

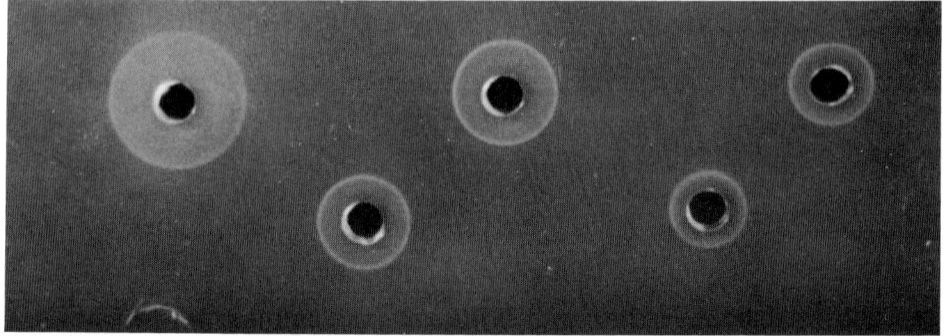

Figure 4.3. Radial immunodiffusion. Quantitation of antigen (in wells) by antibody-containing gel. The area of precipitate is proportional to the antigen concentration. The agarose gel contains anti-human C4. The top wells contain (left to right) normal human serum diluted 1 : 1, 1 : 2, and 1 : 4. The bottom wells contain, at the left, active SLE serum 1 : 1, and at the right, acute hereditary angioedema serum 1 : 1. (From Brestel EP, Delafuente JC, Longley S, Panush RS: Evaluation of patients with immunologic disease, in Waldman RH (ed): *Clinical Concepts of Immunology.* Baltimore, Williams & Wilkins Co, © 1979, p. 230. Reprinted by permission.)

be clinically applied to study further patients with hypogammaglobulinemia and monoclonal gammopathies found on protein electrophoresis. Concentrated urine may be tested for monoclonal light chains. The method is carried out by dissolving gel in a special buffer. A well is cut to receive the sample. An electropotential applied across the gel allows the proteins in the sample to migrate toward the respective electrodes. At the end of the procedure, a trough is cut parallel to the direction of the protein migration and is filled with an antiserum (Fig. 4.4). The size of the arcs and their closeness to the trough depend on the concentration and molecular weight of the particular protein.

Electroimmunodiffusion

The sensitivity of immunodiffusion in agar may be increased by the technique of electroimmunodiffusion. The method of single electroimmunodiffusion (rocket electrophoresis) is performed by electrophoresing antigen of relatively negative charge into an agarose gel containing monospecific antiserum. A rocket-shaped precipitin is formed in the gel. Its length is used to quantitate the antigen concentration (Fig. 4.5). With double electroimmunodiffusion (counterimmunoelectrophoresis), antigens with a relatively negative net charge migrate toward specific antibody in an adjacent well. The value of counterimmunoelectrophoresis is that results can be rapidly obtained (i.e., during the course of a patient's clinic visit) and used promptly for patient management. This method is somewhat less sensitive than others.

Electrofocusing

Electrofocusing allows greater resolution and definition of mixtures of proteins and is largely used in the investigative laboratory to purify proteins. It permits proteins to migrate to their isoelectric points in specially prepared gels.

Radioimmunoassay

The greatest technical advance for measuring antigens or antibodies at concentrations $< \mu g/ml$ is the radioimmunoassay. The radioimmunoassay has been used to measure hormones, drugs, Australia antigen, IgE, antibodies to deoxyribonucleic acid (DNA), and other substances present in low concentration. Commonly, a purified antigen is radioisotope labeled and is used to compete with unlabeled standard or unknown samples for a specific antibody. The degree of competition (and thus concentration of unknown antigen) may be quantitated by radioactive emission. Separation of bound and unbound antibody may be achieved by ammonium sulfate precipitation of the antigen-antibody complex (the Farr assay), precipitation of high-molecular-weight complexes by polyethylene glycol, covalently linking specific antigen or antibody to an insoluble matrix (as cellulose paper disks or Sepharose beads) and washing away unbound radiolabeled material, and by precipitation by the double-antibody method.

Agglutination and Inhibition of Agglutination

Agglutination and hemagglutination reactions may be used to detect antibodies to a variety of antigens, including antinuclear antibodies (ANAs), antigamma

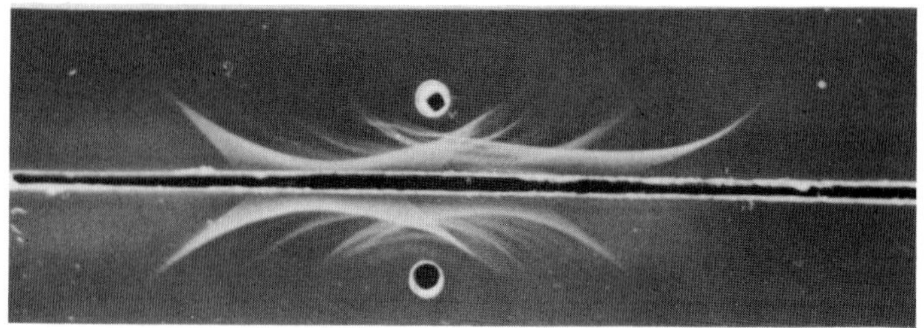

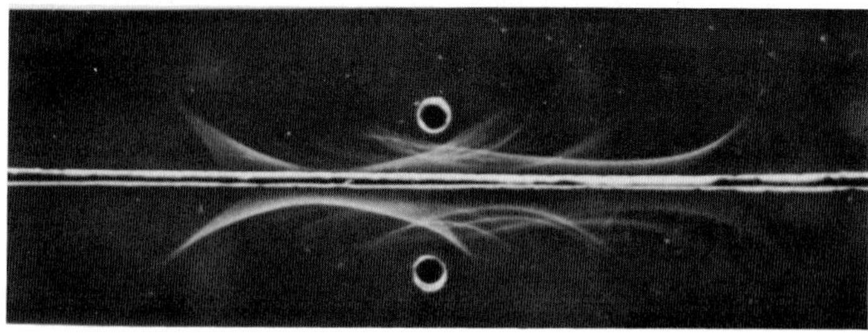

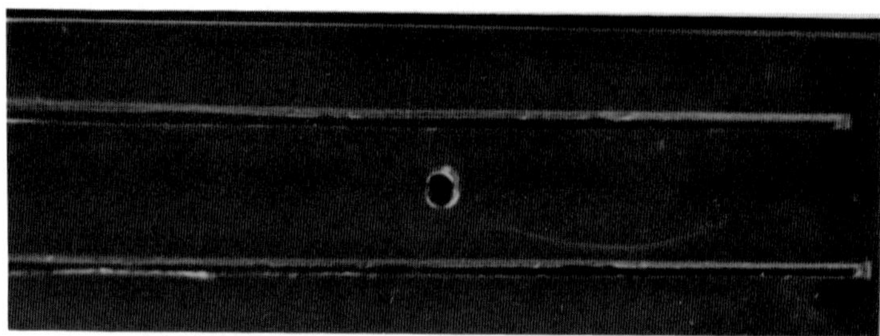

Figure 4.4. Immunoelectrophoresis. The anode is toward the left. (*a*) Top well, normal human serum; bottom well, hypogammaglobulinemic serum; trough, antinormal human serum. Notice the absence of the gamma globulin arc in hypogammaglobulinemic serum (toward the right). (*b*) Top well, normal human serum; bottom well, IgG myeloma serum; trough, antinormal human serum. Notice the broad arc in the gamma region in the myeloma serum (toward the right). (*c*) Well, urine with Bence Jones protein; top trough, antikappa chain; bottom trough, antilambda chain. This urine contains light chains of the lambda type only. (From Brestel EP, Delafuente JC, Longley S, Panush RS: Evaluation of patients with immunologic disease, in Waldman RH (ed): *Clinical Concepts of Immunology*. Baltimore, Williams & Wilkins Co, © 1979, p. 231. Reprinted by permission.)

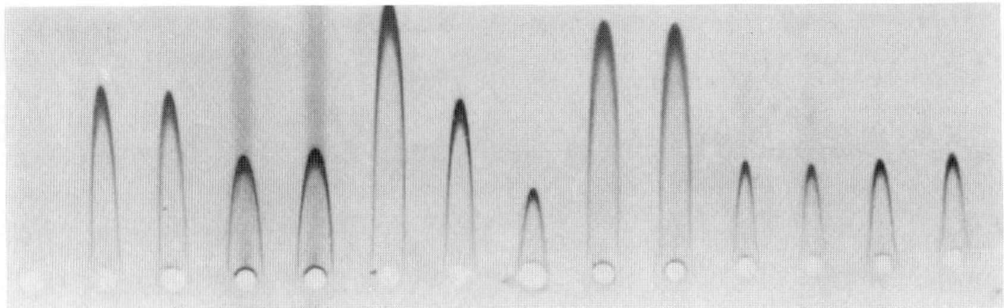

Figure 4.5. Single immunoelectrodiffusion (rocket electrophoresis). The gell contains antiserum to alpha-$_1$ antitrypsin. The fifth, sixth, and seventh wells (left to right) contain 1 : 1, 1 : 2, and 1 : 4 dilutions of standard human serum; the others contain unknown samples. (From Brestel EP, Delafuente JC, Longley S, Panush RS: Evaluation of patients with immunologic disease, in Waldman RH (ed): *Clinical Concepts of Immunology.* Baltimore, Williams & Wilkins Co, © 1979, p 232. Reprinted by permission.)

globulins (rheumatoid factors), anti-red blood cell antibodies, antithyroglobulin, and antimicrobial antibodies. Hemagglutination inhibition detects soluble antigens by their ability to inhibit a standard antibody concentration from agglutinating the sensitized erythrocytes. The method has been used to detect Australia antigen and factor VIII antigen. Agglutination reactions may be direct or indirect. Direct agglutination is used to measure antibodies to some erythrocyte, bacterial, and fungal surface antigens. For indirect agglutination reactions, antigens may be absorbed or covalently linked to insoluble matrices as erythrocytes, bacteria, or polystyrene-latex particles. When serum containing antibodies to these antigens is added, the cells agglutinate and form a visible clump. Quantitation is usually determined by titration.

AUTOANTIBODIES

Rheumatoid Factors

Although rheumatoid factors occur in most patients with rheumatoid arthritis, they are not detected by standard methods in all patients, nor are they necessarily specific for rheumatoid arthritis when found. Rheumatoid factors can be detected in approximately 60%–95% of patients with rheumatoid arthritis but also occur in other diseases as well (Table 11.1).

The presence of rheumatoid factors in the blood of patients with rheumatoid arthritis is associated with progressive, aggressive, and extra-articular disease.

Rheumatoid factors are antibodies to IgG. Rheumatoid factors are usually detected by tests that use the capacity of 19 S IgM rheumatoid factor in serum to agglutinate antigen (IgG) attached to cells (sheep red blood cells) or particles (latex or bentonite). Rheumatoid factors are discussed more fully in Chapter 11.

Antinuclear Antibodies

The lupus erythematosus (LE) cell test is specific for lupus (because these cells occur infrequently in other diseases) but is not very sensitive. It is positive in 60%–90% of patients with SLE. The LE cell phenomenon occurs in vitro (rarely in vivo in pathologic effusions). It is caused by IgG antibody to nucleoprotein (LE factor) reaching cell nuclei, fixation of complement, and engulfment of homogeneous nuclear material by phagocytic cells. Since it is insensitive and because of technical and interpretive difficulties for the routine laboratory, LE cell testing has been supplanted largely by testing for ANAs.

Antinuclear antibodies is a term designating antibodies to a variety of nuclear constituents, not all of which have been well characterized (Table 4.3). These antibodies include native or double-stranded (DS) DNA; denatured or single-stranded (SS) DNA; soluble or insoluble DNA:histone (nucleoprotein); ribonucleic acid (RNA):protein (Mo); acidic nuclear proteins (Sm); extractable nuclear antigen (ENA), which is a composite of Sm and RNP antigens; and histone and nucleolar antigens. The antibodies to these antigens are distributed among all immunoglobulin classes—IgG, IgA, IgM, IgD, and IgE.

Many methods have been developed for detecting ANAs—antiglobulin consumption tests, complement fixation tests, precipitin reactions in gel, hemagglutination reactions (sheep red blood cells, latex, or bentonite particles), hemagglutination inhibition, horseradish-peroxidase-conjugated antibody, binding assays, counterimmunoelectrophoresis, and indirect immunofluorescence techniques. Of these, immunofluorescence is most widely used. It is possible to determine titers and patterns of ANAs when they are detected in serum (Table 4.3). The homogeneous or diffuse pattern is produced by antibodies to nucleoprotein and the peripheral (rim or shaggy) pattern by antibodies to DS-DNA. The speckled pattern results from antibodies to extractable ribonucleoprotein antigens. The nucleolar pattern reflects antibodies to nucleolar antigens, possibly RNA-protein. Additional patterns have also been described.

The incidence of ANAs in certain clinical states is listed in Table 4.4. Test results are positive in about 5% of normal persons, virtually all patients with lupus, approximately 15%–35% of those with discoid lupus, most with drug-induced lupus, 15%–40% of patients with juvenile or adult rheumatoid arthritis, 60% of those with scleroderma, 68% of those with Sjögren's syndrome, all reported patients with mixed connective tissue disease, and infrequently in patients with vasculitis and polydermatomyositis. The titers and patterns of positive ANA

Table 4.3. Correlation of Antinuclear Antibody Fluorescent Staining Patterns and Disease

Pattern	*Antigen*	*Disease*
Peripheral	DS-DNA	Systemic lupus erythematosus
Speckled	Acidic nuclear protein	Rheumatoid arthritis
	Ribonucleoprotein	Systemic lupus erythematosus
	Extractable nuclear antigen	Scleroderma
		Mixed connective tissue disease
Homogeneous	Deoxyribonucleoprotein	Rheumatoid arthritis
	Histone	Systemic lupus erythematosus
		Other
Nucleolar	Nucleolar RNA	Progressive systemic sclerosis
		Other

Table 4.4. Antinuclear Antibodies (ANA) in Health and Disease

Condition	Positive ANA		
	%	Titer	Pattern[a]
Normal subjects	5	Low	—
Systemic lupus erythematosus	90–100	High	P, D, S, N
Discoid lupus erythematosus	15–35	Low	S, D
Drug-induced lupus erythematosus	68–100	Low–high	D
Rheumatoid arthritis	20–40	Low	D
Juvenile rheumatoid arthritis	15	Low	D, S
Scleroderma	60	Low–high	S, N, D
Sjögren's syndrome	68	Low–high	P, S, N
Mixed connective tissue disease	99–100	High	S
Vasculitis	25	Low	—
Polydermatomyositis	30	Low	—

[a] P, peripheral; S, speckled; D, diffuse; N, nucleolar.

test results are helpful clinically (Tables 4.3 and 4.4). High-titer positive test results are seen most commonly in patients with systemic or drug-induced lupus and mixed connective tissue disease but have also been noted in some patients with scleroderma or Sjögren's syndrome. The peripheral pattern (anti–DS-DNA) is seen almost exclusively in patients with idiopathic lupus and is considered to be virtually diagnostic for the disease. The homogeneous pattern is the one most often seen in drug-related SLE. Speckled patterns are common in scleroderma and mixed connective tissue disease.

In addition to fluorescent ANAs, antibodies to DNA can also be specifically tested. Antibodies to DS-DNA are assayed by several methods, including complement fixation, diffusion in gel, hemagglutination, immunofluorescence, and radioimmunoassay. The most widely employed and sensitive procedures use radio-labeled DS-DNA and measure binding of radioactive antigen with anti–DS-DNA by ammonium sulfate precipitation (Farr assay), on nitrocellulose filters, glass-fiber filters, or plastic. Recently, the kinetoplast of the protozoan *Crithidia luciliae,* containing pure DS-DNA, has been used as substrate for an indirect immunofluorescence test. This procedure appears simple, sensitive, and reliable. Antibodies to DS native DNA, present in most patients with idiopathic lupus at some time during the course of disease, are almost always diagnostic of systemic lupus and are rarely seen in other instances.

ANAs are generally thought to be present in sera of all lupus patients but are not diagnostic for the disease, since positive test results often occur in other disease states. A positive test result for anti–DS-DNA is usually diagnostic for lupus but is not necessarily found in all patients. A properly performed and consistently negative ANA test in a patient suspected of having lupus is unusual and suggests several possibilities. Conceivably, a serum might give a negative test result at low dilutions but a positive one at higher dilutions; hemolysis during venipuncture might liberate leukocyte nuclear antigens to bind antibodies; or antigen excess or therapeutic immunosuppression might also give rise to negative test results.

Alternatively, other diagnoses should be carefully considered in an ANA-negative patient with multisystem disease—systemic Weber-Christian disease, vasculitis, cryoglobulinemia, polychondritis, atypical infection, lymphoma, malignancy, Whipple's disease, sarcoidosis, or periodic syndromes.

ANAs not only have diagnostic use but also are of clinical value in following up patients with lupus. Anti–DS-DNA tends to be detectable in increasing titers in sera of patients with disease exacerbations. Titers also correlate with decreased concentrations of serum complement, increased levels of DNA, active nephritis, or active nonrenal lupus. Anti–DS-DNA, together with other serologic abnormalities such as in serum complement levels, can be observed to facilitate the management of patients with lupus.

Other Autoantibodies

A variety of other autoantibodies may be encountered in patients with immunologic diseases. Patients with SLE often have antibodies to RNA, clotting factors, enzymes, cells (red cells, white cells, lymphocytes, and platelets), and tissues (thyroid, neurons, muscles, liver, kidneys, joints, and capillaries). Patients with chronic active hepatitis have antibodies to smooth muscle, and those with primary biliary cirrhosis have antibodies to mitochondria. Antibodies to glomerular basement membrane are present in patients with Goodpasture's syndrome. Approximately 70% of Sjögren's syndrome patients have antibodies to salivary duct antigen. Other antigen-antibody systems that have strong associations with specific diseases are being investigated—nuclear antigens associated with rheumatoid arthritis (RANA), scleroderma (Scl 70 antigen), polymyositis (PM 1 antigen), and Sjögren's syndrome (SS-A and SS-B antigens).

IMMUNE COMPLEXES

Immune complexes have a pathogenetic role in such diseases as the serum sickness prodrome of hepatitis B infection, rheumatoid arthritis, SLE, hypersensitivity pneumonitis, the Arthus reaction, some forms of glomerulonephritis, and vasculitis. A number of methods have been developed to quantify complexes. Most measurements have been based on the high sedimentation velocity of immune complexes or on their interactions with rheumatoid factors, the complement system, platelets, or lymphocyte surface receptors (Table 4.5).

Ultracentrifugal analysis may reveal intermediate-sized or macromolecular complexes of antigens and antibodies. In rheumatoid arthritis, 7 S IgG (antigen) may complex with 7 S IgG or 19 S IgM antigammaglobulins, which produce either 11–14 S or 22 S complexes. This method is not widely available and is relatively insensitive. Immune complexes have also been identified by coupling monoclonal rheumatoid factor with cellulose particles. Immune complexes in test serum compete for the rheumatoid factor with ^{125}I-aggregated IgG complexes. This method has been used to detect immune complexes in the serum and synovial fluid of patients with rheumatoid arthritis and correlates directly with the severity of the disease and inversely with the serum C4 level. This method was not sensitive for detecting immune complexes in SLE and other vasculitides.

Various methods use the ability of C1q to bind to immune complexes. The method of precipitating C1q with aggregated gammaglobulin or immune com-

Table 4.5. Immune Complexes

Methods of detection
  C1q precipitation or binding
  Monoclonal rheumatoid factor (MRF) precipitation
  Ultracentrifugation
  Anticomplementarity
  Tissue immunofluorescence
  Tissue elution
  Cryoprecipitation
  Binding to cells with C receptors
  Platelet aggregation test
  DNAase digestion and anti-DNA titers
Diagnostic value
  Documentation of immune-complex-mediated disease (rheumatoid arthritis, systemic
    lupus erythematosus, glomerulonephritis, others)
  Identification of immunoreactants
Prognostic value
  Correlates with disease severity (RA and SLE) and exacerbations

plexes in agarose gel was used to detect immune complexes in patients with SLE and in joint fluids of patients with rheumatoid arthritis. Immune complexes may also be detected by mixing ^{125}I-C1q with test serum plus disodium ethylenediamine tetra-acetate (EDTA) and precipitating the immune complex–[125]I-C1q with polyethylene glycol. The presence of complexes correlated inversely with the serum C4 level. Additionally, immune complexes may compete with antibody-sensitized erythrocytes for ^{125}I-C1q. The degree of inhibition is measured by separating the soluble immune complex–[125]I-C1q by centrifugation. Immune complexes have also been measured by their ability to compete with radiolabeled aggregated IgG for C1q bound to polystyrene tubes.

Another recently developed method for detecting immune complexes employs the Raji cell. This is a human lymphoblastoid cell with B-cell characteristics but without surface immunoglobulin. Raji cells have receptors for the immunoglobulin (Fc) region and C3b. Immune complexes may be quantitated by reacting patient serum with the Raji cells and then measuring the ability of these cells to take up ^{125}I-antihuman IgG. Results are evaluated by comparing the ability of Raji cells mixed with aggregated human gammaglobulin to take up ^{125}I-antihuman IgG. These methods have been used to detect immune complexes in serum hepatitis and other infections, SLE, rheumatoid arthritis, malignancies, and other diseases.

The assays have proved useful for clinical investigators but remain of uncertain value to the practicing clinician at present.

CRYOPROTEINS

Cryofibrinogens have been observed in association with malignancies and with hematologic and rheumatic disorders, especially scleroderma. Cryoglobulins are

Table 4.6. Cryoproteins

Methods of measurement
  Serum/plasma incubation at 4 C
  Cryocrit
  Quantitative cryoprotein determination
Diagnostic value
  Type I (monoclonal Ig): dysproteinemias
  Type II (monoclonal ab to polyclonal ag): dysproteinemias, malignant, rheumatic,
    infectious diseases
  Type III (mixed polyclonal): malignant, rheumatic, infectious diseases, essential
    cryoglobulinemia

---

present in many infectious, rheumatic, and malignant diseases (Table 4.6). They are thought to consist of immune complexes and may contain a variety of immunoreactants (Ig, complement, antinuclear antibodies, antigammaglobulins, and others). Cryoglobulins have been classified into three types. Type I contains monoclonal Ig. Type II consists of a monoclonal component with antibody activity to a polyclonal component—that is, IgG or IgM antigamma globulin (monoclonal)–IgG (polyclonal). Type III is mixed polyclonal cryoglobulins, usually Ig with or without non-Ig. Cryoproteins may cause damage through their capacity as immune reactants (type II or III) or through their mass or viscosity (e.g., type I, Waldenström's macroglobulinemia). Type I, particularly when IgM is present, may be removed effectively by plasmaphoresis.

Blood to be examined for cryoproteins is drawn into warm syringes at 37 C. For cryofibrinogens the sample is anticoagulated with disodium EDTA or citrate. The serum or plasma is separated by centrifugation at 37 C and is then stored at 4 C for at least 72 hours. A precipitate or gel should be redissolved at 37 C before the presence of the cryoprotein is confirmed. Immunochemical analyses may be performed on the precipitates. Cryofibrinogens are cryoproteins that form in anticoagulated plasma. If the precipitates are washed and redissolved, a mixture of proteins is present and can include albumin and alpha, beta, and gamma globulins.

COMPLEMENT

The details of activation of human complement are discussed in Chapter 8. A brief description of the methods of measurement is included here. Complement values may be increased in many diseases, particularly acute, infectious, or inflammatory states, behaving like an acute-phase reactant. Certain uncommon congenital deficiencies of complement components might be detected by low values of CH50 or individual complement proteins. Hereditary angioneurotic edema is such an entity. It is characterized by functional absence of the C1 inhibitor. Patients usually have low C4 and C2 values and are deficient in C1 inhibitor. Acquired serum hypocomplementemia occurs in many immunologic diseases, such as SLE, glomerulonephritis, cryoglobulinemia, and other immune-complex-mediated processes. Classic complement activation leads to depressions of C1, C4, and C2, as well as C3. Alternative pathway use produces low values for properdin, C3, and later-acting components. Acquired hypocomplementemia also occurs in effusions (synovial, pericardial, and pleural) from patients with rheumatoid arthritis and lupus. Occasionally hypocomplementemia is diagnostically helpful, since it supports a presumption of immune-complex-mediated disease. It may also lead to diagnosis of congenital complement deficiency syndrome. Patterns of abnormalities are sufficiently nonspecific that they are not often useful in trying to establish a specific diagnosis. Once it is clear that a patient has an immune-complex-mediated disease and when complement abnormalities correlate with clinical abnormalities, it is useful to follow complement levels serially. This information is helpful to many clinicians caring for certain patients with SLE, nephritis, and vasculitis.

CH50 Assay

The CH50 assay is used to measure the entire complement system. It is far less sensitive than hemolytic methods for the individual complement components. Sheep erythrocytes (E) are washed and coated with antibody (A) specific for the cell. Dilutions of the serum to be tested are added to a standard number of sensitized cells (EA). A standard serum of known complement content is used as a control. Lysis of the erythrocyte is accomplished by complement activation through the classic pathway. Once C9 is activated, the erythrocytes lyse and release hemoglobin into the supernatant fluid. The degree of lysis is measured by the amount of hemoglobin released and depends on the concentration of complement in the original serum sample. The serum titration that lyses 50% of the sensitized erythrocytes is taken as the CH50.

Measurement of Individual Components

Individual complement components may be titrated by diluting the sample to be tested and adding all other components in excess. For example, to measure C4, purified C1 is added to sensitized sheep erythrocytes (EAC1). Dilutions of the C4 source are incubated with EAC1 cells. After this, C2 and then C3–9 are added in excess and the mixture is incubated for a standard time interval. The degree of hemolysis is measured by the spectrophotometric detection of hemoglobin in the supernatant. These methods require considerable time and expense in maintaining fresh reagents and are not generally available to the clinician.

Extensive consideration of complement abnormalities in disease is beyond the scope of this discussion. Complement levels (C3, C4, and C1 esterase inhibitors) are generally determined by radial immunodiffusion, since the assay is readily available and relatively easy to perform. Hemolytic measurements are technically more difficult and require resources not generally available (Table 4.7).

Complement Fixation

The complement fixation test can detect antigens and antibodies to microbial organisms, nuclear constituents, and others. When fluid-phase antigens and anti-

Table 4.7. Complement

Methods of detection
Hemolytic (functional) assays
Immunochemical (protein) assays

Methods of detection
  Hemolytic (functional) assays
  Immunochemical (protein) assays
Diagnostic value
  Inherited C component deficiencies
  Hereditary angioedema (C1 inhibitor deficiency)
  Decreased (C4, C3) in synovial fluid in rheumatoid arthritis, SLE, glomerulonephritis, cryoglobulinemias, immune-complex diseases
Prognostic value
  ↓ C associated with active immune-complex disease
  ↓ C associated with active severe rheumatoid arthritis, SLE
  ↑ or ↓ C may antedate clinical remission or exacerbation, respectively, of SLE

bodies are allowed to react in the presence of complement (standard fresh serum with a known content of complement), complement components are fixed and activated. After a standard period of incubation, the mixture is diluted and its ability to lyse sensitized sheep erythrocytes (EA) is determined. If large quantities of antibody are present in a patient's serum, a greater quantity of complement will be used in the original incubation. This process will leave less complement to lyse the sensitized sheep cells. Sometimes the result of complement fixation will be reported as "anticomplementary." A number of factors are known to be responsible for this phenomenon, including contamination of the serum sample test reagents with microorganisms, agents that bind calcium and magnesium ions, immune complexes, aggregated immunoglobulin, and prolonged storage of serum.

IMMUNOFLUORESCENCE

Immunofluorescence is clinically practical for examining biopsy specimens for the presence of immunoglobulin and complement and localization of specific antigens. Serum also may be examined for specific antibodies by the indirect immunofluorescence method, as in the fluorescent treponemal antibody absorption and ANA tests. Fluorescein and rhodamine are organic compounds that fluoresce brilliant yellow-green and red, respectively, on absorption of ultraviolet light. These compounds can be covalently linked to macromolecules, such as proteins, for histochemical studies. With direct immunofluorescence the antibody specific to a given antigen is conjugated with a fluorescent compound and applied directly to the tissue or source of antigen to be examined. After a thorough rinsing, the material is examined with a special fluorescent microscope equipped with an ultraviolet lamp. Localization of the antigen in the tissue is detected by fluorescence. With indirect immunofluorescence the tissue or source of antigen to be examined is first incubated with untagged specific antibody. Fluorescein-labeled heterologous antibody specific for the untagged immunoglobulin is then applied and the sample examined for immunofluorescence. This process has also been called the *sandwich technique.*

ERYTHROCYTE SEDIMENTATION RATE

Determination of the erythrocyte sedimentation rate (ESR) has been used to monitor patients with inflammatory diseases. The Westergren method is preferred. Blood anticoagulated with disodium EDTA or citrate is drawn into a 200-mm column, which is allowed to stand vertically for 60 minutes. Normal values are usually 0–10 mm/hr for men and 0–15 mm/hr for women. The ESR may be increased with inflammatory diseases, malignancies, infections, increased fibrinogen or alpha or gammaglobulins, lipemia, fever, increased metabolic activity, thyroid disease, or dysproteinemias. It may also be increased during the third trimester of pregnancy or because the tubes were not precisely vertical or blood was not shaken before being drawn into the tubes. Inexplicably low or normal values may occur with anisocytosis, sickle cell disease, spherocytosis, hypochromasia, viral illness, acute liver disease, or congestive heart failure or because of clotted blood in the tubes. The ESR has its greatest applicability in following the course of patients with rheumatoid arthritis. It is of less value in managing patients with other inflammatory or rheumatic diseases.

CELLULAR IMMUNE FUNCTION

Lymphocytes

Human lymphocytes comprise heterogeneous populations of cells, which may be categorized by their distinctive surface characteristics and functions. The major classes of lymphocytes are T and B cells, with other subpopulations now being delineated. The main functions of lymphocytes are to produce antibodies, to effect cell-mediated immunologic reactions, and to control immune responses. T cells constitute 50%–70% and B cells 5%–20% of the circulating peripheral blood lymphocytes. A detailed discussion of lymphocyte functions appears in Chapter 6.

Purification

Assays of lymphocyte populations or functions require a purified suspension of mononuclear cells from whole blood. Commonly, the suspension is obtained by centrifuging whole blood over a mixture of ficoll-Hypaque. This procedure separates formed elements in the blood according to cell density and yields a highly purified population of mononuclear cells at the interface, consisting of 70%–90% of lymphocytes, suitable for the studies to be described.

T- and B-cell Enumeration

Many in vitro methods are available for determining the percentages of T and B lymphocytes in blood or pathologic specimens (Table 8.2). Lymphocyte populations have been enumerated for many disease states. These studies can help identify immunologic abnormalities in patients with certain diseases but have not been diagnostically helpful for individual patients (Table 4) (Chap. 6).

Table 4.8. Quantitation of Lymphocyte Subclasses

Methods of detection
  B cells: surface Ig, C3b receptor (EAC rosettes)
  T cells: sheep red blood cell (E) rosettes
Diagnostic value
  Lymphoproliferative disorders
  Immunodeficiency diseases

Surface Immunoglobulin

Surface immunoglobulin serves as a marker for B cells. Human T cells have little, if any, immunoglobulin on their surface. Immunofluorescent staining with $F(ab')_2$ antihuman immunoglobulin will detect B cells. When living B cells react with the fluorescein-labeled antisera, the cell surface becomes uniformly stained (Fig. 4.6).

EAC Rosettes

B cells have also been shown to have surface receptors for C3b, C3d, and C4b. The method most used for detecting the receptors consists of coating sheep eryth-

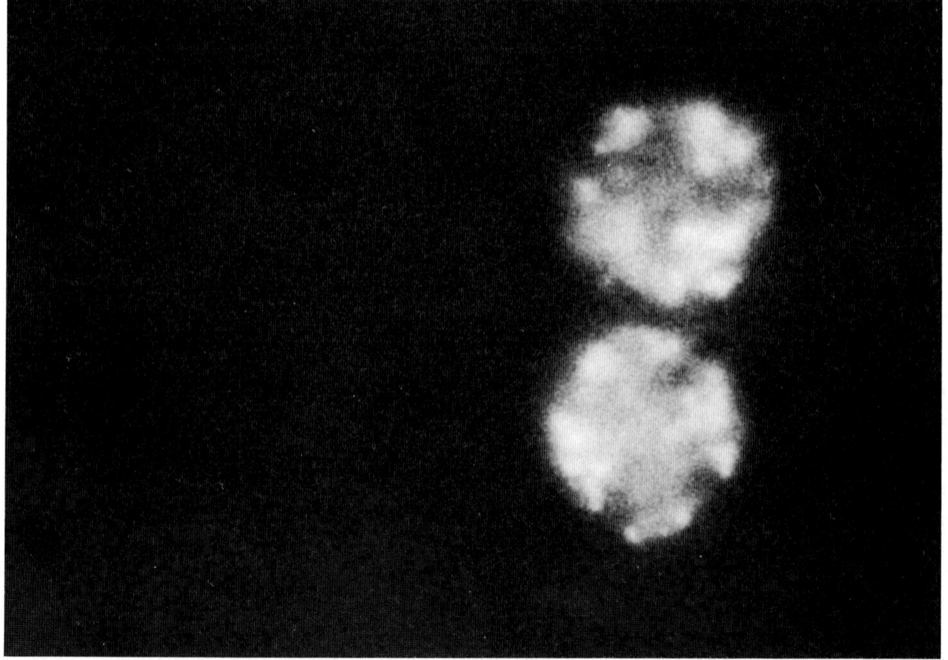

Figure 4.6. Membrane immunofluorescence of human B lymphocytes stained with fluoresceinated goat antihuman Ig (original magnification ×810). (Courtesy of Dr. Perry O. Teague) (From Brestel EP, Delafuente JC, Longley S, Panush RS: Evaluation of patients with immunologic disease, in Waldman RH (ed): *Clinical Concepts of Immunology.* Baltimore, Williams & Wilkins Co, © 1979, p 241. Reprinted by permission.)

rocytes with antibody and complement (C3b, C3d, or C4b). Under appropriate conditions, these coated sheep cells (EAC) will form rosettes with B cells. Since neutrophils and monocytes can also form EAC rosettes, they need to be identified by other procedures.

Anti–B-cell Antibody

Antisera to human B cells can be produced by immunizing animals with B cells. The antibodies produced can be fluorescein-labeled, and immunofluorescence studies can detect these B cells.

Fc Receptors

Another marker on B cells is the Fc receptor. These receptors bind the Fc portion of an immunoglobulin in the form of an immune complex or as aggregated immunoglobulin. The Fc receptor-bearing cells are usually detected by incubating radioisotope or fluorescein-labeled antigen-antibody complexes or heat-aggregated immunoglobulin with lymphocytes and examining cell suspensions by scintillation counting or fluorescent microscopy. Other cells, such as macrophages, T cells, and some null cells, also have Fc receptors.

E Rosettes

Unlike the B cell, most T cells are devoid of Fc and C3b receptors. The T cell is most commonly identified by its ability to form rosettes with normal sheep erythrocytes (Fig. 4.7). The methods are similar to the EAC rosette assay. Thus the E rosette provides a good marker for human T cells.

Anti–T-cell Antibodies

Antisera to human T cells and T-cell subpopulations can be produced by immunizing animals. The antibodies produced can be labeled with fluorescein, and immunofluorescence studies can be done as described for B cells or placed on indicator erythrocytes for rosetting studies.

In Vivo Assays of Lymphocyte Function

Skin testing can be performed in vivo to assess delayed hypersensitivity responses of patients. Cutaneous reactivity is often depressed in the congenital or acquired defects (Table 4.8). When certain antigens are injected intradermally, a delayed type of hypersensitivity reaction will occur. Antigens often used include mumps, streptokinase-streptodornase, purified protein derivative, trichophyton, and *Candida albicans*. Erythema and induration are measured after 48 hours. Contact sensitization to dinitrochlorobenzene can also be tested. More than 90% of normal persons will react to two or more antigens.

In Vitro Lymphocyte Activation

The integrity of cell-mediated immune function in vitro can be assessed by testing lymphocyte activation or lymphokine production (also discussed in Chap. 6). Abnormalities of lymphocyte activation have been seen in many disease states, including malignancies, rheumatic diseases, and infectious diseases. These are usu-

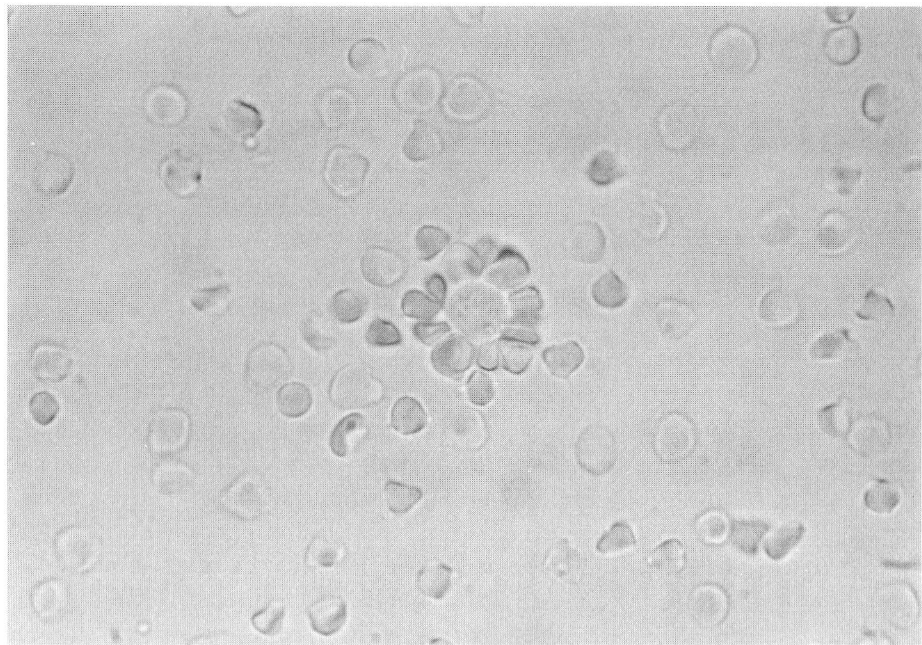

Figure 4.7. Rosette formed by human T lymphocyte with sheep erythrocytes (original magnification ×388). (From Brestel EP, Delafuente JC, Longley S, Panush RS: Evaluation of patients with immunologic disease, in Waldman RH (ed): *Clinical Concepts of Immunology*. Baltimore, Williams & Wilkins Co, © 1979, p 242. Reprinted by permission.)

ally nonspecific and not unique to a single disease. These assays do not usually provide important information to the clinician regarding individual patients.

Lymphokines

When sensitized lymphocytes interact with antigens, many soluble substances are generated. These *lymphokines* are reviewed in detail in Chapter 6 (Table 6.3). Biologic assays for the detection of lymphokines are numerous and difficult to perform. The pertinence of these substances in infectious, immunologic, neoplastic, and other diseases is under active investigation.

NEUTROPHILS

Occasionally, the clinical immunologist will evaluate patients for possible congenital or acquired defects of neutrophil functions (Table 4.9). The primary functions of polymorphonuclear neutrophils (PMNs) are phagocytosis and killing of particulate materials, such as bacteria. The PMNs gain access to the areas of inflammation and invading pathogens by being attracted by chemotactic factors derived from serum complement, lymphocytes, and other sources. Neutrophil phagocytosis, motility, and bacterial killing can be assayed.

Table 4.9. Phagocytosis

Methods of evaluation
  Nitroblue tetrazolium test
  Intracellular killing assays
  Particle ingestion and enumeration
  Lysosomal enzyme release
Diagnostic value
  Congenital disorders (Job's syndrome, Chédiak-Higashi syndrome, chronic granulomatous
    disease, complement deficiency, others)
  Acquired disorders (malignant, infectious, rheumatic diseases, drugs, sickle cell disease,
    others)

Nitroblue Tetrazolium Test

A clinically useful assay for phagocytosis is the nitroblue tetrazolium dye-reduction test. Nitroblue tetrazolium is a water-soluble yellow compound. Reduction of dye in the phagocytic vacuole can be measured photometrically. This is a useful test for determining the metabolic integrity of phagocytes and is diagnostically important in chronic granulomatous disease.

Intracellular Killing Assay

Another useful assay of phagocytosis is the microbial killing technique, in which the ability of the phagocytes to kill ingested bacteria is determined. Phagocytes are incubated with bacteria, and the number of viable ingested organisms is determined from colony counts. This method provides information about the rate of intracellular killing as well as the ability of the phagocyte to kill (Table 4.9). Clinical disorders of phagocytosis are beyond the scope of this chapter.

Chemotaxis

The ability of neutrophils and macrophages to undergo directional migration, known as *chemotaxis,* can be assessed in vitro. Defective chemotactic responses of mononuclear and PMN leukocytes have been described for congenital disorders, such as Wiskott-Aldrich syndrome and chronic mucocutaneous candidiasis, and for acute influenzal infections, rheumatic diseases, cirrhosis, renal disease, and others (Table 4.10). Chemotaxis is usually measured in a Boyden chamber, which has two compartments separated by a filter membrane. The leukocytes are placed in the upper chamber and the chemotactic factors (complement, bacteria, and lymphocyte derived) in the lower chamber. After incubation, the filter membrane is removed, rinsed with saline, and stained. The cells on the underside of the filter are quantitated microscopically.

Other Tests

Other methods to test PMN functions include phagocytosis of lipopolysaccharide emulsified in oil red O, phagocytosis of insoluble particles with microscopic visualization, or assays for lysosomal enzymes.

Table 4.10. Chemotaxis

Methods of evaluation
  Boyden changers
  Agarose gels
  Skin window
  Guinea pig peritoneal cavity
Diagnostic value
  Congenital disorders (Wiskott-Aldrich syndrome, mucocutaneous candidiasis, complement deficiencies, agammaglobulinemia)
  Acquired disorders (infections, malignancy, rheumatic disease, liver disease, renal disease, diabetes, drugs)

MACROPHAGES

Macrophages are mononuclear cells present in various tissues, such as the spleen, lungs, and lymph nodes, and in the blood. Circulating macrophages are known as *monocytes*. Macrophages phagocytose bacteria, viruses, damaged cells, and neoplastic cells. They also affect induction of the immune response through interaction with T and B lymphocytes (Chap. 6).

Macrophages from humans are usually obtained from surgical specimens of tonsils, thymus, spleen, lymph nodes, and synovium. Tests have not yet been standardized for evaluating macrophage functions and their relevance to human disease. The nitroblue tetrazolium test, intracellular killing assay, and chemotaxis assays described for PMNs can be applied to macrophages and blood monocytes.

HLA TYPING

Recognition of familial associations of many rheumatologic and immunologic diseases has been confirmed by HLA testing. HLA, or human leukocyte antigens, occur on cell surfaces, are involved in cell-cell recognition and interactions, and are under genetic control. The presence of these antigens can be assayed by microcytotoxicity testing of donor cells with appropriate antisera and complement. The striking association of HLA B27 with spondyloarthritis is reviewed in Chapter 13. HLA typing for the presence of B27 is not necessary in clinically recognizable syndromes, but it may be helpful when the diagnosis is uncertain or for genetic counseling. The clinical and immunopathologic significance of lymphocyte-defined D, Dr, and Ia antigens in rheumatic diseases is being investigated (see Chaps. 11, 13, and 17). Available information is summarized in Table 4.11.

TISSUE BIOPSY

Biopsies of tissues help in the diagnosis of many rheumatic diseases. The value of muscle (this chapter) and synovial biopsy (Chap. 3) has been discussed. The biopsy of other tissues will be described in the appropriate sections. The biopsy of normal and involved skin, with immunofluorescence, is helpful in establishing a

Table 4.11. Human B-cell Alloantigens and Rheumatic Diseases

Disease	*B-cell Alloantigens*
Rheumatoid arthritis	↑DRW 4 × 7, ↓DRW1, ↓DRW3
Juvenile rheumatoid arthritis	↑DW7, ↑DW8, ↑DRW4
Pauciarticular juvenile rheumatoid arthritis	↑TMD
SLE	↑DR2, ↓DRW 4 × 7
Systemic sclerosis	↑DRW3, ↓DRW 4 × 7
Idiopathic thrombocytopenic purpura	↑DRW2

diagnosis of SLE because complement and Ig at the dermoepidermal junction are present in the involved skin of approximately 80%–90% of patients and in the uninvolved skin of 40%–60%. Similarly, uninvolved skin may contain a deposition of immunoreactants in a small percentage of patients with other forms of vasculitis. Biopsy of the skin also aids in confirming a diagnosis of progressive systemic sclerosis, of minor salivary glands in Sjögren's syndrome; of vasculature in vasculitis; of kidney in vasculitis, lupus, Goodpasture's syndrome, progressive systemic sclerosis, or amyloidosis; of temporal artery in giant cell arteritis; and of the rectum, gingiva, or liver in amyloidosis.

CONCLUSION

This chapter has summarized methods, particularly immunologic, used to evaluate rheumatic diseases and has reviewed their underlying principles. Specific abnormalities in certain conditions and their importance in the pathogenesis, manifestations, course, and treatment of diseases were briefly discussed.

The material in *Humoral Immune Function, Antinuclear Antibodies, Immune Complexes, Cryoproteins, Complement, Cellular Immune Function, Macrophages,* and Tables 4.3–4.10 appears in similar form in the following two publications: Brestel EP, Delafuente JC, Longley S, Panush RS: Immunologic techniques, in Lockey RF (ed): *Allergy and Clinical Immunology.* Garden City, NY, Medical Examination Publishing Co, Inc, an Excerpta Medica company, © 1979, pp 556–572; Prestel EP, Delafuente JC, Longley S, Panush RS: Evaluation of patients with immunologic disease, and Panush RS: Autoantibodies and human diseases, in Waldman RF (ed): *Clinical Concepts of Immunology.* Baltimore, Williams & Wilkins Co, © 1979, p 141–146, 227–246. Reprinted by permission.

BIBLIOGRAPHY

Chess L, MacDermott RP, Sondel PM, et al: Isolation and characterization of cells involved in human cellular hypersensitivity, in Brent L, Holborow J (eds): *Progress in Immunology,* vol 3. New York, American Elsevier Publishing Co, 1974, p 125.

Cohen AS (ed): *Laboratory Diagnostic Procedures in the Rheumatic Diseases,* ed 2. Boston, Little, Brown & Co, 1975.

Editorial. Testing neutrophil function. *Lancet* 2:1391, 1976.

Fernandez-Madrid F, Mattioli M: Antinuclear antibodies (ANA): Immunologic and clinical significance. *Semin Arthritis Rheum* 6:83, 1976.

Fessel WJ: Muscle diseases in rheumatology. *Semin Arthritis Rheum* 3:127, 1973.

Greaves MF, Owen JJT, Raff MC: *T and B Lymphocytes, Origins, Properties and Roles in Immune Responses.* New York, American Elsevier Publishing Co, 1974.

Laurell CB: Electroimmunoassay. *Scand J Clin Lab Invest* 29 (suppl 124):21, 1972.

Mancini G, Carbonara AO, Heremans JF: Immunochemical quantitation of antigens by single radial immunodiffusion. *Immunochemistry* 2:235, 1965.

Ouchterlony O: Antigen-antibody reactions in gels. *Acta Pathol Microbiol Scand* 26:507, 1949.

Panush RS, Bianco NE, Schur PH: Serum and synovial fluid IgG, IgA and IgM anti-gammaglobulins in rheumatoid arthritis. *Arthritis Rheum* 14:737, 1971.

Rapp HJ, Borsos T: *Molecular Basis of Complement Action.* New York, Appleton-Century-Crofts, 1970.

Reichlin M, Mattioli M: Antigens and antibodies characteristic of systemic lupus erythematosus. *Bull Rheum Dis* 24:756, 1974.

Rocklin RE, MacDermott RP, Chess L, et al: Studies on mediator production by highly purified human T and B lymphocytes. *J Exp Med* 140:1303, 1974.

Rose NR, Friedman H (eds): *Manual of Clinical Immunology.* Washington, DC, American Society for Microbiology, 1976.

Ruddy S, Gigli I, Austen KF: The complement system of man. *N Engl J Med* 287:489, 545, 592, 642, 1972.

Stage DE, Mannik M: Rheumatoid factors in rheumatoid arthritis. *Bull Rheum Dis* 23:720, 1972–1973.

Tannenbaum H, Schur PH: The role of lymphocytes in rheumatic diseases. *J Rheumatol* 1:392, 1974.

Territo MC, Cline MJ: Monocyte function in man. *J Immunol* 118:187, 1977.

Theofilopoulos AN, Wilson CB, Dixon FJ: The Raji cell radioimmunoassay for detecting immune complexes in human sera. *J Clin Invest* 57:169, 1976.

Zubler RH, Lambert PH: Detection of immune complexes in human diseases. *Prog Allergy* 24:1, 1978.

5

Radiology of Rheumatic Diseases

Terry M. Hudson

RADIOGRAPHIC EXAMINATION

Roentgenologic examination of the patient with rheumatic disease may serve to confirm the clinical impression, to evaluate the progression of disease, or to identify important abnormalities not suspected clinically, such as atlantoaxial subluxation or chondrocalcinosis.

Early roentgenographic abnormalities are subtle and nonspecific in most rheumatic diseases. With progression the abnormalities become more diagnostic, but in late stages severe destruction may obscure specific diagnostic patterns.

The physician may order roentgenograms of clinically abnormal joints only, or of those joints likely to be diseased. A general survey might include views of the flexed lateral cervical spine, hands and wrists, pelvis (to show sacroiliac and hip joints), knees, feet, and ankles. When radiographic signs are nonspecific or confusing, the distribution of abnormalities may be of considerable diagnostic help and the roentgenographic survey may be extremely useful.

Although rheumatic diseases are complex, roentgenograms reflect the limited number of ways tissues can respond to injury and disease. Therefore a manageable but thorough systematic roentgenographic evaluation is readily possible. A useful sequence for examining roentgenograms is: (1) soft tissues (swelling, atrophy, calcifications), (2) articular cartilage, (3) bone, (4) overall configuration (size, shape, alignment), (5) distribution of abnormalities, and (6) correlation with clinical and laboratory data. Specific abnormalities will be discussed under the individual diseases, and salient features are summarized in Table 5.1.

Sometimes roentgenographic abnormalities are so characteristic that a specific diagnosis can be made with great confidence. However, roentgenograms are often less specific or even confusing, and in such instances, the history, physical examination, and laboratory data are obviously essential.

Table 5.1.   Radiographic Features of Rheumatic Diseases

Disease	Soft Tissues	Articular Cartilage	Juxta-articular Bone	Alignment and Shape	Distribution
Rheumatoid arthritis	Swelling of joints, other synovial areas; subcutaneous nodules	Destroyed in months to years; ankylosis common	Juxta-articular osteoporosis; marginal erosions, subarticular cysts; minimal proliferative response, but late secondary hypertrophic changes	Common, typical malalignments (swan neck, boutonniere); subluxations (e.g., atlantoaxial)	Any synovial joint: hands, feet, knees, hips, elbows, ankles; cervical spine; symmetric
Juvenile rheumatoid arthritis	Like adult RA	Like adult RA	Periosteal reaction common; erosions later, less prominent than in adult RA	Growth abnormalities: short bones, bulbous epiphyses, protrusio acetabuli	Monoarticular or pauci-articular disease; often large joints: knee, wrist, ankles, tarsal, hip
Ankylosing spondylitis (axial skeleton)	Involved by bone proliferation	Narrowing, anky-losing of SI joints; end stage: complete spinal ankylosis	Proliferation is hallmark: paravertebral ossification, syndesmophytes, enthesopathy	Abnormal spinal curves	SI disease earliest; invariably seen with spinal disease
(peripheral joints)	Synovial joint swelling	Uniform loss; ankylosis	Normal density; marginal periosteal reaction; erosions, but smaller than in RA	Depends on extent of disease	Larger joints: hip, shoulder; less frequently smaller joints
Psoriatic arthritis (peripheral joints)	Synovial joint swelling	Uniform loss in affected joint	Osteoporosis not prominent; erosions common; widespread, often profuse, thick periosteal reaction	May have subluxations, malalignment	Often more distal joints: DIPs
(spondylitis)			Paravertebral ossification: coarse, asymmetric, often nonmarginal syndesmophytes		Always SI disease (asymmetric) with spondylitis
Reiter's spondylarthritis	Peripheral joint swelling	Uniform loss in affected joint	Erosions usually mild may be severe; periosteal reaction common	May have subluxations, malalignment	Predilection for lower extremities, SI; asymmetric
DISH	Usually no swelling	Usually normal	Thick, asymmetric paraverte-bral ossification with normal	No typical abnormalities	Spine, pelvis, other

			disc heights; bony proliferation at many musculotendinous insertions		
SLE	Joint swelling	Preserved	No erosions	Severe malalignment, subluxations may occur	Hands; occasionally feet
PSS	Atrophy of finger tips; subcutaneous calcification	Occasionally narrowed	Resorption of distal phalanges	Variable	Hands predominantly
MCTD	Joint swelling; occasional distal atrophy, subcutaneous calcification	Often narrowed	Osteoporosis; marginal erosions; occasional distal phalangeal resorption	Variable	Hands especially
DJD	Occasional swelling	Narrowed early; asymmetric loss	Marginal osteophytes; subarticular hypertrophy	Malalignment due to asymmetric cartilage loss	Hips, knees, DIPs of fingers, thumb CM
Paget's disease	Not involved	May be narrow with DJD	Enlarged, with thick, coarse trabecular pattern	Bowing, distortion	Pelvis, skull, femur
Gout	Joint swelling; later, tophi	Uniform loss in affected joint	Typically not osteoporotic; well-marginated erosions	When severe, late destruction, deformity	Distal joints, especially lower extremity: great toe MTP
CPPD	Joint swelling; calcification occasionally in capsule tendon, bursa	Calcification (not detectable in 10%)	Osteophytes; carpal cysts; irregular para-articular proliferation occasionally	Flexion contractures	Wrist, knee (3 compartments), elbow, ankle
Septic arthritis (usual pyogenic)	Joint swelling	Rapid destruction (days)	Osteoporosis, marginal erosions, indistinct subarticular cortex	Severe destruction may end in gross deformity	Any synovial joint
Septic arthritis (TB, GC, brucella)	Joint swelling	Destruction in weeks to months	Osteoporosis, erosions	Slow development of deformity	Any synovial joint
Neurotrophic	Joint swelling, often massive; multiple fragments, calcified debris late	Slow or rapid destruction	Hypertrophy, osteophytes	Gross deformity and malalignment	Depends on distribution of sensory deficit

RADIOGRAPHIC FEATURES OF RHEUMATIC DISEASES

Rheumatoid Arthritis and Related Diseases

Rheumatoid Arthritis (RA)

The earliest radiographic abnormality of RA is swelling within one or more joints (Fig. 5.1). Soft tissue swelling may also be due to tenosynovitis, rheumatoid nodules, or olecranon, retrocalcaneal, or subacromial bursitis. Later, soft tissue atrophy may result from debilitation and disuse.

Articular cartilage destruction occurs uniformly within an involved joint and appears months to years after the onset of disease, at about the same time as detectable bone erosion. The cartilage may eventually be completely destroyed, and end-stage bony ankylosis commonly involves carpals, tarsals, and interphalangeal (IP) joints.

Juxta-articular osteoporosis appears after soft tissue swelling. Marginal erosions soon follow, detected earliest at the styloid process of ulna, radial side of heads of metacarpals, and bases of proximal phalanges and carpal bones (Figs 5.1, 5.2). The erosions may be poorly marginated, with no reactive bony rim and the "rat bite" appearance, or they may develop rims of reactive bone, the "punched-out" appearance. Erosion can extend to subchondral bone and may lead to severe resorption, as seen in the "opera glass hand."

After subchondral bone is denuded of cartilage, pressure erosion may produce a ball-in-socket appearance (Fig. 5.2). Erosions may also affect nonarticular bone (tips of lower cervical spinous processes, posterior ribs, clavicles). Subarticular cysts may become quite large.

Although bone atrophy and erosion predominate, RA elicits some bone proliferation even in early stages, when thin marginal osteophytes are found along the dorsum of the foot or at the elbow. Later, secondary hypertrophic degenerative changes may simulate primary degenerative joint disease.

Malalignment is common and characteristic, with the hand often severely involved. Ulnar deviation at the metacarpophalangeal (MCP) joints, boutonniere and swan-neck deformities (Fig. 5.3), and subluxations at MCP and other joints are common. In the feet, lateral deviation at the metatarsophalangeal (MTP) joints, "cock-up" toes, flat feet, spreading of the metatarsals, and hallux valgus occur.

Atlantoaxial subluxation is common but may be detectable only with the spine flexed (Fig. 5.4). Although this subluxation may be asymptomatic and not evident on physical examination, it is potentially very hazardous.

RA characteristically is bilaterally symmetric and involves all compartments of an affected joint uniformly. Most commonly involved are the wrist, hand (especially MCP and proximal interphalangeal (PIP) joints), foot (especially subtalar, talocalcaneonavicular, and MTP joints), knee, hip, elbow, ankle, and cervical spine, including apophyseal joints and discs. However, any peripheral joint may be involved.

When swelling, cartilage loss, osteoporosis, erosions and malalignments are found in typical distribution, the radiologic diagnosis is straightforward, but many patients have atypical radiographs.

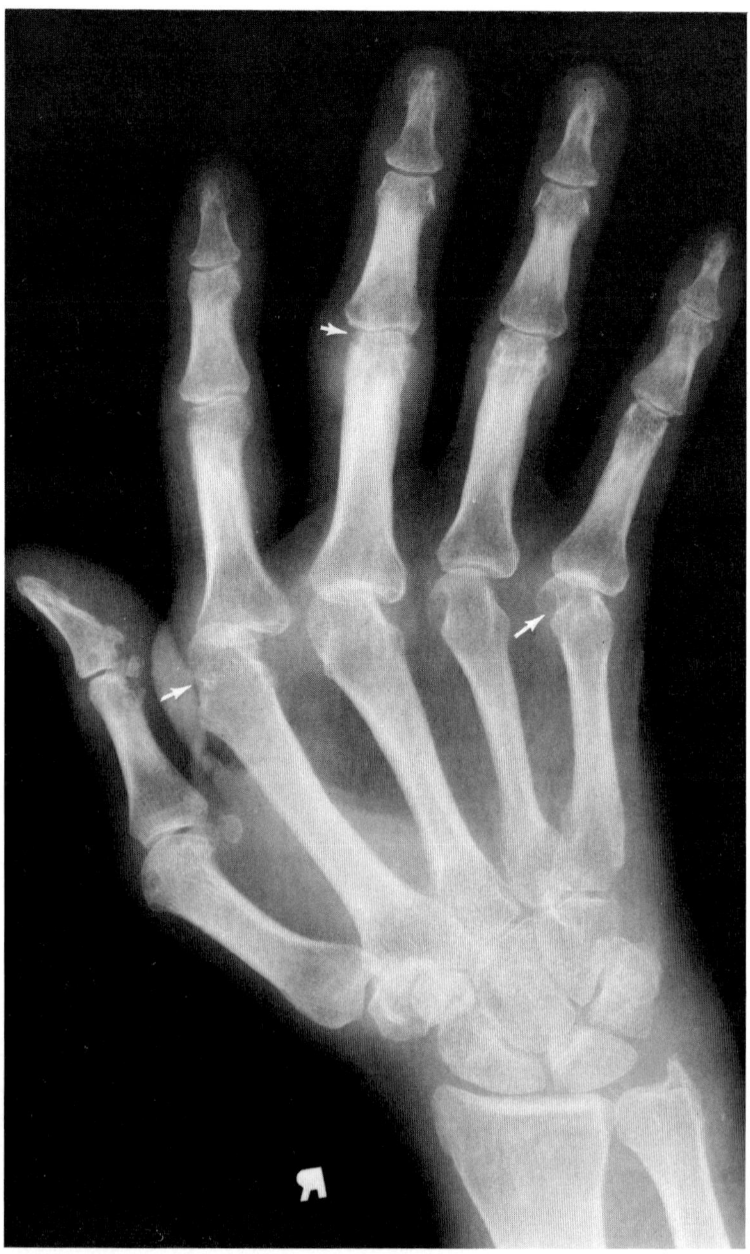

Figure 5.1. Rheumatoid arthritis with synovial swelling adjacent to the ulnar styloid and within IP and MCP joints, erosions of ulnar styloid and at margins of joints (arrows), juxta-articular osteoporosis, ulnar deviation of fingers, and subluxations of MCPs, worse toward the radial side of the hand.

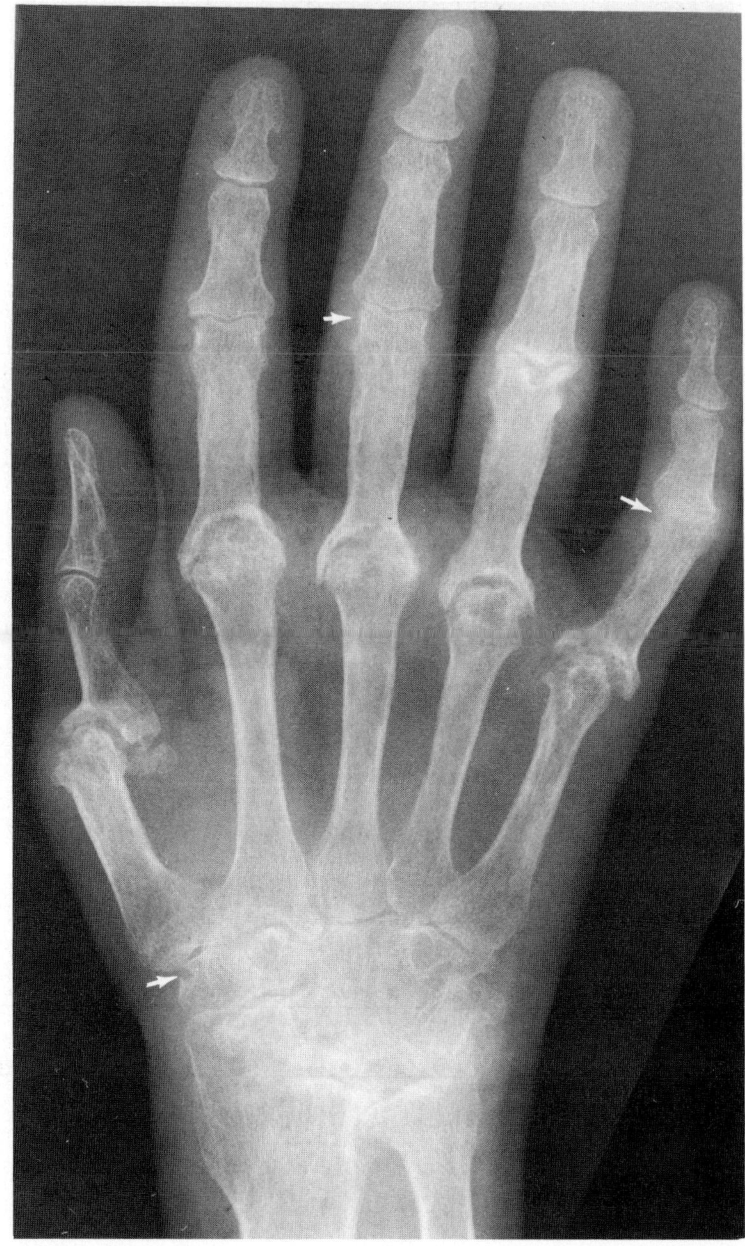

Figure 5.2. Advanced rheumatoid arthritis with both marginal erosions (arrows) and pressure erosions of bases of the proximal phalanges. There is also severe cartilage destruction of IP, MCP, and intercarpal joints and diffuse osteoporosis.

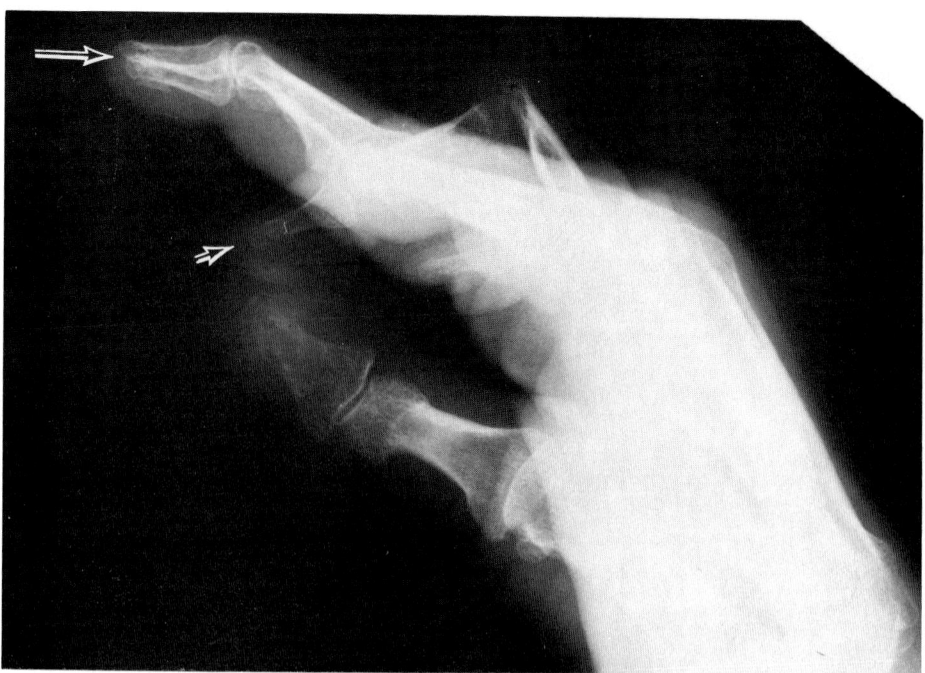

Figure 5.3. Rheumatoid arthritis with boutonniere deformity of the index finger (short arrow) and swan-neck deformity of the ring and long fingers (long arrow).

Juvenile Rheumatoid Arthritis (JRA)

Children with classic seronegative JRA have a disease that is clinically and radiographically different from adult RA. Radiographic abnormalities that distinguish JRA from adult disease include growth disturbances, periosteal reaction, different distribution of involvement, pauciarticular disease, delayed onset of both radiographically evident cartilage loss and juxta-articular erosions, more common joint ankylosis, and metaphyseal bands of osteoporosis.

Joint disease is asymmetric in approximately one-fifth of the children. Knees, wrists, and ankles are commonly involved, and temporomandibular joint disease with micrognathia occurs in about one-fifth of patients.

Early roentgenographic abnormalities may be subtle, including swelling of joints and other synovial structures, juxta-articular osteoporosis, and periosteal reaction. In late stages, soft tissue atrophy and undergrowth of bone may be seen. Calcifications are found adjacent to affected joints in about 6% of JRA patients.

Usually 2 years of disease are required before significant cartilage loss becomes evident. If the disease becomes inactive, fibrocartilage reconstitution of the joint may occur. However, ankylosis of joints is common, especially involving the wrist and carpometacarpal (CM) joints of the second through fifth fingers and the upper half of the cervical spine (Fig. 5.5).

Marginal erosions are not detected radiographically until they involve bone and, since JRA bone is protected by a thicker layer of cartilage than in an adult (due to incomplete epiphyseal ossification), they are detected later in the disease.

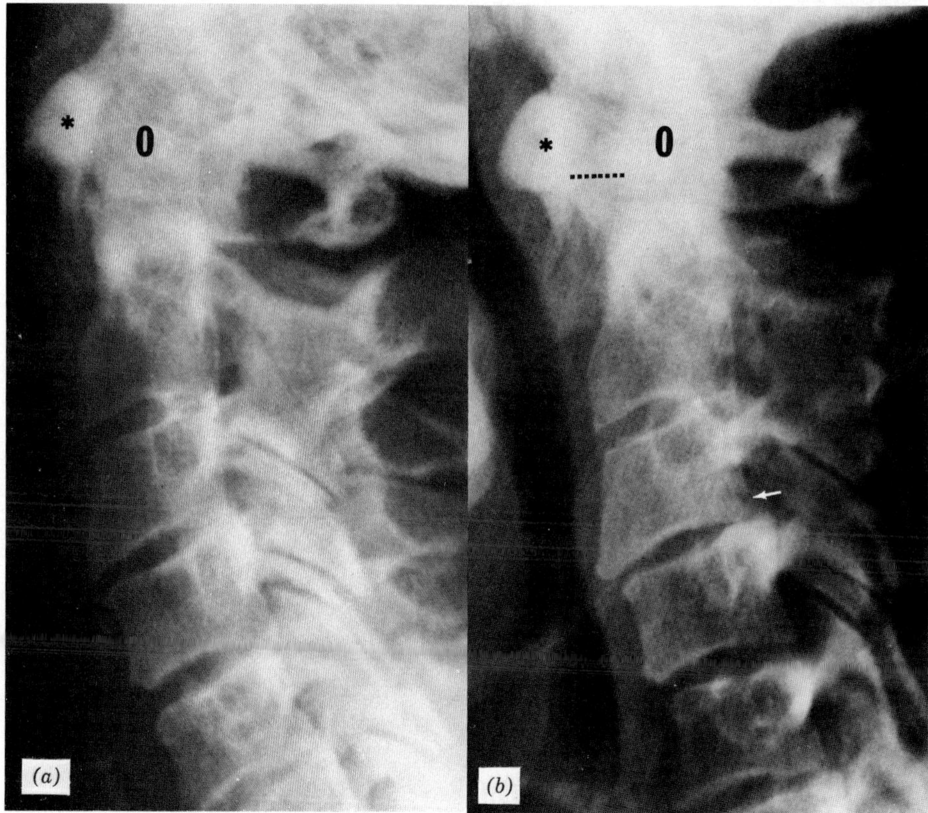

Figure 5.4. (*a*) Rheumatoid arthritis affecting the cervical spine with mild disc narrowing. Note the close apposition of the atlas (asterisk) and odontoid (O). (*b*) Flexion view shows marked anterior subluxation of the atlas away from the onontoid. The distance measured 7 mm (dotted line) on the original radiograph (normal adult up to 3 mm). There is also subluxation of C-3 on C-4 (arrow).

Furthermore, preexisting erosions in epiphyseal cartilage may become radiographically evident only after the epiphysis ossifies.

Joint subluxations frequently involve small joints of the hands and feet, the cervical spine, and even larger joints.

Abnormal skeletal growth is common in JRA, in contrast to adult RA. Premature fusion of epiphyseal growth plates frequently results in short bones, but overgrowth may also occur, leading to bulbous and enlarged epiphyses.

Spondylarthritides
The spondylarthritides are systemic rheumatic disorders with prominent and often characteristic spinal involvement.

Ankylosing Spondylitis (AS).   AS is predominantly a disease of the spine and sacroiliac (SI) joints, primarily affecting paravertebral soft tissues and their bony insertions (entheses), but it frequently also involves peripheral large joints such as hips and shoulders.

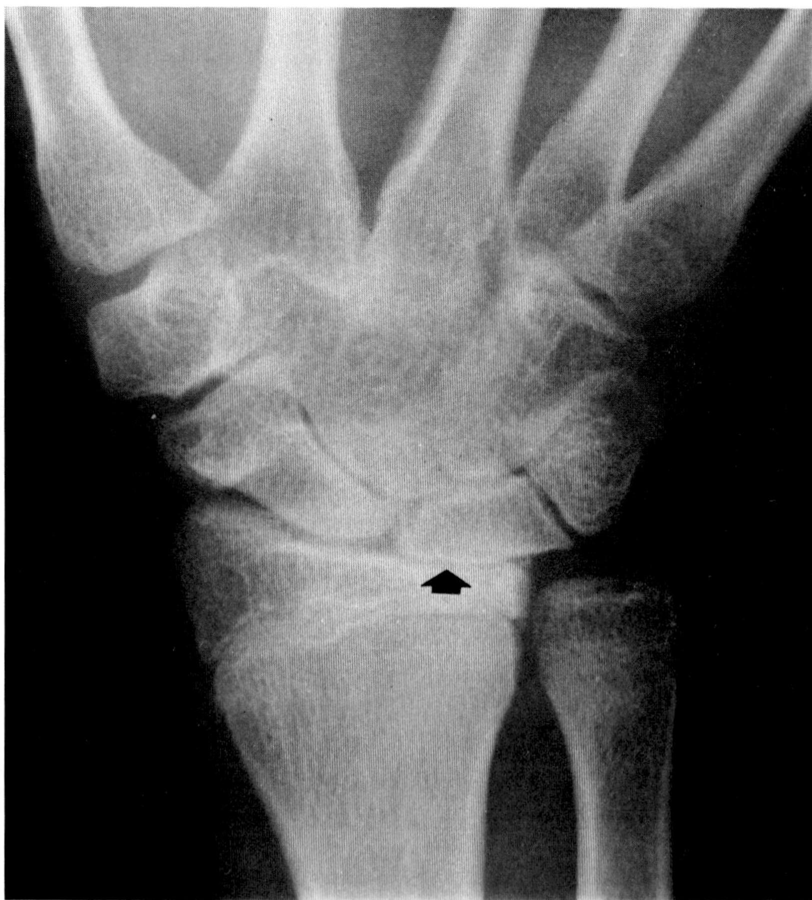

Figure 5.5. Late stage of JRA affecting the wrist. Three carpal bones and one or two metacarpals are fused into a single bony mass. There is cartilage loss in the radiocarpal joint (arrow).

Bony proliferation is prominent and characteristic. Thin, smooth marginal syndesmophytes arise within the peripheral fibers of the annulus fibrosis and extend vertically from the vertebral bodies (Fig. 13.4). They are diffuse and symmetric, usually appear first in the lumbar region, and extend later to the thoracic or cervical spine (Fig. 5.6). About half of the patients also have nonmarginal syndesmophytes that arise from the vertebral body farther from the end plate. Ossification of interspinous ligaments and apophyseal joint capsules combined with the syndesmophytes progresses to bony ankylosis. Bone also proliferates at various musculotendinous insertions of axial and peripheral skeleton.

Erosions of the corners of vertebral bodies produce a flat anterior surface rather than the normal concavity (Fig. 13.4). Reactive bone may give this eroded corner a dense, "white" appearance. Osteoporosis is common and often severe, and intervertebral discs and apophyseal joints may be narrowed late in the disease. Straightening of the cervical and lumbosacral curves, thoracic kyphosis and scoliosis, and atlantoaxial subluxation may also occur.

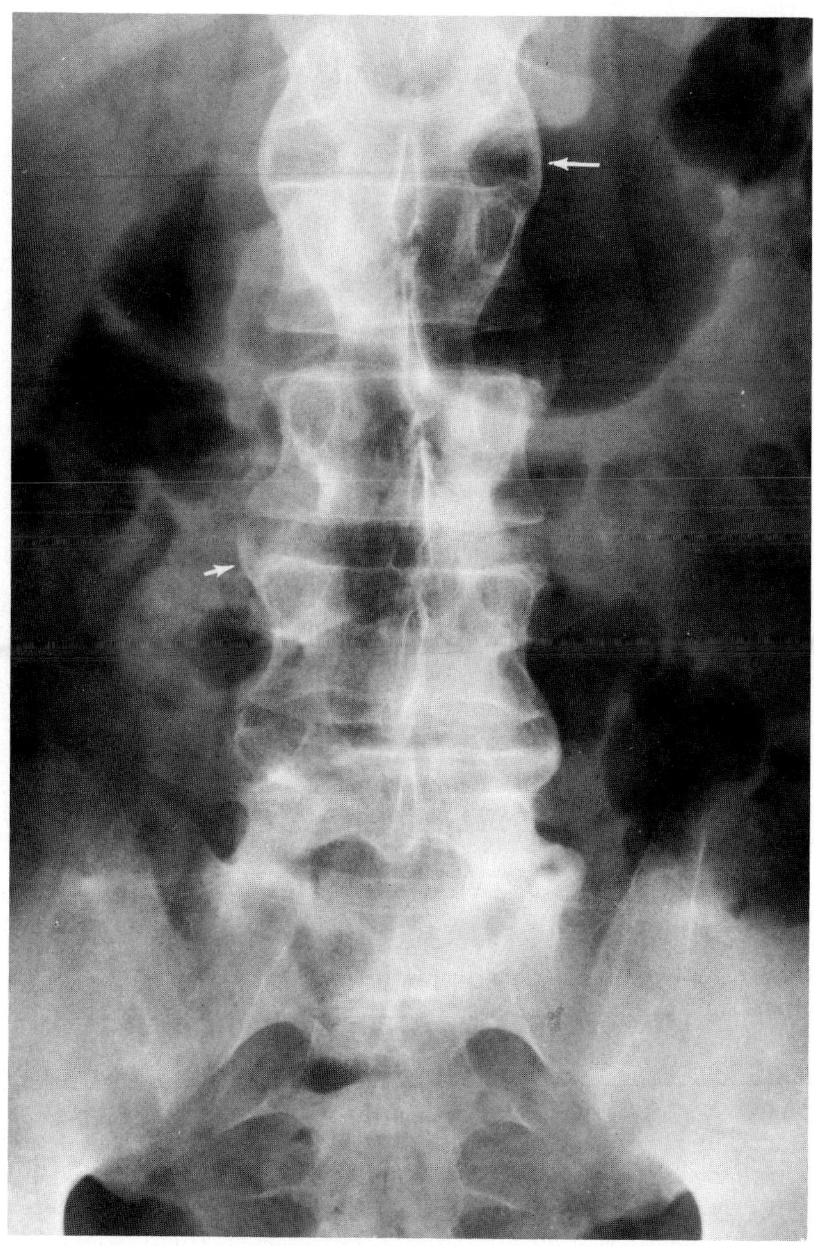

Figure 5.6. Ankylosing spondylitis with obliterated SI joints due to advanced sacroiliitis, and syndesmophytes (arrows). (Radiograph courtesy of Dr. Forrest Clore, Veterans Administration Medical Center, Gainesville, Florida)

Sacroiliitis invariably accompanies spinal disease and is often the earliest radiographic abnormality, indicated by marginal reactive bone formation, later widening of the joints, and finally ankylosis (Figs. 13.2, 13.3). Pubic symphysitis is common.

Juvenile AS differs little from the adult form except that peripheral joint involvement occurs earlier and affects up to 90% of patients.

AS can usually be distinguished from psoriatic arthritis or Reiter's syndrome by its association with marginal erosions of vertebral bodies, apophyseal ankylosis, symmetric SI and spinal disease, marginal syndesmophytes, and by the type of peripheral joint disease when it occurs. Unlike psoriatic arthritis, AS has no predilection for distal interphalangeal (DIP) joints. Unlike Reiter's disease, AS involves hips and upper extremity joints. The peripheral joint disease of AS differs from RA. AS is asymmetric, lacks juxta-articular osteoporosis, has small erosions, and more often elicits periosteal reaction.

Enteropathic Arthritis.   Arthritis occurs in about 20% of patients with ulcerative colitis or regional enteritis. Peripheral arthritis is usually transient, and radiographic abnormalities may include only soft tissue swelling and juxta-articular osteoporosis. When spondylitis occurs, its radiographic appearance is identical to that of AS, including the invariable association of sacroiliitis.

Psoriatic Arthritis.   Both psoriatic arthritis and Reiter's disease differ significantly from RA by demonstrating less juxta-articular osteoporosis, more extensive bony proliferation, frequent sacroiliitis and spondylitis, involvement of DIP joints, frequent asymmetric or oligoarticular disease, and less characteristic patterns of deformity and subluxation.

Patients with psoriasis and arthritis may have different forms of the disease, and arthritis may precede skin manifestations. Joint and soft tissue swelling in classic psoriatic arthritis resembles that of RA except for distribution and the absence of subcutaneous nodules. Cartilage destruction commonly occurs, but widening of joints is sometimes seen even with advanced articular cartilage destruction. Although early juxta-articular osteoporosis is unusual, erosion of bone is common, often severe, and can lead to marked deformity, with tapered ("penciled") and shortened bones (Fig. 5.7). Severe late stage abnormalities may closely resemble those of RA.

Widespread, exuberant proliferation of new bone is characteristic. Periosteal reaction along the shafts of small bones may be linear but is more often fluffy and irregular. Joint disease is often asymmetric and frequently includes malalignment and subluxation of IP and atlantoaxial joints. Spinal involvement is common and nearly always accompanied by sacroiliitis. In contrast to AS, the syndesmophytes are mostly nonmarginal (arising from the vertebral body away from the endplate) and more asymmetric. Coarse, irregular masses of paravertebral ossification, separated from the vertebrae, are also common.

Reiter's Syndrome.   Except for its predilection for the lower extremities, Reiter's syndrome arthritis strongly resembles psoriatic arthritis. Therefore, the distribution of joint involvement is often a helpful diagnostic feature. Joint and soft tissue swelling is often the only radiographic abnormality, and juxta-articular os-

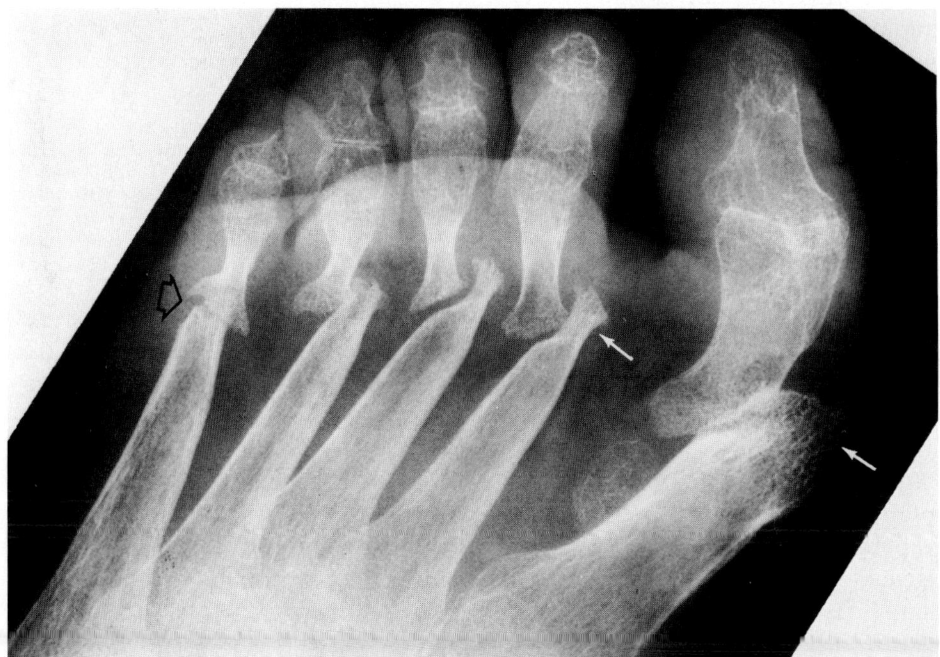

Figure 5.7. Psoriatic arthritis shows severe destruction of MTP joints with "penciled" erosions (small arrows) and a "pencil-in-cup" appearance (large open arrow).

teoporosis, as in psoriatic arthritis, is usually not prominent but is occasionally severe. Although juxta-articular erosion is usually mild, it can be severe and may affect the small joints of the feet, the knees, and the SI joints. Severe destruction of some joints with nearly complete sparing of immediately adjacent ones is a fairly characteristic pattern. Even with severe destruction of cartilage, however, joints do not typically ankylose.

Linear or fluffy periosteal bone proliferation occurs in Reiter's disease, although it is not usually as exuberant as in psoriasis. Bone proliferation is common in the foot, typically involving the calcaneus. Spinal abnormalities resemble those of psoriasis, with asymmetric nonmarginal and marginal syndesmophytes, paravertebral ossification, and sacroiliitis (Fig. 5.8).

Diffuse Idiopathic Skeletal Hyperostosis (DISH)

DISH is also called *ankylosing hyperostosis* or *Forestier's disease*. It is not an inflammatory arthropathy but is conveniently discussed here because of its predominant involvement of the spine, although it involves both axial skeleton and peripheral joints.

New bone formation in para-articular soft tissues is characteristic and most striking anterior and slightly to the right of the vertebral bodies, where it may progress to ankylosis (Fig. 5.9). The disc heights remain normal, in contrast to degenerative disc disease. Other features are ossification or calcification at ligamentous insertions, large, well-defined osteophytes adjacent to hips and SI joints,

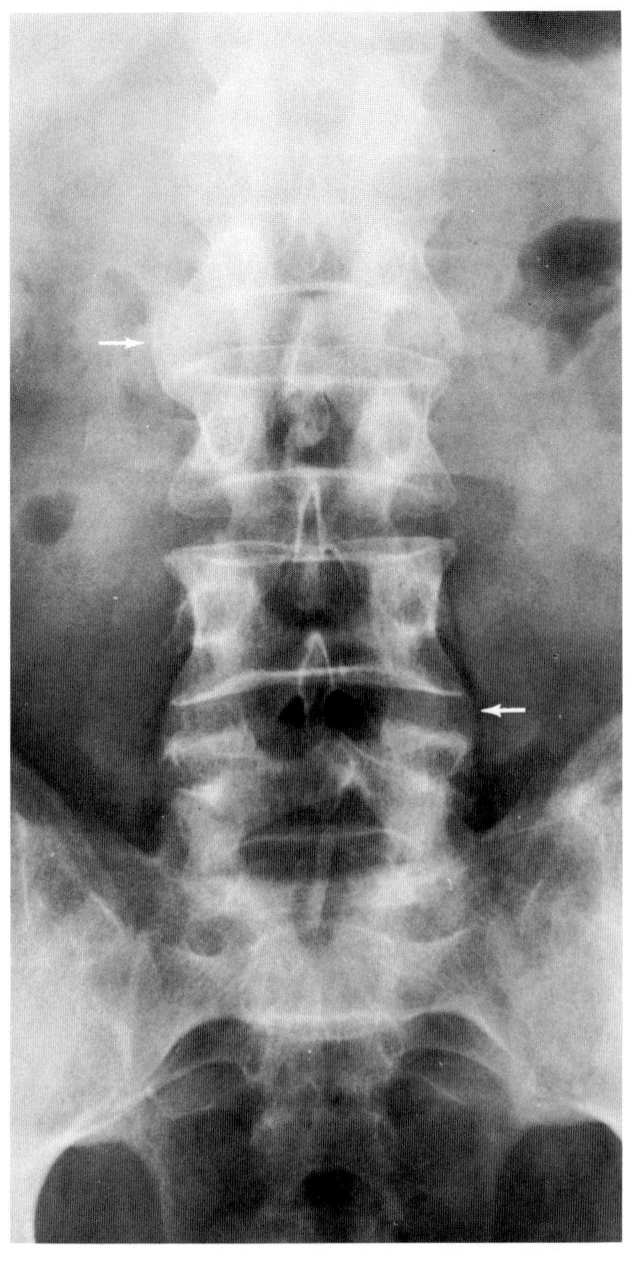

Figure 5.8. Reiter's spondylarthritis with obliteration of SI joints due to severe sacroiliitis and asymmetric syndesmophytes (arrows), both thin and coarse.

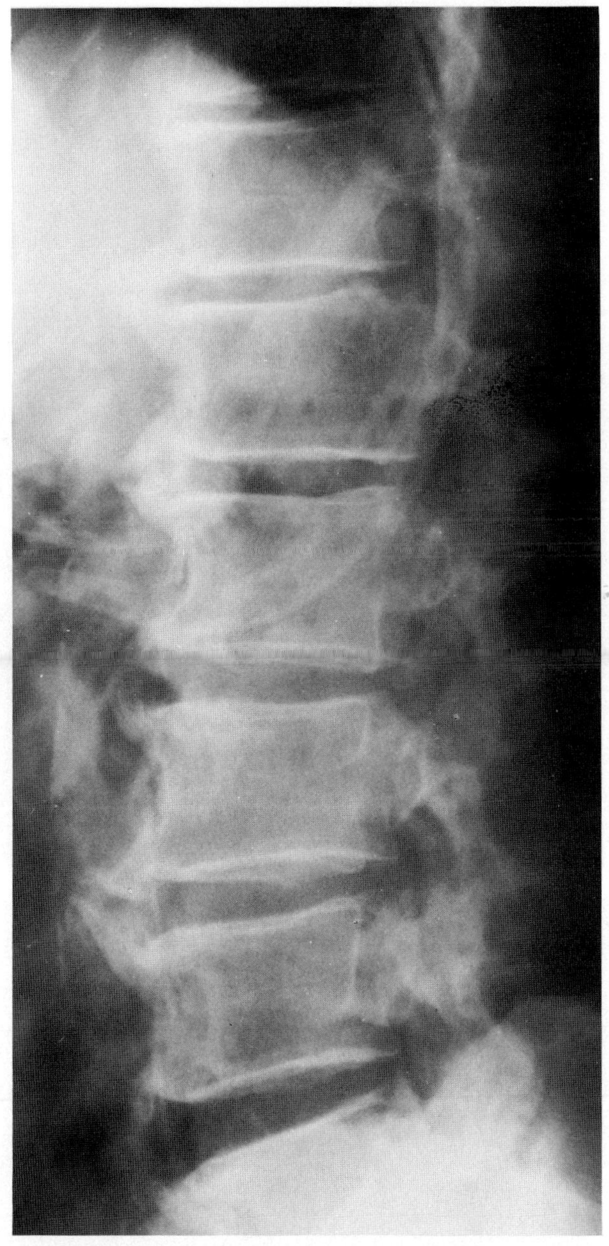

Figure 5.9. DISH (ankylosing hyperostosis) with coarse, prominent paravertebral ossification but normal intervertebral disc heights. There was less prominent ossification at the musculotendinous insertions of the pelvis and hands, and the patient's symptoms were consistent with the DISH syndrome.

and irregular bony proliferation in the form of "whiskering" or spurs at many musculotendinous or capsular insertions.

Since similar but milder abnormalities are frequent in older asymptomatic individuals, it is often difficult to decide whether the radiographic abnormalities really represent DISH.

Systemic Lupus Erythematosis (SLE)

More than half of patients with SLE have radiographic musculoskeletal abnormalities, usually consisting of swelling in or around joints, mild juxta-articular osteoporosis, and occasional deformities. Severe malalignment or hyperextension deformities may occur, but without erosions or cartilage loss (Fig. 5.10). A few

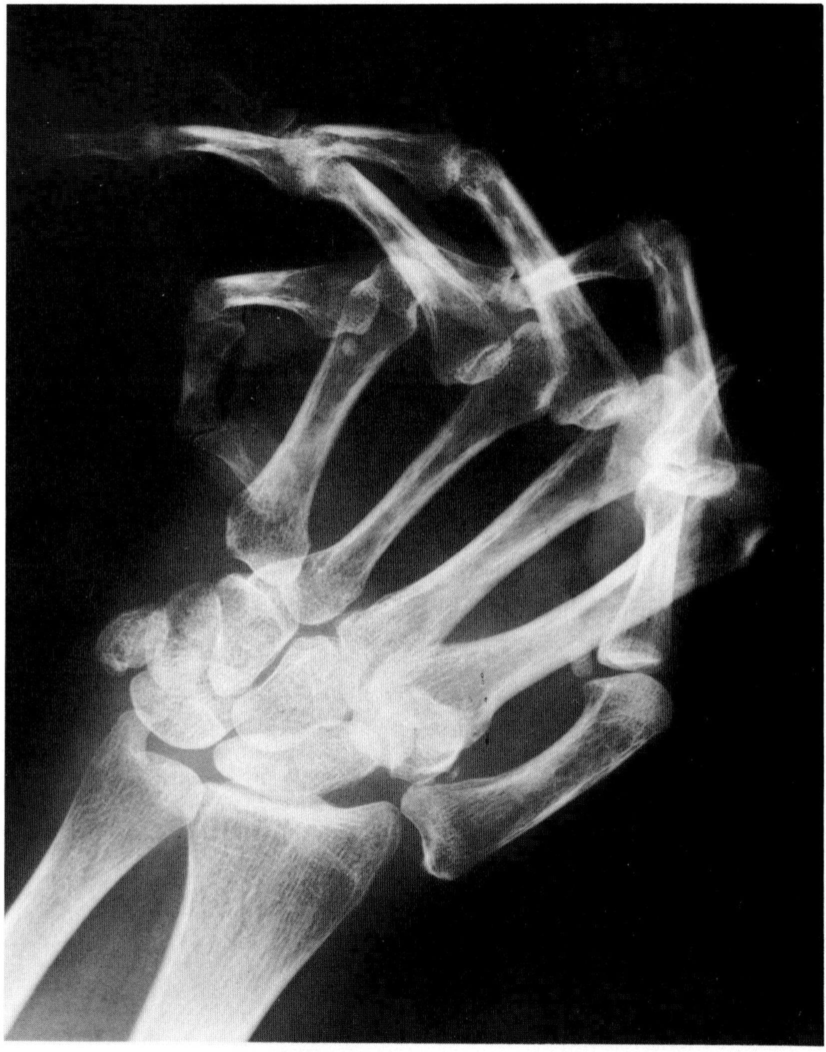

Figure 5.10. Severe hand deformity due to SLE with dislocated MCP and thumb CM joints and flexion deformities of fingers. There is diffuse osteoporosis but, in contrast to RA, there are no erosions.

patients develop aseptic necrosis, particularly of the femoral head, usually following steroid treatment.

Progressive Systemic Sclerosis (PSS)

The most common radiographic abnormalities in PSS are soft tissue atrophy (especially of the finger tips), subcutaneous calcifications, and resorption of distal bony tufts (usually occurring in patients with Raynaud's phenomenon). Some patients have thickened periarticular tissues, juxta-articular osteoporosis, erosions, cartilage narrowing, or joint destruction.

Mixed Connective Tissue Disease

Mixed connective tissue disease is accompanied by radiographic evidence of inflammatory, erosive arthritis. Most patients have swelling around the joints, juxta-articular or diffuse osteoporosis, or marginal erosions. Many have carpal or PIP cartilage loss, soft tissue calcifications, soft tissue atrophy, distal bony tuft resorption, or deformities of DIP joints. Others have radiographic features typical of PSS, SLE, or RA.

Other Systemic Rheumatic Diseases

In rheumatic fever, joint effusion may be seen. The joints usually return to normal but in rare cases evolve to Jaccoud's arthropathy—alignment abnormalities at the MCP joints and volar subluxation of proximal phalanges or hyperextension of PIP joints without cartilage loss.

In Sjögren's syndrome, about half the patients have RA, SLE, or PSS and display radiographic abnormalities of those diseases. Patients with polymyositis or dermatomyositis occasionally have widespread calcification of skin, subcutaneous tissue or muscle, so-called calcinosis universalis. In amyloidosis, soft tissue masses or large, well-demarcated marginal erosions associated with amyloid infiltration of the synovial tissue may be seen.

Degenerative Joint Disease (DJD)

DJD (osteoarthritis) is characterized by articular cartilage loss and hypertrophic bone reaction. Since DJD is not primarily inflammatory, soft tissue swelling is not prominent, although intermittent effusions may occur. Articular cartilage loss is usually the earliest sign and is typically nonuniform within the involved joint. Subarticular cysts are common, especially at the hip, and they occasionally precede perceptible cartilage loss.

Bone proliferation comprises both marginal osteophytes and hypertrophy (increased density) of subarticular bone. Osteophytes occasionally break off to form loose bodies in the joint. Calcification of fibrocartilage is occasionally found. Alignment abnormalities depend on eccentricity of cartilage loss.

Large joints are usually affected, particularly hips and knees (Fig. 5.11), but DIP joints of the fingers (Fig. 5.12) and the joints of the base of the thumb are also commonly involved. Erosive or inflammatory osteoarthritis occurs with abrupt onset, affects middle-aged, postmenopausal women, and involves the IP joints of the fingers.

Degenerative disease of the intervertebral discs leads to disc narrowing, increased density of adjacent vertebral end plates, sometimes the "vacuum sign" (a transient collection of gas within clefts of the degenerated disc), and marginal osteophytes adjacent to the protruding annulus fibrosis (Fig. 5.13). These osteophytes are thick, coarse, and predominantly horizontal, in contradistinction to syndesmophytes. True DJD affects the apophyseal joints and may be associated with disc degeneration or spinal instability.

Metabolic Bone and Joint Disease

Paget's Disease

Bones affected by Paget's disease are enlarged and display coarse, prominent trabeculae and areas of lytic destruction (Fig. 5.14). The disease always involves subarticular bone (except in the skull or tibia) and predisposes to early DJD in adjacent joints.

Gout

The diagnosis of gout should be established years before the characteristic radiographic features develop. Early in the disease, acute joint inflammation is manifested by articular swelling and sometimes juxta-articular osteoporosis, but little else. Later, uniform articular cartilage loss is frequently seen, while bone density usually remains normal. Bone erosions commonly begin at the joint margin and progress centrally, although erosions beneath tophi may occur distant from joints. Erosions are typically well marginated (punched out) in gout (Fig. 5.15), but such erosions are also seen in RA. Very characteristic of gout is the "overhanging edge"—a thin bony shelf that develops at the margin of an erosion and partially extends over it. Erosion occasionally progresses to severe destruction and the end stage opera glass hand. Late ankylosis occasionally occurs in IP or carpal joints. The distribution of involved joints is variable and asymmetric, but distal joint disease predominates, involving especially the lower extremities. The great toe MTP joint is the most frequently involved.

There is occasional malalignment or subluxation, and secondary degenerative changes are frequently superimposed on the primary disease, as in most inflammatory arthritides.

Calcium Pyrophosphate Dihydrate (CPPD) Crystal Deposition Disease

CPPD strongly resembles DJD radiographically, although CPPD disease differs in the distribution and variability of osteophyte formation and often displays numerous subarticular lucencies or "cysts." The earliest sign may be joint swelling alone.

Chondrocalcinosis (articular cartilage calcification) is the most characteristic abnormality and, when detectable, will be found in the knees in 90% of patients, in the knees or symphysis pubis in 98%, and in the knees, symphysis, or wrists in 100% (Fig. 5.16). Elbows and hips are other common sites. Chondrocalcinosis is roentgenographically detectable in 90% of joints from which CPPD crystals are recovered by aspiration, but good-quality, fine-detail, or magnification radiographs may be required. Calcification may also be found in joint capsules, tendons, or bursae; bizarre, irregular bone proliferation or para-articular ossification about various joints is sometimes seen. Erosions do not occur, but flexion contractures may involve the elbow or knee and narrowing of intervertebral discs occasionally occurs, especially in the cervical spine.

Abnormalities resembling DJD in an unusual distribution (wrist, all three knee compartments, elbows, ankles), especially with multiple carpal cysts, strongly suggest CPPD disease even without demonstrable chondrocalcinosis. CPPD arthropathy is sometimes severe and rapidly progressive, both resembling and associated with neuropathic joint disease.

The arthropathy commonly affects knees, wrists, MCPs, elbows or ankles, and occasionally the trapezioscaphoid and thumb CM joints. Almost always more than two groups of joints are involved, commonly bilaterally and fairly symmetrically.

Other Bone Diseases

When musculoskeletal symptoms are due to osteoporosis, osteomalacia, hyperparathyroidism, or bone tumors, radiographic signs of these entities may be ob-

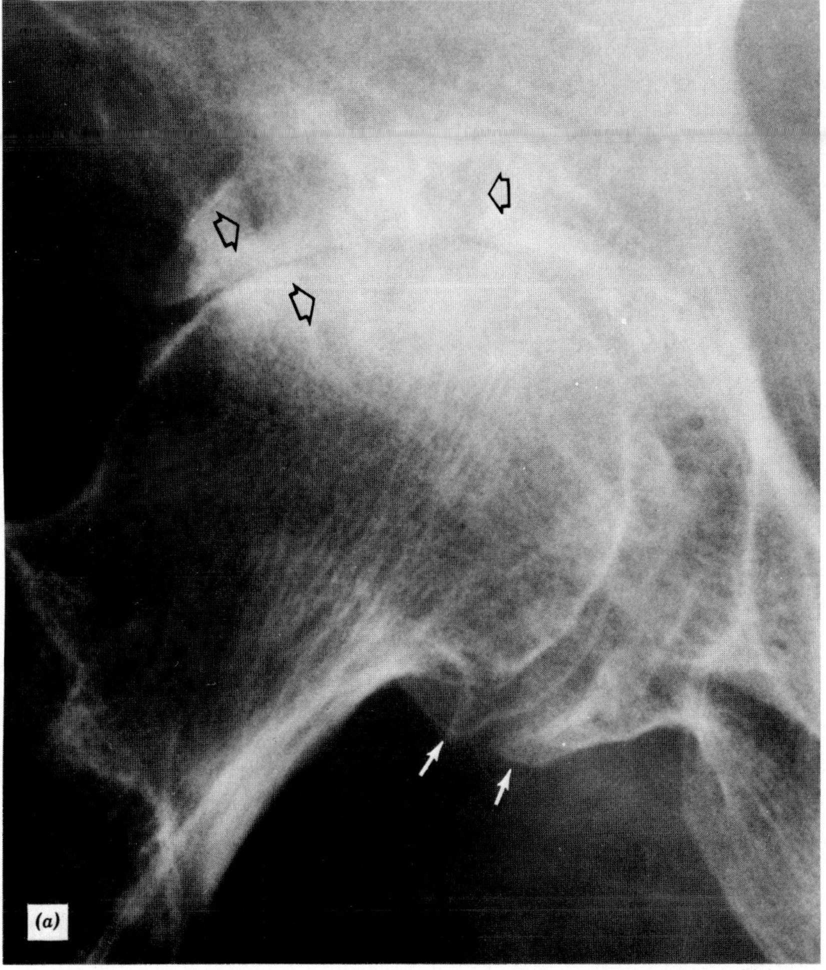

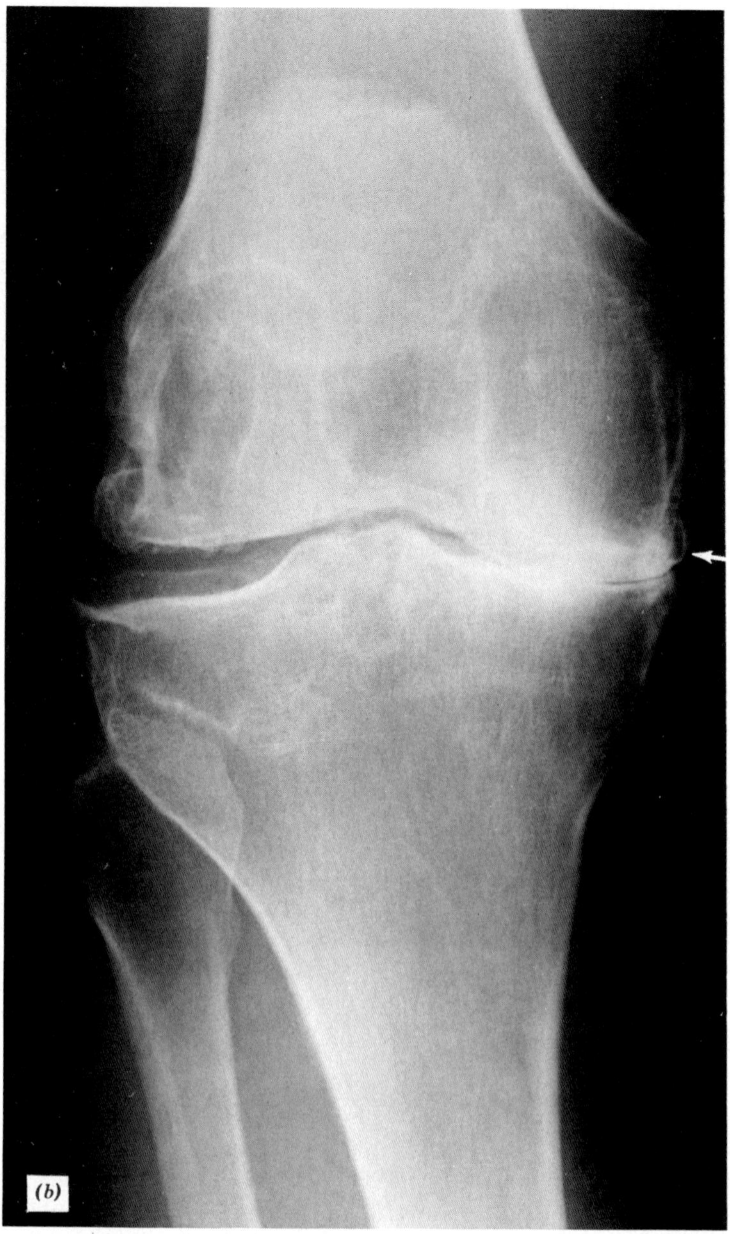

Figure 5.11. (*a*) DJD of the hip with asymmetric cartilage loss in the superolateral quadrant, subarticular bone hypertrophy or "sclerosis," subarticular cysts (open arrows), and large medial osteophytes arising from the femoral head and acetabulum (white arrows). (*b*) Standing AP view of the knee shows DJD with severe medial compartment cartilage loss resulting in varus malalignment. There are osteophytes (arrows) and subarticular bone hypertrophy.

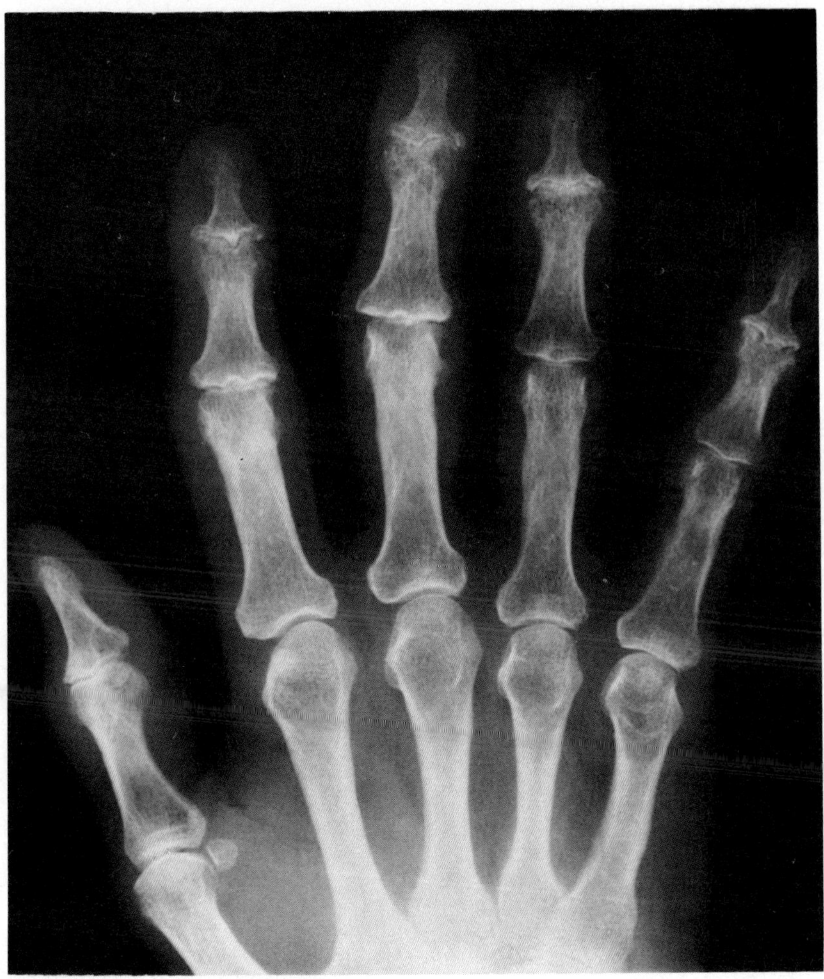

Figure 5.12. Degenerative joint disease of fingers. Typical distribution involving DIP and PIP joints with cartilage loss, irregular subchondral cortex, and moderate hypertrophic osteophyte formation.

served in juxta-articular bone. Chondroblastomas, giant cell tumors, and osteoid osteomas are commonly subarticular. Children with metastatic neuroblastoma, leukemia, or Ewing's tumor may appear with fever, systemic illness, arthritis, and destructive bone lesions. Renal dialysis patients may develop painful uremic peri-arthritis with rapid calcification of soft tissues. Occasionally, marginal erosions of hyperparathyroidism simulate erosive arthritis.

Infectious Arthritis

In pyogenic infections, joint destruction occurs within days or weeks. The first radiographic sign is soft tissue swelling. Then, 7–10 days after symptoms begin, osteoporosis and small marginal and subarticular erosions appear, and articular

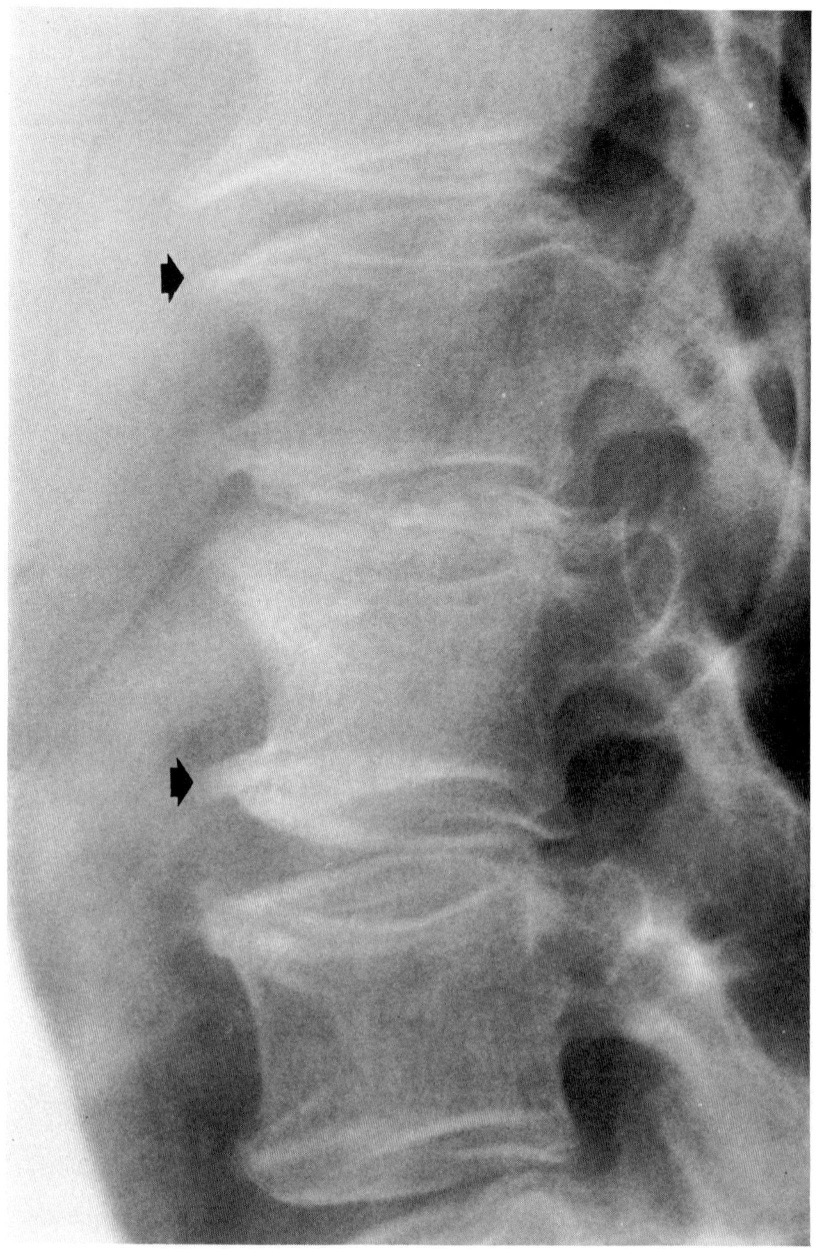

Figure 5.13. Degenerative intervertebral disc disease. Discs are narrowed. Osteophytes (arrows) are coarse and extend horizontally from the margins of vertebral bodies.

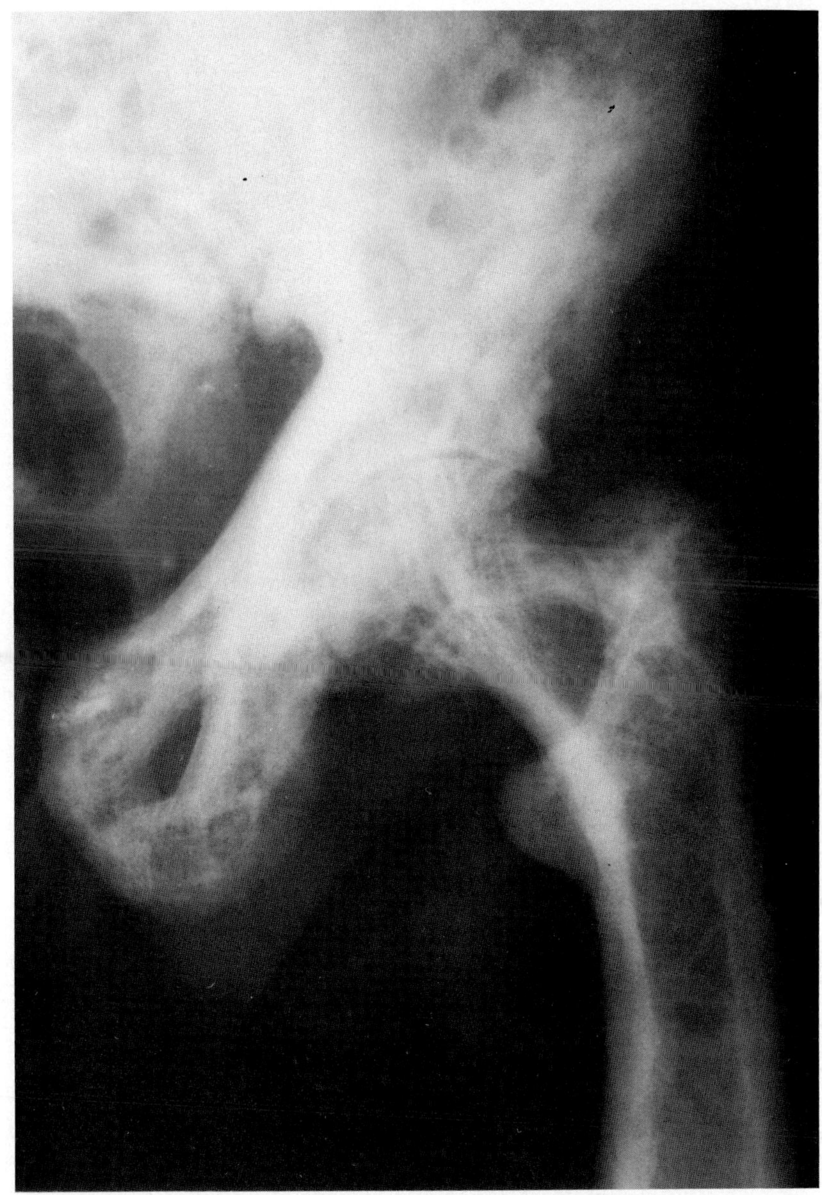

Figure 5.14. Advanced Paget's disease with enlargement of bones, coarse prominent trabeculae, and bowing of femur. There is secondary DJD of the hip with cartilage narrowing.

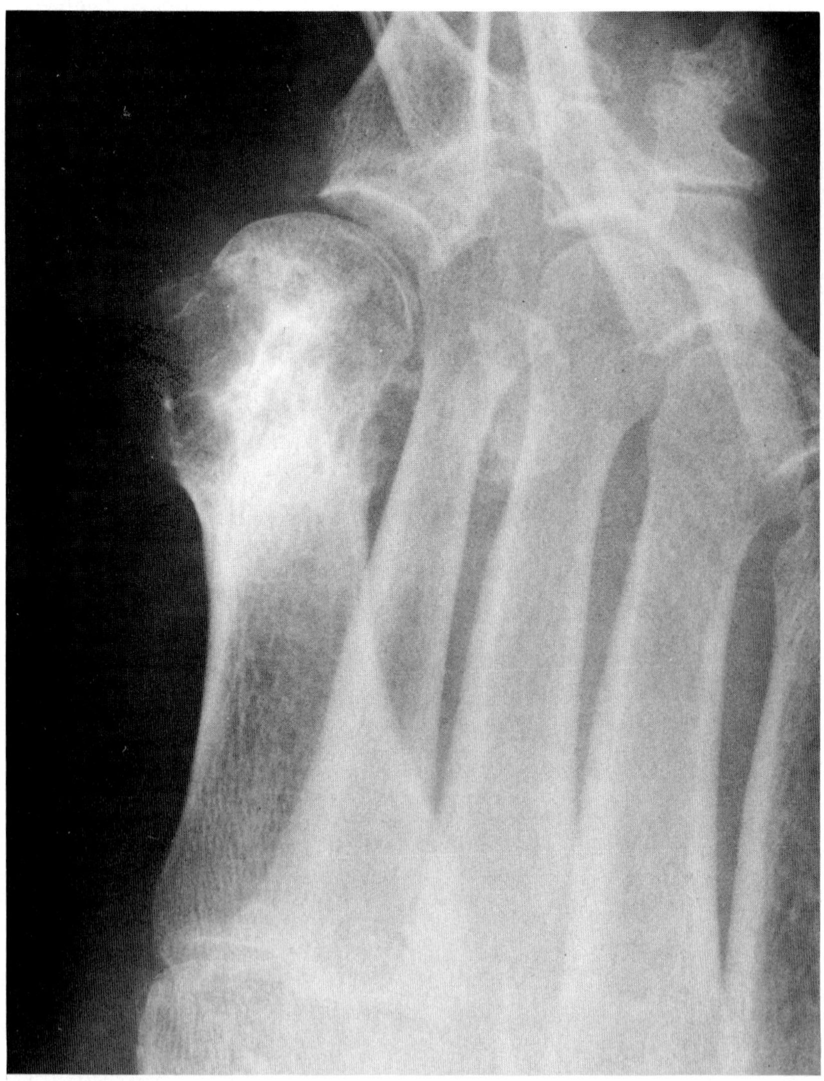

Figure 5.15. Gout with classic involvement of the great toe MTP joint. There is soft tissue swelling and marked erosion of the metatarsal head.

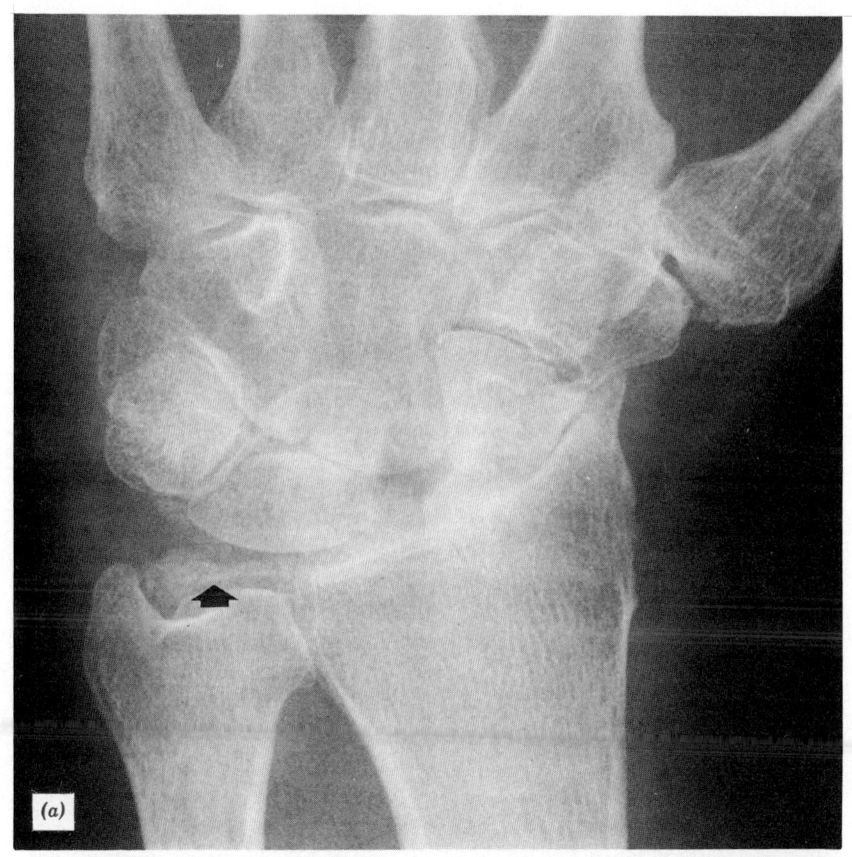

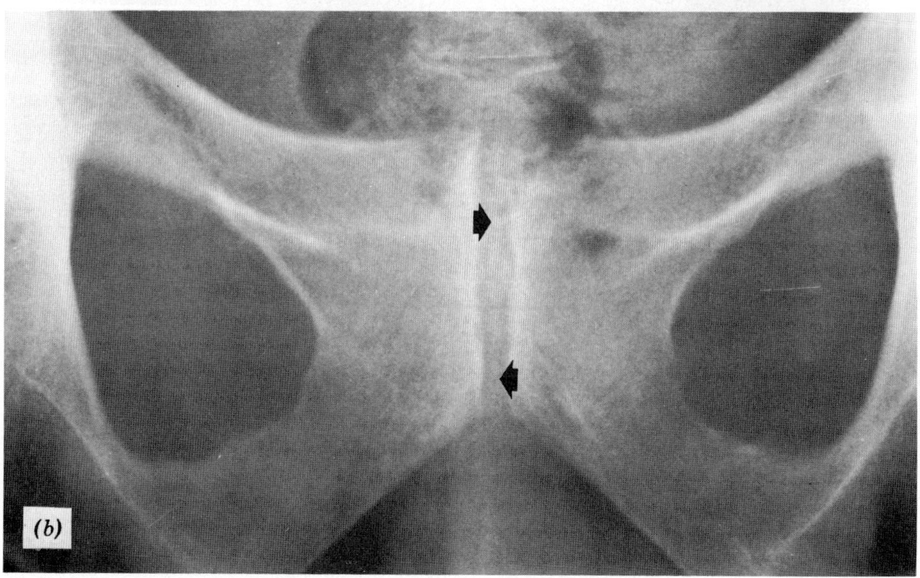

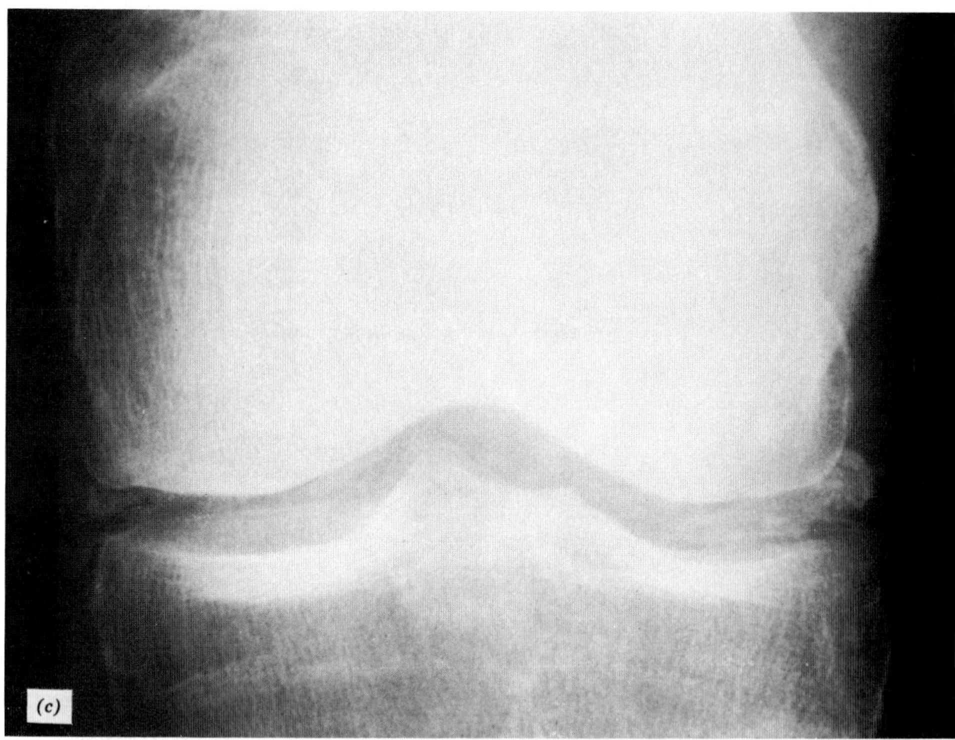

Figure 5.16. (*a*) Chondrocalcinosis of CPPD disease. Wrist with degenerative changes of the radiocarpal joint (cartilage narrowing and subarticular bone hypertrophy) and dense calcification of triangular fibrocartilage (arrow). (*b*) Calcification within fibrocartilage of the symphysis pubis (arrows). (*c*) Heavy calcification of fibrocartilaginous menisci and articular cartilage of both compartments of the knee.

cartilage loss rapidly follows (Fig. 5.17). After infection has subsided, there may be considerable reactive bone and osteophyte formation. The end stage resembles DJD but if all the cartilage is destroyed, bony ankylosis occurs.

Slowly progressive joint infections (tuberculous, brucellar, or gonococcal) feature joint swelling, followed gradually by juxta-articular osteoporosis and slow destruction of articular cartilage leading to end stage DJD, with uniformity of involvement suggesting the inflammatory etiology. Pyogenic infections of the spine begin in the vertebral end plate, but the first radiographic sign is narrowing of the disc, followed by rapid destruction of the disc and the adjacent vertebrae.

Other Musculoskeletal Disorders

Synovial Chondromatosis

In synovial chondromatosis, metaplastic cartilage nodules form and grow in the synovial tissue, and may eventually separate to form numerous loose bodies of varying size within the joint (Fig. 5.18). When these nodules are not calcified (one-third of instances), radiographic diagnosis may require arthrography. Swell-

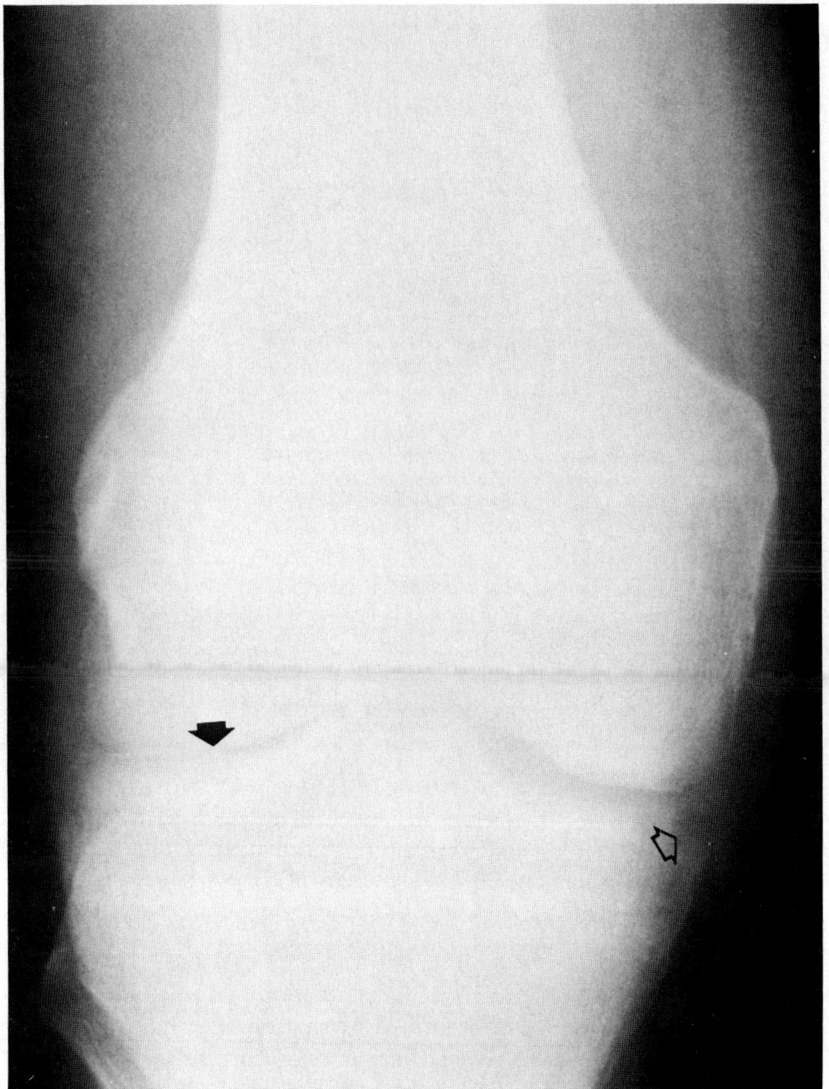

Figure 5.17. Septic arthritis of the knee with indistinct subarticular cortex (closed arrow), cartilage loss both medially and laterally, and large marginal erosion of the tibia (open arrow).

ing within the joint is seen due to the multiple loose bodies and associated effusion. Secondary DJD develops after many years. The knee and hip are affected most commonly. When there are only a few loose bodies, other etiologies must be considered, such as DJD, osteochondritis dissecans, trauma, or neuropathic joint.

Pigmented Villonodular Synovitis

Pigmented villonodular synovitis features marked synovial hypertrophy with consequent swelling and effusion. The disease may extend beyond the normal limits

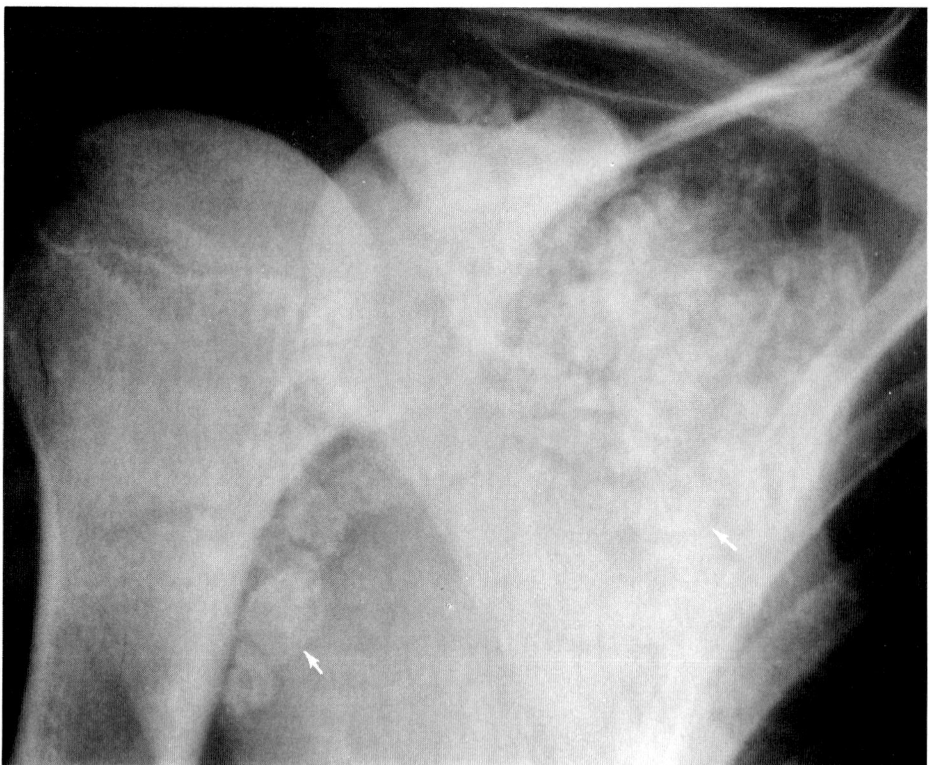

Figure 5.18. Synovial chondromatosis of the shoulder with countless dense osteocartilaginous loose bodies within the joint (arrows).

of the joint, dissecting into the calf from the knee, for example. Articular cartilage is preserved at first, but destruction of cartilage and adjacent bone may occur later. The disease is usually monarticular and most often involves the lower limb, especially the knee, but ankle, hip, elbow, shoulder, tarsal, and carpal joints are sometimes affected.

Hemophilia

Joint involvement is a prominent feature of hemophilia, radiographically resembling JRA. Joint swelling is followed by cartilage destruction, marginal bone erosions, diffuse osteoporosis, subarticular cysts, and premature fusion or overgrowth of epiphyses and secondary DJD. The disease chiefly involves hinge joints—wrist, elbow, knee, and ankle. Bleeding into bone may result in lytic areas, periosteal reaction, and even extensive destruction simulating a malignant tumor (pseudotumor).

Multicentric Reticulohistiocytosis

Multicentric reticulohistiocytosis, a rare disease with multiple histiocytic nodules involving skin and mucous membranes, may produce a severely mutilating and deforming arthropathy with cartilage destruction, extensive resorption of adjacent bone, and striking late deformities.

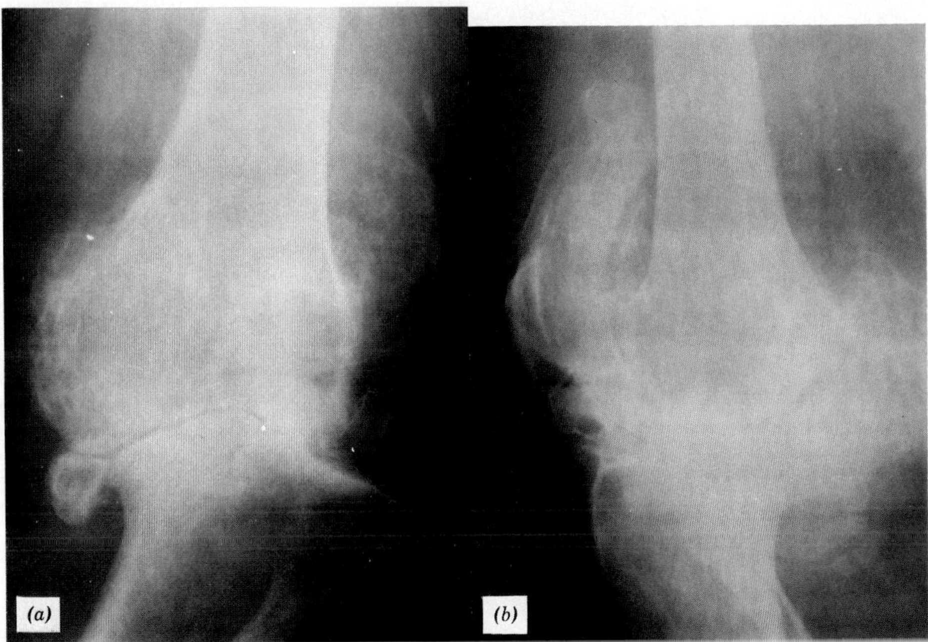

Figure 5.19. Neuropathic knee with subluxation, cartilage destruction, huge osteophytes, and bony fragments in soft tissue.

Neuropathic Joint Disease

The early radiographic abnormalities of neuropathic joint disease look like those of DJD. However, rapidly progressive destruction, gross instability, and subluxation are characteristic (Fig. 5.19). Joint swelling is followed by gradual cartilage loss, osteophytes, subarticular bone hypertrophy, severe destruction of juxtaarticular bone, multiple loose bodies, and calcified debris within the joint and capsule.

Aseptic Necrosis

Aseptic necrosis most commonly involves the femoral head. The earliest radiographic abnormality is a subtle mottling of medullary bone. Gradually a rim of reactive bone then forms around the infarcted area (Fig. 5.20a). Pathologic fracture follows but may be radiographically obscure. When it becomes evident, a thin rim of subarticular cortex is separated from infarcted bone by the irregular fracture line—the "crescent sign." This line may be visible only on a "frog-leg" lateral radiograph or on tomograms (Fig. 5.20b). End stage DJD may obscure the characteristics of osteonecrosis.

Osteochondritis Dissecans

Osteochondritis dissecans consists of a wedge of infarcted subarticular bone, probably secondary to trauma, and most commonly seen on the lateral aspect of the medial condyle of the distal femur. A small segment of the subarticular bone is separated from surrounding normal bone by a thin lucent line. Gradually the fragment may become looser but remain attached by a flap of articular cartilage, or may separate entirely to become a loose body in the joint.

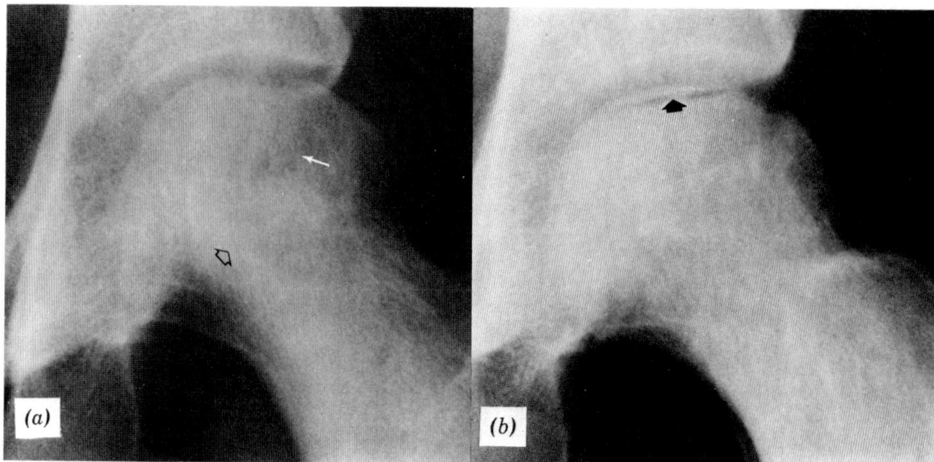

Figure 5.20. (*a*) Aseptic necrosis of the femoral head. The early stage shows subtle radiographic abnormalities. The bone is mottled with lucent areas (white arrow) and dense areas (open arrow). (*b*) Later, pathologic fracture results in the "crescent sign" of subarticular bone (arrow) on a frog-leg lateral view.

Sarcoid

Granulomatous bone involvement most commonly causes an osteoporotic, reticular trabecular pattern with multiple rounded lucencies. The small bones of the hands and feet, especially middle and distal phalanges, are most susceptible, and the disease may progress to extensive bone destruction.

Hypertrophic Pulmonary Osteoarthropathy (HOA)

HOA begins with soft tissue proliferation of distal tufts of fingers. Later, thick periosteal bone formation profusely involves the distal paired bones of the extremities and sometimes more proximal long bones or metacarpals, metatarsals, and phalanges (Fig. 5.21).

Reflex Sympathetic Dystrophy Syndromes

In reflex sympathetic dystrophy syndromes, painful extremities with trophic changes radiographically show diffuse and localized periarticular swelling of the involved limb and striking osteoporosis. Radionuclide bone scans may be abnormal even before radiographic abnormalities appear. After symptoms subside, the radiographs may return to normal or some osteoporosis may persist. Transient painful (migratory) osteoporosis is a similar entity (Fig. 5.22).

OTHER RADIOGRAPHIC STUDIES

Arthrography

Injection of contrast medium into joints is useful for demonstrating synovial disease, articular cartilage surfaces (as in osteochondritis dissecans), loose bodies, meniscal tears of the knee, and synovial cysts that may be clinically confused with thrombophlebitis (Fig. 5.23).

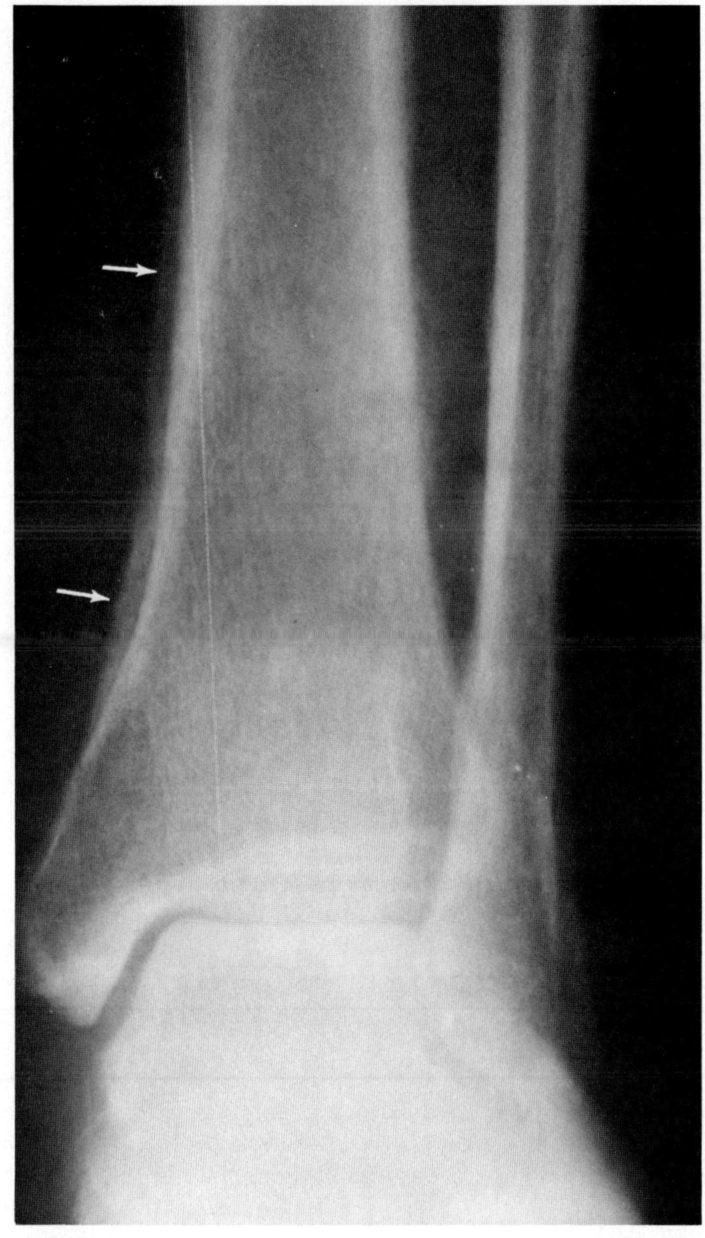

Figure 5.21. Hypertrophic osteoarthropathy with a thick periosteal reaction along the distal tibia and fibula (arrows) in a patient with lung cancer.

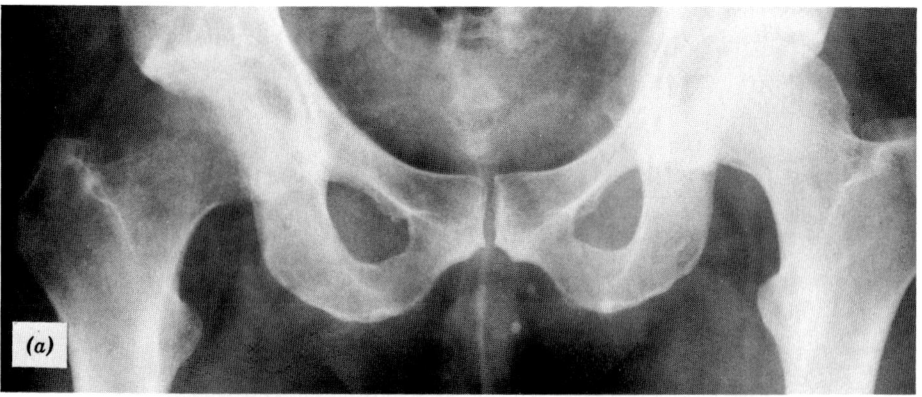

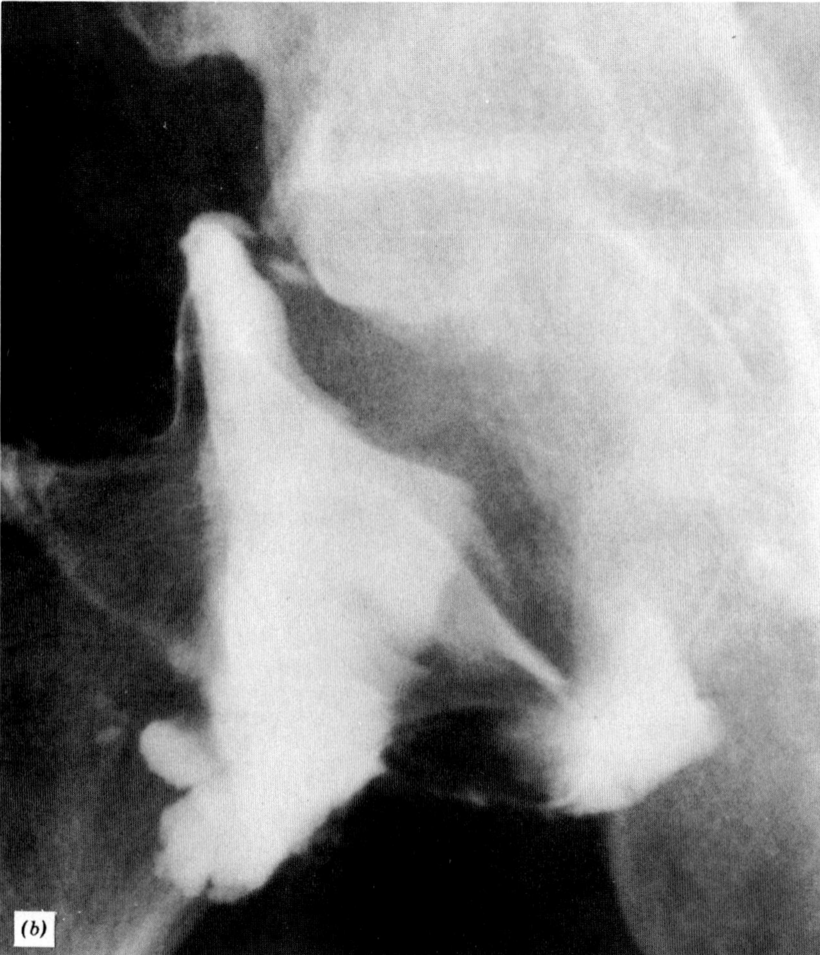

Figure 5.22. (*a*) Transient painful osteoporosis. Striking osteoporosis around the right hip. (*b*) Aspiration yielded 8 cc of clear synovial fluid. The hip arthrogram shows preservation of articular cartilage. Symptoms and osteoporosis resolved with no specific treatment.

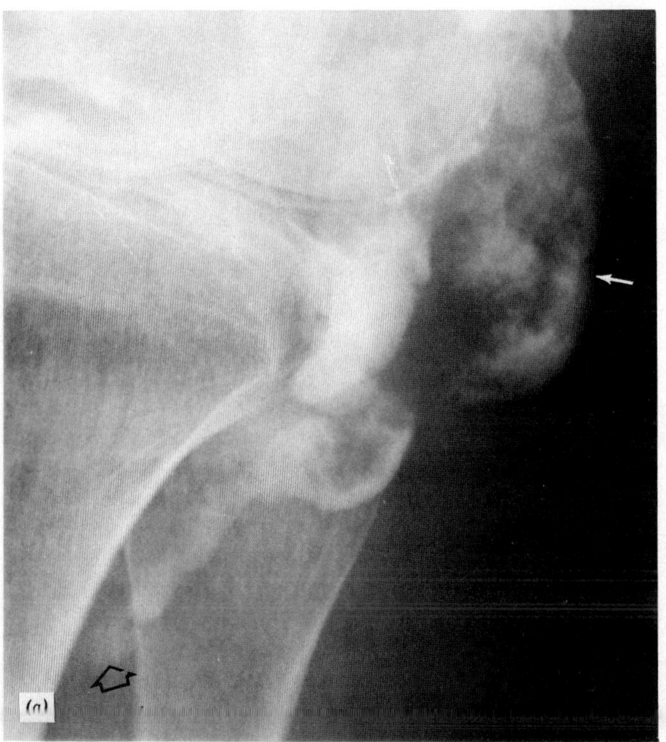

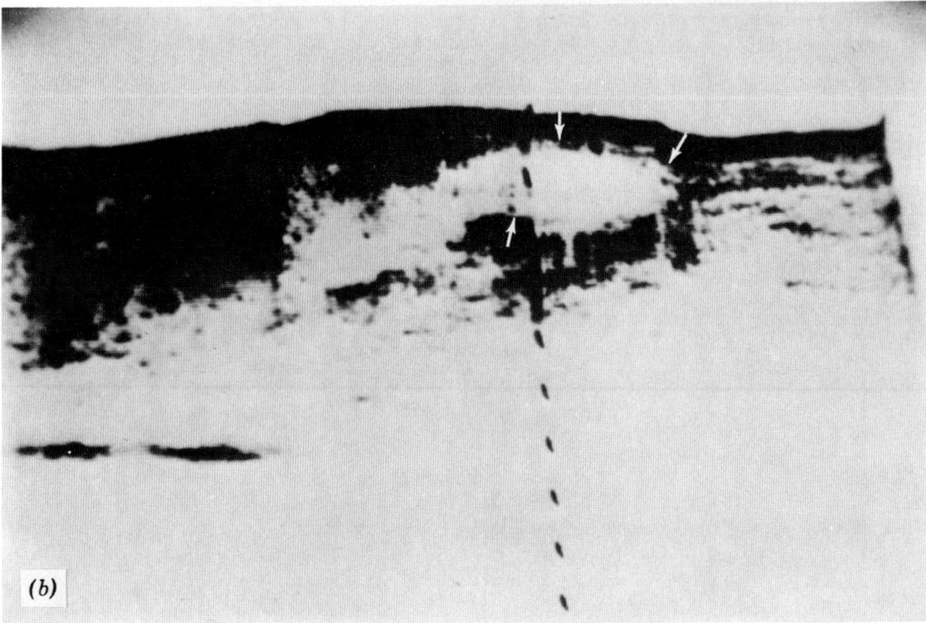

Figure 5.23. (*a*) Dissecting popliteal cyst due to RA. The cyst has been opacified by injection of radiopaque material into the knee joint. It protrudes into the popliteal space (white arrow) and dissects distally into the calf (open arrow). Filling defects in the cyst are due to fibrin or hypertrophic synovial tissue. (*b*) Ultrasound image of the cyst (arrows) clearly shows it dissecting distally into the calf. Longitudinal scan with patient prone. The dotted line indicates the popliteal crease.

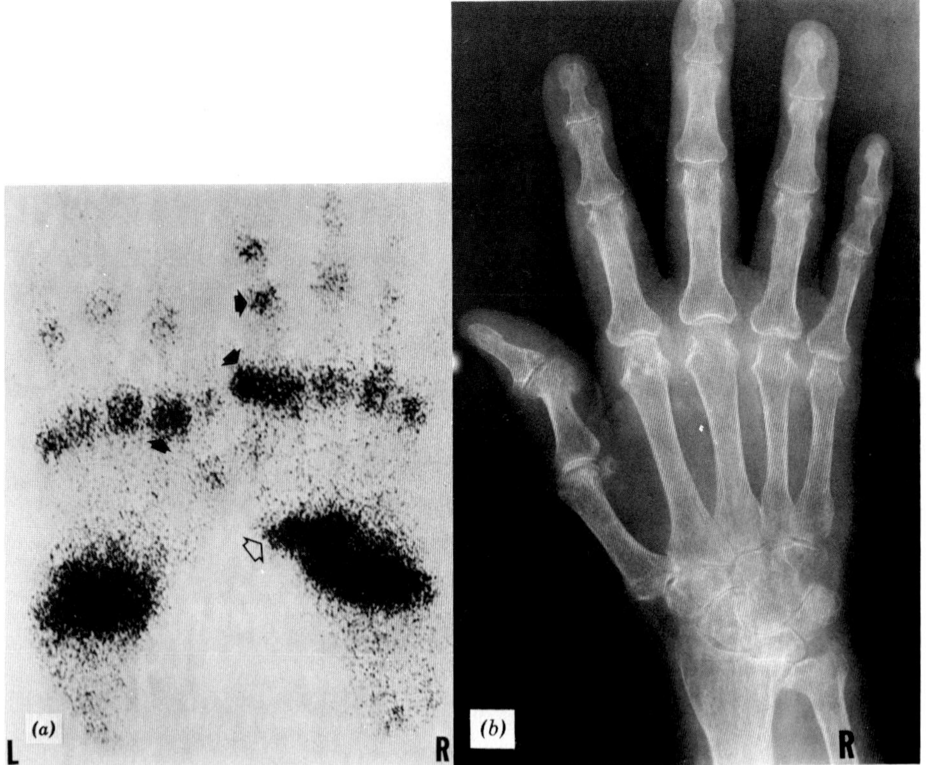

Figure 5.24. (*a*) Radionuclide bone scan of the hands of a patient with RA shows abnormally intense uptake at both wrists, right CM joints (open arrow), and several MCP and IP joints (closed arrows). (*b*) Radiograph of the right hand shows swelling, cartilage loss, and erosions typical of RA. Bone scans can show areas of active synovitis even before typical radiographic abnormalities appear. (Courtesy of Dr. Susan Curry, Department of Radiology, University of Florida)

Radionuclide Scanning

Whole body scans using bone-seeking phosphate agents labeled with technetium 99m are nonspecific but quite sensitive in detecting joint involvement by systemic rheumatic disease, and they are sometimes used for initial evaluation and follow-up (Fig. 5.24). Bone scanning may also detect early aseptic necrosis when radiographic abnormalities are subtle.

Angiography

Microaneurysms in patients with polyarteritis nodosa (Fig. 5.25) or small vessel disease associated with Raynaud's phenomenon may be demonstrated by arteriography. In Takayasu's arteritis, characteristic irregular narrowing of large vessels is found.

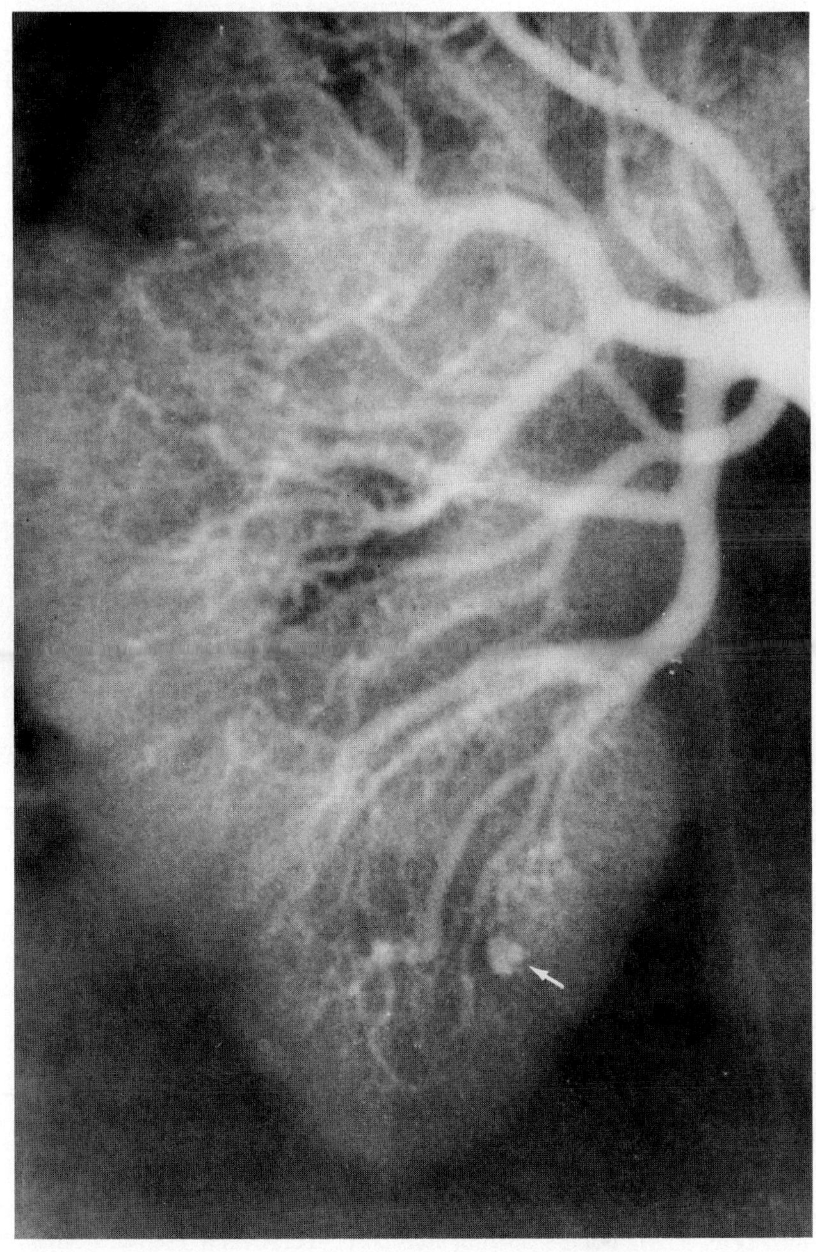

Figure 5.25. Renal arteriogram of a patient with polyarteritis nodosa showing typical microaneurysms (arrow). (Angiogram courtesy of Dr. Irvin F. Hawkins, Jr., Department of Radiology, University of Florida)

Computed Tomography

Computed tomography, a recent innovation, has found application to the musculoskeletal system primarily in the imaging of focal neoplastic or inflammatory lesions and in the evaluation of spinal stenosis. Recently it has shown promise in the early evaluation of sacroiliitis.

BIBLIOGRAPHY

Ansell BM, Kent PA: Radiological changes in juvenile chronic polyarthritis. *Skeletal Radiol* 1:129, 1977.

Berens DL, Lin RK: *Roentgen Diagnosis of Rheumatoid Arthritis.* Springfield, Ill, Charles C Thomas, Publisher, 1969.

Edeiken J, Hodes PJ: *Roentgen Diagnosis of Diseases of Bone,* ed 2. Baltimore, Williams & Wilkins Co, 1973, pp 662–839.

Forrester DM, Brown JC, Nesson JW: *The Radiology of Joint Disease,* ed. 2. Philadelphia, WB Saunders Co, 1978.

Greenfield GB, Schorsch HA, Shkolnik A: The various roentgen appearances of pulmonary hypertrophic osteoarthropathy. *Am J Roentgenol* 101:927, 1967.

Kleinman P, Rivelis M, Schneider R, et al: Juvenile ankylosing spondylitis. *Radiology* 125:775, 1977.

Martel W, Braunstein EM, Borlanza G, et al: Radiologic features of Reiter disease. *Radiology* 132:1, 1979.

Martel W, Champion CK, Thompson GR, et al: A roentgenologically distinctive arthropathy in some patients with the pseudogout syndrome. *Am J Roentgenol* 109:587, 1970.

Martel W, Holt JF, Cassidy JT: Roentgenologic manifestations of juvenile rheumatoid arthritis. *Am J Roentgenol* 88:400, 1962.

Martel W, Sitterley BH: Roentgenologic manifestations of osteonecrosis. *Am J Roentgenol* 106:509, 1969.

McEwen C, DiTata D, Lingg C, et al: Ankylosing spondylitis and spondylitis accompanying ulcerative colitis, regional enteritis, psoriasis and Reiter's disease. *Arthritis Rheum* 14:291, 1971.

Meszaros WT: The regional manifestations of scleroderma. *Radiology* 70:313, 1958.

Peterson CC Jr, Silbiger ML: Reiter's syndrome and psoriatic arthritis. *Am J Roentgenol* 101:860, 1967.

Resnick D: The radiographic manifestations of gouty arthritis. *CRC Crit Rev Diagn Imaging* 9:265, 1977.

Resnick D, Niwayama G, Goergen TG, et al: Clinical, radiographic and pathologic abnormalities in calcium pyrophosphate dihydrate deposition disease (CPPD): Pseudogout. *Radiology* 122:1, 1977.

Resnick D, Shaul S, Robins JM: Diffuse idiopathic skeletal hyperostosis (DISH): Forestier's disease with extraspinal manifestations. *Radiology* 115:513, 1975.

Udoff EJ, Genant HK, Kozin F, et al: Mixed connective tissue disease: The spectrum of radiographic manifestations. *Radiology* 124:613, 1977.

Weissman BN, Rappoport AS, Sosman JL, et al: Radiographic findings in the hands in patients with systemic lupus erythematosus. *Radiology* 126:313, 1978.

Weissman BN, Sosman JL: The radiology of rheumatoid arthritis. *Orthop Clin North Am* 6:653, 1975.

Part 2

IMMUNOLOGY AND INFLAMMATION

6
Cellular Immunity

Jeffrey C. Delafuente

Andrea Dlesk

Richard S. Panush

There are two broad limbs of immune responses. Humoral immunity is mediated by plasma cell production of immunoglobulins (antibodies) (Chap. 7). It may also be considered to include other mediator systems such as complement, kinins, prostaglandins, and products of clotting and fibrinolysis (Chap. 8). Cell-mediated immunity (CMI) is that specific immune response to antigens mediated by sensitized lymphocytes and macrophages, with minor participation by neutrophils, eosinophils, basophils, and platelets. CMI responses may follow exposure of the immune system to diverse antigens—protein, polysaccharide, chemical, bacterial, viral, transplantation, or autologous.

Lymphocytes encountering specific antigens participate in intricate interactions that (1) process antigen, (2) regulate immune responses, and (3) effect CMI. These processes are mediated by both cell-to-cell interactions and cell-derived soluble substances. Cellular immunity is responsible for (1) delayed-type hypersensitivity, (2) foreign graft rejection, and (3) resistance to certain kinds of infection (e.g., viral, bacterial, protozoan and metazoan, parasitic, and fungal). Derangement of CMI may lead to (1) congenital or acquired immunodeficiency diseases, (2) autoimmune disease, (3) tumor growth, (4) contact dermatitis, and (5) drug reactions. This chapter discusses the roles and interactions of participants in the cellular immune response. Clinical application of CMI testing is discussed in Chapter 4.

CELLULAR CONSTITUENTS OF CELL-MEDIATED IMMUNITY

Lymphocytes

The lymphoid system can be divided into three compartments: (1) the stem cell pool, (2) the primary lymphoid organs (thymus and bursa or bursa equivalent), and (3) the secondary lymphoid organs (lymph nodes, spleen, and Peyer's patches). Stem cells are pluripotent cells capable not only of extensive self-replication but also of differentiation into more mature forms (Fig. 6.1). These cells originate in

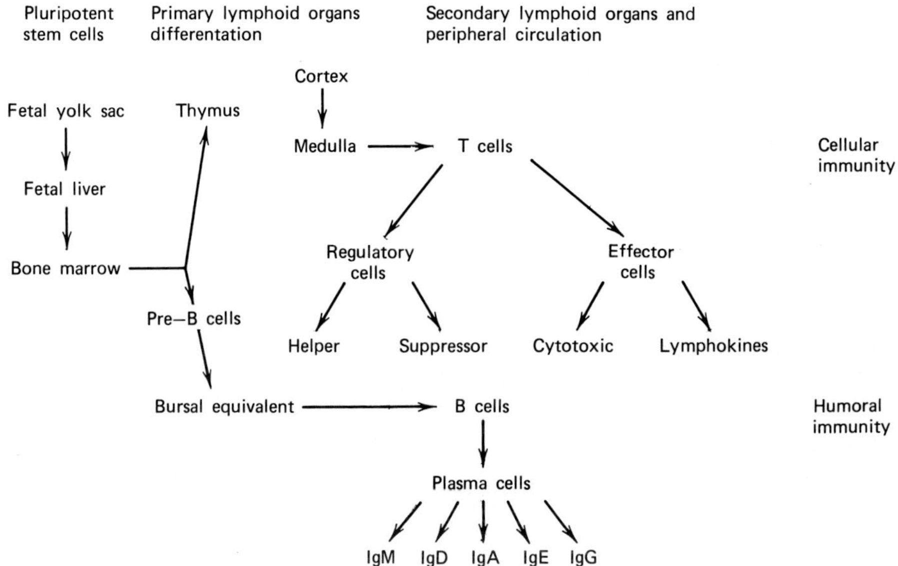

Figure 6.1. Lymphocyte differentiation. Pluripotential stem cells differentiate into T or B cells upon being influenced by the thymus or bursa equivalent, respectively. T cells are largely concerned with so-called cellular immunity or delayed-type hypersensitivity, while B cells participate in humoral immune processes.

blood islands of the embryonic yolk sac, then in the fetal liver, and finally in adult bone marrow. They may become programmed to differentiate into T or B cells that have distinctive surface markers and functional characteristics.

T Lymphocytes

The T lymphocyte is the major cell type responsible for CMI. T lymphocytes originate in the thymus, an epithelioid organ derived from the third and fourth pharyngeal pouches. During the second half of embryogenesis, stem cells migrate first into the thymic cortex and then into the medulla. At this time, prethymocytes undergo stepwise differentiation into immunocompetent T cells. A large portion (80%–90%) of T cells never leave the thymic medulla. The remainder migrate to the peripheral circulation and populate secondary lymphoid organs. Specific subpopulations of human T cells with unique surface characteristics and functions are now being identified.

T lymphocytes comprise approximately 80% of adult human peripheral blood lymphocytes (PBL). They can first be demonstrated in the fetus at 10 to 16 weeks of gestation. At birth, T cells represent only 50%–60% of PBLs and are functionally immature. Patients with a congenital absence of the thymus have greatly reduced or absent T-cell populations. Patients with agammaglobulinemia have normal numbers of T cells.

T lymphocytes play a primary role in effecting CMI responses such as delayed-type hypersensitivity, contact sensitivity, acquired resistance to infections, allograft rejection, and tumor immunity. Tissue injury caused by cellular mechanisms is mediated by (1) effector lymphocytes, (2) soluble cell-derived products, lymphokines (see below), and (3) cytotoxic lymphocytes. Cytotoxic T cells can lyse target cells via a cell-to-cell interaction in the absence of complement and antibody. Another recently described cytotoxic lymphocyte is the K or killer cell. This lymphocyte has surface receptors for the Fc portion of immunoglobulin (Ig) and can carry out antibody-dependent, complement-independent, cell-mediated cytotoxicity. Other subpopulations of T cells exert regulatory control over antibody production by B cells in response to certain antigens and over cellular effector responses. These cells have been termed *helper* or *suppressor* T cells (see below).

B Lymphocytes

B cells are the cell type directly responsible for the synthesis of antibody. They are now also known to (1) produce lymphokines, (2) act as effector cells in CMI, and (3) possibly exert regulatory effects as well. The precise location of human B lymphocyte differentiation is unknown. In chickens, B cells differentiate in the bursa of Fabricius, an area of epithelial tissue in the gut. A bursa equivalent has never been clearly identified in human beings, but current evidence favors bone marrow, fetal liver, or spleen as likely sites.

Like T cells, pre-B cells undergo stepwise differentiation, beginning in the second half of embryogenesis, into immunocompetent cells bearing characteristic surface determinants. In contrast to T cells, the majority of B-cell differentiation occurs in the periphery. Pre-B cells synthesize IgM, which is then inserted into the cell membrane. During subsequent differentiation, the density of IgM on the cell surface diminishes and is replaced by IgD. These cells may serve as precursors for IgG- and IgA-secreting plasma cells.

Neonates have numbers of B cells comparable to adults. However, production of substantial amounts of IgG and IgA does not occur until 1 and 6 years of age, respectively, perhaps due to T-cell suppression of B-cell differentiation. In the adult, B cells comprise 10% of the peripheral blood lymphocyte pool. Less than 1% of these cells bear surface IgG or IgA, the majority carrying IgM or IgD. B cells are absent in most cases of congenital agammaglobulinemia but not in patients with thymic aplasia.

Lymphocyte Surface Markers

Lymphocyte subpopulations can be identified by their cell surface characteristics. Table 6.1 lists distinctive surface markers and assays used to identify lymphocyte subpopulations. These markers and assays are discussed more fully in Chapter 4.

Human T cells have a unique receptor on their surface that allows them to bind to sheep erythrocytes (E) to form E rosettes, providing a means to identify T lymphocytes (Fig. 4.1). Approximately 80% of human PBLs form E rosettes. Subsets of human T cells, similar to those recognized in mice, with unique surface markers and distinctive functions, are now recognized. A subpopulation of T cells bears surface receptors for the Fc portion of immunoglobulins. These receptors are demonstrated by their ability to rosette with sheep red blood cells (SRBC) coated with anti-SRBC antibodies (EA rosettes). The Fc receptor will not bind native Ig but will bind the Fc portion of an immunoglobulin in the

Table 6.1. Surface Receptors of Lymphocytes

Receptor	*T Cells*	*B Cells*	*Null Cells*
Sheep red blood cells (E rosettes)	80[a]	0	0
Fc portion of immunoglobulins (EA rosettes)	5–70	10	6
Surface immunoglobulin	0	10	0
Complement (C3b) (EAC rosettes)	0	3	7
% of total peripheral lymphocytes	80	10	10

[a] Numbers refer to the percent of total peripheral blood lymphocytes.

form of an immune complex or as aggregated antibody. Most T cells, however, are devoid of Fc and complement receptors and surface Ig. Fc receptor-bearing cells have been estimated to include anywhere from 5% to 70% of human T cells. T cells with Fc receptors for IgG (T gamma) appear to be suppressor lymphocytes, whereas those with IgM Fc receptors (T mu) are helper lymphocytes.

B cells bear surface immunoglobulins, the majority (90%) of which are IgM or IgD (Fig. 4.6). In addition, these cells have Fc receptors for specific antibody or antigen-antibody complexes. Approximately 10% of human PBLs are B cells. Three percent of these cells have surface receptors for C1q, C3b, or C4b. C3b receptor-bearing cells are detected by rosetting with sheep erythrocytes coated with IgM anti-SRBC antibody and complement (EAC rosettes).

Other cell surface markers, first detected among B cells and thus termed *B cell alloantigens,* have been recently identified. These surface determinants are coded at the D locus of the major histocompatibility complex of the sixth chromosome in humans (human leukocyte antigen [HLA] D), closely linked to the major transplantation antigens. They are analogous to the I region-associated (Ia) antigens of the mouse coded for by the murine major histocompatibility complex (MHC) located in the seventeenth chromosome. In humans these antigens exist on B cells, macrophages, spermatozoa, epithelial cells, and some T cells. As discussed in other chapters (4, 11, 12, 13, 15, 17), susceptibility to certain rheumatic diseases can now be linked to particular B-cell alloantigens.

Between 2% and 10% of PBLs lack surface receptors for SRBC as well as surface immunoglobulin. These non-T, non-B cells are termed *null* cells. Approximately 4% of null cells bear surface receptors for complement alone, 3% for the Fc portion of immunoglobulins, and 3% for both. There is evidence that 20%–30% of null cells may represent B-cell precursors.

Macrophages also possess distinctive cell surface receptors, including receptors for the Fc portion of IgG and for C3b. They may have adsorbed immunoglobulin. It is therefore important to control for the presence of these cells when assessing the relative frequency of T, B, and null cells by separating out adherent or phagocytic macrophages.

Table 6.2. In Vitro Functional Activity of Human
T and B Lymphocytes

Response	*T Cells*	*B Cells*
Proliferative response to		
Mitogens (PHA, PWM, Con A)[a]	+	+
Sodium periodate	+	−
Anti-immunoglobulin	−	+
Lipopolysaccharide	−	±
Antigen	+	−
Mixed lymphocyte culture	+	+
Lymphokine production		
Migration inhibitory factor	+	+
Blastogenic factor	+	−
Lymphotoxin	+	+
Chemotactic factors	+	+
Interferon	+	+
Ig production	−	+
Cytotoxicity	+	±
Suppressor/helper function	+	±

[a] PHA, phytohemagglutinin; PWM, pokeweed mitogen; Con A: concanavalin A.

Lymphocyte Functional Responses

T and B cells can be activated in vitro by both specific antigenic and nonspecific (plant mitogens, allogeneic cells) stimuli. Many in vitro responses mirror in vivo delayed-type hypersensitivity and are useful in correlating cellular responses and hypersensitivities. As is illustrated in Table 6.2, lymphocytes can be induced to proliferate, release soluble mediators, and exhibit cytotoxicity, or immunoregulatory functions. Certain responses seem unique to T or B cells. However, experimental conditions vary greatly, so that these assays are not well standardized. Specificities of responses for cell types must be interpreted with caution.

Mononuclear Phagocytes

The mononuclear phagocyte system plays an integral part in CMI. This system is composed of three major cell types: (1) monocytes, precursors of the inflammatory macrophage, (2) normal macrophages (including histiocytes, Kupffer cells, alveolar macrophages, sinusoidal lining cells, osteoclasts, and microglial cells), and (3) inflammatory macrophages, including epithelioid giant cells. These cells have similar morphologic characteristics, a high phagocytic capability, and the ability to attach firmly to glass surfaces. Mononuclear phagocytes originate in the bone marrow. The bone marrow progenitor cell is the monoblast, which differentiates to form the promonoblast. These cells mature and migrate into the periphery, where they constitute 1%–8% of the total white blood cell count (280–550 cells/cu mm). In addition, they migrate to the connective tissue, liver, lung, spleen, synovial lining, sinus cavities, bone, and nervous system to become normal macrophages.

Monocytosis occurs normally in neonates and in adults with (1) infections (tuberculosis, syphilis, subacute bacterial endocarditis, typhoid fever, rickettsial and protozoal disease), (2) rheumatic diseases (rheumatoid arthritis, systemic lupus erythematosus, and rheumatic fever), (3) inflammatory diseases (ulcerative colitis and regional enteritis), (4) neoplastic diseases, and (5) other disorders (cirrhosis, drug reactions, sarcoidosis, hemolytic anemia, and postsplenectomy).

Tissue macrophage lysosomes contain many hydrolytic enzymes, including phosphatases, esterases, beta-glucuronidase, lysozyme, and arysulfatase. Macrophages also secrete elastase, collagenase, plasminogen activator, complement, prostaglandins, and other enzymes important in inflammatory responses. Circulating monocytes contain many of these enzymes, but in smaller amounts. These cells have receptors for the Fc portion of IgG (IgG1 and IgG3) and for the third component of complement, C3. Macrophages participate in (1) phagocytosis and killing, (2) antigen processing, (3) cytotoxic reactions, and (4) regulation of T- and B-cell responses. They carry out these functions by both direct cell-to-cell interactions and elaboration of soluble mediators (monokines), as will be discussed.

Monocytes and macrophages engulf particulate materials by pinocytosis and phagocytosis. When foreign material enters the body, it is rapidly taken up by these phagocytes. Antigen molecules entering lymphoid tissue are taken up by macrophages and degraded. Antigen bound to macrophages is highly immunogenic and is important in initiating immune responses.

Polymorphonuclear Leukocytes

Polymorphonuclear leukocytes (neutrophils) are phagocytic cells that also participate in immune and inflammatory responses. Neutrophil granules contain many enzymes, such as acid hydrolases, myeloperoxidase, proteases, and lysozyme. The enzymes are capable of degrading microbes, immune complexes, Ig, and injured cells. They also augment inflammation, initiate other cellular functions, and may injure normal tissue. Once localized at the inflammatory site, neutrophils are capable of binding and ingesting opsonized materials. In all delayed-type hypersensitivity reactions neutrophils are present to some extent, probably in response to specific chemotactic factors produced by lymphocytes, complement, kinins, and other immunologic systems. These and other experimental observations suggest neutrophil-lymphocyte interactions in the cellular immune response. Neutrophil-derived factors that modulate lymphocyte migration and activation are under study.

Basophils

Basophils are known to be involved in immediate hypersensitivity reactions but may have a role in CMI. In guinea pigs, cutaneous basophil hypersensitivity reactions occur in response to an intradermal injection of certain proteins. This reaction differs from a delayed-type hypersensitivity reaction. The basophil-mediated lesion displays little induration and is characterized by intense infiltration of basophils as well as by mononuclear cells. Cutaneous basophil hypersensitivity is antibody independent, and its pathogenesis is poorly understood.

Basophils contain vasoactive amines (serotonin), as do platelets and mast cells. It has been proposed that activation of lymphocytes by a specific antigen may release a factor that causes nearby cells to release their vasoactive amines. The released amines may then increase postcapillary venule permeability, allowing egress of circulating inflammatory cells that augment and localize the cellular immune response.

Eosinophils

It has long been known that eosinophilia is associated with many allergic reactions and parasitic infections. Evidence suggests that eosinophils may also have a role in CMI. Eosinophils have surface receptors for the complement components C3b, C3d, and C4, which are similar to those found on B lymphocytes and monocytes. They also have Fc receptors that probably aid in phagocytosis of immune complexes.

The functional role of eosinophils is poorly understood. Although eosinophils do phagocytize, they are less efficient than neutrophils in ingesting, degrading, and killing. Eosinophils contain many hydrolytic enzymes, including ribonuclease (RNAase), cathepsin, arylsulfatase, catalase, and trypsin. Eosinophil-derived arylsulfatase can inactivate the slow-reacting substance of anaphylaxis, a potent mediator of acute allergic reactions. Animal models suggest the possibility of eosinophil-lymphocyte interactions. Immunologically induced peritoneal eosinophils are often associated with a mononuclear infiltrate. The exact nature of this interaction is not known, but the eosinophils may be involved in antigen processing.

Eosinophil chemotactic factor of anaphylaxis (ECF-A) is one of several substances that cause eosinophils to accumulate at the site of an acute inflammatory response. ECF-A has been found in human lung, leukemic human basophils, and rat mast cells. Sera from patients with various inflammatory disorders contain a chemotactic factor for eosinophils that appears to be identical to the fifth component of complement, C5a.

SOLUBLE MEDIATORS OF CELL-MEDIATED IMMUNITY

When sensitized lymphocytes interact with antigen, a number of soluble substances may be produced. These nonimmunoglobulin products of activated lymphocytes possess in vitro biological activities that mediate, in part, cellular immune responses. These substances have been termed *lymphokines*. Many lymphokines are glycoproteins that range in molecular weight from 20,000 to 100,000.

In the laboratory, lymphokines are present in the supernatant from sensitized lymphocytes cultured with an antigen or nonspecific mitogen (plant-derived substances that activate lymphocytes). Table 6.3 lists some of the soluble products of lymphocytes that have been described. Certain of these products have received much investigative attention and will be discussed.

Table 6.3. Soluble Mediators of Cellular Immunity

Factors affecting lymphocytes
  Blastogenic (mitogenic) factor (LBF, LMF, LTF)
  Transfer factor
  Lymphocyte chemotactic factor
  Helper factor(s)
  Suppressor factor(s)
Factors affecting macrophages
  Migration inhibitory factor (MIF)
  Macrophage-activating factor (MAF)
  Macrophage chemotactic factor
  Macrophage-aggregating factor (MAF)
  Macrophage-spreading factor
Factors affecting neutrophils
  Leukocyte inhibitory factor (LIF)
  Leukocyte chemotactic factor
Factors affecting eosinophils
  Eosinophil chemotactic factor (ECF)
  Eosinophil-promoting factor
Factors affecting cell growth
  Lymphotoxin (LT)
  Proliferation inhibitory factor (PIF)
  Clonal inhibitory factor (CIF)
  Inhibitor of DNA synthesis (IDS)
Other
  Osteoclast-activating factor (OAF)
  Basophil chemotactic factor
  Interferon
  Ig binding factor
  Complement-activating factor (CAF)
  Fibroblast chemotactic factor

Lymphocyte-derived Mediators (Lymphokines)

Factors Affecting Lymphocytes

Lymphocyte Mitogenic Factors. Lymphocyte mitogenic factor (LMF) (also termed *blastogenic [LBF]* or *transforming [LTF] factor*) induces normal lymphocytes to undergo blast transformation and to incorporate increased amounts of ³H-thymidine into newly synthesized cellular DNA. LMF produced from specific antigen stimulation is effective in inducing blastogenesis of nonsensitized lymphocytes. Investigations with thymectomized and bursectomized chickens support the view that both T and B lymphocytes may produce LMF, but B-cell production of this factor requires the presence of T cells. Human LMF, however, seems to be secreted by T, not B, cells. LMF acts like a polyclonal B-cell activator, resulting in B-cell proliferation and morphologic and functional changes, such as the appearance of endoplasmic reticulum, loss of surface C3 receptors, and antibody synthesis.

LMF may have considerable biologic importance. It could explain how small numbers of sensitized lymphocytes can recruit nonsensitized cells, resulting in an enhanced immune response. By stimulating nonsensitized lymphocytes, LMF probably induces the secretion of other lymphokines from these recruited cells. LMF is resistant to treatment with RNAase, DNAase, and proteolytic enzymes. It has a molecular weight of 20,000 to 30,000.

Transfer Factor. Cellular immunity and delayed-type hypersensitivity can be transferred from a sensitized person by means of a lymphocyte extract termed *transfer factor*. Transfer factor may be more than one molecular moiety and is as effective as viable lymphocytes in transferring immunity. Transfer factor is a dialyzable molecule with a molecular weight of 2,000 to 4,000. It is resistant to DNAase, RNAase, and proteolytic enzymes.

When transfer factor is given to a nonsensitized person, the recipient's lymphocytes will undergo blast transformation and lymphokine secretion when exposed to the specific antigen to which the transfer factor donor is sensitive. Transfer factor has been used successfully to initiate or restore cellular immunity in selected patients with a wide range of immunodeficiencies, tumors, viral and fungal infections, and rheumatic diseases.

The mechanism by which transfer factor can induce recipient cellular responses is unknown. In vitro and in vivo data suggest that transfer factor may act by uncovering or causing the de novo appearance of specific receptor sites on recipient lymphocytes. After administration, transfer factor may initiate a new population of circulating lymphocytes with appropriate antigen receptors.

Lymphocyte Chemotactic Factor. Lymphocytes can also respond to chemotactic stimuli. Lymphotactin, an extract from the thymus of immunized guinea pigs and calves, is chemotactic for rabbit lymphocytes. Antigen-stimulated rat lymph node cells also produce a chemotactic factor. Lymphocyte chemotactic factors may attract nonsensitized lymphocytes to reaction sites to become involved in cellular immune responses, such as that seen in delayed-type hypersensitivity skin-test reactions.

Helper and Suppressor Factors. Soluble substances have been detected in culture supernatants that can enhance or suppress lymphocyte functions and are discussed below.

Factors Affecting Macrophages
Macrophage Migration Inhibitory Factor. Lymphocytes stimulated by specific antigens or nonspecific mitogens secrete migration inhibitory factor (MIF), which acts upon macrophages to inhibit their in vitro migration out of capillary tubes. Production of MIF is dependent on the presence of T cells, but both T and B cells can produce MIF. Supernatants from antigen-stimulated human peripheral lymphocyte cultures also have been shown to increase macrophage adherence to culture vessels as well as glucose oxidation. The molecule(s) responsible for these effects are in the same molecular weight range as MIF and are not immune complexes.

The production of MIF by human lymphocytes stimulated by antigens is closely associated with the presence of in vivo cellular hypersensitivity of the host to the stimulating antigen. MIF production by antigen-stimulating lymphocytes is specific; macrophage response to MIF is not.

Human MIF has a molecular weight of approximately 25,000 and is indistinguishable from a factor that activates the defense capacities of macrophages, macrophage-activating factor (MAF). MIF activity is not altered by treatment with RNAase or DNAase but is inactivated by proteolytic enzymes. MIF synthesis can be blocked by inhibiting lymphocyte protein synthesis.

Macrophage Chemotactic Factor.   Delayed hypersensitivity-type reactions in the skin of guinea pigs are associated with the appearance of a lymphocyte-derived chemotactic factor for monocytes. Chemotactic factors may be responsible for macrophage- and lymphocyte-rich inflammatory exudates characteristic of cellular immune reactions.

Guinea pig lymph node lymphocytes, cultured in the presence of specific antigens, secrete a substance that is chemotactic for homologous and heterologous mononuclear cells. This factor differs electrophoretically from guinea pig MIF.

Other lymphocyte-derived factors affect macrophage aggregation, spreading, and other functions. Their distinction from MIF and/or chemotactic factors is uncertain.

Factors Affecting Neutrophils

Leukocyte Chemotactic Factor.   Human lymphocytes stimulated with mitogens and antigens release soluble substance(s) chemotactic for mononuclear and polymorphonuclear cells. In vitro data indicate that the production of these factors precedes lymphocyte blastogenesis.

In an avian model, leukocyte chemotactic factors have been shown to be a T-lymphocyte product. Lymphocytes from chickens rendered agammaglobulinemic by bursectomy have no demonstrable B-cell function, although T-cell functions are normal. These chicken lymphocytes produce normal amounts of chemotactic factors.

Leukocyte Inhibitory Factor.   Polymorphonuclear leukocyte migration is inhibited by another soluble material, termed *leukocyte inhibitory factor (LIF)*. LIF may act to immobilize neutrophils once they have been induced to migrate to the site of an immunologic/inflammatory reaction. LIF is secreted by human PBLs cultured with a specific antigen or nonspecific mitogens. Lymphocytes from donors lacking the delayed-type hypersensitivity to a specific antigen do not produce LIF in response to that antigen. LIF does not inhibit the migration of human monocytes or guinea pig macrophages. LIF is yet another link between the lymphocyte and the other cell types involved in the inflammatory process.

Human LIF has a molecular weight of approximately 69,000. It has a buoyant density similar to that of pure protein and is inactivated by chymotrypsin. It is also irreversibly inactivated by treatment with esterase inhibitors, suggesting that LIF has esterase properties.

Factors Affecting Eosinophils

Stimulated human peripheral leukocytes also produce an eosinophil chemotactic factor (ECF). ECF is released from neutrophils during phagocytosis and basophils stimulated with IgE immune complexes. Unlike ECF-A, which is stored preformed in mast cells, ECF is generated during cell activation and is not stored in the leukocytes. Other lymphocyte-derived factors that affect eosinophils, such as an eosinophil stimulation promoter, have also been described.

Factors Affecting Cell Growth

Lymphotoxin. Activation of lymphocytes by mitogens, antigens, or allogeneic cells results in the release of another soluble factor or factors, lymphotoxin(s) (LT). LT can lyse certain target cells in the absence of lymphocytes. There are several assay systems that detect LT. Generally, the supernatant from stimulated lymphocyte cultures is incubated with the target cells, such as the mouse L cell (fibroblast). Cytotoxicity of the target cell is determined by enumerating viable cells, measuring reduction of radiolabeled amino acid incorporation into cellular protein, or release of ^{51}Cr from labeled target cells. Secretion of LT by activated lymphocytes serves as an in vitro model of CMI in which tissue destruction occurs. These immune responses are often seen in delayed-type hypersensitivity disease.

LT has been detected in plasmas from patients with rheumatoid arthritis, multiple sclerosis, neoplasia, and renal transplants. No LT activity was found in healthy control subjects. Lymphocytes from children with severe combined immunodeficiency disease do not produce LT. In vitro LT production is diminished in common variable hypogammaglobulinemia and Bruton's disease. Following thymus or bone marrow transplant in these immunodeficient patients, LT appears in culture supernatants.

Human lymphotoxin has an estimated molecular weight of 80,000–150,000 and is inactivated by proteolytic enzymes. Other lymphocyte-derived factors inhibiting cell growth in certain culture systems have also been described (Table 6.3).

Other Soluble Mediators

Osteoclast-activating Factor. A lymphokine known as *osteoclast-activating factor (OAF)* is elaborated after in vitro lymphocyte stimulation. This mediator is capable of activating osteoclasts in bone. It is chemically different from parathyroid hormone and does not produce hypercalcemia in vivo.

Production of OAF is dependent upon macrophage-lymphocyte interactions. OAF may play an important role in bone lesions associated with chronic inflammation (Chap. 11) and neoplasia. Bone marrow cells from patients with myeloma produce a substance similar to OAF, whereas bone marrow cells from patients with other hematologic neoplasms do not. OAF from myeloma bone marrow may lead to local bone destruction. The myeloma cell is the most likely source of this bone resorbing factor.

Fibroblast Chemotactic Factor. Human peripheral blood lymphocytes produce an antigen-specific chemotactic factor for human dermal fibroblasts. This fibroblast chemotactic factor does not exert an effect on monocyte or mononuclear cell migration. Likewise, chemotactic factors for monocytes are not chemotactic for fibroblasts.

Lymphocyte-derived chemotactic factors for fibroblasts may have biologic significance. Cell-mediated reactions to tubercle bacilli result in granulomas characterized by an increased number of fibroblasts. Fibroblast chemotactic factor released by sensitized lymphocytes may be responsible for attracting connective tissue fibroblasts into these granulomas. The increase in collagen formation characteristic of progressive systemic sclerosis may also be the consequence of fibroblast chemotactic factor (see Chap. 20).

Monocyte-Derived Mediators (Monokines)

Macrophages have roles in immune response regulation that have not yet been fully defined. Macrophages and monocytes elaborate numerous soluble products that regulate other cell types and augment inflammatory responses. These soluble mediators are referred to as *monokines*. They include lymphocyte-activating factors, colony-stimulating factor, substances modulating lymphocyte responses, and probably others. Macrophages also produce plasminogen activator, prostaglandins, collagenase, and complement proteins and secrete other enzymes in response to appropriate stimuli. Two monokines will be briefly discussed.

Lymphocyte-activating Factor (LAF)

Lymphocyte-activating factor (LAF) is a product secreted by stimulated macrophages. Although LAF is not mitogenic, it enhances DNA synthesis of mitogen-activated T lymphocytes. LAF has a molecular weight of approximately 15,000. A high-molecular-weight ($\sim$ 85,000) LAF has been described. Mechanisms of action of LAF are not clear.

Colony-Stimulating Factor (CSF)

Macrophages secrete products known as *colony-stimulating factors (CSF)*, which are required for in vitro clonal proliferation of B lymphocytes. CSF is demonstrable in normal sera and is often elevated in conditions associated with granulopoiesis, as well as during viral and bacterial infections. The physical-chemical properties of CSF have not yet been fully delineated.

THE NORMAL IMMUNE RESPONSE

The immune response involves recognition of an antigen as foreign and generation of a humoral and/or cellular effector response. Antigen is recognized as foreign by T or B cells possessing appropriate surface receptors in the presence of macrophages (Fig. 6.2). Mechanisms of antigen processing, generation of the immune response, and regulatory interactions between the cellular and soluble participants are exceedingly complex.

Antigen Recognition and Cellular Interactions

A variety of mechanisms have been proposed to explain how cellular constituents of immune responses interact. T and B lymphocytes, as well as macrophages, are required to initiate an immune response to most antigens. Figure 6.2 schematically summarizes some of the hypothesized cellular interactions involved in CMI. These interactions may occur by direct cell-to-cell contact, through lymphocyte- or macrophage-derived soluble factors, or a combination of events.

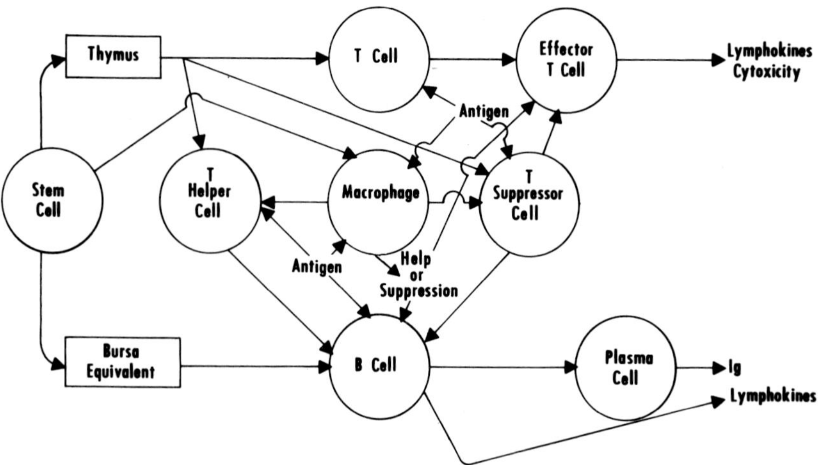

Figure 6.2. Possible cellular interactions in CMI. T and B lymphocytes derive from stem cells influenced by the thymus or bursa equivalent, respectively. T cells may (1) affect cellular immunity by direct cellular reactions or elaborating lymphokines, (2) regulate (help or suppress) B-cell or effector T-cell responses, and (3) help process antigen. B cells may (1) secrete Ig or (2) lymphokines. Antigen may initially come in contact with either a T cell, a B cell, or a macrophage. Antigen may form a bridge between two cells, bringing them into close proximity. Antigen may directly activate T or B cells or interact with surface receptors on T cells or macrophages, which then trigger the release of soluble substances, signaling responder cells appropriately.

Macrophages present antigens to reactive lymphocytes. Interactions between T cells, B cells, and macrophages are mediated by complementary cell surface receptors and soluble cell products. The antigen receptor on T cells seems analogous, in part, to that on B cells; it contains a portion of the variable Ig light chain region of the immunoglobulin antigen-combining site. This may permit clonal expansion of T and B cells appropriate to the antigen. Normally, the immune response to an antigen intensifies initially and then stabilizes at a somewhat higher basal level. Reexposure induces an anamnestic response with greater production of antibody than in the primary response.

Generation and Regulation of the Immune Response

A number of mechanisms, not all well understood, precisely control the immune response. One means of regulating the immune response is by regulatory cells and their signals.

Regulatory Cells

Lymphocytes.   A subpopulation of T lymphocytes that are required for B-cell immunoglobulin production are known as *T helper cells*. These cells are characterized by surface receptors for the Fc portion of IgM. T helper cells react with the carrier molecule of a hapten to induce antibody formation. Carrier molecules are usually proteins. Other effective carriers that react with carrier-reactive T helper cells include subunits on protein molecules or determinants on allogeneic erythrocytes. Some antigens will induce antibody responses without T helper cells, but these thymus-independent antigens are usually large molecules with repeating antigenic determinants.

Recently, a subset of T helper cells has been described in mice. These *amplifier cells* act synergistically with T helper cells in primed antibody responses. Whereas T helper cells are long-lived after thymectomy in adult mice, amplifier cells are short-lived. Evidence suggests that two distinct T–B interactions occur: T-helper–B-cell interactions, followed by T-amplifier–B-cell interactions.

Supernatants of antigen-stimulated T cells can replace T helper cells for in vitro antibody response by B cells. Two classes of T helper cell factors found in T-cell supernatant cultures have been demonstrated: nonspecific factors and antigen-specific factors. The nonspecific factors generated by T cells act like polyclonal B-cell activators, causing B cells to proliferate and produce immunoglobulin to a variety of antigens. Antigen-specific factors induce production of antibodies directed only to that antigen used to elicit the factor.

T lymphocytes, with surface receptors for Fc fragments of IgG, exert a suppressive regulatory effect on antibody synthesis. Suppressor T cells have a role in (1) antibody regulation, (2) prevention of autoimmunity, (3) genetically determined unresponsiveness to certain antigens, (4) prevention of reaginic hypersensitivity, and (5) inhibition of tumor immunity. Abnormal suppressor T-cell function has been identified in certain diseases, such as systemic lupus erythematosus, agammaglobulinemia, selective IgA deficiency, sarcoidosis, Hodgkin's disease, and others.

In mice, suppressor T-cell factors have been identified. These factors are specific for antigen, are not immunoglobulin, and have a molecular weight of 35,000–55,000. They also contain determinants coded for in the I region of the major histocompatibility complex. Other nonspecific suppressor factors have also been described. Mitogen-treated mouse T cells secrete a nonantigen-specific soluble immune response suppressor substance that will suppress antibody formation to T cell-dependent and independent antigens in vitro. This suppressor substance appears to act through macrophages.

Macrophages.   There is much evidence that macrophages interact with lymphocytes not only to initiate but also to regulate certain immune responses (Fig. 6.2). In vitro experimentation indicates that macrophages play an important role in modulating both T- and B-lymphocyte responses. Even in the presence of antigen bound to macrophage surface membranes, T helper cells are still required for B-cell functions. The macrophage-bound antigen may serve to bridge T and B lymphocytes. Culture supernatants derived from antigen-pulsed macrophages do not induce an immune response, suggesting that a direct physical interaction between macrophages and lymphocytes is required. For this interaction to occur, the interacting cells must share their identity at some portion of the major histocompatibility complex.

Regulatory Control Mechanisms
Network Theory.   One of the most promising conceptual frameworks of regulation has been proposed by Jerne—the so-called network theory of idiotypes. Idio-

types are distinct antigenic determinants present in the hypervariable regions of immunoglobulin light and heavy chains. That is, they are the specific structures of the antigen-combining site of an antibody molecule. Idiotypes are identical for B-cell surface immunoglobulin, plasma cell-secreted immunoglobulin, and (probably) T-cell receptors that recognize a given antigen. An anti-idiotype is a cell surface receptor that recognizes a specific idiotype.

For example, a B cell and a T cell that have the capacity to bind antigen "Z" might do so through receptors with identical idiotypes. The B-cell anti-Z would have the same idiotype as the interacting T-cell surface receptor. One could then take this anti-Z antibody, use it as an immunogen, and create an anti–anti-Z. The anti–anti-Z (anti-idiotype) would react not only with the anti-Z but also with the surface receptors of the T and B cells involved in the original anti-Z immune responses. It must be appreciated that a given antibody, possessing an idiotype, may react not only with its specific immunizing antigen but also with other structurally similar molecules. Thus every antibody molecule, every surface immunoglobulin B-cell antigen receptor, and every T-cell antigen receptor is both an idiotype and an anti-idiotype capable of interacting with some other idiotype in the immune system itself. It is thought that this idiotype–anti-idiotype network allows the generation of both helper and suppressor functions and closely regulates immune responses.

Immune Response Genes.   Immune response (Ir) genes constitute another important element in the regulation of immune responses to specific antigens. These genes are located in the major histocompatibility complex. The presence of an appropriate Ir gene is required for immune responses to specific antigens. It may be that the Ir gene product stimulates T helper cell activity, while its absence leads to T suppressor cell activity that prevents specific antibody formation. In humans, the HLA-D locus may contain the Ir genes, linking autoimmune and immune deficiency diseases with histocompatibility phenotypes (Chap. 4).

CLINICAL ASPECTS OF CELL-MEDIATED IMMUNITY

CMI is not only responsible for host protection against invading pathogens and tumor cells but is also involved in many acute and chronic illnesses. Aberrations in cellular immunity accompany a variety of immunodeficiencies and clinical disorders. Cellular involvement and pathogenesis of various inflammatory and autoimmune diseases are discussed in the appropriate chapters. An evaluation of immunocompetent cells is presented in Chapter 4.

Clinical disorders associated with impaired cellular immunity fall into two broad categories: congenital (Table 6.4) and acquired (Table 6.5). Congenital disorders include (1) stem cell defects, (2) B-cell defects, (3) T-cell defects, and (4) other atypic states. Numerous disorders of stem cell maturation and proliferation have been described, leading to severe combined immunodeficiencies. Both T- and B-cell functions are abnormal or absent in these diseases, which are characterized by agammaglobulinemia, lymphopenia, absence of cellular immunity, and recurrent bacterial, viral, and fungal infections resulting in death, usually

Table 6.4. Congenital Disorders with Impaired Immunity

Stem cell defects
  Severe combined immunodeficiency
    X-linked
    Autosomal recessive
B-cell defects
  Agammaglobulinemias
    X-linked
    Somatic
  Dysgammaglobulinemias
  Agammaglobulinemia with B cells present
  Common variable hypogammaglobulinemia
T-cell defects
  Di George syndrome
  Nezelof syndrome
Others
  Wiskott-Aldrich syndrome
  Hereditary ataxia-telangiectasia
  Chronic mucocutaneous candidiasis
  Phagocyte functional deficiencies
    Chédiak Higashi syndrome
    Lazy leukocyte syndrome

Table 6.5. Acquired Immunodeficiency States

Primary
  Physiologic hypogammaglobulinemia
  Idiopathic hypogammaglobulinemia
Secondary
  Lymphoproliferative disorders
  T-cell disorders
    Mycosis fungoides
    Sézary syndrome
  B-cell disorders
    Multiple myeloma
    Paraproteinemias
  Others
    Hodgkin's disease
    Lymphomas
    Anemia
  Myeloproliferative disorders
  Metabolic disorders
    Kwashiorkor
    Uremia
    Diabetes mellitus
    Hypothyroidism

Table 6.5. (Continued)

Iron deficiency
Vitamin C deficiency (scurvy)
Infectious diseases
  Subacute bacterial endocarditis
  Malaria
  Viral diseases (rubella, hepatitis,
    infectious mononucleosis, others)
  Fungal infections
  Syphilis
  Leprosy
  Whipple's disease
Chronic inflammatory disorders
  Systemic lupus erythematosus
  Rheumatoid arthritis
  Sjögren's syndrome
  Mixed connective tissue disease
  Polymyositis
  Pernicious anemia
  Biliary cirrhosis
Granulomatous disorders
  Sarcoidosis
  Wegener's granulomatosis
  Inflammatory bowel disease
Hypercatabolic states
  Nephrotic syndrome
  Burns
  Protein-losing enteropathy
  Malignancy
  Myotonia dystrophica
  Surgery
Others
  Aging
  Pregnancy
  Drugs
  Atopic diseases
  Amyloidosis
  Cirrhosis

---

by the age of 2 years. These diseases are transmitted as autosomal recessive or X-linked traits. Normal immunologic reactivity has been restored in affected infants with histocompatible bone marrow transplants.

B-cell defects appear between three and six months after birth, at which time protective maternal immunoglobulin disappears. Infants with these diseases develop recurrent pyogenic infections of the skin and respiratory and alimentary tracts. These diseases are often X-linked. Variants have been described with a total absence of B cells, selective deficiencies of immunoglobulin subclasses, and normal numbers of B cells that do not synthesize immunoglobulins. Successful

Robbins DL, Gershwin ME: Identification and characterization of lymphocyte subpopulations. *Semin Arthritis Rheum* 4:245, 1978.

Rosenthal AS, Lipsky PE, Shevach EM: Macrophage-lymphocyte interaction and antigen recognition. *Fed Proc* 34:1743, 1975.

Tada´ T, Taniguchi M, Takemiri T: Properties of primed suppressor T cells and their products. *Transplant Rev* 26:106, 1975.

Waksman BH, Namba Y: On soluble mediators of immunologic regulation. *Cell Immunol* 21:161, 1976.

Ward PA: Biological aspects of leukotactic factors. *J Allergy Clin Immunol* 58:224, 1976.

Wedner HG, Parker CW: Lymphocyte activation. *Prog Allergy* 20:195, 1976.

Weksler ME: Autologous immune reactions as regulatory mechanisms (symposium). *Fed Proc* 37:2360, 1978.

7
The Humoral Immune System

Jacques R. Caldwell

The humoral immune system is concerned with the production, function, control, and biologic interaction of antibodies. All antibodies are immunoglobulins, but not all immunoglobulins necessarily have antibody activity. Immunoglobulins are specialized glycoproteins produced by cells derived from B lymphocytes. This chapter will discuss their structure, function, the role of antigen in their production, and their control by other cells of the immune response.

STRUCTURE OF IMMUNOGLOBULINS

Immunoglobulins (Ig) contain one or more subunits consisting of two pairs of polypeptide chains linked together by interchain disulfide bonds, electrostatic forces, hydrogen, and hydrophobic binding. A schematic representation of the immunoglobulin G (IgG) molecule is presented in Figure 7.1. The basic subunit is Y shaped and is composed of two identical heavy polypeptide chains (H chains) and two identical smaller chains (light chains or L chains). The heavy chains have a molecular weight varying from 51,000 to 72,000. Each light chain has a molecular weight of approximately 22,000.

The amino-terminal ends of the heavy and light chains are situated in the "arms" of the Y-shaped immunoglobulin subunit and contain the antigen-combining portion of the molecule. One-quarter of the amino-terminal end of the heavy chain and one-half of the amino-terminal portion of the light chain are highly variable (V region) and are extremely heterogeneous as to their amino acid sequence and content. The carboxy-terminal end of the light chains and heavy chains are much less variable and are referred to as the *constant* or *C regions* of the molecule. The physiologic properties of any given immunoglobulin class are determined by the structure of the C-terminal end.

In the human, there are five major classes of immunoglobulins. Each class is determined by its heavy chain content and designated as *gamma, mu, alpha, delta,* and *epsilon* present in the classes IgG, IgM, IgA, IgD, and IgE, respectively. There are only two types of light chains—kappa, which composes about

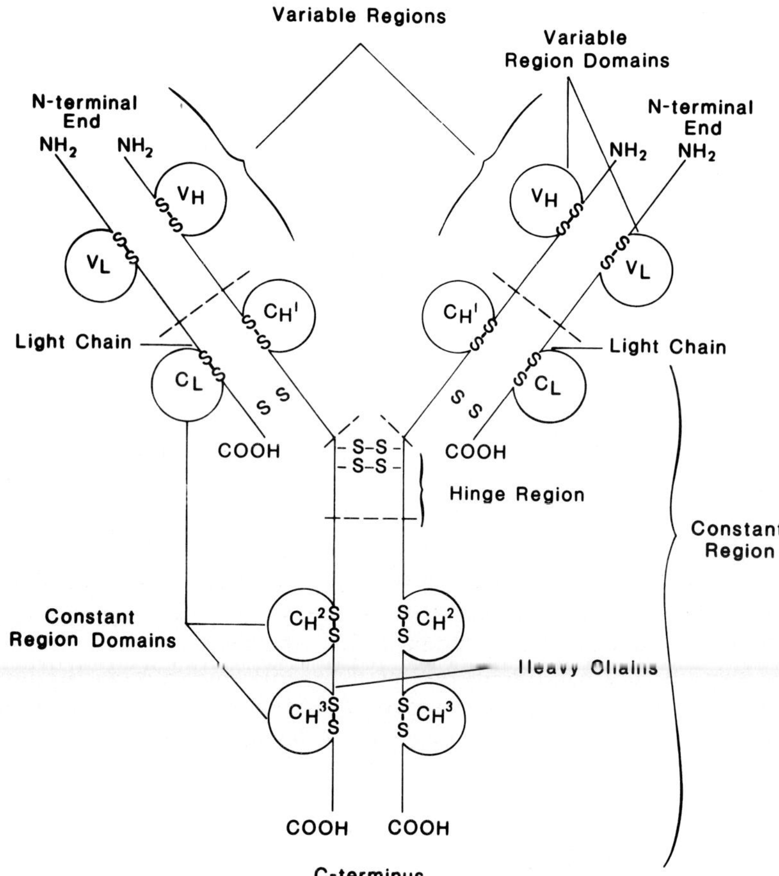

Figure 7.1. Schematic representation of the immunoglobulin structure of an IgG molecule. Each molecule contains two chains, two heavy and two light chains. The disulfide bonds are represented by -s-s. The number of disulfide bonds between heavy chains varies with the immunoglobulin class and subclass. Polymeric forms of antibody (e.g., IgA and IgM) are joined in the Fc region near the carboxyl terminus. In addition to -s-s interchain links, noncovalent forces such as hydrogen and hydrophobic bonding and electrostatic forces (not shown) bind polypeptide chains together.

The domain regions are loops within the polypeptide bonds. Each loop has an intrachain disulfide bond. CH1, CH2, and CH3 are the domains in the constant portion of the heavy chain. VH is the domain in the variable portion of the heavy chain. VL is the variable domain of the light chain. Domains contain large concentrations of antiparallel arranged beta-pleated sheets.

70% of the light chains, and lambda. Each heavy and each light chain contains amino acid regions with similar amino acid composition and spatial configurations called *domains*. Each domain consists of a polypeptide loop containing about 60 amino acids whose two ends are connected by an intrachain disulfide bond. The chains in the domain are folded in an antiparallel beta-pleated sheet array. The specific physiologic characteristics of a given immunoglobulin class can be localized to certain domains within the constant region of the heavy or light chains.

IMMUNOGLOBULIN CLASSES

Immunoglobulin G

The most common type of immunoglobulin is IgG, which is extraordinarily critical in defending the host against certain viral and bacterial antigens. Its absence in Bruton-type agammaglobulinemia subjects the affected person to recurrent pyogenic infections with pneumococcus, staphylococcus, and streptococcus. Macrophages and polymorphonuclear leukocytes are capable of binding its Fc portion, thereby enhancing phagocytosis of bacteria, particulate matter, or antigen-antibody complexes. Antibodies of the IgG class are transported across the placenta from mother to fetus and thereby supply the newborn with normal humoral immunity during the early weeks of life. After a primary antigenic challenge, IgG molecules appear in serum after IgM antibodies. However, they are the major antibody class stimulated by secondary antigenic challenge. IgG molecules are secreted by plasma cells and have a molecular weight varying from 146,000 to 165,000.

There are four subclasses of IgG—IgG1, IgG2, IgG3, and IgG4. The amino acid composition of the constant region of the heavy chains varies among the subclasses slightly, but the constant regions of the heavy chains of any one subclass are identical. Some biologic differences exist among the different subclasses. Complement is efficiently activated by IgG1 and IgG3, poorly by IgG2, and not at all by IgG4. Staphylococcal protein A is bound by the Fc portion of each subclass except IgG3. The serum half-life of IgG1, IgG2, and IgG4 is about 23 days, but it is only 16 days for IgG3.

Immunoglobulin M

The immunoglobulin M (IgM) class consists of a large (19 S) molecule with a molecular weight of approximately 970,000. It is a polymer consisting of five basic subunits linked together by disulfide bonds. IgM contains two subclasses of molecules; each subclass varies in its ability to activate the complement system. IgM contains another highly specialized immunoglobulin chain called the *J chain,* which has a molecular weight of 20,000 but whose function is not known.

Following a primary antigenic challenge, IgM antibody is the first class to be detected in serum. IgM antibodies in human blood function as anti-blood group A and anti-blood group B isohemagglutinins. IgM is the most common form of rheumatoid factor. It can fix complement very efficiently. Its large size limits it primarily to the intravascular space.

Monomeric subunits of IgM (7 S IgM) are found in certain disease states such as systemic lupus erythematosus or rheumatoid arthritis accompanied by small vessel vasculitis, and in illnesses characterized by the symptom complex of acquired C1 inhibitory deficiency, low levels of the complement components, C1, C4, and C2, angioedema, and lymphosarcoma. The 7 S IgM subunit is also found on the surface of a high percentage of circulating B lymphocytes and may play a role as an antigen receptor on these cells.

Immunoglobulin A

Immunoglobulin A (IgA) exists in three forms in the human. One is a monomeric IgA consisting of two alpha and two light chains. Another is a polymeric molecule consisting of two or more subunits, each containing two alpha and two light chains linked together by a J chain. The third form is secretory IgA that is the predominant immunoglobulin in the respiratory, salivary, and intestinal secretions. This form contains both a J chain and a specialized glycoprotein moiety called the *secretory component*. The function of the secretory component is apparently to facilitate the transport of the IgA across the epithelial cells into secretions and to protect IgA against degradation by proteolytic enzymes. Secretory IgA arises from plasma cells resident in the subepithelium and usually consists of a dimer, subunits of which contain two alpha and two light chains. Monomers, pentamers, and certain other polymeric forms are present in smaller amounts. The secretory IgA system functions independently of the serum IgA system.

Mucosal secretory IgA production can be induced by direct presentation of the antigen to gastrointestinal or respiratory surfaces, while little or no concomitant IgA appears in the serum. Whether or not IgA antibodies can mediate biologic activities other than antigen combination is unknown. They cannot activate complement by the classic pathway, although artificially aggregated secretory IgA complexes can activate the alternative complement pathway. Their ability to facilitate opsonization by attachment to phagocytic cells is uncertain. In the respiratory secretions and gastrointestinal tract, they prevent molecules from penetrating the mucosal lining.

The absence of IgA is fairly common and occurs in approximately 1 in 700 persons. Such persons may have an increased incidence of upper respiratory tract infections, gastrointestinal disorders, or autoimmune disorders and frequently experience allergic responses to respiratory antigens or to milk or egg proteins. Many persons with IgA deficiency are asymptomatic. Forty percent of IgA-deficient people produce antibodies to IgA and are susceptible to anaphylactic reactions when transfused with blood products.

Two subclasses of IgA have been identified in humans: IgA1 and IgA2; 93% of human IgA is IgA1.

Immunoglobulin E

Immunoglobulin E (IgE) exists in the serum in very low concentrations. The major locale and site of action is on the cell membrane of circulating basophils or tissue mast cells. IgE molecules contain two heavy chains and two light chains arranged as structures similar to the IgG molecules. They bind to basophils and mast cells by their Fc portion by means of a specific Fc receptor on the cell membrane. The bridging of two adjacent IgE receptors by two molecules of IgE interacting with antigen will trigger the release of histamine and other mediators of the anaphylactic or allergic reaction. The physiologic role of IgE has been debated. It may be important in the gastrointestinal tract in the expulsion of parasites from the body and in the protection of the host against parasitic organisms. IgE-mediated inflammation may be the first step in eliciting the participation of other immunoglobulins and complement in the inflammatory response. The concentration of IgE is elevated in the serum of patients with atopic (allergic) disease. IgE may also play a role in promoting capillary permeability and facilitating immune complex deposition on endothelial membranes.

Immunoglobulin D

Immunoglobulin D (IgD) is present in very low concentrations of human serum. Each molecule consists of the basic subunit of two heavy and two light chains—a structure analogous to the IgG molecule. IgD is characterized by a very short serum half-life of approximately 2.8 days, has an unknown function in serum, and can be found on the membrane surface of about 3% of human peripheral blood lymphocytes, where it frequently shares space with membrane-bound IgM molecules. Apparently, IgD and IgM molecules on the same B cell are produced by that cell, have identical light chain and heavy chain domains, and share identical antigen-binding specificities and idiotypic determinants. On the cell surface, IgD may function as an antigen receptor, but it can replace or augment membrane-bound IgM in providing the initial signal for the induction of the antibody response.

CARBOHYDRATE CONTENT OF IMMUNOGLOBULINS

Immunoglobulins contain carbohydrates that compose 2.5%–12% of their weight. Carbohydrate moieties are present in both the constant and variable domains of the molecules. Their function is unknown, but it has been postulated that they may participate in the secretion of the protein from the producing cell.

IMMUNOGLOBULIN FRAGMENTS

Much of our knowledge of antibody function has come from the study of immunoglobulin fragments produced by chemical dissociation and cleavage of the antibody chains. Most studies of antibody structure and function have been performed on myeloma proteins, which are homogeneous immunoglobulin molecules produced in unusually large amounts. Individual polypeptide chains can be produced by cleavage of the interchain disulfide bonds with mercaptoethanol or dithiothreitol.

Treatment of the intact immunoglobulin molecule with pepsin results in the generation of a single $(Fab')_2$ plus two Fc′ pieces of the heavy chain. The $(Fab')_2$ fragment contains two antigen-combining sites. Treatment of the immunoglobulin molecule with papain or trypsin cleaves the heavy chains in the intact immunoglobulin molecule in a region closer to the amino-terminal end than does treatment with pepsin, so that the interheavy chain disulfide bond no longer links the heavy chain fragments. Such treatment generates two Fab fragments, each containing a portion of the heavy chain and the entire light chain, plus an Fc fragment composed of the residual portions of the two heavy chains connected with the interchain disulfide bond. The term *Fd fragment* has been applied to that portion of the heavy chain contained within the Fab fragment (Fig. 7.2). Cyanogen bromide cleaves polypeptide chains at methionine sites. Additional fractions can be obtained by further treatment with plasmin or subtilisin.

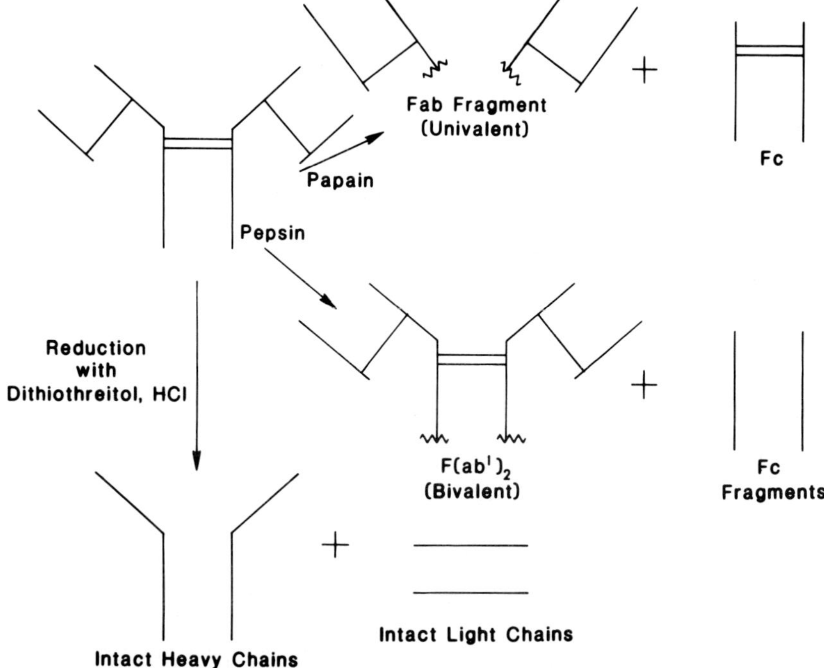

Figure 7.2. Production of immunoglobulin fragments by chemical manipulation of homogeneous immunoglobulins. Papain splits the heavy chain into Fab and Fc fragments. Each Fab contains a single antigen-combining site consisting of the N-terminus portion of the heavy chain connected by a disulfide bond to the entire light chain. The Fc fragment consists of the remainder of the heavy chains interconnected with the disulfide bond.

Pepsin cleavage converts the intact molecule into an F(ab')₂ fragment that contains both antigen-combining sites. The interheavy chain disulfide bonds persist. Multiple dialyzable Fc' fragments are also produced.

Reduction with sulfhydryl reducing agents in an acid pH can disrupt interchain disulfide bonds to leave intact heavy and light chains.

ANTIGENIC DETERMINANTS OF IMMUNOGLOBULINS

Immunoglobulins can be injected into animals and stimulate antibody production against certain structures of the molecule. Isotypic antigens are those that designate the major class of a polypeptide chain and are contained in the constant regions of the molecule, primarily in the C_H2 and C_H3 domains. Allotypic determinants are genetically coded antigenic markers present on the heavy and light chains that often reflect a single amino acid substitution in the constant portion of the chain. These markers are codominantly inherited and indicate the presence within a given animal species of several alleles at a given genetic locus. Their presence provides a means of typing immunoglobulin molecules in a manner analogous to the typing of human erythrocytes by determining ABO blood groups. The allotypic markers have been found on IgG1, IgG2, and IgG3 subclasses and have been designated *Gm markers*. A single allotypic marker (Am) has been found on IgA2 antibodies. Three different allotypic markers have been found on human kappa chains.

Idiotypes are distinct antigenic determinants present in the hypervariable regions of immunoglobulin light and heavy chains. Antibodies directed against the idiotypic markers of a given myeloma protein will not react with another myeloma protein of the same class or subclass. A common idiotype occurring in several different humans has been identified in IgM cold agglutinins recovered from the serum of several unrelated patients. All these cold agglutinins were directed to the antigen of the erythrocytes. Similar homogeneous idiotypes have been identified on several rheumatoid factors.

ROLE OF THE ANTIGEN IN THE ANTIBODY RESPONSE

Antigens are foreign substances that have the capacity to elicit an immune response. They are usually macromolecules; the antigenic determinant is the portion of the molecule that specifically interacts with the antigen-binding component of a cellular receptor or an antibody. The remaining part of the antigenic molecule has been called the *carrier*. Both parts of the molecule are important in inducing an immune response. Haptens are simple chemical compounds that are unideterminant. They cannot induce antibody synthesis alone, but they can interact with an antibody molecule. When haptens are attached to macromolecular carriers, they can incite antibody production.

When an animal is challenged by antigen, the antigen usually combines with a membrane receptor of a macrophage-related cell called an *antigen-presenting cell*. These cells are found in inflammatory exudates, spleen, lymph nodes, and skin and subsequently are partially internalized. Antigen may be biochemically altered and subsequently presented to the antigen-specific T cell by direct physical interaction. The interaction of the antigen-presenting cell with the T cell occurs only between cells sharing the same major histocompatibility structures on their surface.

The ability of an antigenic determinant to stimulate antibody production is dependent upon several factors.

1. The genetic background of the animal is important. Some antibody-combining structures on macrophages and T lymphocytes are directly determined by immune response genes. The capacity of a given antigen to stimulate antibody varies among the different species and even among animals of one species. A close association has been demonstrated between the specific histocompatibility gene (H-2) haplotypes of the mouse and the immune response to a number of synthetic protein or allelic antigens.

2. The route of antigenic challenge effects subsequent immune responses, that is, challenge by intradermal, intravenous, or mucosal routes will elicit a different quality and quantity of antibody. The optimal route for antigen administration is by subcutaneous or intramuscular injection, in which antigen is released slowly from the tissues and transferred by the lymphatics to the local lymph nodes. Antigens given intravenously are distributed widely throughout the body and cleared rapidly from the circulation by the spleen and may not evoke a good antibody response. Intravenous administration of antigen in small doses may produce an exclusive IgM response. Antigens applied to the skin or given intradermally can bind skin proteins and produce a strong IgE response or a strong cel-

lular immune response. Subcutaneous and intramuscular routes favor an IgG response, while presentation of the antigen to the mucosal surfaces stimulates secretory IgA production. Introduction of the antigen through the respiratory tract frequently facilitates the development of IgE antibodies.

3. The concentration of antigen is important. High concentrations can generate large amounts of antibody with low binding affinity; low concentrations generate small amounts of antibody with high affinity.

4. The presentation of an antigen along with an adjuvant will affect the antibody response. Adjuvants are substances that increase the host response to a given antigen. Most adjuvants are lipids such as water and oil emulsions (as in Freund's adjuvant). Insoluble particles such as alum, bentonite, or carbon particles, bacterial products such as endotoxin, bacteria such as *Bordetella pertussis*, BCG vaccine and mycobacteria have been used as adjuvants. Adjuvants probably function by retarding antigen destruction, facilitating phagocytosis by macrophages, and promoting local inflammatory responses that enhance the accumulation of phagocytic and antibody-producing cells.

5. The chemical structure of the antigen is important. The antigenic determinant must be solvent-accessible. The more structurally complex a compound, the greater its antigenicity. For instance, polypeptides of single amino acids are poor antigens. The addition of different amino acids into the structure of such synthetic antigens renders the macromolecule antigenic.

6. The optical configuration of macromolecules is important. In general, cross-reactivity between D and L isomers does not occur.

7. The size of the antigen also determines the antibody response. In general, an amino acid chain consisting of a minimum of seven units is the smallest size that can induce humoral immunity in guinea pigs. When combined with Freund's adjuvant, however, antigens containing a hapten with as few as two lysine residues can incite antibody production. Proteins with a molecular weight exceeding 10,000 are good immunogens. Those with molecular weights of less than 1,000 are usually nonimmunogenic.

8. The three-dimensional confirmational appearance of the antigen will also affect antibody specificity, affinity, and quantity. Macromolecules with multiple chains will contain multiple antigenic determinants.

9. The chemical class of antigen, too, is important. Proteins such as serum proteins, bacterial toxins, or enzymes; lipoproteins derived from some membranes or serum; glycoproteins such as occur in blood group substances or the human leukocyte antigens (HLA); polysaccharides such as the capsules of bacteria or dextrans; lipopolysaccharides such as the endotoxins derived from Gram-negative bacteria; polypeptides such as insulin, ACTH, and growth hormone; and nucleic acids such as the nuclear proteins and DNA are all excellent antigenic substances. Substances such as synthetic polymers of D-amino acids or polyvinylpyrolidone are generally nonimmunogenic. Autologous tissues and proteins are not generally antigenic unless altered by chemical, bacterial, or viral action.

FATE OF ANTIGEN IN THE HOST

After an intravenous injection, antigen is distributed widely through the body, with large amounts deposited in the liver, spleen, lungs, lymph nodes, and bone marrow. The spleen is the major site of antibody synthesis, while the liver is the major site of antigen degradation. Local antigen challenge, for example, via the skin, results in local lymph node antibody production. Subcutaneous injection of antigen delays its appearance in the blood, since the antigen is carried to local lymph nodes. The antigen-stimulated lymph node responds by blocking the output of lymphocytes during the first several hours. Simultaneously, there is a heightened ingress of lymphocytes to the stimulated node that results in a three-fold increase in the mass of the node. Within 24 hours, the lymph node begins to release large amounts of lymphoblastoid cells into efferent lymph that produces antibody to the specific antigen. This increased output continues for about 1 week.

Antigen, after entry into the host, can be taken to antibody-producing cells in the lymph nodes and spleen by several mechanisms. First, antigens can bind directly to macrophages in blood or to macrophage-like dendritic cells within lymph node follicles. Second, lymphocytes can bind antigen directly by specific receptors that have an immunoglobulin-like structure specific for the antigen. Third, antigen can combine with antibody, and the resultant immune complex can activate complement and attach C3b. C3b can adhere to receptors on B lymphocytes and macrophages. When entering a lymph node, an antigen concentrates in the immediate subcortical tissue. Next, it is transported to follicles—often by dendritic cells that are highly specialized to retain the antigen along their surface dendritic processes for a prolonged period. Germinal centers form around dendritic cells in the follicles. The function of the germinal centers seems to be differentiation of B cells. Antibodies formed in the germinal centers account for only a small portion of the total amount of antibody produced. Daughter progeny of germinal center cells are plasma cells and migrate into the medulla of the lymph node, where the majority of antibody production occurs.

ANTIBODY MEMORY

Approximately 10 days after a primary immunization, memory B cells appear in the circulation. These cells are short-term memory lymphocytes that consist of several subpopulations differing in size, surface immunoglobulin class, life span, and recirculating properties. Eventually, they are replaced in the circulation with small, long-term memory cells that continuously recirculate from the blood to the lymph. Upon reencounter with the antigen, the circulation becomes transiently depleted of these antigen memory lymphocytes, presumably due to trapping by lymph nodes in the region of the antigenic challenge.

Booster immunization in humans results in the appearance of at least three types of memory cells. Initially, human lymphoblastoid cells appear in the circulation that are capable of synthesizing IgG in a T cell-independent fashion. Although only 1 circulating lymphocyte in 10,000 is of such a type, 10%–60% of the total immunoglobulin synthesis by peripheral blood B cells can be accounted for by antibody of such recently stimulated memory cells. The rate of antibody synthesis by these cells ranges from 10 to 50 pcg/cell/hr.

Ten days after booster immunization in humans, a second subset of memory B cells appears, at which time the initial lymphoblastoid response has waned. These cells can be stimulated by pokeweed mitogen and are T cell-dependent.

They persist for approximately 4 weeks in the circulation and account for approximately three to five cells per 10,000 peripheral blood B lymphocytes.

Additionally, a third type of memory cell appears in the human circulation—the IgM memory cell. These cells persist in the circulation for indefinite periods and are not dependent on booster immunization. These IgM-producing memory cells probably represent long-term memory cells and are distinct from the other two subpopulations described above.

CELLULAR ASPECTS OF ANTIBODY SYNTHESIS

Immunoglobulin molecules are produced by B cells and their progeny, plasma cells. The primordial B cell appears to arise in the bone marrow, where it contains IgM antigenic markers and demonstrates specificity for antigen but does not have the potential for producing antibody. B cells that exit the bone marrow to enter the peripheral tissues enter a second stage of differentiation. During this second stage, IgD appears on the surface of the cell, often together with IgM, and a receptor for the C3b component of complement also appears. The IgD on the surface may be the antigenic receptor. Differentiation of the B cell is independent of antigenic stimulation. The next stage of B-cell differentiation is initiated by antigenic challenge and results in B-cell proliferation and antibody production. The production of antibodies is directly related to proliferation of the antibody-producing cells. Antibody production usually occurs in the late G1 or early S phase of the cell cycle; it is markedly reduced at the time of metaphase.

Each immunoglobulin polypeptide chain, a given immunoglobulin polypeptide chain, or a given immunoglobulin molecule is produced in a single cell and is translated from a single messenger RNA molecule. The heavy and light chains are secreted into the cisternae of the endoplasmic reticulum, where they are assembled into disulfide-linked molecules and are joined to carbohydrate by glycosylation. They are then secreted from the cell. The whole process of assembly and secretion takes only 20–30 minutes. The mechanism by which the variable and constant portions of the heavy and light chains are assembled is controversial.

The differentiation of the B cell to an antibody-producing cell depends upon at least two signals. The first is the interaction of the B-cell membrane receptor with the antigen. The second signal is provided by either T cells (called *T helper* cells) or perhaps by the interaction of T helper cells with macrophages or products derived from macrophages. In mice, several soluble helper factors have been described. One such factor has a molecular weight of 150,000, contains light and heavy immunoglobulin chains, and is antigen specific. After interaction with antigen, it binds to the surface of macrophages. B-cell activation is brought about after macrophage attachment to the B cell. A second helper factor has been described that also specifically binds antigen, but there is no resemblance to immunoglobulin. It seems to be a gene product of the I region of the mouse H-2 complex. Additionally, soluble, nonspecific T-cell helper factors have been described that can replace the role of the T cell in the activation of the B lymphocyte (Chap. 6).

B-cell activation can be T-cell independent. Large carbohydrates, such as the capsular carbohydrates of the pneumococcus or molecules with numerous repeating molecular units, are thymus independent and can stimulate B cells directly. Such stimulation usually results in the production of a limited number of antibody species that are almost exclusively of the IgM class. Most B cells undergo an immunoglobulin class switch. Originally, all B cells have IgM on their surface, but peripheral tissue B cells are capable of producing immunoglobulins of all other antibody classes. The exact cause of this switch is not understood.

Antibody production is also under careful homeostatic control. It has been known that injection of antibody into an animal will prevent proliferation in germinal centers after challenge with a specific antigen. Additionally, the phenomenon of antigenic competition has been observed. When an animal is immunized with a single antigen and challenged several days later with a different antigen, the antibody response to the second antigen is inhibited. A subclass of T lymphocytes, T suppressor cells, exists that is capable of secreting antigen-specific and antigen-nonspecific factors that limit both the activation and subsequent proliferation of B lymphocytes. Macrophages also may play a role in the inhibition of B cell antibody production (Chap. 6).

ANTIBODY DIVERSITY

One of the major concerns of immunologists has been the capacity of the body to produce antibodies to potentially large numbers of different antigenic substances; yet at the same time, each antibody produced demonstrates a high degree of specificity for the given antigen. For instance, animals immunized with a hapten trinitrophenol will react specifically with the trinitrophenol group but will show no or little cross-reaction to a similar chemical substance, dinitrophenol. It has been estimated that there are approximately 1 to 2 million distinct haptens currently available, so the potential number of antigenic determinants is indeed large. Furthermore, the antibody response to a given antigen is markedly heterogeneous, that is, multiple different antibody species of all antibody classes will arise to a single stimulus with a single antigen.

The binding affinity between antibody and a given antigen will vary markedly, even within a given antibody class or subclass. In 1959, Burnet advanced his clonal selection theory, which has been supported by a huge amount of experimentation since that time. In essence, the clonal selection theory proposes that antibody-forming cells become randomly diversified during development so that each cell can make only one type of antibody. Antibody-forming cells respond to specific antigens either by replicating or by dying. It can be mathematically determined that the host animal cannot respond to every antigen with a distinctly different antibody-producing clone of cells. In the last several years, evidence has demonstrated that individual immunoglobulin molecules combine a number of structurally different antigens and that such binding is physiologically functional. When two dissimilar antigens bind to one antibody cell, either antigen can stimulate the production of the immunoglobulin molecular species derived from that cell. From a physiologic viewpoint, antibody affinity is very important. Many antibodies will bind to multiple antigenic determinants with low binding affinities. Interaction of immunoglobulins with antigens with binding constants in the order of 1×10^3 L/mole is extremely common; any given antibody molecule might bind with one of 20–25 antigen molecules presented to it with a binding affinity in the range of 1×10^3 L/mole. Interactions of antigens with antibody with higher binding affinities, on the order of 1×10^5 L/mole, are less common and occur approximately once in 140 compounds presented to a given antibody species. Low binding affinities of antigen and antibody are probably functionally insignificant. For example, complement activation by antibody-antigen complexes will not occur unless the binding affinity between the antibody-combining site and the antigen is relatively high.

The marked diversity with which a single immunoglobulin reacts with multiple structurally different antigens can be explained by the presence in the hypervariable regions of the antibody-combining site of several highly diverse regions of amino acid sequence. Since there are many such hypervariable sequences within the antigen-combining site of the molecule, a large amount of antibody diversity is permitted.

BIBLIOGRAPHY

Ada GL: Antigen binding cells in tolerance and immunity. *Transplant Rev* 5:105, 1970.

Benacerraf B, Dorf ME: Genetic control of specific immune responses. *Prog Immunol* 2:181, 1974.

Capra JD, Kehoe JM: Structure of antibodies with shared idiotypy: The complete sequence of the heavy chain variable regions of two immunoglobulin M anti-gamma globulins. *Proc Natl Acad Sci USA* 71:4032, 1974.

Capra JD, Kehoe JM: Hypervariable regions, idiopathy, and the antigen-combining site. *Adv Immunol* 20:1, 1975.

Davies DR, Padlan EA: Three-dimensional structure of immunoglobulins. *Ann Rev Biochem* 44:639, 1975.

Dreyer WJ, Bennett JC: The molecular basis of antibody formation, a paradox. *Proc Natl Acad Sci USA* 54:864, 1965.

Frangione B, Franklin EC: Heavy chain disease: Clinical features and molecular significance of the disordered immunoglobulin structure. *Semin Hematol* 10:53, 1973.

Gally JA, Edelman GM: The genetic control of immunoglobulin synthesis. *Ann Rev Genet* 6:1, 1972.

Hood L, Barstad P, Loh E, et al: Antibody diversity: An assessment, in Sercarz EE, Williamson AR, Fox CF (eds): *The Immune System.* New York, Academic Press Inc, 1974, p 119.

Low TLK, Liu Y-S V, Putnam FW: Structure, function and evolutionary relationships of Fc domains of human immunoglobulins A, G, M, and E. *Science* 191:390, 1976.

Mage R, Lieberman R, Potter M, et al: Immunoglobulin allotypes, in Sela M (ed): *The Antigens,* vol 1. New York, Academic Press Inc, 1973, p 299.

Mitchison NA: Antigen recognition. *Cold Spring Harbor Symp Quant Biol* 32:431, 1967.

Natvig JB, Kunkel HG: Human immunoglobulin: Classes, subclasses, genetic variants, and idiotypes. *Adv Immunol* 16:1, 1973.

Padlan EA, Davies DR: Variability of three-dimensional structure in immunoglobulins. *Proc Natl Acad Sci USA* 72:819, 1975.

Poljak RJ: The three-dimensional structure, function and genetic control of immunoglobulins. *Nature* 256:373, 1975.

Tada T, Takemore T: Selective roles of thymus-derived lymphocytes in the antibody response: I. Differential suppressive effect of carrier-primed T cells on hapten-specific IgM and IgG antibody responses. *J Exp Med* 140:239, 1974.

Tomasi TB Jr, Bienenstock J: Secretory immunoglobulins. *Adv Immunol* 9:1, 1968.

Vitetta ES, Uhr JW: Immunoglobulin-receptors revisited. *Science* 189:964, 1975.

Weil E, Felix A: Quoted in Richards FF, Konigsberg WH, Rosenstein RW, et al: On the specificity of antibodies. *Science* 187:130, 1975.

8

Mediators of the Acute Inflammatory Response

Jacques R. Caldwell

The acute inflammatory response is characterized by dilatation of small capillaries and venules, by an increase in vascular permeability, and by the appearance of neutrophils, eosinophils, lymphocytes, and macrophages at the site of the inflammatory response. Initiation of inflammation depends upon activation of one of several protein or biochemical cascades. This process generates mediators capable of acting upon target end organs such as vascular smooth muscle, endothelial cells, or the inflammatory cells themselves. This chapter will review the details of these systems and offer certain clinical-pathologic correlations.

THE COMPLEMENT SYSTEM

The complement system is a group of at least 21 protein substances that interact upon appropriate stimulation to generate several biologically active substances (Fig. 8.1). Complement activation can induce lysis of hematopoietic cells, tumors, bacteria, or viruses; generate chemotactic factors and vasoactive peptides; and participate in the pathogenesis of infectious and autoimmune diseases. There are at least two pathways for activation of the complement system.

The Classic Pathway of Complement Activation

The classic pathway consists of nine proteins, designated C1 through C9, and contains three functional units—the C1 unit, the C423 unit, and the C56789 membrane attack unit. The second pathway of complement activation is the alternative pathway and will be described subsequently.

The classic complement pathway can be activated in at least two ways. The first is by the interaction of two IgG molecules or one IgM molecule with antigen. The second is directly by RNA tumor viruses (oncoronaviruses) independent of antiviral antibody. Historically, the sole function of complement was thought to be immune lysis of bacteria or susceptible hematopoietic cells. Thus, measurement of the functional integrity of the classic complement pathway components is dependent upon the lysis of antibody-coated sheep erythrocytes by dilu-

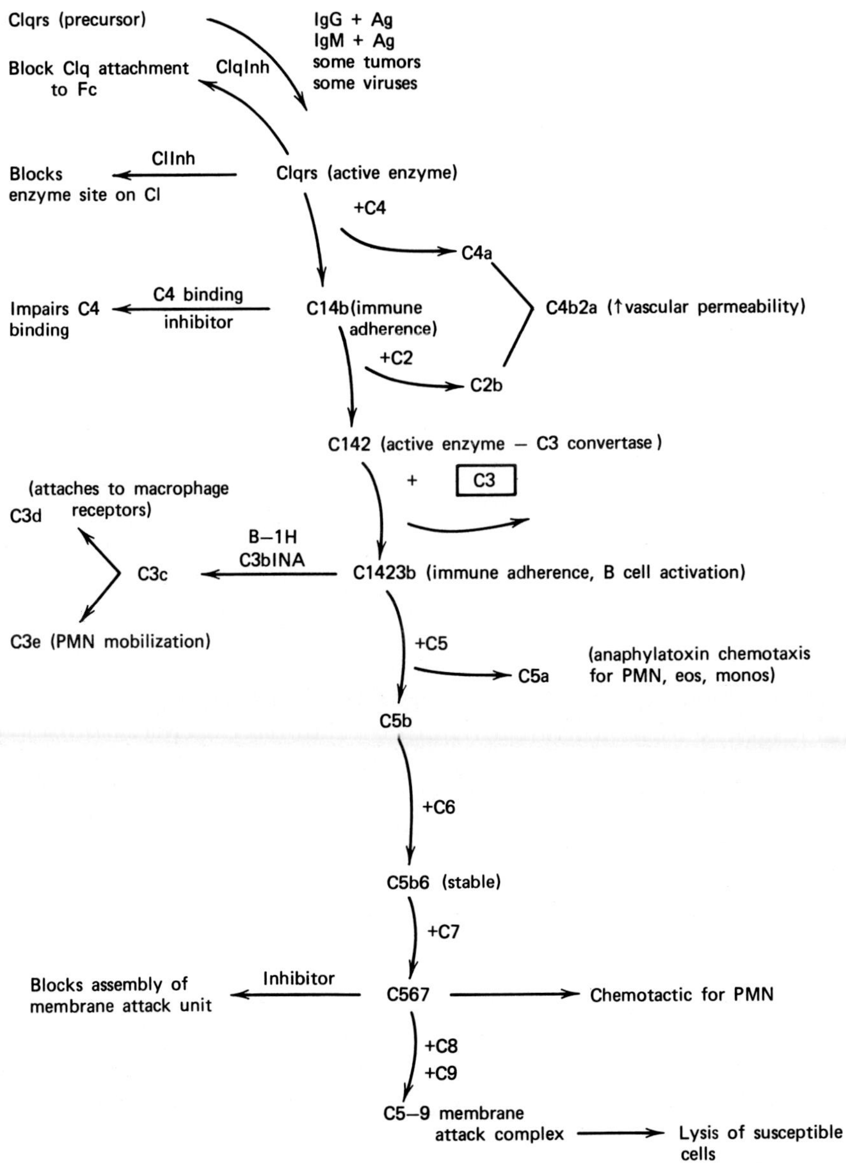

Figure 8.1. The components of the classic complement pathway together with inhibiting proteins and biologic activities generated by cleavage and activation of proteins within the cascade. See text for details. Ag, antigen; PMN, neutrophils; eos, eosinophils; monos, mononuclear cells.

tions of serum or body fluid (Chap. 4). The presence on the erythrocyte membrane of a single IgM molecule, or two sterically apposed IgG molecules, allows binding and activation of the first functional unit of complement, the C1 macromolecular complex. C1 consists of a tricomponent complex that has a molecular weight of about 1 million and contains three subunits designated *C1q, C1r,* and *C1s.* The interaction of IgM or IgG with specific antigen alters the Fc regions of these immunoglobulin molecules so that C1q can bind to the Fc region. Thus bound, C1q becomes sterically altered so that the second subunit, C1r, is converted to an active enzyme that subsequently cleaves C1s and generates another active enzyme—a serine esterase denoted C1s̄.

C1s̄ rapidly acts upon its two natural substrates, C4 and C2. One molecule of C1 can cleave hundreds of molecules of C4, such cleavage generating two fragments from C4. The larger-molecular-weight fragment, C4b, can bind to biologic membranes such as an antibody-coated red blood cell or tumor cell. Less than 10% of the C4b generated becomes cell bound. C4a, the smaller piece, enters the tissue fluid. After splitting of C4, C2 is cleaved by C1s̄. C2 cleavage can occur directly by C1s̄ action or progress in an enhanced fashion by the action of C1s̄ in the presence of C4b.

A large piece of C2, C2a, combines with C4b and forms the C4b-C2a complex (also called *C3 convertase*). This process further propagates the complement cascade by fragmenting C3 into C3a and C3b. C3a is a low-molecular-weight cleavage product that remains in the tissue fluid phase, while the large fragment, C3b, becomes membrane or particle bound. C3b can be randomly positioned on the cell membrane. When it is positioned in close proximity to the C42 complex, it forms the final enzyme of the classic complement pathway, C4b-C2a-C3b, which is capable of splitting C5.

A large fragment of C5, C5b, interacts with C6 to form a stable complex. Attachment of C7 forms a trimolecular complex that combines with C8 and C9 to form a membrane attack unit capable of lysing cells.

The sequential activation–cleavage process of the nine classic complement components—generates several biologically active substances (Table 8.1). The interaction of IgM antibody and certain viruses with C1, C4, C2, and C3, or C1 and optimal amounts of C4 alone, results in neutralization of the virus.

Data exist demonstrating that the smaller split products from C4 and C2, C4a and C2b, can combine to form a highly vasoactive substance that may be important in hereditary angioedema.

Cleavage of C3 produces several biologically reactive materials, of which C3b is the most important. The attachment of C3b to a cell membrane proximal to C4b and C2a generates a C5-cleaving enzyme. The attachment of C3 to a circulating immune complex, bacteria, virus, or other cell allows this target cell to adhere to C3b receptors on human neutrophils, monocytes, B lymphocytes, or erythrocytes (a phenomenon termed *immune adherence*).

The immune adherence phenomenon has been utilized in the laboratory for identification and enumeration of B lymphocytes and monocytes in peripheral blood. C3b attached to antibody-coated erythrocytes will form a rosette around a leukocyte containing C3b receptors. The adherence of immune complexes to cellular C3b receptors markedly facilitates the phagocytosis of such complexes. Anti-

Table 8.1. Biologic Activities of the Complement System

Activity	Components or Cleavage Fragments Involved	Comments
Virus neutralization	Ab[a] C1 C4	Herpes simplex
	Ab C1 C4 C2 C3b	Herpes simplex, Newcastle disease virus Murine leukemic virus
Virus lysis	Ab C1–9	
Vasodilation and increased vascular permeability	C42 kinin C3a C5a	
Immune adherence	C3b C3d C4b	Immune complex + PMN, macrophages, B-lymphocyte receptors, immune complex + macrophages
B-lymphocyte activation	C3b	Split product of C3b → C3c + C3c
PMN[b] leukocytosis	C3e	↓ C3e
Chemotaxis	C3a	Monocytes, neutrophils, eosinophils
	C5a	Monocytes, neutrophils, eosinophils
	C5, C6, C7	Specific for PMN
	Ba	Neutrophils
Macrophage activation	Bb	Alternative pathway activation
Regulation of cell-mediated immunity	C4 and C2 split products	
Antibody-dependent cytotoxicity	C5–9 membrane attack unit	Part of K-lymphocyte surface membrane structure
Schistosome destruction	C3a, C5a	Eosinophils

[a] Ab, antibody.
[b] PMN, polymorphonuclear neutrophil.

body production to T-dependent antigen is also facilitated by the presence of C3b on the antigenic surface.

The cleavage product of C3, C3a, which does not bind to the cell membrane surface, has two biologic functions. First, it is a potent anaphylatoxin—discharging histamine from tissue mast cells and peripheral blood basophils and increasing the permeability and dilatation of small blood vessels. More importantly, C3a is chemotactic for neutrophils, eosinophils, and monocytes. Chemotactic factors are substances that can stimulate the unidirectional migration of inflammatory cells to the site of chemotactic generation. A second anaphylatoxic and chemotactic factor activity also resides in the smallest split product of C5, C5a. C5a is a more potent chemotactic factor for neutrophils, eosinophils, and monocytes than C3a.

A third chemotactic factor, specific for neutrophils but with no effect on eosinophils and monocytes, results from the formation of the trimolecular complex composed of C5b, C6, and C7.

A split product of C3b, C3c, mobilizes neutrophils from bone marrow and is responsible for the leukocytosis noted in many inflammatory diseases.

The five terminal components of the complement system, C5b, C6, C7, C8, and C9, combine on the membrane surface to form a specific, highly sterically organized molecule with the ability to insert into the lipoprotein structure of certain cell membranes, thereby interrupting the osmotic integrity of the cell and promoting lysis. Cell lysis proceeds with the attachment of C5–8 to the membrane. The addition of C9 to the C5–8 complex markedly accelerates the lytic process.

Complement plays a role in biologic activities other than those outlined here. Components of the classic pathway, such as C4 and C2, modulate cell-mediated immune responses. Components of the membrane-attack complex (C5b–9) are produced by K lymphocytes that destroy antibody-coated target cells in antibody-mediated cytotoxicity. Antibody-independent lysis of tumors can result from direct C1 activation by certain tumors and discharge of the entire complement sequence. Similarly, schistosomes can also activate complement in an antibody-independent fashion, releasing the eosinophilic chemotactic factors from C3 and C5 and generating a marked eosinophilic response. Eosinophils rapidly ingest and destroy the schistosomes.

The Alternative Pathway of Complement Activation

The alternative pathway of complement activation (Table 8.2) is an antibody-independent system in which the nonimmune host can generate the biologically

Table 8.2. Alternative Complement Pathway

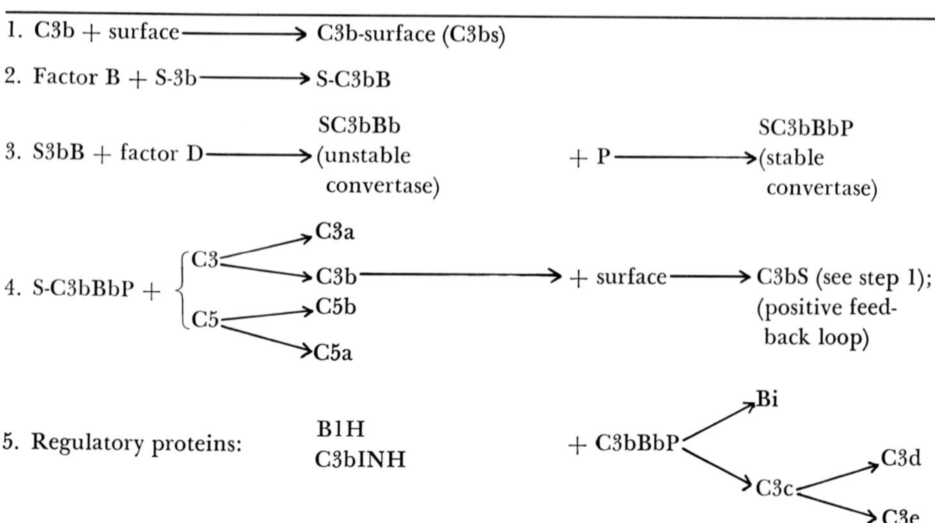

C3b combines with factor B. Factor B is converted into Bb by factor D. The C3Bb complex becomes attached to membrane and can spread more C3 and C5. The addition of properdin stabilizes the C3Bb complex. The C3Bb complex is broken down by the synergistic activity of beta 1H and C3b inactivator.

active molecules derived from the terminal (C3–9) complement components. The alternative pathway enters the cascade at the C3 step and does not involve C1, C4, or C2. It is dependent upon the biochemical characteristics of particles that bind the major cleavage product of C3, C3b. Polysaccharides such as zymosan from yeast, lipopolysaccharides from Gram-negative bacteria, human lymphoblastoid cells, and teichoic acid from pneumococci can activate this pathway.

The C3b complexes with factor B at the particle surface. Factor B is cleaved by activated factor D and generates an alternative pathway C3 convertase, C3bBb. This convertase splits C3 and C5 and initiates the steps involving C5–9. The efficiency of this pathway is dependent upon the resistance of the C3bBb convertase to inactivation by two serum proteins, beta 1H and C3b inactivator (C3bINA). Beta 1H dissociates a piece of factor B from the convertase, and C3bINA digests C3b. These regulatory proteins work synergistically to destroy the C3bBb enzyme. Partial resistance to the inhibitory effects of beta 1H and C3bINA is provided by properdin, another serum protein that attaches to and stabilizes C3bBb. Cleavage of native C3 is (markedly) accelerated and amplified as more C3b is generated. The alternative pathway-activating mechanism thus contains a positive feedback loop, dependent upon generation of C3b and its interaction with factor B and regulated by beta 1H and C3bINA.

Additional biologic activities have been described for the alternative pathway proteins. A factor B split product, Ba, is chemotactic for neutrophils. The major split product of factor B, Bb, can activate macrophages (Table 8.1).

Controlling Enzymes of the Complement Pathway

Multiple different molecules regulate complement activation. A C1q inhibitor (C1Inh) interferes with the attachment of the first complement component to the Fc portion of antibody and blocks activated C1r and C1s̄. A C4-binding inhibitor impairs C4 binding to membrane surfaces. C3bINA cleaves the C3c fragment from C3b (impairing alternate pathway activation of C5–9 by C3bBb, C3 convertase) and also cleaves C4b. The anaphylatoxin activities of C3a and C5a are inhibited by carboxypeptidase-B, which cleaves arginine from the C-terminal ends of these molecules, but maintain their chemotactic activities. An inhibitor of the membrane attack unit is not well characterized but exists. Also, antithrombin III can inhibit the membrane attack unit.

Immune Complexes

Circulating complexes of antigen and antibody can be trapped on endothelial surfaces, where they generate a local inflammatory response and cause focal destruction of the blood vessels and surrounding tissues. Animals that respond to an antigenic stimulus with high-affinity, high-titer antibody production rapidly eliminate the antigen from the circulation and destroy it in the tissues. The production of low-affinity antibody, blockade of the reticuloendothelial system, or the presence of intermediate-sized antigen-antibody complexes predisposes to persistence of the antigen in the circulation. Such complexes are deposited on endothelial surfaces. Deposition is dependent upon the release of certain vasoactive amines by interaction of the complex with platelets, mast cells, or basophils. Activation of complement by the immune complex leads to attachment of the C3b portion to the complex, which interacts with platelet C3b receptors, causing release of serotonin. When the antigenic component of the immune complex interacts with IgE on tissue basophils, platelet-activating factor and other vasoactive amines are released from the basophils.

The vasoactive amines, such as histamine and serotonin, act directly to cause endothelial cell shrinkage and produce a cleft between contiguous cells. The immune complex can be trapped along the exposed basement membrane, or the epithelial cells can attach directly to the C3b of the complexes via specific C3b receptors. Complement is activated locally, chemotactic factors are generated, and a polymorphonuclear leukocyte response ensues. The inflammatory response is amplified by release of lysosomal enzymes from the polymorphonuclear leukocytes—collagenase, elastase, neutral proteases, additional chemotactic factors, factors that release kinins from kininogen, and other tissue-destructive enzymes. Such mechanisms have been proposed for the tissue injury of immune complex diseases such as systemic lupus erythematosus (Chap. 17), rheumatoid arthritis (Chap. 11), vasculitis, and serum sickness (Chap. 18), and for the noncardiac vascular complications of subacute bacterial endocarditis.

Complement and Human Disease: Acquired Complement Abnormalities

Complement is implicated as an important mediator system in several acquired diseases. This conclusion is based on a reduction of serum concentration of complement, the presence of complement fragments resulting from component activation in blood or body fluids, component deposition at sites of tissue injury, and increased metabolism of individual components. Immunologic aspects of systemic lupus erythematosus, rheumatoid arthritis, and vasculitis are discussed elsewhere (Chaps. 11, 17, 18).

Complement abnormalities can be found in the serum of patients with certain infectious diseases. The prodromal phase of hepatitis B virus infection is associated with a serum sickness-like disorder in about 20% of patients. Affected persons may demonstrate urticaria, arthritis or arthralgias, glomerulonephritis, or cutaneous vasculitis several days to weeks before the onset of clinical hepatitis. During this prodromal phase, decreased concentrations of C4 and circulating immune complexes can be detected in the serum. In patients with chronic hepatitis B infections, clinical glomerulonephritis may develop in which complement can be found in the kidney lesions. In such persons, serum complement levels are usually normal. Marked reductions in complement components of C1–5 and factor B have been found in children with dengue hemorrhagic shock.

Complement participates in several hematologic diseases. Patients with disseminated intravascular coagulation (DIC) have reduced serum C3 levels.

Most patients with autoimmune hemolytic anemia have a positive Coombs' test result for erythrocyte membrane C3 and C4, but serum complement levels are normal. Patients with paroxysmal nocturnal hemoglobinuria have platelets, neutrophils, and erythrocytes that are extremely susceptible to lysis by the alternative complement pathway. Some patients with lymphosarcoma exhibit low levels of C1, C4, and C2, decreased levels of the C1 inhibitor, and occasionally autoimmune diseases such as rheumatoid arthritis or systemic lupus erythematosus. Such

is seen in infants with Leiner's syndrome (seborrheic dermatitis, severe intractable diarrhea, recurrent local and systemic infections, marked wasting and dystrophy, and susceptibility to Gram-negative bacterial infections). Patients with deficiencies of C6, C7, and C8 have increased susceptibility to meningococcal or gonococcal infections.

HAGEMAN FACTOR, KALLIKREIN, BRADYKININ SYSTEM

Hageman factor, factor XII of the clotting system, participates in the activation of the coagulation cascade, the fibrinolytic (plasmin) pathway, and in the generation of kallikrein and bradykinin from their precursors in plasma. It is thus a protein central to several enzyme pathways. It is activated upon contact with negatively charged materials such as glass, collagen, basement membrane components, crystals, human sebum, and endotoxin. Activation depends upon the participation of kallikrein and a high-molecular-weight form of kininogen. Once activated, Hageman factor dissociates into several subunits that subsequently participate in clotting, fibrinolysis, or the kallikrein-kinin pathway (Fig. 8.2).

Activated Hageman factor generates a biologically active substance—kallikrein. Kallikrein is a proinflammatory substance that is chemotactic for neutrophils and monocytes. Prekallikrein exists in noncovalent linkage with high-molecular-weight kininogen. Kallikrein, once activated, cleaves the nonapeptide, bradykinin, from the kininogen moiety. Bradykinin is a highly active, smooth muscle contractor that acts directly on blood vessels to increase vascular permeability and stimulate small nerve fibers to produce severe pain.

Activated Hageman factor also interacts with plasminogen activator to release plasmin from plasminogen. Plasmin can split bradykinin from kininogen, convert the precursor form of C1 to C1s, and cleave C3b from C3, and is the major enzyme of the fibrinolytic pathway.

Discharge of the coagulation cascade by activated Hageman factor ultimately leads to the generation of fibrinopeptides A and B. These fibrinopeptides are chemotactic for neutrophils, eosinophils, and monocytes and potentiate the vasoactive properties of bradykinin. Thus, activated Hageman factor is a critical protein in the inflammatory cycle.

There are multiple regulatory proteins for these various Hageman factor pathways, but one, C1, is common to several. C1Inh directly inhibits plasmin, the action of activated C1 on C4 and C2, activated Hageman factor, and kallikrein. The role of the Hageman factor–kallikrein–kinin system in immunologic disease has not been firmly demonstrated.

PROSTAGLANDINS

Prostaglandins (PGs) are 20-carbon, monocarboxylic, unsaturated fatty acids with a single five-membered ring (Fig. 8.3). The PG precursors are released from cell membranes by the action of phospholipase A. The stimulus for release can be trauma, contact with crystals, interaction with immune complexes, or virtually any perturbation of the cell membrane. Arachidonic acid can be converted

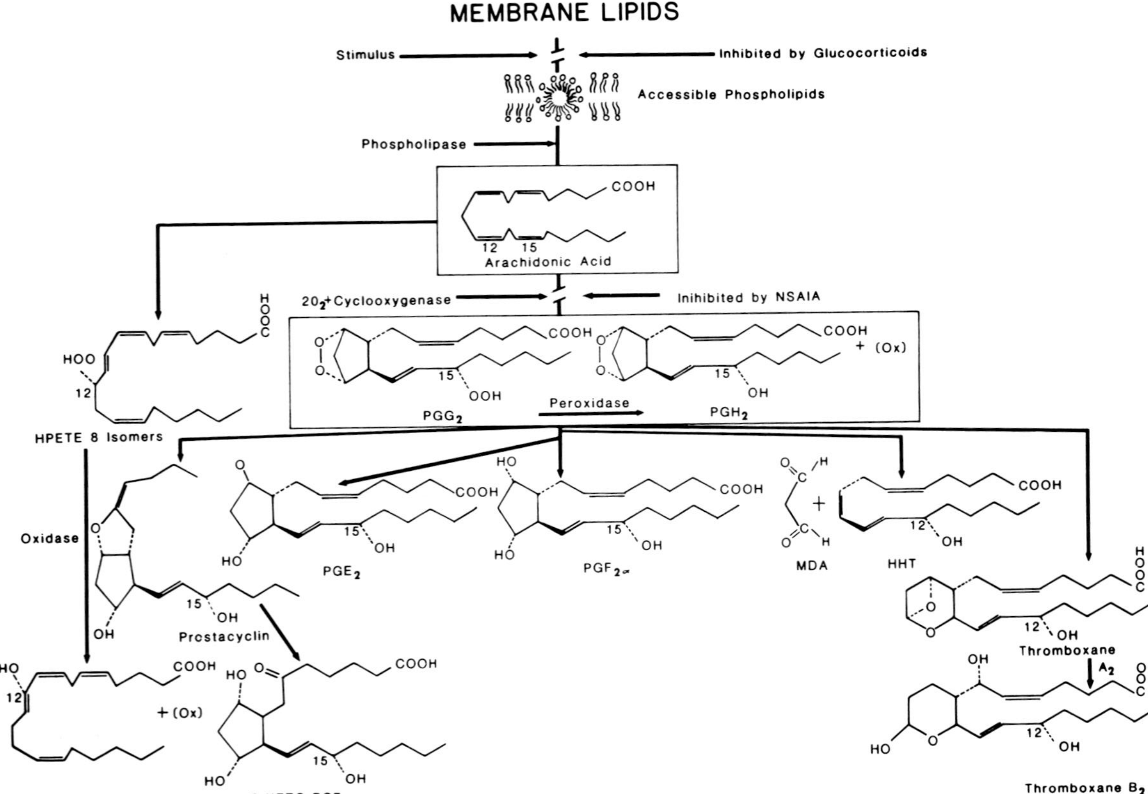

Figure 8.3. Arachidonic acid metabolism. Arachidonic acid is released by perturbation of cell membranes by the action of phospholipase A. It is catabolized by two pathways: by cyclooxygenase and by lipoxygenase. Prostaglandins are generated by the cyclooxygenase pathway, but other substances, such as thromboaxanes and prostaclyclins, may be more important biologically than prostaglandins. NSAIA, nonsteroidal anti-inflammatory agents.

into PG by all mammalian cells except erythrocytes. This conversion progresses by two pathways. The first employs cyclooxygenase and oxygen, which transform arachidonic acid into the cyclic endoperoxides PGG_2 and PGH_2, labile substances having half-lives of less than 5 minutes. The conversion of arachidonic acid to the endoperoxide releases charged oxygen radicals called *super oxides,* which produce an inflammatory reaction in tissues. The endoperoxides are subsequently altered into a group of products with different biologic activities— prostacyclin (which inhibits platelet aggregation and dilates blood vessels), PGE, PGF_{2a}, a C_{17}-hydroxy acid (HHT), and thromboxane.

PGs within the E or F family have been studied most extensively. Their precise role in the inflammatory response is confusing. Their action varies markedly from tissue to tissue in the same host and varies within homologous tissues of different species. Their role in inflammation has been inferred from certain observations. For example, PGE_1 in low doses is chemotactic for neutrophils. PGs are released at the site of an acute inflammatory reaction. During the third phase of carrageenan-induced paw edema in the rat, PG concentrations closely parallel the release of neutrophil lysosomal enzymes. When injected into the skin, PGs induce erythema with a duration longer than that produced by bradykinin, histamine, or mecholyl. PGS enhance, in a synergistic fashion, the pain and edema-forming responses of skin to bradykinin and histamine. PGs also inhibit lymphocyte transformation, DNA, protein, and RNA synthesis. They can also prevent lymphocyte-mediated cytotoxicity. Under certain conditions, they can either enhance or suppress T-cell responses. By increasing intracellular cyclic AMP, they inhibit release of mediators from mast cells. When injected into experimental animals, they can prolong homograft survival. PGE_2 can increase cyclic AMP in macrophages, stimulate macrophage activation, and propagate the release of certain tissue-destroying enzymes such as collagenase.

A second pathway for arachidonic acid metabolism is by conversion by lipoxygenase into HPETE and HETE, which are hydroperoxide and hydroxy fatty acids. HETE has a molecular weight of 340, is chemotactic for eosinophils and neutrophils, and enhances random migration of these cells.

Nonsteroidal anti-inflammatory drugs, such as aspirin, indomethacin, and ibuprofen, inhibit the cyclooxygenase enzyme system, thereby preventing the formation of the stable PGs PGE_{2a} and PGE_2 in addition to inhibiting prostacyclin and thromboxane formation.

The difficulties in assessing the role of the PGs in the inflammatory response are multiple; most studies have focused on the role of PGs of the E and F series in inflammation. However, these substances probably represent only 10% of the endoperoxide breakdown products (resulting from the cyclooxygenase conversion of arachidonic acid). Ninety percent of the biochemical derivatives of this pathway are thromboxanes or prostacyclin—compounds with profound activities on the vasculature and platelets. The role of prostacyclins and thromboxanes on the cellular components of inflammation is unknown.

A second difficulty is that measurement of arachidonic acid metabolites in tissues is impaired because of the very short half-lives of the biologically reactive intermediates and because any laboratory manipulations of tissues can activate the arachidonic acid release system. Further knowledge of arachidonic acid metabolism depends upon more sophisticated technology.

THE MAST CELL, IgE, AND MEDIATORS
OF THE ACUTE INFLAMMATORY RESPONSE

The anaphylaxis phenomenon was first described by Richet and Portier in the study of dogs reacting to the poison of the sea anemone. The use of horse antiserum for the treatment of diphtheria in the 1920s led to the recognition of clinically significant anaphylaxis in humans. Prausnitz and Küstner discovered that allergic persons had a substance in their serum that could passively transfer hypersensitivity, as measured by a wheal and flare skin reaction, from the affected person to a skin site of a normal person. This material subsequently was called *reaginic antibody* (Fig. 8.4).

IgE

In 1967, Ishizaka and others identified reaginic antibody as belonging to a unique class of immunoglobulins—immunoglobulin E (IgE). It is present in normal serum in a concentration of 1–300 ng/ml, is rapidly metabolized, and has a serum half-life of 2–3 days. It has a molecular weight of 190,000 and a configuration similar to that of IgG, composed of two light chains and two heavy (epsilon) chains. Unlike IgG, however, IgE has four instead of three domains in the constant region of the molecule. It is heat labile and has the unique property of fixing to tissues for prolonged periods of time. Its persistence at tissue sites contrasts notably to its short half-life in the serum. IgE attaches to specific receptors on blood basophils or tissue mast cells. Each cell surface contains 40,000 to 100,000 receptors, and the average cell has about 10,000 to 40,000 IgE molecules affixed to it. The Fc portion of the IgE molecule binds the receptors in a reversible, noncovalent fashion. When two IgE molecules on the membrane surface interact with specific antigen, the membrane IgE surface receptors are crosslinked and a series of molecular events is triggered, resulting in the discharge of histamine and multiple other mediators from the mast cell.

IgE levels are increased in the nasal and respiratory secretions of patients with atopic disease. It is apparent that there are T-cell-derived materials that either suppress or enhance IgE antibody synthesis. Normal IgE production is controlled by a damping mechanism. This damping mechanism may be altered transiently by a change in homeostatic balance, such as by exposure to an antigen, irradiation, or viral infection. When IgE-enhancing activity exceeds suppressor activity, large amounts of IgE are produced and the animal develops an allergic diathesis.

Histamine

The tissue mast cell or blood basophil contains large numbers of mediators of the acute allergic reaction. Histamine (beta-imidazolylethylamine) is associated with the granules of these cells. Histamine is also found in the gastrointestinal tract and central nervous system. It is synthesized in the cell from L-histidine by histidine decarboxylase and has multiple proinflammatory functions. It dilates small postcapillary venules by contracting adjacent endothelial cells, thereby increasing the intercellular cleft size to allow transudation of intravascular proteins into adjacent tissue spaces. It causes vasodilatation of these same blood vessels. It contracts bronchial smooth muscle and has direct chemotactic activity for eosinophils. All these proinflammatory effects occur at low concentrations in tissues. In concentrations 10 to 100 times higher, histamine has anti-inflammatory effects. It can inhibit T-lymphocyte cytotoxic activity, macrophage migration inhibitory factor (MIF) production by guinea pig T lymphocytes, and guinea pig delayed hypersensitivity skin responses, and can even inhibit further histamine release from human basophils and the chemotactic responsiveness of human neutrophils. In terms of human pathology, histamine usually manifests a proinflammatory effect. Elevated blood levels are detected in anaphylaxis, during bronchial challenge with antigen, and in several types of urticaria. It can be found in the urine of patients suffering from Gram-negative septicemia.

Slow-reacting Substance of Anaphylaxis (SRS-A)

SRS-A is an acidic sulfate ester with a molecular weight of approximately 400 that causes slow contraction of smooth muscle. It powerfully contracts human bronchiole muscle and produces increased vascular permeability. There is a possibility that it is derived from lipoxygenase metabolism of arachidonic acid in the PG cycle. It is not stored in the mast cell but is synthesized de novo, after antigenic challenge of sensitized cells. It is possible that SRS-A is not produced only by the mast cell, since other inflammatory cells may participate in its production and secretion at the site of the inflammatory stimulus.

Eosinophilic Chemotactic Factor of Anaphylaxis (ECF-A)

ECF-A is a hydrophobic acidic tetrapeptide that is released during the acute anaphylactic reaction. Two tetrapeptides account for ECF-A activity—val-gly-ser-glu and ala-gly-ser-glu. It is preformed and stored in human mast cells. In basophils, it appears to be generated rapidly after cell stimulation. It also can attract neutrophils but is relatively selective for eosinophils. Additional, slightly larger oligopeptides with eosinophilic chemotactic activity are also present in mast cell granules.

Neutrophil Chemotactic Factor (NCF)

NCF is a substance with a molecular weight of about 750,000. At neutral pH, it is chemotactic for neutrophils. It is preformed in mast cells and released upon antigenic challenge.

Platelet-Activating Factor (PAF)

PAF is a lipid-like substance with a molecular weight of 300 to 500. It induces platelet aggregation in the presence of fibrinogen and triggers the release of serotonin and other amines from platelets. It is not stored in mast cells but is generated after release of other mediators from these cells.

HETE (12-1-hydroxy-5,8,10,14-Eicosatetraenoic Acid)

HETE is a chemotactic factor derived from the lipoxygenase pathway of arachidonic acid metabolism. It attracts both neutrophils and eosinophils and stimulates random motion of these cells.

Serotonin (5-hydroxytryptamine)

Serotonin is present in the mast cells of several animal species but is absent from human mast cells. In humans, it is stored in platelets. Serotonin causes smooth muscle contraction and produces vasodilatation and increased vascular permeability of small venules. Its precise role in the acute inflammatory response is unknown.

Heparin and Other Mast Cell Substances

Heparin is a macromolecular acidic proteoglycan that has a molecular weight of about 750,000 and forms an integral part of the granule structure. It imparts a metachromatic appearance to the mast cell granule and is released by IgE-mediated mechanisms upon antigenic challenge. Its function in acute inflammation is unknown.

Other Enzymes

Other enzymes are released from mast cells. A chymotrypsin-like enzyme, chymase, with a molecular weight of 25,000, is one. Its activity is not certain, but it may participate in fibrinolysis, plasminogen activation, kinin inactivation, and of degradation of protein portions of cartilage and other connective tissue. Arylsulfatase has a molecular weight of 115,000, is preformed in granules, and is capable of inactivating SRS-A.

Biochemical Mechanism of Mediator Release from Mast Cells and Basophils

The release mechanism of mast cell mediators after immunologic challenge is poorly understood. The combination of bivalent or multivalent antigens with membrane IgE bridges adjacent Fc receptors within the membrane structure. This event is the signal for the activation of intracellular enzymatic steps that lead to microtubule organization, granule discharge, and secretion of mediators from the cell. The initial step seems to be the influx of calcium ions followed by the activation of a precursor enzyme, poorly defined, that is inhibitable by diisopropyl fluorophosphate. A second, energy-requiring, calcium-dependent event proceeds, cyclic AMP levels fall, microtubule assembly occurs, and the mediators are released into the extracellular fluid.

Regulation of Mediator Release

Mediator release is regulated by substances arising directly from the mast cell, from materials arising from other cells, or by drugs. Agents such as the beta-adrenergic drugs epinephrine or isoproterenol increase intracellular cyclic AMP by stimulation of adenyl cyclase. Adenyl cyclase stimulation and increased cyclic AMP concentrations result from the interaction of released histamine with H2 receptors or by attachment of E-PGs to receptors distinct from the beta-adrenergic receptors. Other substances such as theophylline, which inhibit cyclic AMP catabolism by phosphodiesterase, also elevate cyclic AMP levels.

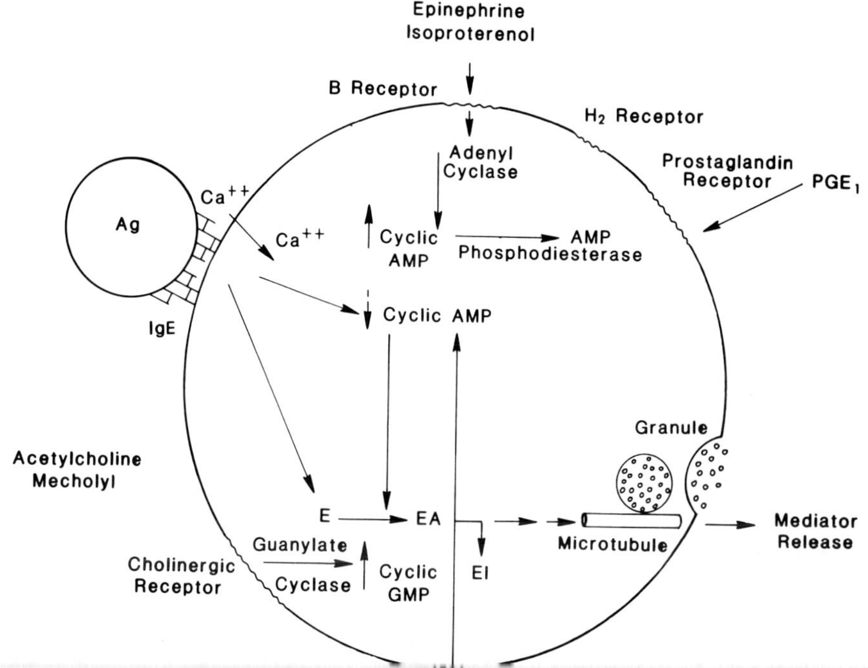

Figure 8.4. Release of mediators from mast cells. The interaction of IgE with antigen bridges IgE Fc receptors within the membrane substance. This process causes an influx of calcium and activation of a poorly understood enzyme (E) system dependent upon the glycolytic pathway. The end results of activation are the assembly of microtubules and the secretion of granules and inflammatory mediators from the cell. Modulation of this process is effected by cyclic AMP. Increased intracellular cyclic AMP by synthesis mediated by adenyl cyclase or by prevention of catabolism by phosphodiesterase will inhibit mediator secretion. Increased cyclic GMP enhances mediator secretion, as does stimulation of the cell membrane with alpha-adrenergic agents. EA, activated enzyme; EI, inactivated enzyme.

Stimulation of guanylate cyclase by the reaction of a cholinergic receptor with agents such as acetylcholine will increase cyclic GMP within the cell. This increased cyclic GMP enhances mediator release. Stimulation of alpha-adrenergic receptors can, under special circumstances, also enhance the release of mediators from the mast cell. Once released, mediators are inactivated by products of other cells. The eosinophil is particularly effective in this regard. It secretes histaminase, arylsulfatase-B, and phospholipase-D, which biodegrade histamine, SRS-A, and PAF, respectively.

Role of the Immediate Hypersensitivity Reaction in Other Phases of Inflammation

Immediate-type hypersensitivity occurs within minutes after antigenic challenge. It may function to propagate the intermediate (4–6 hour) and delayed hypersensitivity reactions. For instance, chemotactic factors, NCF, and HETE, can attract polymorphonuclear leukocytes into the reaction milieu. Vasoactive substances such as histamine and serotonin can incite local vasodilatation and promote increased vascular permeability. This heightened permeability will increase local blood flow and allow an outpouring of complement and antibodies into the reaction site. Local generation of chemotactic factors from complement can attract additional neutrophils and mononuclear cells so that the inflammatory process is further prolonged.

Thus the mast cell phase of inflammation, although usually studied in terms of a noxious (allergic) reaction, is probably in reality the initial phase of host defense to pathologic challenge. It has the potential of triggering and promulgating the subsequent cellular phases of inflammation.

In summary, the inflammatory process recruits several different enzymatic pathways. Each of these pathways can proceed independently of one another, but they also can share certain functional interrelationships, thereby providing the host with multiple mechanisms of protection against alien substances.

BIBLIOGRAPHY

Austen KF: Structure and function of chemical mediators derived after the activation of mast cells, in Lichtenstein LM, Austen KF (eds): *Asthma: Physiology, Immunopharmacology and Treatment, Second International Symposium*. New York, Academic Press, Inc, 1977.

Bennich H, Ishizaka K, Ishizaka T, et al. A comparative antigenic study of E-globulin and myeloma-IgND. *J Immunol* 102:826, 1969.

Biological Aspects of the Acute Allergic Reactions. New York, Plenum Publishing Corp, 1976.

Fearon DT: Activation of the alternative complement pathway by Escherichia coli: Resistance of bound C3b to inactivation by C3bINA and β1H. *J Immunol* 120:1772, 1978.

Fearon DT, Daha MR, Strom TB, et al: Pathways of complement activation in membranoproliferative glomerulonephritis and allograft rejection. *Transplant Proc* 9:729, 1977.

Fearon DT, Austen KF: Activation of the alternative complement pathway due to resistance of zymosan bound amplification convertase to endogenous regulatory mechanisms. *Proc Natl Acad Sci USA* 74:1683, 1977.

Gewurz H, Shin HS, Mergenhagen SE: Interactions of the complement system with endotoxic lipopolysaccharide: Consumption of each of the six terminal complement components. *J Exp Med* 128:1049, 1968.

Goetzl EJ: Mast cell-mediated reactions of host defense and tissue injury: The regulatory role of eosinophil polymorphonuclear leukocytes. *Inflammation* 2:239–256, 1977.

Ishizaka K: Cellular events in the IgE antibody response. *Adv Immunol* 23:1, 1976.

Kaplan AP: Urticaria and angioedema, in Middleton Jr E, Reed CE, Ellis, EF (eds): *Allergy: Principles and Practice*. St Louis, CV Mosby Co, 1978.

Katz DH, Bargatze RF, Bogowitz CA, et al: Regulation of IgE antibody production by serum molecules, I.V. Complete Freund's adjuvant induces both enhancing and suppressive activities detectable in the serum of low and high responder mice. *J Immunol* 122:2184–2190, 1979.

Marcus RL, Shin HS, Mayer MM: An alternate complement pathway: C3 cleaving activity, not due to C4, 2a on endotoxic lipopolysaccharide after treatment with guinea pig serum; relation to properdin. *Proc Natl Acad Sci USA* 68:1351, 1971.

Muller Eberhard HJ: Complement abnormalities in human disease. *Hosp Pract* 65–76, 1978.

Weissmann G: The inflammatory process and tissue injury: *Curr Con Wel Trends Rheumatol* 1:6–7, 1979.

9

The Inflammatory Response

Jacques R. Caldwell

The final outcome of an immune reaction or the mammalian response to any noxious encounter is the generation of an inflammatory response. If the host survives, the noxious agent, such as a bacterial or virus pathogen, is either eradicated or at least isolated from the host's internal milieu. In most instances, inflammation results in some damage to healthy tissue. Normally, this is of little biologic consequence unless the site of inflammation is a critical area, such as the eye, brain, or heart valve. Certain genetic defects, such as the absence of a critical complement component or an immunoglobulin class, render the host more susceptible to development of immunologic disease.

Inherited defects or deficiencies of one or two inflammatory pathway proteins are rarely fatal to the host since the inflammatory mechanism of the affected pathway can usually be assumed by another pathway.

INTERACTIONS AMONG INFLAMMATORY PATHWAYS

Some of the interstices among the inflammatory pathways are summarized in Tables 9.1 and 9.2. The Hageman factor–kallikrein–bradykinin pathway interfaces with complement in two ways. Kallikrein interacts directly to activate C1. Plasmin, which is derived from the enzymatic cleavage of plasminogen by kallikrein, also activates C1. The Hageman factor–kallikrein–bradykinin pathway also initiates the clotting cascade by the action of Hageman factor (factor XII) on factor XI. Plasmin disrupts the end product of the clotting system—the fibrin clot—and releases fibrinopeptides A and B, which are chemotactic and potentiate bradykinin activity. Complement can activate the mast cell system via the generation of C3a and C5a, anaphylatoxins that release mast cell mediators. The prostaglandins interact with bradykinins and promote pain (Chap. 8).

MECHANISMS OF IMMUNOLOGIC TISSUE INJURY

The clinical immunologist is concerned more with the control of excess and chronic inflammation than with deficiencies of inflammatory enzymes. "Immune diseases" such as the allergic and autoimmune diseases are manifested as chronic

Table 9.1. Summary of the Immune Inflammatory Response

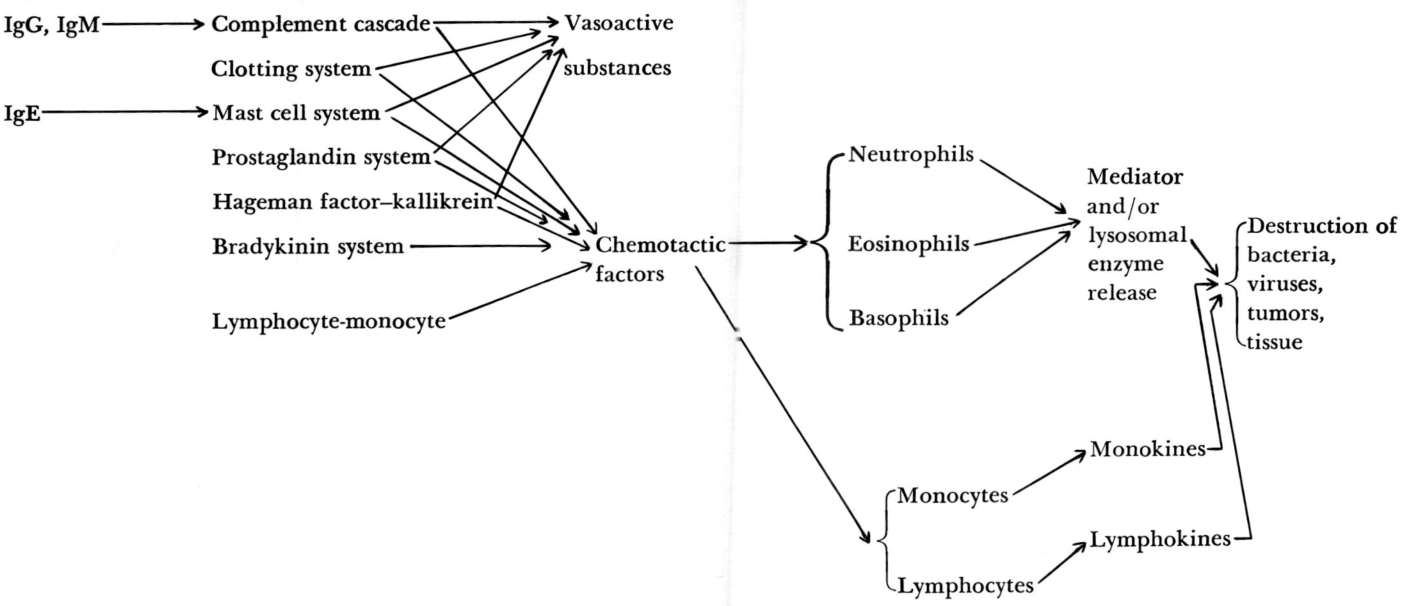

Table 9.2. Interactions among the Inflammatory Pathways

Hageman factor–kallikrein–bradykinin
  With complement
    Plasmin activates C1
    Kallikrein enhances enzymatic potency of C1
  With clotting
    Via factor XII and factor XI
    Bradykinin's activity potentiated by fibrinopeptides
    Plasmin lyses fibrin clot and releases fibrinopeptides
Complement
  With mast cells
    Via anaphylatoxic activity of C3a and C5a
  With Hageman factor–kallikrein–bradykinin
    Via plasmin and kallikrein
  With lymphocytes—enhance and inhibit various functions
Mast cells
  With complement via C3a and C5a
Prostaglandins
  With bradykinin → pain

---

inflammatory states in one or more organ systems and frequently result in an insidious destructive process of the affected tissues.

Pathologic immune responses have been divided into four types. Type I responses are produced by the interaction of IgE or other homocytotropic antibodies on the surface of the mast cells with antigen that stimulates release of mast cell inflammatory mediators. Urticaria (hives), allergic rhinitis, asthma, and anaphylactic shock are clinical examples of type I responses.

Type II reactions are caused by cytotoxic, complement-activating antibodies reacting with components of the host's own tissues. Goodpasture's syndrome, myasthenia gravis, rheumatic fever, and pemphigus vulgaris reflect type II hypersensitivity.

Type III reactions are characterized by the presence of circulating immune (i.e., antigen-antibody) complexes. Such complexes are deposited on endothelial surfaces of any tissue, elicit an inflammatory response (usually by activation of the complement system), and attract inflammatory cells to the site. Disgorgement of tissue-disruptive enzymes by phagocytic cells accompanies ingestion of the immune complexes and promotes tissue destruction. Type III reactions are operative in systemic lupus erythematosus, rheumatoid arthritis, the vasculitic lesions of subacute bacterial endocarditis, and serum sickness.

Type IV reactions are mediated by sensitized lymphocytes and macrophages—either by a direct cell-to-cell effect or by release of lymphokines and monokines. The tissue injury seen in tuberculosis, leprosy, contact dermatitis, polydermatomyositis, or graft rejection is the result of type IV reactions.

This division of hypersensitivity reactions into four types may be conceptually helpful but is highly artificial biologically. In many immune diseases, one type of response may evolve into another type. For instance, some IgE-mediated (type I) skin reactions may be temporally followed by local type III and later type IV reactions. The pathologic phenomena that accompany some illnesses may represent several hypersensitivity responses. For example, in certain lymphomas, anaphylaxis or hives results from mast cell-fixed IgE interactions with tumor antigen, vasculitic lesions arise from circulating tumor antigen-IgG complexes, and skin eruptions occur that are characterized by type IV (cell-mediated) responses.

AUTOIMMUNITY

A wealth of knowledge concerning the mechanisms of ·the immune response and inflammatory processes has been derived from study of the autoimmune diseases. The concept of autoimmunity has undergone dramatic alterations during the past century and particularly during the past decade. Paul Ehrlich considered autoimmunity as a biologic absurdity—as a "horror autotoxicus." Burnet, when presenting his clonal selection theory in 1959, proposed that autoantibodies were normally prohibited by the destruction of clones capable of producing antibodies reactive with self-antigens during early ontogenetic development. Burnet recognized the presence of autoantibodies in certain instances and explained them as products derived from renegade cells that escaped elimination during fetal development of the immune system.

During the 1950s and 1960s, autoantibodies were discovered in a plethora of diseases, such as systemic lupus erythematosus, rheumatoid arthritis, scleroderma, Sjögren's syndrome, myasthenia gravis, thyroiditis, adrenalitis, chronic liver disease, and many others. The role of autoantibodies in the pathogenesis of these diseases was vigorously researched, and the hypothesis that autoimmune diseases represent aberrant immune hypersensitivity states became accepted.

The 1970s witnessed the retreat of these previous theories of autoimmunity. Some types of autoimmune illness were associated with immune deficiency states. These included the appearance of rheumatoid arthritis and dermatomyositis in people with agammaglobulinemia; increased incidence of systemic lupus erythematosus in patients with deficiencies of C1r, C1s, C4, C2, and C5; and cellular immune defects in patients who coincidentally have an autoimmune disease and a lymphoma. These observations cast doubt on the concept of autoimmune disease as simply a reflection of an immune hypersensitivity state.

Furthermore, autoantibodies were discovered frequently in many "normal" people and in patients with no evidence of autoimmune disease. For example, small amounts of antinuclear antibody or rheumatoid factor are detected in many healthy persons with certain infections, such as subacute bacterial endocarditis, brucellosis, or osteomyelitis, up to 50% of whom develop rheumatoid factor; antinuclear antibodies appear in many persons treated with hydralazine, procainamide, or anticonvulsants; and cold agglutinins reactive with the I antigen of autologous erythrocytes appear after mycoplasma infections. Not all such persons develop autoimmune disease.

More recently, autoimmunity has become recognized as a normal homeostatic property of the immune response. Peripheral blood lymphocytes express surface receptors for multiple autologous antigens. The induction of the normal immune response by antigen depends upon the interaction of two cell types—T and B cells. The interacting cells must share two common attributes—a receptor for the antigen and surface determinants derived from the major histocompatibility complex through which they can communicate (Chap. 6).

The host defense against viruses and tumors uses autoimmune reactivity. Certain virus infections are eradicated by the destruction of infected cells by cytotoxic T lymphocytes that possess identical major histocompatibility complex surface markers with virus-infected target cells. Certain lymphoblastic tumors are lysed by the recognition and interaction of a cytotoxic lymphocyte with shared antigenic determinants on the tumor cell.

The normal humoral immune response is partially controlled by the production of anti-idiotypic antibodies that react with the antigen-combining site of antibody molecules resident on cell surfaces and in tissue fluids (Chap. 6).

This autoimmunity is not the horror autotoxicus of Ehrlich or the consequence of renegade clones of cells. It is a normal biologic process. Autoimmune disease in which an exuberant, uncontrolled expression of autoimmunity appears is abnormal.

Studies in mice support the theory that autoimmune disease arises from defects in immune regulation. New Zealand black/white F_1 hybrid mice develop a high incidence of systemic lupus erythematosus and demonstrate marked immunoregulatory defects (Chap. 17). MRL mice develop a lupus-like disease often accompanied by a lymphoproliferative disorder. The antibody-forming cells of such mice fail to respond to the negative feedback signals of suppressor T cells. Moth-eaten (ME) mice express hyperimmunoglobulinemia and immune complex glomerulonephritis. These animals demonstrate two defects—an increased number of T helper cells and a dearth of T suppressor cells.

The importance of immune regulatory defects in the expression of murine autoimmune disease can be seen by depleting normal mice of all T cells and dividing these mice into two groups. The first group is immunologically reconstituted by injection of a mixture of all types of T cells obtained from normal untreated syngeneic mice. This group subsequently lives free of autoimmune disease. The second group receives only T helper cells from syngeneic untreated mice. (T suppressor cells are lacking.) This second group develops an autoimmune disease characterized by the appearance of autoantibodies against erythrocytes, thymocytes, and thyroglobulin and the glomerular deposition of immune complexes.

IMMUNE DEFICIENCY

The relationship between human autoimmune disease and immune deficiency states or the hypothesized viral infection remains conceptually unclear. We can speculate that immunoglobulin deficiency states are accompanied by an absence of anti-idiotypic antibodies. Since anti-idiotypic antibodies provide a negative feedback control for antibody production, their absence leads to unbridled production of autoantibodies.

The relationship between a complement component deficiency (particularly deficiences of Clr, Cls, and C4) and a predisposition to autoimmune disease has been attributed to the importance of the early-reacting complement components in the host defense against viruses. The absence of one of these components may permit the persistence of virus infection. Since virus infections can profoundly

10

Rheumatoid Arthritis: Clinical Aspects

Richard S. Panush

This chapter will discuss clinical features, laboratory findings, radiologic changes, pathologic abnormalities, and management of rheumatoid arthritis. Immunologic aspects of disease will be presented in Chapter 11.

CLINICAL FEATURES

Rheumatoid arthritis may represent a single disease entity or a syndrome that reflects similar entities with etiologic and pathogenetic differences. Since there is no single feature reliably pathognomonic of rheumatoid arthritis, diagnostic criteria have been suggested by the American Rheumatism Association (Table 10.1). Criteria include (1) pain on motion or tenderness in at least one joint, (2) swelling in at least one joint, (3) swelling in at least one other joint, (4) symmetric swelling for at least 6 weeks, (5) morning stiffness, (6) subcutaneous nodules, (7) positive rheumatoid factors (RF) test, (8) poor synovial fluid mucin clot formation, (9) radiologic abnormalities, and typical pathologic changes in (10) synovium or (11) subcutaneous nodules. There should be no features of other rheumatic diseases. A diagnosis of "classic" rheumatoid arthritis is made when at least seven criteria are fulfilled. "Definite" rheumatoid arthritis requires five and "probable" rheumatoid arthritis three criteria. Possible rheumatoid arthritis can be considered when any two of the following have been present for at least 3 weeks: (1) morning stiffness, (2) pain on motion or tenderness, (3) joint swelling, (4) subcutaneous nodules, (5) increased erythrocyte sedimentation rate (ESR) or C-reactive protein, or (6) iritis. These criteria are most useful in standardizing clinical studies. They are also helpful in patient evaluation and should be reviewed when establishing a diagnosis of rheumatoid arthritis.

PREVALENCE

Rheumatoid arthritis afflicts nearly 2%–3% of the population when estimated by population criteria. When more stringent criteria are used, the prevalence is

Table 10.1. American Rheumatism Association Criteria for the Diagnosis of Rheumatoid Arthritis

Pain on motion or tenderness in one joint
Swelling in one joint for 6 weeks
Swelling in one other joint
Symmetric swelling
Morning stiffness exceeding 1 hour
Positive rheumatoid factors test
Subcutaneous nodules
Poor synovial fluid mucin clot formation
Typical radiologic changes
Characteristic synovial membrane histology
Characteristic nodule histology

closer to 1%. Approximately two to three times more women than men acquire this illness.

COURSE

Rheumatoid arthritis occurs in all races and at all ages, with peak incidence in the fourth and fifth decades. Its natural history is variable; this fact may reflect, in part, difficulties in defining rheumatoid arthritis in population studies. Estimates are that 35% of patients have a monocyclic course with lasting remission occurring within 2 years of onset, 50% of patients have progressive polycyclic disease with superimposed exacerbations, and another 15% of patients have progressive unremitting disease. Most patients retain fair to good functional capacity. About 25% are restricted in activities, and fewer than 10% are significantly disabled. A poorer prognosis is associated with older age, insidious onset, early rapid progression, extra-articular disease, positive RF test, hypocomplementemia, circulating cryoglobulins or immune complexes, and abnormal cell-mediated immune function.

CLINICAL MANIFESTATIONS

Articular

The most prominent clinical manifestation is symmetric polyarthritis. Occasionally, however, the initial appearance may be atypic with oligoarticular, monoarticular, or anarticular rheumatoid disease. The joints most commonly affected are the proximal interphalangeals (PIP), metacarpophalangeals (MCP), wrists, elbows, shoulders, knees, spine, hips, ankles, and small joints of the feet. Inflammatory synovitis occurs with erythema, pain, stiffness, and swelling. Less often involved, and less often recognized, may be the temporomandibular, sternoclavicular, acromioclavicular, and cricoarytenoid joints.

It is beyond the scope of this chapter to review all the ways that individual areas may be involved by the rheumatoid process. However, certain of the more commonly encountered instances bear emphasis. In the hand, swan neck and boutonniere deformities of PIP and MCP joints may be seen, in addition to the fusiform appearance of digits caused by PIP swelling. Swan neck deformities reflect hyperextension at PIPs and flexion at distal interphalangeal joints (DIPs); boutonniere deformities reflect hyperextension at DIPs and flexion at PIPs. Volar wrist tenosynovitis may accompany carpal tunnel syndrome. Dorsal wrist tenosynovitis frequently occurs. At the elbow, olecranon bursitis often accompanies and may be confused with synovitis. Uncommonly, elbow synovium herniates with ulnar or interosseous nerve entrapment. Synovial cysts may also be found at the shoulder. Cricoarytenoid arthritis may cause morning hoarseness or, rarely, laryngeal obstruction.

Cervical spine involvement is frequent (approximately 15%–50%) but is not always recognized. Involvement of C1–2 at the atlantoaxial joints is also common (approximately 25%–70%) and potentially hazardous. Symptoms of this condition may be neuralgias, headaches, occipital pain, nerve compression, vertebral artery insufficiency, anterior spinal artery embarrassment, medullary compression and respiratory depression and may lead to sudden death. The remainder of the spine and even sacroiliac joints may be affected by rheumatoid arthritis, but this condition is not usually clinically important.

Rheumatoid arthritis at the hip may be associated with osteoporotic collapse or aseptic necrosis and secondary degenerative changes. The knees also may exhibit superimposed degenerative changes. Popliteal cysts, with or without dissection or rupture, occur. Edema over inflamed ankles may be seen; it is important to realize that this condition occurs with rheumatoid arthritis and need not be the result of circulatory, renal, metabolic, or other disorders. Subluxation and "cock-up" deformities are frequent at the metatarsophalangeal joints.

Extra-articular

Rheumatoid arthritis is a systemic disease. Indeed, *rheumatoid disease* may be a more appropriate term than *rheumatoid arthritis*. Although common, extra-articular manifestations of rheumatoid disease are often subtle and less dramatic than those of other systemic rheumatic diseases (juvenile rheumatoid arthritis, systemic lupus erythematosus (SLE), vasculitis, or scleroderma). Many patients will manifest symptoms of low-grade fever, weight loss, malaise, fatigue, anorexia, and tachycardia. Such symptoms usually require a number of other systemic diseases to be considered in the differential diagnosis of rheumatoid arthritis; when the other diseases are excluded, it must be appreciated that constitutional symptoms certainly can accompany articular disease (Table 10.2).

Cutaneous involvement usually reflects subcutaneous nodules or manifestations of vasculitis. Rheumatoid nodules are generally firm, nontender, and appear in subcutaneous tissues of approximately one-fourth to one-third of patients. These nodules are most commonly located over extensor surfaces of joints, particularly the elbow, but may occur virtually anywhere in the body. It has usually been thought that subcutaneous nodules are associated with severe disease, although this conclusion has recently been questioned. Occasionally, linear subcutaneous bands rather than nodules may be seen. Cutaneous rashes, livido reticularis, splinter hemorrhages, gangrene, purpura, capillary changes, digital vasculitis (approxi-

Table 10.2. Extra-Articular Manifestations of Rheumatoid Arthritis

Constitutional	Fever, weight loss, malaise, fatigue, anorexia, tachycardia
Skin	Vasculitis, nodules, linear subcutaneous bands, rash, livido reticularis
Neurologic	Myasthenia, neuropathy, vasculitis, central nervous system involvement
Musculoskeletal	Bursitis, tendinitis, entrapment syndromes, myositis
Pulmonary	Pleuritis, pleural effusion, granulomata, interstitial fibrosis, Caplan's syndrome
Cardiac	Granulomata, pericarditis, myocarditis, aortic regurgitation, mitral valve abnormalities
Renal	Amyloidosis, interstitial nephritis (Sjögren's syndrome), renal tubular acidosis (Sjögren's syndrome), analgesic nephropathy, glomerulitis (vasculitis), membranous nephropathy
Gastrointestinal	Xerostomia, amyloidosis, vasculitis, peptic ulceration, bleeding, abnormalities of liver function
Hematologic	Anemia, eosinophilia, Felty's syndrome, hyperviscosity syndrome, adenopathy, malignancy
Endocrinologic	Thyroiditis
Vascular	Hyperviscosity syndrome, Raynaud's phenomenon, vasculitis, gangrene
Other	Keratoconjunctivitis sicca, scleritis, choroiditis

mately 15%), and skin ulcerations (approximately 15%) may be present as manifestations of vasculitis.

The nervous system may also be involved. Central nervous system vasculitis has been documented in rare instances. Intracranial granulomata have also occurred. Peripheral neuropathy, "stocking-glove," or mononeuritis multiplex often accompany rheumatoid vasculitis. Myasthenia too has been reported with rheumatoid arthritis.

Besides the articular abnormalities described previously, bursitis, tendinitis, and nerve entrapment syndromes, such as carpal tunnel syndrome, often coexist with rheumatoid arthritis. Muscle weakness or myopathy is not uncommon but is usually obscured by synovitis.

Pulmonary abnormalities may prevail in nearly half of patients with rheumatoid arthritis. Interstitial fibrosis has been reported in approximately 20%. However, as many as 40% may exhibit subtle abnormalities of pulmonary diffusion in the absence of symptoms or radiologic findings. Pleurisy has been reported in approximately 20% of patients, and pleural effusion occurs in about 3%. Rheumatoid pleural effusions occasionally contain cholesterol crystals. More typically, they contain rheumatoid arthritis cells (or *ragocytes*—large neutrophils that have ingested immune complexes represented as coarse cytoplasmic granules), hypocomplementemia, and low glucose. Rheumatoid pneumoconiosis (Caplan's syndrome—multiple pulmonary nodules in coal miners with rheumatoid arthritis) has been described. Rheumatoid nodules or granulomata may be found within the lung parenchyma.

Similarly, nodules or granulomata may form in the heart—on the valves or myocardium. Asymptomatic pericarditis or effusions have been detected in approximately one-half of patients. Echocardiography may detect mitral valve abnormalities in 10%–30% of patients. Occasionally, patients have been described with myocarditis or coronary arteritis. Aortic regurgitation in rheumatoid arthritis has also been described.

Renal disease is not usually associated with uncomplicated rheumatoid arthritis. It is usually thought to be secondary to amyloidosis, interstitial nephritis, or the renal tubular acidosis of Sjögren's syndrome, analgesic nephropathy, glomerulitis secondary to another cause (SLE, vasculitis, scleroderma), membranous nephropathy secondary to gold therapy, or the effects of nonsteroidal antiinflammatory agents on renal perfusion and function. It has recently been suggested that a few patients with rheumatoid arthritis may have membranous nephropathy.

Uncomplicated rheumatoid arthritis does not commonly involve the gastrointestinal tract. Many patients may develop xerostomia as part of Sjögren's syndrome. Occasional patients may have esophageal motility abnormalities. Peptic ulceration and gastrointestinal bleeding are often encountered but are difficult to separate from drug-related problems. Abnormalities of liver function are frequent, but these too may reflect a combination of disease- and drug-associated abnormalities. Complications of rheumatoid arthritis, such as amyloidosis and vasculitis, may involve the gastrointestinal tract.

Anemia, eosinophilia, leukopenia, leukocytosis, and thrombocytosis may all prevail among patients with rheumatoid arthritis. Approximately 12% of patients will have lymphadenopathy. Hyperviscosity syndrome, secondary to circulating intermediate-sized immune complexes, has been described. Interestingly, the overall incidence of malignancies in patients with rheumatoid arthritis was somewhat less than that of a control population. However, plasma cell dyscrasias and lymphoreticular malignancies have been associated with rheumatoid arthritis. The combination of splenomegaly, neutropenia, and rheumatoid arthritis is termed *Felty's syndrome.* Approximately 5% of patients with rheumatoid arthritis have splenomegaly without granulocytopenia. Patients with Felty's syndrome may also have anemia and thrombocytopenia and are susceptible to pyogenic infection and leg ulcerations. Lithium carbonate administration or splenectomy may benefit selected patients with Felty's syndrome.

Vasculitis may complicate rheumatoid arthritis in approximately 1%–2% of patients. This condition may be manifested by peripheral neuropathy (mononeuritis multiplex, 10%–24% of patients), necrotic skin ulcers, digital gangrene, nail bed vascular changes, or arteritis with other symptoms (depending on the vascular beds and viscera involved) and is often associated with extra-articular symptoms. Immune complexes in the serum and deposits in the skin and other tissues can be detected. An association of cutaneous necrotizing venulitis with HL-A antigens A11 and Bw35 has been described. In addition, cryoglobulinemia has been described in most patients with rheumatoid vasculitis.

Other manifestations associated with rheumatoid arthritis include Raynaud's phenomenon, scleritis, episcleritis (approximately 9% of patients), keratoconjunctivitis sicca, thyroiditis, susceptibility to infections (particularly intra-articular), choroiditis, and amyloidosis (approximately 20% of patients).

LABORATORY FINDINGS

Anemia is common among rheumatoid arthritis patients (Table 10.3) and is usually normocytic, hypochromic, or normochromic. Its cause is usually multifactorial and reflects blood loss, iron loss, or deposition in inflamed tissues, impaired iron use, mild hemolysis, decreased red cell survival, and possibly low erythropoetin levels, low colony-stimulating factor levels, and low folate levels. Leukocytosis occurs in some patients and leukopenia in others. Both can be secondary to drugs, and the latter is associated with Felty's syndrome. Neutropenia can also occur with Felty's syndrome. Possible mechanisms are reticuloendothelial system sequestration and destruction, impaired production, or antibody-mediated removal of neutrophils. Eosinophilia is often associated with severe rheumatoid arthritis with extra-articular manifestations as well as drug hypersensitivities.

The ESR is a reliable indicator of inflammation and is elevated in patients with active disease. Serum proteins may be abnormal, but patterns are not specific. Alpha-2 globulin, fibrinogen, complement, and IgA may rarely be absent and albumin or IgD decreased. Cryoglobulins may be found in up to one-fourth of patients and in all or most with rheumatoid vasculitis. Rheumatoid factors are present in 60%–95% of patients (see Table 11.1). Biologic false-positive serologic test results occur in fewer than 10%. Positive lupus erythematosus (LE) cell reactions occur in fewer han 20%–30% of patients, and antinuclear antibody tests (ANA) are positive in 20%–40% and are usually in a low-titered homogeneous pattern. Antibodies to double-stranded DNA are rarely detected.

Abnormalities of liver function occur, and their relationship to disease or therapy in adult rheumatoid arthritis is not entirely clear. Renal function is usually

Table 10.3. Laboratory Abnormalities in Patients with
Rheumatoid Arthritis

Nonspecific
    Anemia
    Leukocytosis/leukopenia
    Granulocytopenia
    Eosinophilia
    Increased erythrocyte sedimentation rate
    Increased alpha-2-globulin
    Increased fibrinogen
Immunologic
    Positive rheumatoid factors test (60%–95%)
    Serum hypercomplementemia (31%) or
        hypocomplementemia (4%)
    Reduced synovial fluid complement
    Increased serum IgG, IgA, and IgM
    Absent serum IgA (< 1%–2%)
    Biologic false-positive serologic test result for syphilis (< 10%)
    Positive lupus erythematosus cell test result (< 30%)
    Positive antinuclear antibodies test result (20%–40%)
    Depressed cutaneous delayed-type hypersensitivity
    Impaired in vitro lymphocyte responsiveness

normal. Increases or decreases of serum uric acid values occur—and may confuse the diagnosis—but are usually the result of medication affecting urate metabolism. Serum histidine values are low. Levels of various trace metals have been abnormal, but their relationship to disease pathogenesis and diagnosis is uncertain.

Synovial fluid from patients with rheumatoid arthritis is characteristically inflammatory and noninfectious in type. The fluid is yellow to green and cloudy; it has poor viscosity and a poor mucin clot test and contains 10,000–30,000 WBC/cu mm, 50%–80% polymorphonuclear cells, and phagosomal cells (see Chap. 3). The fluid has reduced whole hemolytic complement (CH50), complement (C) C1, C4, C2, C3, properdin, factor B, and increased C9 and gives positive results for ANA and RF tests (in patients who have positive serum tests), and cryoproteins (see Chap. 11). Major clinical and laboratory features of rheumatoid arthritis are summarized and compared with other rheumatic diseases in Table 10.4.

RADIOLOGIC CHANGES

Since the responses of joints to tissue injury are limited, the pattern as well as the type of x-ray finding in rheumatic diseases is important. The joints commonly affected in rheumatoid arthritis have been mentioned. The earliest changes are soft-tissue swelling and juxta-articular osteoporosis. Loss of articular cartilage is seen as "joint-space" (cartilage) narrowing. Invasive pannus leads to subchondral erosions. Early erosions and loss of cortical bone are best perceived near the attachment of the joint capsule—that is, the proximal side of PIPs and the radiovolar aspect of metacarpal heads. Further destruction is seen as malalignment, subluxation, or bony or fibrous ankylosis. These conditions are detailed in Chapter 5.

PATHOLOGIC CHANGES

Rheumatoid synovitis is characterized by exudation, cellular infiltration, and proliferation. There is vasculitis of the small vessels with infiltration of neurophils, lymphocytes, plasma cells, or mononuclear cells; hyperplasia of synovial lining cells; and fibrinous exudation. Although these conditions are characteristic of rheumatoid arthritis, smiliar changes are also seen in other arthritides. Rheumatoid nodules have a central zone of necrosis surrounded by palisading granulation tissue. Muscles may show atrophy and foci of mononuclear inflammatory cells. Granulomatous inflammation may be apparent in tendons and ligaments. Rheumatoid vasculitis may involve terminal arteries or be indistinguishable from polyarteritis nodosa. Granulomata, foci of inflammatory cell infiltrates, or fibrosis may occur at virtually any site.

MANAGEMENT

General

Patient evaluation and formulation of therapeutic programs are facilitated by determining the functional classification, anatomic stage, and disease activity.

Table 10.4. Major Features of Rheumatoid Arthritis Contrasted to Other Rheumatic Diseases

Feature	Rheumatoid Arthritis	Osteoarthritis	Gout	Systemic Lupus Erythematosus	Spondyl- arthritides	Rheumatic Fever	Pyogenic Arthritis
Sex	F > M	M ≅ F	M > F	F > M	M > F	M ≅ F	M = F
Age	20–45 yr	> 50 yr	> 35 yr	20–45 yr	18–30 yr	5–15 yr	Any age
Onset	Insidious	Insidious	Abrupt	Insidious	Insidious	Abrupt	Abrupt
Family history	±	±	+	±	+	−	−
Constitutional symptoms	+	−	±	+−+	±	+++	++
Extra-articular manifestations	++	−	−	+−+	+	++	±
Spine/sacroiliac	+/±	+/±	−	−	+++/+++	−	−
Peripheral joints	Small, symmetric, upper ≅ lower extremity	DIPS,^{a} large, symmetric, lower > upper	1 MTP^a	Small, symmetric, nondeforming	Large, oligoarthritis, asymmetric, lower > upper	Migratory, additive, large joint, lower > upper	Monoarthritis
Subcutaneous nodules	++	−	−	−	−	+	−
Tophi	−	−	++	−	−	−	−
Serum uric acid	Normal-↓	Normal	↑	Normal	Normal	Normal	Normal
Rheumatoid factor	60%–95%	< 20%	< 10%	20%–30%	< 5%	< 5%	< 5%
Antinuclear antibody	20%–40%	< 20%	< 5%	99%–100%	< 5%	< 5%	< 5%
Serum complement	Normal-↑	Normal	Normal-↑	↓ - Normal	Normal	Normal-↑	Normal-↑
Synovial fluid	Inflammatory, ↓ complement	Noninflam- matory	Inflammatory, urate crystals	Inflammatory	Inflammatory	Inflammatory	Infectious
Radiographs	Cartilage loss, osteoporosis, erosions, deformities	Sclerosis, cartilage loss, hypertrophic changes	Punched-out erosions	Soft-tissue swelling	Sacroiliitis/ spondylitis	Soft-tissue swelling	Soft-tissue swelling, late destruction

^{a} Abbreviations used: DIP, distal interphalangeal joints; MTP, metatarsophalangeal joints.

↑ increased, ↓ decreased, ± rare, + occasionally, ++ common, +++ very common.

Patients are classed I–IV, depending on their ability to function: class I, complete function; II, normal but with discomfort; III, limited; IV, incapacitated. They are staged I–IV according to the anatomic and radiologic severity of disease: stage I, early (osteoporosis, no destruction); II, moderate (slight cartilage destruction, osteoporosis, no deformities, extra-articular disease); III, severe (cartilage or bony destruction, deformity, muscle atrophy, extra-articular disease); IV, terminal (ankylosis and criteria of III). Patients have active rheumatoid arthritis if three of the following criteria are met: sedimentation rate (Westergren) exceeding 28 mm/hr, morning stiffness exceeding 45 minutes, and the presence of six tender or three swollen joints.

In formulating a treatment program, one should consider the class, stage, course, duration, and activity of disease; age, sex, occupation, and responsibilities of the patient; and response to prior therapy. The goal of therapy is to preserve or restore musculoskeletal function, thus enabling the patient to maintain physical comfort and financial independence. Available therapeutic modalities are drugs, physical (physical and occupational therapy, rest, hospitalization, splinting, bracing), and surgical (prophylactic and reconstructive operations) (Table 10.5).

It cannot be emphasized too strongly that rheumatoid arthritis is a treatable, manageable disease. Under proper care, the overwhelming majority of patients will respond to therapy and enjoy an improved quality of life. Patients, their families, and the physician must, however, recognize that they are together making a commitment to ameliorate a chronic disease. Cures and complete remission are unusual; improvement often occurs slowly. Attention to details (e.g., drug dosage, time medications are taken, occupational therapy devices, metatarsal bars) is important because seemingly trivial changes may greatly alter patients' functional abilities.

The prognosis, expectations, medical insurance, occupation, vocational retraining, daily activities, and other family, social, economic, and medical considerations should all be explored and candidly discussed with patients and their families. Only by appreciating these factors can the physician effectively initiate and individualize the treatment program and the patient realistically cooperate and participate.

Medical

Most of the available antirheumatic drugs provide symptomatic benefit to patients in varying and often striking degrees. They do not usually induce remission of disease. These agents include salicylates and substituted salicylates, such as aspirin, choline salicylate, sodium salicylate, and magnesium-choline salicylate. A variety of nonsteroidal anti-inflammatory agents continue to be introduced for clinical use. At present, many of these agents are structurally proprionic acid derivatives. They include ibuprofen (Motrin), naproxen (Naprosyn), and fenoprofen (Nalfon). Others are indolacetic acids—indomethacin (Indocin), tolmetin (Tolectin), and sulindac (Clinoril). The pyrazalones include phenylbutazone (Butazolidin) and oxyphenbutazone (Tandearil). Some information about these newer medications is summarized in Table 10.6. In general, the newer nonsteroidal anti-inflammatory agents have proved at least as effective as aspirin in the treatment of rheumatoid arthritis and induce fewer adverse effects. It is not yet clear

Table 10.5. Management of Patients with
Rheumatoid Arthritis

Basic program
   Patient education
   Rest
   Adequate nutrition
   Physical and occupational therapy
Anti-rheumatic drugs
   Palliative
      Anti-inflammatory
         Salicylates
         Phenylbutazone
         Indomethacin
         Ibuprofen
         Fenoprofen
         Naproxen
         Tolmetin
         Sulindac
         Corticosteroids (systemic or intra-articular)
      Analgesic
         Acetaminophen
         Propoxyphene
   Remission-inducing
      Gold salts
      Antimalarials
      d-Penicillamine
Surgery
      Synovectomy
      Reconstructive operations
Investigational approaches
   Immunosuppressive drugs (azathioprine,
      cyclophosphamide, methotrexate, others)
   l-histidine
   Other nonsteroidal anti-inflammatory drugs
   Transfer factor
   Bacillus Calmette-Guerin immunization
   Thoracic-duct drainage
   Intra-articular radioactive colloids
   Levamisole
   Lympho- or plasmaphoresis

---

whether any of these agents is consistently superior to another. Patients respond individually and unpredictably to a given agent, making it necessary in practice to try a number of different drugs for each patient.

Most of these agents are used after a trial of aspirin has proved either ineffective or poorly tolerated. Most clinicians will initiate therapy with acetylsalicylic acid. Treatment is usually begun with two or four tablets (5 grains each) taken with meals and at bedtime. Patients are instructed to increase the dosage by one or two tablets each every 1–4 days until tinnitus occurs (approximately 16–20

Table 10.6. Comparison of Certain Nonsteroidal Anti-inflammatory Drugs

Drug	Dosage	GI	Skin	CNS	Liver	Blood	Approx. Cost/ Month
Acetylsalicylic acid (aspirin)	10–20 grains pc and hs	+	±	±	+	+	$2.60
Choline salicylate (Arthropan)	10–20 mg qid	±	—	±	—	—	9.50
Phenylbutazone (Butazolidin)	100 mg bid–qid	+	+	—	—	+	9.50
Indomethacin (Indocin)	25–50 mg tid–qid	+	—	+	—	—	14.00
Ibuprofen (Motrin)	400–800 mg tid–qid	±	±	±	—	—	23.00
Fenoprofen (Nalfon)	600–900 mg qid	±	±	±	—	—	28.00
Naproxen (Naprosyn)	250 mg qam and 250–500 mg qhs	±	±	±	—	—	17.00
Tolmetin (Tolectin)	400–600 mg tid	±	±	±	—	—	29.00
Sulindac (Clinoril)	150–200 mg bid	±	±	±	—	—	21.00

tablets daily). They continue taking the dosage of aspirin that maintains them just below the threshold of tinnitus. It is often useful to confirm that levels of salicylate have reached the therapeutic range, 20–30 mg/100 ml, approximately 2 hours after a dose of aspirin. If patients complain about the gastrointestinal effects of aspirin, these can sometimes be minimized by initiating therapy with suboptimal dosages of aspirin and increasing the dosage slowly, by adding antiacids to the therapeutic regimen or by substituting various buffered aspirin preparations. If acetylsalicylic acid is still poorly tolerated but has been clinically effective, then one of the substituted salicylates should be considered (Table 10.6).

In those patients who have found salicylates to be either ineffective or intolerable, one of the newer nonsteroidal anti-inflammatory drugs may be tried (Table 10.6). These drugs, like salicylates, should be used in dosage adequate to produce clinical effects.

Additional palliative drugs include analgesics, such as acetaminophen, propoxyphene, or ethoheptazine. Reliance on stronger analgesics or narcotics for treatment of an inflammatory disorder is to be discouraged. Drugs containing codeine or codeine-like derivatives should be used only in carefully selected circumstances, if at all.

Judicious use of systemic or intra-articular corticosteroids may also provide considerable relief to patients. Intra-articular injections of corticosteroids are beneficial to patients with persistent involvement or exacerbation of a small number of accessible joints. Injections are not usually repeated more than three to four times annually. Oral corticosteroids, 5–15 mg prednisone per day or every

Table 10.7. Remission-inducing Drugs Used in the Treatment of Rheumatoid Arthritis

Drug	Dosage	Indications	Major Side Effects
Antimalarials (chloroquine, hydroxychloroquine)	Chloroquine, 1–2 mg/kg/day; hydroxychloroquine, 3–4 mg/kg/day	Active, progressive rheumatoid arthritis	Hematologic, alopecia, GI, skin, ocular, myopathy
Gold salts (Myochrysine, Solganol)	50 mg/wk until 1,000 mg total, then 50 mg every 2–4 weeks	Active, progressive rheumatoid arthritis	Renal, hematologic, skin, mucosal, GI, "nitratoid (vasomotor) reactions," other
d-Penicillamine	250 mg qd; increase 250 mg qd/month up to 750 mg qd	Active, progressive rheumatoid arthritis patients who are gold failures	Renal, hematologic, skin, mucosal, GI, immunologic (SLE, Goodpasture's disease)

other day, are added to a patient's medical regimen only after considerable deliberation. They are usually used to supplement a program for patients who have not responded to simpler agents; who require prompt amelioration of symptoms to function effectively; or who have begun receiving drugs with a delayed onset of action, such as gold, antimalarials, or d-penicillamine.

Those drugs that are capable of inducing remission of disease include the antimalarials, gold salts, and d-penicillamine (Table 10.7). Chloroquine and hydroxychloroquine have been shown to be effective in treating rheumatoid arthritis and occasionally achieving remission of the disease. In general, the antimalarial agents are not thought to be as potent or consistent as gold or d-penicillamine in ameliorating disease. They are particularly useful for those patients who have slowly progressive disease and have not responded well to a more conservative program and for whom the physician cannot or does not yet wish to initiate therapy with gold salts or d-penicillamine. The antimalarials provide the advantage of oral use and do not require frequent monitoring for toxicity of gold and d-penicillamine. The recommended dosage of chloroquine is 1–2 mg/kg per day and 3–4 mg/kg per day of hydroxychloroquine. When these dosages are used, retinal toxicity now seems rare. Nonetheless, it is still recommended that patients obtain baseline and 4- to 6-month ophthalmologic examinations. Other problems infrequently encountered with antimalarials are corneal deposits, myopathy, rash, gastrointestinal intolerance, blood dyscrasias, or alopecia. Therapeutic effects are not usually apparent until after several months of therapy.

A number of studies have established beyond doubt that gold salt therapy can improve and cause remission of rheumatoid arthritis (Table 10.7). As with antimalarials, the onset of action is often delayed several months. Gold salts are generally indicated for patients with progressive, unresponsive disease of more than 6–12 months' duration. Gold salts must be given intramuscularly and are administered in weekly injections up to a total of 1,000 mg. Injections are then continued indefinitely at less frequent intervals, usually every 2–4 weeks if patients have benefited. Adverse reactions—cutaneous, hematologic, renal, mucosal, hepatic—are monitored continually by patient interviews, urinalyses, blood chemistries, and complete blood counts. Approximately 20%–30% of patients must discontinue gold therapy because of side effects.

d-Penicillamine has now been approved for use in rheumatoid arthritis. Its mechanism of action is unknown, but it has proved to be as effective as gold in treating this disorder (Table 10.7). It also often acts only after months of therapy. It is usually reserved for patients with active, progressive disease unresponsive to gold or for patients unable to continue taking gold. *d*-Penicillamine therapy usually begins with 250 mg orally per day for the first month. The drug may be increased by 250 mg per day each month, if necessary, to 750 mg per day for the third month and thereafter, for approximately 6 months, to obtain improvement. Major side effects are frequent (20%–60% of patients) and are similar to those of gold. They include rashes, gastrotoxicity, thrombocytopenia, and proteinuria. Patients should be monitored regularly for adverse actions. The efficacy of *d*-penicillamine appears comparable to that of gold or immunosuppressive agents.

Immunosuppressive agents, including azathioprine, cyclophosphamide, chlorambucil, methotrexate, nitrogen mustard, and others, have all been used in the treatment of rheumatoid arthritis. Although effective, they are not yet recommended for widespread use, and their proper place in treating patients with rheumatoid arthritis remains to be determined. Antimalarials, gold salts, *d*-penicillamine, and immunosuppressives often produce delayed and incomplete remissions. Patients will usually require concomitant therapy with nonsteroidal, or even steroidal, anti-inflammatory agents.

Other investigational therapies have included acupuncture, 1-histidine, a number of experimental nonsteroidal anti-inflammatory drugs, bacillus Calmette-Guérin immunization, transfer factor, thoracic duct drainage, intra-articular radioactive colloids, levimasole and lympho- or plasmaphoresis (Table 10.5).

Surgical

Surgical procedures are also available and useful for selected patients with rheumatoid arthritis. For certain instances of synovitis refractory to appropriate medical management, early synovectomy may retard the progression of disease. When extensive destruction of the bone has occurred, surgical restoration of the joint is often coupled with synovectomy. These procedures are indicated for patients with more advanced disease. The importance of close collaboration with orthopedic surgeons in a team fashion should be stressed. A detailed discussion of surgical management of rheumatoid arthritis is beyond the scope of this chapter and may be found elsewhere.

Physical

A program including physical measures is important for most patients with rheumatoid arthritis. These measures include physical therapy, such as the application of heat, ultrasound, paraffin baths, and home exercise programs. Activities of daily living should be reviewed with a qualified occupational therapist and assistance provided where indicated. In addition, splinting and bracing can provide significant relief when appropriate.

Overall Management Program

Considering the preceding modes of therapy, a few generalizations can be made about the treatment of arthritis (Table 10.8). For symptomatic patients, a conservative treatment program is usually instituted when the diagnosis is made and consists of salicylates to tolerance and appropriate physical measures. Other drugs are added or substituted as needed to increase symptomatic improvement. If disease progresses for 6–12 months despite proper conservative therapy, antimalarials, gold, or d-penicillamine may be added. Intra-articular corticosteroids are used to ameliorate inflammation localized to a small number of joints. Small doses of steroids, orally administered daily or on alternate days, are occasionally added while anticipating delayed benefit from gold, antimalarials, or d-penicillamine or when other symptomatic measures have been inadequate for patient needs. Early synovectomy may afford substantial relief and arrest localized disease. Reconstructive surgical approaches are indicated for patients with progressive joint destruction despite medical management or for appropriate stage III–IV patients. d-Penicillamine or immunosuppressive agents may aid patients with rheumatoid vasculitis. If the attendant risks are recognized, immunosuppres-

Table 10.8. Management of Rheumatoid Arthritis

	Stage I[a]	Stage II[b]	Stage III[c]	Stage IV[d]
Education	+	+	+	+
Physical therapy	+	+	+	+
Occupational therapy	+	+	+	+
Vocational retraining	+	+	+	±
Nonsteroidal anti-inflammatory drugs	+	+	+	+
Analgesics	+	+	+	+
Oral steroids	−	±	±	−
Intra-articular steroids	±	±	±	−
Antimalarials	±	+	+	±
Gold salts	±	+	+	±
d-Penicillamine	−	+	+	−
Immunosuppressive drugs	−	±	±	−
Synovectomy	±	+	±	−
Reconstructive surgery	−	±	+	+

[a] Early disease.
[b] Progressive, reversible disease.
[c] Progressive, active, partially reversible disease.
[d] Severe, irreversible disease.

sive agents may also be considered in selected patients with progressive disease that has not responded to other therapy.

Material in *Clinical Features, Prevalence, Course, Management,* and Tables 10.2, 10.3 and 10.5 appears in similar form in Panush RS: Immunologic aspects of rheumatoid arthritis and related diseases, in Lockey RF (ed): *Allergy and Clinical Immunology,* Garden City, NY, Medical Examination Publishing Co, Inc, an Excerpta Medica company, © 1979, pp 182–188. Reprinted by permission.

BIBLIOGRAPHY

Baum J: Infection in rheumatoid arthritis. *Arthritis Rheum* 14:135, 1971.

Gordon DA, Stein JL, Broder I: The extra-articular features of rheumatoid arthritis: A systematic analysis of 127 cases. *Am J Med* 54:445, 1973.

Gupta VP, Ehrlich GE: Organic brain syndrome in rheumatoid arthritis following corticosteroid withdrawal. *Arthritis Rheum* 19:1333, 1976.

Hollingsworth JW: *Management of Rheumatoid Arthritis and Its Complications.* Chicago, Yearbook Medical Publishers, Inc, 1978.

Huskisson EC: Anti-inflammatory drugs. *Semin Arthritis Rheum* 7:1, 1977.

Jaffe IA: The technique of penicillamine administration in rheumatoid arthritis. *Arthritis Rheum* 18:513, 1975.

Kaye RL, Pemberton RE: Treatment of rheumatoid arthritis. *Arch Intern Med* 136:1023, 1976.

Khan AH, Spodick DH: Rheumatoid heart disease. *Semin Arthritis Rheum* 1:327, 1972.

Mongan ES, Cass RM, Jacox RF, et al: A study of the relation of sero-negative and seropositive rheumatoid arthritis to each other and to necrotizing vasculitis. *Am J Med* 47:23, 1969.

Moore CP, Wilkens RF: The subcutaneous nodule: Its significance in the diagnosis of rheumatoid disease. *Semin Arthritis Rheum* 7:63, 1977.

Mowat A: Hematologic abnormalities in rheumatoid arthritis. *Semin Arthritis Rheum* 1:195, 1971.

Multicentre Trial Group: Controlled trial of D(−) penicillamine in severe rheumatoid arthritis. *Lancet* 1:275, 1973.

Samuels B, Lee JC, Engleman EP, et al: Membranous nephropathy in patients with rheumatoid arthritis: Relationship to gold therapy. *Medicine* 57:319, 1977.

Short CL, Bauer W, Reynolds WE: *Rheumatoid Arthritis.* Cambridge, Mass, Harvard University Press, 1957.

Sienknecht CW, Urowitz MB, Pruzanski W, et al: Felty's syndrome. *Ann Rheum Dis* 36:100, 1977.

Sigler JW, Bluhn GB, Duncan H, et al: Gold salts in the treatment of rheumatoid arthritis: A double-blind study. *Ann Intern Med* 80:21, 1974.

Steinberg AD, Plotz PH, Wolff SM, et al: Cytotoxic drugs in treatment of nonmalignant diseases. *Ann Intern Med* 76:619, 1972.

Talbott JH (ed): Surgical treatment in rheumatology. *Semin Arthritis Rheum* 1:1, 1971.

Walker WC, Wright V: Pulmonary lesions and rheumatoid arthritis. *Medicine* 47:501, 1968.

Zvaifler NJ: Anti-malarial therapy of rheumatoid arthritis. *Med Clin North Am* 52:759, 1968.

11
Rheumatoid Arthritis: Immunologic Aspects

Richard S. Panush

This chapter will review experimental models of rheumatoid arthritis, immuno-genetic aspects of the disease, etiologic possibilities, humoral and cellular immune abnormalities, and cartilage and collagen abnormalities. It will then present an integrated scheme of the current concepts of the pathogenesis of rheumatoid arthritis. This topic is particularly exciting to review because study of this disease has provided many important insights into the immune pathogenesis of other human diseases and basic concepts of autoimmunity and immunologic inflammation.

EXPERIMENTAL MODELS

Until recently there were no known appropriate nonhuman models for the study of rheumatoid arthritis. Several infectious diseases in animals are associated with chronic inflammatory arthritis—pleuropneumoniae-like organism infections in goats, poultry, rats, and mice; *Erysipelothrix insidiosa* infection in swine, *Mycoplasma hyorhinis* in swine; *Mycoplasma pulmonis* in mice; *Hemophilus influenzae suis* in swine; *Corynebacterium pyogenes* in cattle; and *Streptobacillus moniliformis* in rodents. Certain of these diseases resemble rheumatoid arthritis and are associated with the presence of rheumatoid factor (RF). Adjuvant arthritis in the rat, induced by repeated injections of myobacterial products, also bears many similarities to rheumatoid arthritis and other rheumatic diseases. However, this is largely a cell-mediated immune process, whereas rheumatoid arthritis manifests both humoral and cell-mediated immune abnormalities. Other model systems have also been studied. These systems include homologous disease (induced by transfer of lymphoid cells in rats), systemic injection of antigen and intra-articular injection of antibody, intra-articular injection of antigen-antibody complexes, intra-articular injection of antigen into immunized animals, or injection of zymosan into joints. These examples suggest the importance of both infectious and immunologic factors in the pathogenesis of rheumatoid arthritis. These models have not, however, been generally accepted as animal equivalents of humans with rheumatoid arthritis.

A spontaneous polyarthritis occurs in dogs. This condition closely resembles rheumatoid arthritis in humans and provides an attractive and probably unique model for future studies. Rheumatoid arthritis in canines is characterized by spontaneity, female predominance, peripheral inflammatory polyarthritis, constitutional symptoms, radiologic and pathologic changes similar to those described in humans, and the presence of RF. Experiments in progress suggest transmission of synovitis by homogenized and sonicated synovium.

IMMUNOGENETICS

Epidemiologic studies of rheumatoid arthritis have shown instances of increased prevalence of disease or serologic abnormalities among families or monozygotic twins of patients. It is now appreciated that human leukocyte antigens (HLA) at the cell surface are under genetic control and may regulate immune responses. With the recognition of immunologic and possible genetic aspects of rheumatoid arthritis, associations between HLA antigens and rheumatoid arthritis were sought. No consistent associations have been found at the A or B loci, which are easily typed by serologic methods (see Chap. 4). More recent work has revealed the presence of a lymphocyte-defined D locus antigen, HLA DRw4, occurring in approximately 25%–70% of rheumatoid arthritis patients. DRw4 occurs in approximately 10%–30% of normal persons. Preliminary studies suggested that rheumatoid arthritis patients with DRw4 were more likely to have severe disease than those without. Patients with rheumatoid arthritis were also reported to have an increased prevalence of the HLA C series determinant, Cw3, probably because Cw3 exists in linkage disequilibrium with DRw4. The HLA D complex is thought to be the gene region that links the human histocompatibility antigens and immune response. It is responsible for B-lymphocyte cell surface alloantigens similar to immune response gene-associated (Ia) antigens in mice. Ia alloantigens have also been examined in patients with rheumatoid arthritis, whose cells reacted with particular Ia alloantisera in patterns distinctly different from those of normal subjects and patients with lupus. All of these observations suggest that genetic and immunologic factors interrelate in the pathogenesis of and susceptibility to rheumatoid arthritis through mechanisms that are not now completely understood.

ETIOLOGY

The cause (or causes) of rheumatoid arthritis remains unknown. Hereditary, endocrinologic, psychologic, and perhaps nutritional and metabolic factors may all influence rheumatoid arthritis, but they do not seem to be the cause. Environmental influences also may be important. There is little historical evidence that rheumatoid arthritis existed before the seventeenth century. Thus it may be a "new" disease. An increased prevalence has been found among pet owners. As reviewed earlier, rheumatoid arthritis also occurs in familial aggregations. The most attractive idea is that immunologic abnormalities are triggered by an antigenic stimulus, perhaps an infectious agent, in susceptible persons. Besides the infectious arthritides in animals, a variety of further evidence in support of this concept has accumulated: occasional isolation of *Mycoplasma* organisms from patients, cellular immune response to *M. fermentans,* resistance of cultured synovial cells to rubella virus infection, isolation of diphtheroids from filtrates of rheumatoid synovium, increased DNA polymerase in synovial cells, and increased rubella antibody titers. Other investigators have been unable to isolate microorganisms from specimens or to find significantly elevated antibody titers to infectious agents. Since this remains a compelling hypothesis, investigators continue to search for infectious agents or their products that may participate in the pathogenesis of rheumatoid arthritis.

IMMUNOLOGIC ASPECTS

Rheumatoid Factor

Rheumatoid arthritis has long been characterized by the presence of an abnormal autoantibody, namely, RF. Rheumatoid factors are antibodies to immunoglobulin. They may, therefore, be directed against IgG, IgA, IgM, IgD, or IgE. Usually only those antibodies directed against IgG are referred to as RF in patients with rheumatoid arthritis. The presence of these antibodies in patients with rheumatoid arthritis has been recognized since 1922. Early studies identified RF as 19 S IgM antibodies. Subsequent work revealed that RFs are not restricted to the 19 S IgM class but also occur as IgG, IgA, IgD, and 7 S IgM antibodies. To detect RF, many test systems have been developed, most of which use the capacity of 19 S IgM RF in serum to agglutinate antigen (IgG) attached to cells (sheep red blood cells) or particles (latex or bentonite). Other assays, available only to investigative laboratories, employ additional immunochemical methods to detect RF of other Ig classes. Although RFs occur in most patients with rheumatoid arthritis (60%–95%), they are not detected by standard methods in all patients, nor are they necessarily specific for rheumatoid arthritis when found. RF can be detected in approximately the following percentages of patients (Table 11.1): Sjögren's syndrome, 80%–95%; polydermatomyositis, 50%; subacute bacterial endocarditis, 50%; scleroderma, 25%–30%; systemic lupus erythematosus, 20%–30%; hepatic disease, 20%–30%; juvenile rheumatoid arthritis, 20%; chronic infectious diseases, 15%–20%; sarcoidosis, 15%–20%; patients over 60 years of age, 10%–20%; ankylosing spondylitis, < 5%; normal individuals, < 5%; and osteoarthritis, 5%–20% (comparable to age-matched normal subjects).

The presence or absence of RF in the blood of patients with rheumatoid arthritis provides useful clinical, as well as diagnostic, information (Table 11.2). The presence of RF, particularly in a high titer, has often been associated with a poor prognosis, progressive and unremitting disease course, significant functional impairment, the presence of subcutaneous nodules, a high erythrocyte sedimentation rate (ESR), a large number of actively inflamed joints, radiologic evidence of joint destruction, cryoglobulinemia, low synovial fluid complement, and frequent extra-articular complications such as vasculitis, pleuropulmonary disease, pericarditis, or ocular disease. Tests for RF that are positive usually remain so during the course of the disease. Titers do not tend to fluctuate with disease activity. They may be decreased during sustained remission or after plasma-

Table 11.1. Prevalence of Rheumatoid Factors in Rheumatic and Other Diseases

Disease	Positive Rheumatoid Factor Test	Titer
Rheumatoid arthritis	60–95	High
Sjögren's syndrome	80–95	Low–high
Polydermatomyositis	50	Low
Subacute bacterial endocarditis	50	Low
Progressive systemic sclerosis	25–30	Low
Systemic lupus erythematosus	20–30	Low
Hepatic diseases	20–30	Low
Juvenile rheumatoid arthritis	20	Low
Chronic infectious diseases	15–25	Low
Sarcoidosis	15–20	Low
Aged individuals (> 65 years)	10–20	Low
Spondylitides	< 5	Low
Osteoarthritis	5–20	Low

pheresis or treatment with steroids, d-penicillamine, gold, or antimalarial or immunosuppressive agents.

Synovial fluid or other effusion fluid RF usually occurs in those patients seropositive for RF. However, RFs also occur in nonrheumatoid effusions. Because of the lack of specificity, testing effusions for the presence of RF is not widely recommended.

There have been many efforts to define biologic activities of RF in vitro and in vivo, in hopes of clarifying mechanisms of disease production (Table 11.3). In vivo, injected RF or antigen-antibody complexes induced mesenteric vasculitis in rats; transfusions of RF(+) plasmas did not induce disease in recipients;

Table 11.2. Clinical Associations of Rheumatoid Factors in Patients with Rheumatoid Arthritis

Poor prognosis
Progressive disease
Unremitting course
Significant functional impairment
Presence of subcutaneous nodules
High erythrocyte sedimentation rate
Many actively inflamed joints
Radiologic evidence of joint destruction
Cryoglobulinemia
Low synovial fluid complement
Frequent extra-articular complications

Table 11.3. Biologic Activities of Rheumatoid Factors

Neutralize infectivity of virus-antibody complexes

Interact with IgG to activate complement

Serum and synovial fluid IgM anti-IgG, and IgG
   anti-IgG:IgG are inversely proportional to complement levels

Facilitate immune complex phagocytosis

Enhance elimination of immune complexes

Influence Ig catabolism and antibody responses

? Activate kinin system

? Mitogenic for lymphocytes

---

autologous IgG injected into the knees of patients with rheumatoid arthritis
(usually RF[+]) provoked inflammation; and passive administration of human
RF reduced mouse antibody responses to subsequent immunization with human
IgG and has influenced Ig catabolism. In vitro, IgM RF has neutralized virus-
antibody complex infectivity; IgG and IgM RF interacted with aggregated IgG,
activated the classic complement system, and generated chemotactic factor activity;
addition of RF to immune complexes enhanced their precipitation and phagocytosis; IgM RF converted soluble complexes to complement-fixing aggregates;
RF has been weakly mitogenic to lymphocytes; and RF-IgG complexes may activate the kinin system.

Other Antibodies

Other antibodies have been detected in serum and synovial fluids from patients
with rheumatoid arthritis. A few patients have antinuclear (20%–40%) or hetero-
phile antibodies. These antigen-antibody systems, as well as RF-IgG, may be involved in the pathogenesis of joint inflammation. Also described have been antibodies to a rheumatoid arthritis-associated nuclear antigen in about two-thirds of
patients.

Immune Complexes

Circulating immune complexes have been detected by a number of methods in
serum, synovial fluid, and tissues of patients wih rheumatoid arthritis. It has been
shown that 22 S complexes circulate and consist of 19 S IgM RF and 7 S IgG. Intermediate-sized complexes consist of IgG RF-IgG or (less often) IgA RF-IgG.
Cryoprecipitates, presumably immune complexes containing IgG, IgM, RF, antinuclear antibody, nuclear antigen, or complement, have been consistently found
in synovial fluid and occasionally in serum of patients with rheumatoid arthritis.
Immunofluorescence and elution techniques have shown Ig, RF, or complement
localized to synovial fluid phagosomes, synovial membrane, or certain tissues in
patients with rheumatoid vasculitis. A "rheumatoid biologically active factor,"
thought to be an immune complex but incompletely characterized, has also been
found in serum and synovial fluid of patients. Recently, complexes have been

detected in 20%–80% of sera and synovial fluid from rheumatoid arthritis patients by using C1Q, monoclonal RF, and platelet interaction assays. Concentrations of detectable complexes were directly related to the severity of disease, measured by anatomic stage, functional class, RF level, number of involved joints, ESR, grip strength, and extra-articular disease. The amounts of the complexes were inversely proportional to concentrations of CH50, C4, and C3d. Sensitivities differ in the various methods of assaying immune complexes in patients with rheumatoid arthritis. This fact suggests that complement-fixing and noncomplement-fixing complexes of various sizes and constituents circulate. More study is required to identify those complexes unique to rheumatoid arthritis and important to disease pathogenesis.

Complement

Complement abnormalities have been well studied in patients with rheumatoid arthritis. Synovial fluid concentrations of CH50, C1, C4, C2, C3, properdin, and factor B are all absolutely reduced, and C9 is relatively depleted. C3d, C4d, and Ba (breakdown products of C3, C4, and factor B, respectively) were increased in synovial fluid. These changes were usually more pronounced in patients who were RF(+) than RF(−). Synovial fluid complement measurements are generally corrected for synovial fluid protein concentration and compared with serum measurements as well as with similar determinations for control groups. Synovial fluid values below 30%–50% of serum are usually considered to be depressed. The synovial fluid complement system was thought to be immunologically activated based on the following observations: hypercatabolism of C3 in patients; identification of C4 and C3 cleavage products (C3c and C3d); production of conversion products of factor B; the presence of chemotactic activity derived from C3, C5, and $C\overline{567}$; and detection of intracellular inclusions of complement and Ig. Depressed synovial fluid C levels have correlated with values of synovial fluid IgG and IgM RF, the amount of IgG RF-IgG complexes, the severity of radiologic and pathologic changes, unremittent disease, subcutaneous nodules, and extensive clinical disease.

Serum complement values in patients tend to be normal or increased. A few patients—those with severe and active disease, circulating immune complexes, often with extra-articular or vasculitic complications—will have serum hypocomplementemia. Increased catabolism of serum C3 has been found in some patients. Immunologic activation and consumption of complement are thought to occur in the synovium and cause low measurable levels. If synovial or tissue use increases with increasingly severe disease, the serum concentration may also be reduced. Activation of complement generates a number of molecules that are potentially of biologic importance in the inflammatory response—C3a, C5a, and $C\overline{567}$ polymorphonuclear chemotactic factors; C3a and C5a anaphylatoxins; C3b-enhanced immune adherence and phagocytosis; and C42 kinin. The participation of these molecules in immunologic inflammation will be discussed subsequently.

Other Humoral Systems

Other humoral systems that may participate in the inflammatory response in rheumatoid arthritis remain to be thoroughly studied. Fibrin deposition occurs in the synovium and at other sites of tissue injury. Although RF or RF-IgG were thought to activate kinins, more recent studies have shown that synovial fluid concentrations of kininogen and bradykinin were unaltered. Synthesis of prostaglandin E_2 (PGE_2) is stimulated by a monocyte-derived soluble factor that acts on adherent rheumatoid synovium. PGE_2 may be important in bone resorption.

Polymorphonuclear cells that are phagocytizing Ig and complement release lysosomal hydrolases into synovial fluid. Lysosomal enzymes have caused synovitis in rabbits, can produce biologically active materials from C5 and the kinin system, partially degrade gamma globulin, induce collagenase and plasminogen activator secretion by fibroblasts, and modulate lymphocyte responses—all potentially important events in intra-articular inflammation.

Connective tissue-activating peptides have been extracted from a variety of human cell types. These peptides activate connective tissue fibroblasts to produce hyaluronic acid and lactic acid and use glucose. Peptide concentrations were increased in rheumatoid synovial cells. This increase may be an important part of the proliferative process in the rheumatoid synovium.

Lymphocytes: Cell-mediated Immunity

There is increasing evidence that cellular immunologic events participate in the pathogenesis of rheumatoid arthritis: (1) It is likely that humoral and cellular responses interrelate, as they do in normal immune events and in other immunologic diseases. (2) Rheumatoid-like arthritis develops in agammaglobulinemic children. (3) The pathologic picture of the rheumatoid synovium reveals a prominent mononuclear cell proliferation. (4) Studies of patients have usually revealed abnormal cell-mediated responses.

Both in vivo and in vitro cell-mediated immunity are generally abnormal in patients with rheumatoid arthritis. Discrepancies result from methodologic differences, different patient populations, and possibly the effects of certain drugs on immunologic responses. Cutaneous reactivity to common antigens and responses to the contact sensitizer dinitrochlorobenzene have been reduced. In the systemic circulation, numbers of T and B lymphocytes were usually normal, but increases or decreases were noted. Null cells were usually increased. In vitro responses to phytomitogenic or antigenic stimulation were often reduced, and dissociation of in vivo and in vitro reactivity to antigens occurred. In vitro mixed lymphocyte reactivity (rheumatoid arthritis cells as both stimulator and responder cells) was reduced in some patients with rheumatoid arthritis. Rheumatoid peripheral lymphocytes have exhibited cytotoxicity to fibroblast monolayers. Rheumatoid arthritis serum may modulate lymphocyte responses by virtue of enhancing or inhibiting activities. Rheumatoid arthritis peripheral blood lymphocytes have reacted weakly to RF and occasionally to IgG.

In the synovial fluid, numbers of T and null cells tended to increase and B cells to decrease, but reports varied. T lymphocytes have also been prominent in the synovial membrane. Synovial fluid lymphocytes showed cytotoxicity to other cell lines. Responses of synovial fluid lymphocytes to phytomitogens tended to be as expected or to be reduced. Cultures of synovial lymphocytes or synovial membrane cells demonstrated the "spontaneous" incorporation of radiolabeled thymidine or the production of blastogenic factor, migration inhibitory factor, or lymphotoxin. Abnormal antibody (RF) production and spontaneous lymphokine production suggest that regulator and effector functions of lymphocytes are abnormal in rheumatoid arthritis.

Cartilage and Collagen

One of the consequences of rheumatoid synovitis is joint erosion with damage to cartilage and bone. The processes leading to articular destruction are not yet completely understood. Prostaglandin E, lymphocyte-derived osteoclast-activating factor, and enzymes (cathepsins, elastase, and collagenase) all participate in these events. The rheumatoid synovium produces collagenase, which is possibly complexed with an inhibitor. Proteases and products of activated mononuclear cells induce secretion. Proteinase activates latent collagenase. Since rheumatoid synovial cultures also produce plasminogen activator, it may be that plasmin, after activation by plasminogen activator, could activate collagenase. Collagenase could then participate in remodeling or destroying connective tissue and cartilage.

Patients with rheumatoid arthritis have antibodies to types I, II, and III collagen and cellular hypersensitivity to types II and III collagen. It is possible that autoantibodies to collagen contribute to the rheumatoid inflammation.

PATHOPHYSIOLOGY

When all these observations are considered, an attempt can be made to construct an integrated scheme of the pathogenesis of adult rheumatoid arthritis (Fig. 11.1). An inciting event or microorganism initiates disease under certain environmental circumstances or in certain susceptible persons. Antigens may localize to articular and periarticular collagenous tissue and may remain there, protected against easy immune elimination. A series of intra-articular immune events follows. IgG may undergo alteration—as a result of lysosomal enzyme degradation, aggregation, or interaction with putative infectious antigen—and itself become antigenic. Rheumatoid factors are produced against the IgG. IgG and IgM anti-IgG together with IgG activate the classic complement sequence and begin to generate the necessary ingredients of an inflammatory reaction—vasoactive substances, chemotactic factors, anaphylatoxins, and adherence- and phagocytosis-promoting activities. Polymorphonuclear leukocytes are recruited into the joint space and phagocytize immune complexes of RF-IgG-C. Leukocytes then release lysosomal enzymes and collagenase (which cause synovitis), modulate lymphocyte responses, and contribute to joint destruction. Lysosomal enzymes can partially degrade IgG, which may increase its antigenicity. The rheumatoid synovium can synthesize IgG and complement and thereby provide immunoreactants needed to perpetuate the inflammation.

Inflamed synovium also produces an activator peptide, which is thought to promote a transition from exudative to proliferative synovitis. Lymphocytes and other mononuclear cells appear in the synovial fluid and synovial membrane and are activated, perhaps by hypothetical antigen, altered Ig, RF, complement, complexes, enzymes, or other substances, to produce lymphokines. Macrophage migration inhibitory factor, blastogenic factor, and lymphotoxin—mediators that have

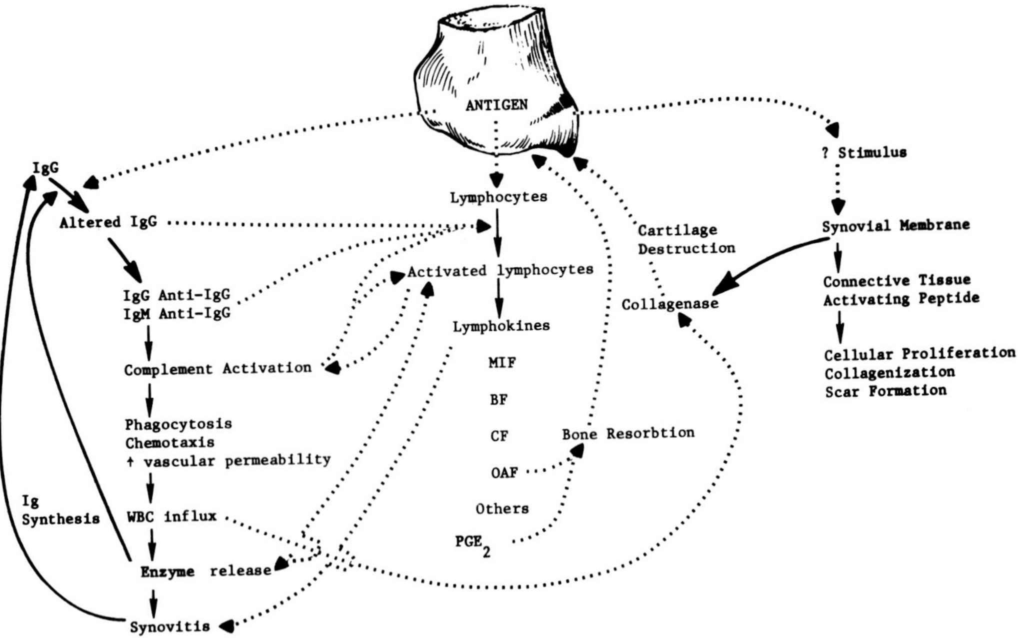

Figure 11.1. Possible pathogenesis of rheumatoid arthritis. (From Panush RS: Autoantibodies and human disease, in Waldman RH (ed): *Clinical Concepts of Immunology.* Baltimore, Williams & Wilkins Co, © 1979, p 150. Reprinted by permission.)

produced arthritis in animals—have been found in rheumatoid arthritis synovial fluid or synovial cell culture supernatants. It seems likely that activated lymphocytes recruit other lymphocytes and macrophages to the site of inflammation, activate them to become cytotoxic, and produce yet other substances capable of contributing to tissue injury. Humoral and cell-mediated pathways interact. Lymphocytes contain a factor capable of activating complement, and complement molecules in turn can modulate lymphocyte reactivity. Defective immunoregulation as the cause of the excessive humoral and cellular effector responses is under study.

IMMUNOLOGIC EFFECTS OF ANTIRHEUMATIC DRUGS

Many processes in the immune response are theoretically amenable to therapeutic modification: antigen recognition, antigen processing, primary and secondary antibody, responses, immune complex formation, clearance of complexes, complex deposition, complement activation, chemotaxis, phagocytosis, lysosomal enzyme release, enzyme activities, lymphocyte activation, lymphokine production, lymphokine activities, and macrophage activation and functions, to name but a few. The study of drug effects on these many immunologic events promises to be important in developing effective therapy and understanding the mechanisms of drug actions.

Nonsteroidal anti-inflammatory drugs, steroids, and other antirheumatic agents

Table 11.4. Effects of Antirheumatic Drugs[a]

Effect	ASA	PBZ	IND	GOLD	OH-CQ	HC	D-PEN	CP	AZA	MTX
Affect amino acid metabolism	+	+		+	+	+				
Affect carbohydrate metabolism	+	+		+	+	+				
Inhibit mucopolysaccharide synthesis	+	+	+		+	+				
Inhibit collagen formation		+		+	+	+	+			
Inhibit oxidative reactions	+	+			+	+				
Uncouple oxidative phosphorylation	+	+	+							
Inhibit ATPase				+	+					
Activate ATPase	+	+	+			+				
Inhibit nucleic acid polymerase	+				+					
Inhibit pyridoxal-dependent enzymes	+	+					+			
Chelate metals							+			
Protein binding	+	+	+	+	+	+				
Stabilize lysosomes—inhibit lysosomes	+	+	+	+	+	+				
Inhibit prostaglandin synthesis	+	+	+	+	+	+				
Inhibit Ag-Ab interaction	+									
Decrease circulating immune complexes								+		
Decrease Ab response	+						+	+	+	+
Decrease reverse passive arthus	+									
Decrease Schwartzman reaction	+									
Reduce serum sickness	+									
Inhibit immune hemolysis	+									
Reduce C levels						+				
Inhibit complement activation				+						
Reduce Ig levels						+	+	+	+	
Depolymerize Ig							+			
Reduce protein synthesis	+	+	+		+	+		+		+
Inhibit blastogenesis	+	+	+	+	+	+	+	+	+	+
Inhibit lymphokine production						+			+	+
Inhibit phagocytosis						+				
Inhibit chemotaxis					+	+				

Table 11.4. (Continued)

Effect	ASA	PBZ	IND	GOLD	OH-CQ	HC	D-PEN	CP	AZA	MTX
Reduce skin-test reactivity	+					+		+	+	+
Inhibit macrophage responsiveness						+				
Inhibit cytotoxicity	+	+	+		+	+			+	
Inhibit connective tissue activation	+	+	+		+	+				

a ASA, salicylate; PBZ, phenylbutazone; IND, indomethacin; OH-CQ, hydroxychloroquine, antimalarials; HC, hydrocortisone, corticosteroids; *D*-PEN, *d*-penicillamine; CP, cyclophosphamide; AZA, azathioprine; MTX, methotrexate.

have important and varied effects on many metabolic and enzymatic pathways. Similarly, these drugs have been recognized to affect many immunologic functions summarized in Table 11.4. Immunosuppressive drugs have now been widely used in treating rheumatic diseases. General effects of alkylating agents (chlorambucil, cyclophosphamide, phenylalanine mustard, and triethylenemelamine), purine antagonists (6-mercaptopurine, azathioprine, 6-thioguanine, 8-azaguanine), and folic acid antagonists (methotrexate, aminopterin) are also shown in Table 11.4. Effects of drugs vary, however, depending on experimental or clinical circumstances, dosage, route of administration, and other factors.

Although it is difficult to extrapolate in vitro or animal data to clinical settings, immunologic effects of these drugs may be pertinent to their antirheumatic properties. The effects of drugs must also be carefully considered during the clinical investigation of immune responses of patients receiving therapy.

Material in *Experimental Models, Rheumatoid Factor, Pathophysiology, Immunologic Effects of Antirheumatic Drugs,* and Tables 11.1–11.4 appears in similar form in Panush RS: Immunologic aspects of rheumatoid arthritis and related diseases, in Lockey RF (ed): *Allergy and Clinical Immunology,* Garden City, NY, Medical Examination Publishing Co, Inc, an Excerpta Medica company, © 1979, pp 188–195, 207–210, and Panush RS: Autoantibodies and human disease, in Waldman RH (ed): *Clinical Concepts of Immunology,* Baltimotre, Williams & Wilkins Co, 1979, pp 146–151. Reprinted by permission.

BIBLIOGRAPHY

American Rheumatism Association Symposium: Cytotoxic drugs in rheumatic diseases. *Arthritis Rheum* 16:77, 1973.

Castor CW: Connective tissue activation. III. Observations on the mechanism of action of connective tissue activating peptide. *J Lab Clin Med* 79:285, 1972.

Clot J, Sany J (eds): Immunological aspects of rheumatoid arthritis. *Rheumatology,* vol 6. Basel, S Karger, 1975.

Gabriel A Jr, Agnello V: Detection of immune complexes. *J Clin Invest* 59:990, 1977.

Harris ED Jr, Vater CA, Mainard CL, et al: Cellular control of collagen breakdown in rheumatoid arthritis. *Agents Actions* 8:36, 1978.

Huskisson ED: Antiinflammatory drugs. *Semin Arthritis Rheum* 7:1, 1977.

Jasin HE, Cooke TD, Hurd ER, et al: Immunologic models used for the study of rheumatoid arthritis. *Fed Proc* 32:147, 1973.

Lloyd TM, Panush RS: Cell-mediated immunity in rheumatoid arthritis. Studies of patients off therapy and correlation with clinical status. *J Rheumatol* 4:231, 1977.

Panush RS: Effects of certain antirheumatic drugs on normal human peripheral blood lymphocytes. Inhibition of mitogen- and antigen-stimulation of tritiated thymidine. *Arthritis Rheum* 19:907, 1976.

Panush RS, Bianco NE, Schur PH: Serum and synovial fluid IgG, IgA, and IgM antigammaglobulins in rheumatoid arthritis. *Arthritis Rheum* 14:737, 1971.

Perper RP (ed): Mechanisms of tissue injury with reference to rheumatoid arthritis. *Ann NY Acad Sci USA* 256:5, 1975.

Ruddy S, Austen KF: Activation of the complement system in rheumatoid synovitis. *Fed Proc* 32:134, 1973.

Ruddy S, Fearon DT, Austen KF: Depressed synovial fluid levels of properdin and properdin factor B in patients with rheumatoid arthritis. *Arthritis Rheum* 18:289, 1975.

Scheinberg MA, Mendes NF, Kopersztych S, et al: Clinical applications of T, B and K cell determinations in rheumatic disease: A review. *Semin Arthritis Rheum* 6:1, 1976.

Stage DE, Mannik M: Rheumatoid factors in rheumatoid arthritis. *Bull Rheum Dis* 23:720, 1973.

Stastny P: HLA-D and Ia antigens in rheumatoid arthritis and systemic lupus erythematosus. *Arthritis Rheum* 21:S139, 1978.

Van Boxel JA, Paget SA: Predominantly T-cell infiltrate in rheumatoid synovial membrane. *N Engl J Med* 293:517, 1975.

Weissmann G: Lysosomal mechanisms of tissue injury in arthritis. *N Engl J Med* 286:141, 1972.

Yu DTY, Peter JB: Cellular immunological aspects of rheumatoid arthritis. *Semin Arthritis Rheum* 4:25, 1974.

Zvaifler NJ: Immunopathology of joint inflammation in rheumatoid arthritis. *Adv Immunol* 16:265, 1973.

12

Juvenile Rheumatoid
Arthritis

Jean M. Jackson

Juvenile rheumatoid arthritis (JRA) was appreciated as a distinct entity by George Frederic Still in 1896 with his original report of 22 cases of chronic joint disease in children. This group included the one that still bears his name; this separate set of 12 patients had "sudden attacks of hyperpyrexia," lymphadenopathy, and splenomegaly, in addition to joint enlargement. Growth retardation was apparent, and pericarditis was a postmortem finding in three cases.

PREVALENCE AND ETIOLOGY

Population studies based on the 1972 census estimate the prevalence of JRA to be 5 childhood cases per 100 adults with rheumatoid arthritis, or 200,000 patients in the United States. Implicated etiologic factors have been heredity, trauma, and infection, but none has been substantiated.

DIAGNOSIS

The disease had been defined in 1959 by Ansell and Bywaters with their report of 216 cases. Their criteria required disease onset before the age of 16 years and involvement of at least four joints, or if only one joint was involved for at least 3 months, then biopsy evidence was needed to support the diagnosis of rheumatoid arthritis. Evidence of other disease entities that may be associated with arthritis excluded those patients from the study.

Criteria have since been revised by the JRA Criteria Subcommittee to allow categorization and multicenter evaluation with regard to treatment response or prognosis. The diagnosis of JRA requires that the arthritis be persistent in one or more joints for at least 6 weeks and that other disease entities be first excluded. Arthritis is defined by swelling or limitation of motion of a joint with heat, pain, or tenderness. The three onset subtypes are determined by manifestations during the first 6 months of disease, although other subtype features may occur later. Systemic or acute febrile onset is associated with persistent intermittent daily temperature elevations to 103 F or more, with or without the rheumatoid rash, an evanescent, macular, erythematous lesion ranging in size from 2 to 10 mm. Pauci- or oligoarticular onset limits the number of involved joints to four or less. Polyarticular onset requires arthritis in at least five joints, with the systemic onset being excluded.

CLINICAL SUBTYPES

Arthritis may be initially absent in the systemic onset subtype, which tends to appear between the ages of 1 and 3 years and to be equally distributed between boys and girls. The most striking feature is the temperature, which may be as high as 105 F; a daily spike and return to normal or even subnormal levels is characteristic. The rheumatoid rash may accompany the fever and tends to be transient, with a distribution over the trunk, upper extremities, thighs and, less often, the face. Generalized lymphadenopathy and hepatosplenomegaly are frequently found. Pleuritis and/or pericarditis have been reported in 36% of the cases. Pain, stiffness, and limitation of motion of the cervical spine are seen in 50% of patients, with other joint involvement being prominent in the wrists, knees, ankles, and elbows.

Pauci- or oligoarticular JRA typically occurs before age 13 and characteristically involves the knee, ankle, elbow, or wrist. Iridocyclitis, or uveitis, is the most outstanding nonarticular feature and may be seen in 25% to 39% of this subgroup with an associated antinuclear antibody positivity. These patients, when young, require slit-lamp examination every 3 to 4 months, as they do not have symptoms of eye pain, photophobia, decreased vision or headache, and insidious visual loss may develop. Moreover, the activity of the uveitis does not parallel the activity of the arthritis. Joint manifestations may lead to leg length discrepancy because of bony overgrowth at the sites of active synovitis.

Polyarticular disease symmetrically involves the wrists, knees, ankles, and hips, as well as the small joints of the feet and hands, particularly the proximal interphalangeal joints. Micrognathia and cervical spine fusion are clinically apparent, and long-term functional disability is seen in 10% of the group overall. Subcutaneous rheumatoid nodules may occur but to a lesser extent than in the adult rheumatoid, which this subgroup most closely approximates. Constitutional symptoms, lymphadenopathy, and splenomegaly are seen in a significant proportion of the patients.

DIFFERENTIAL DIAGNOSIS

Acute rheumatic fever is still a major consideration in the differential diagnosis of the child presenting with an acute polyarthritis; Jones criteria, the fever pattern, and the age of onset all assist in its exclusion. Systemic lupus erythematosus is often accompanied by a facial rash and urinary abnormalities, with the lupus erythematosus cell phenomenon or a highly positive antinuclear antibody titer. The dermatologic features of scleroderma, dermatomyositis, and psoriasis corroborate these entities, and HLA B-27 typing assists in recognizing the asymmetric appearance of the oligoarthropathies seen with ankylosing spondylitis and post-dysenteric or granulomatous bowel disease. Leukemic infiltrates in the periarticular periosteum may be mistaken for arthritis before the appearance of peripheral hematologic abnormalities. Infectious agents are initially invoked by a monarticular presentation, as may be pigmented villonodular synovitis. Nonrheumatologic entities presenting with articular symptoms tend to involve the joints of the lower extremity more often than those of the upper extremity, for example, aseptic necrosis, chondromalacia patellae, and slipped capital femoral epiphysis.

LABORATORY FEATURES

Rheumatoid factor (RF) in JRA tends to be positive in those patients with a later onset of disease and increases with the duration of follow-up. Up to age 4 years, only 12% of patients were seropositive, while 42% in the 10 to 14 age group acquired RF. Similarly, at each 5-year increment of disease duration, the presence of RF increased from 18% to 20% to 27%. Seropositivity increased in the polyarticular onset subtype, as contrasted to the acute febrile and pauciarticular groups. Antinuclear antibody presence was detected in 0%–22% of patients with acute febrile and polyarticular onset and in 20%–41% of 83 oligoarticular onset patients. Leukocytosis is virtually always present in the systemic onset subtype. Anemia is found in approximately half of the children. Antistreptolysin titers are elevated in 22%–34% of patients. Of patients with severe disease, 20% had albumin levels of less than 3.5 g and 51% had elevated gamma globulin fractions above 1.2 g; erythrocyte sedimentation rates are elevated in 81% of patients at some time during the disease.

Also found are elevated Ig levels IgA deficiency (2%–4%), normal to elevated serum complement levels, and occasional abnormal liver (or other organ) function depending on disease manifestation. Synovial fluid findings are similar to those in adult rheumatoid arthritis. Synovial fluid CH50, C1, C4, and C3 were reduced in children with positive RF test results, and occasional phagosomal inclusions of Ig, or complement have been noted.

PATHOLOGY

Synovial tissue has been obtained at the time of joint arthroplasty or by biopsy. The pathology varies with the duration of disease and the presence or absence of RF. Light and electron microscopic findings corroborate the presence of those features seen in the adult rheumatoid synovium, that is, synovial cell hyperplasia and hypertrophy with lymphocytic and plasma cell infiltration and a paucity of neutrophils. Synthetic or B cells are most common in the normal juvenile synovium, with phagocytic or A cells rarely seen. A cells are most numerous in the synovium of the juvenile rheumatoid. Joints themselves are eroded marginally with pannus reflection. Cartilage regeneration may occur to a greater extent than in adults.

The subcutaneous nodule closely resembles that of rheumatic fever, with a fibrinoid lattice, vascular "islands," and the absence of necrosis without the zones seen in the typical adult rheumatoid nodule. The rash of JRA, with its sparse neutrophilic infiltration in the subepithelial layer, contrasts to the florid lesions seen in erythema marginatum.

Visceral involvement is comparatively uncommon, although hepatic histology shows nonspecific periportal collections of mononuclear cells and Kupffer cell hyperplasia. Amyloidosis has been documented by rectal biopsy in 6% of those patients developing proteinuria in the British series.

RADIOLOGY

Radiographic features of JRA tend to increase in severity with disease duration, seropositivity, prior steroid treatment, and mode of onset. The early manifestation of soft tissue swelling is seen in all subtypes. Periosteal new bone formation and metaphyseal rarefaction are noted in the systemic and polyarticular groups. Advanced changes occur in both polyarticular and systemic onset JRA and include cartilage and bone destruction, large joint subluxation, bony ankylosis, and both epiphyseal and vertebral compression fractures. Bony ankylosis is most common in the wrist and may be associated with prior periosteal new bone formation. Growth abnormalities and overgrowth or undergrowth of long bones adjacent to the arthritis occur in 5%–50% of the patients. Spondylitis occurs uniquely, and almost pathognomonically, in the cervical region at the upper apophyseal joints (Fig. 12.1). Sacroiliac disease has been reported in 24% of Still's disease patients; HLA typing was not carried out then, but obvious variants were excluded. Additional consideration of radiologic aspects of JRA may be found in Chapter 5.

MANAGEMENT

The principles of medical management have long identified the need for basic supportive measures that begin with education of the family to enable the child with arthritis to live as normal a life as possible. Rest, splinting, medications, physical and occupational therapy, orthopedic and ophthalmologic consultations, and psychosocial assessments are all relevant facets of a child's treatment program.

Physical therapy, with parental assistance in the young child, is directed at maintaining strength and increasing joint range of motion through assistive, then active, and finally resistive exercises when the synovitis is quiet. Hydrotherapy allows mobility in many children in whom exercises would be impossible because of contractures or muscle loss. Splinting aids in preventing deformities in the acute or active phase. Serial casting may relieve contractures.

Drug therapy is initiated with anti-inflammatory agents. Remission-inducing drugs are added should disease activity persist. Salicylates, whether plain, buffered, coated, or liquid, continue to be the drugs of choice, for toxicity can be monitored by readily obtained serum levels. Therapeutic levels of 25–30 mg/dl are achieved with 3 g/sq m, rather than 100 mg/kg body weight/day, in children weighing more than 40 kg. Of the other nonsteroidal anti-inflammatory agents, only tolmetin has been approved for use in children. Indomethacin,

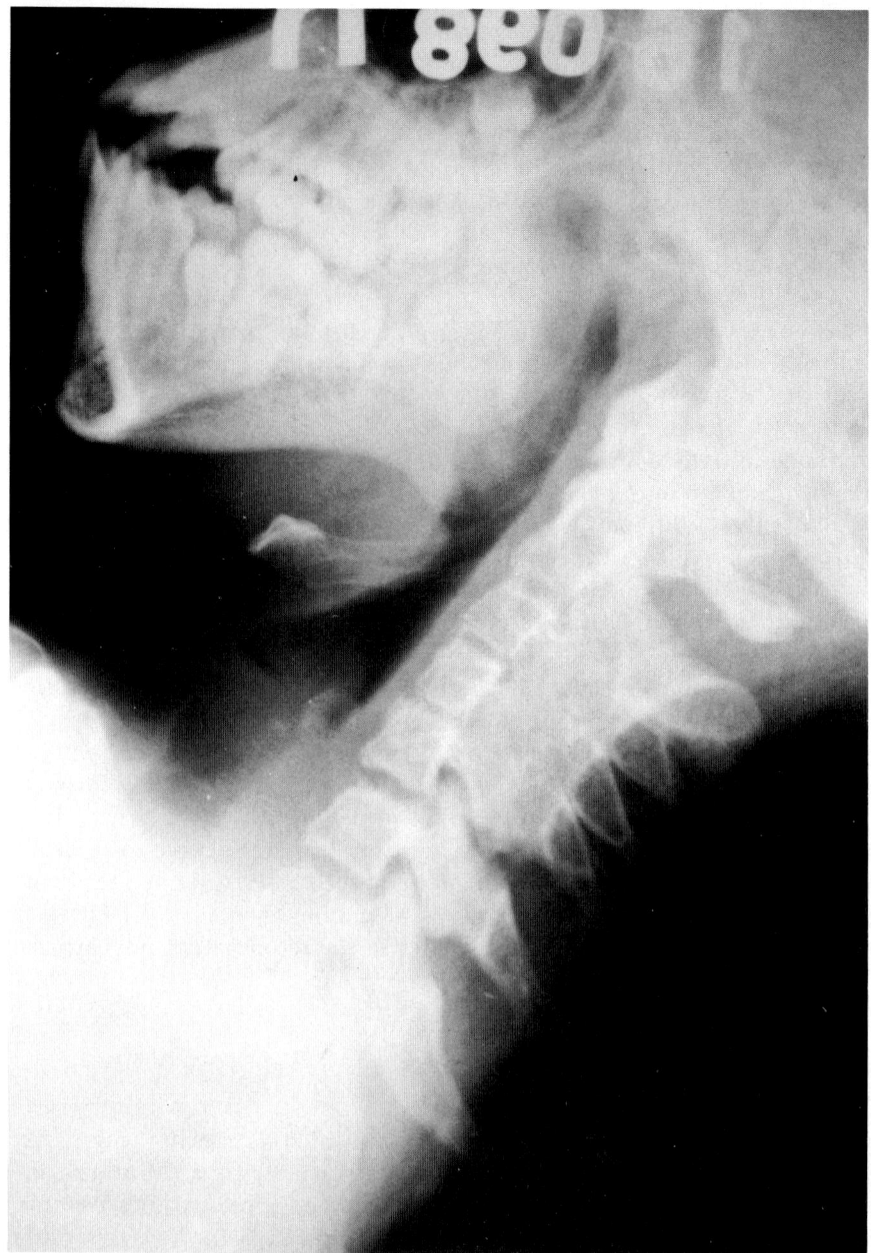

Figure 12.1. Cervical spine apophyseal joint involvement in a patient with JRA.

phenylbutazone, ibuprofen, naproxen, and fenoprofen are not recommended for children less than 15 years of age, although indomethacin may occasionally be used for fever control.

Antimalarials, specifically hydroxychloroquine (Plaquenil), are considered in those patients who fail to respond to salicylates. Ocular keratopathy was not seen in children in whom 5–7 mg/kg/day (120–150 mg/sq m) was not exceeded. Routine ophthalmologic examination for potential retinal toxicity is still mandatory.

Adverse effects to chrysotherapy are no greater in children than in adults. Therapy is initiated with either the water-soluble gold sodium thiomalate (Myochrysine) or the oil-base aurothioglucose (Solganal) in 1 mg/kg body weight/wk parenteral dosages, not to exceed 50 mg/wk. Follow-up hematologic and urinary studies are done initially on a weekly basis; then they are decreased to alternate weeks and ultimately to once monthly. A critical assessment of the drug's efficacy is undertaken at the sixth month of treatment. Penicillamine use in children has been inadequately reported with regard to remission induction and is presently being studied. Systemic glucocorticoids now tend to be reserved for those children whose constitutional symptoms cannot be controlled by other means. Topical steroids and mydriatics are initially used in the treatment of iridocyclitis. Alkylating agents and antimetabolites are rarely warranted in JRA, but chlorambucil has been used in those British patients developing amyloidosis.

Total joint replacement has played a dramatic role in mobilizing the wheelchair-bound child whose epiphyses have closed. Unique problems are encountered with the small skeletal size and the need to design fitting prostheses. Soft tissue releases may relieve contractures that have not been responsive to medical or physical intervention; however, the long-term success rate is not greater than 50%. Synovectomy has yielded a better range of motion than in a comparable joint in the adult, but here too results are better in the seronegative, oligoarticular onset patient.

PROGNOSIS

Long-term prognosis has been favorable in the majority of patients with JRA reported from various centers in the United States and Europe. Mortality in earlier series ranged to 9%; this proportion may have been related to complications from medical therapy. Function has been well preserved in the series cited in Table 12.1. A better outcome was noted with earlier referral after disease onset and a greater functional impairment when the disease appeared before age 6 years. Amyloidosis was present in 6 of 18 deaths but is less common in the United States.

IMMUNOLOGIC ASPECTS

The pathogenesis of rheumatoid arthritis in children has been assumed to be similar to that in adults. It is relatively recently that children have been studied as thoroughly as have adults. Familial aggregations of the disease suggested ge-

Table 12.1. Prognosis of JRA

Author	Number of Patients	Male:Female	% with Severe Crippling	Number of Deaths
Schaller (1972)	124	38:86	13	2
Goel (1974)	100	48:52	16	9
Calabro (1976)	100	38:62	13	3
Stillman (1976)	200	51:149	12	1
Ansell (1976)	243	101:142	19	18

netic influences. An increased incidence of HLA type B27 among patients with juvenile rheumatoid arthritis may reflect children with spondylitis. HLA-D typing has revealed a significant positivity of DW7 and DW8 in JRA patients, as contrasted to the increased frequency of DW4 in the adult patient. The antigen TMo occurs in 46% of those with persistent pauciarticular disease and may represent a susceptibility or resistance factor.

JRA may be more than a single disease and have an infectious etiology. One group reported increased rubella virus antibodies, persistent IgM rubella antibodies, and localization of rubella virus antigen in the synovial fluid of some patients.

By agglutination tests, RF occurs in about 10%–20% of juvenile patients and increases in incidence with age. Cold-reactive (4 C) RFs were detected in an additional 22% of patients seronegative at 37 C. When immunoabsorption techniques were used. IgG RFs were found in virtually all and IgA in most patients with JRA. Seropositivity (at 37 or 4 C) and the presence of IgM RF or elevated levels of IgG RF correlated with progressive active disease, an unfavorable course, and relative depression of complement. Antinuclear antibodies, but rarely anti-DNA, occur in fewer than 20% of patients. Synovial fluid has also been shown to contain elevated levels of IgG, IgA, and IgM RF. Synovial fluid antinuclear antibodies were seen in some patients with positive serum test results.

Complement values (CH50, C1Q, C4, C2, C3, C3 activator, C9) in serum have usually been normal or increased. Values tended to be higher when disease was active, in RF-negative rather than RF-positive patients, decreasing with clinical improvement or seropositivity. Synovial fluid CH50, C1, C4, and C3 were reduced in RF-negative patients. Deposition of complement and Ig in synovial membrane and intra-articular leukocytes has been noted in some patients, suggesting phagocytosis or deposition of immune complexes, as in adults.

Cell-mediated immunity was depressed in those children with active or severe disease. Findings included blunted cutaneous reactivity to common antigens, impaired in vitro proliferative responsiveness to phytomitogens or antigens, impaired migration-inhibitory factor production, or a dissociation of in vivo and in vitro responses. Patients with JRA had decreased peripheral and synovial fluid T lymphocytes and increased null cells.

Immunologic abnormalities in JRA seem qualitatively similar to those noted in adults. There are quantitative differences that may reflect differing etiologies, ages of patients, or milder disease in children. Some event causes anti-IgG (predominantly IgG) formation and presumably the formation of intrasynovial immune complexes. This process leads to complement activation and synovitis. Cellular events probably also participate in this process, as in adults.

ADULT-ONSET STILL'S DISEASE

A pattern of Still's disease in the adult has been appreciated since 1971, when Bywaters reported 14 female patients with a constitutional illness similar to that seen in children and characterized by an elevated temperature (104–105 F), transient rash, synovitis, and occasionally ankylosis in the cervical spine. Wrists and knees were the joints predominantly involved, and pericarditis was present in four. Laboratory features included only an elevated sedimentation rate with absent rheumatoid and antinuclear factors. The prognosis was felt to be good with regard to function. A second series in 1973 from the National Institutes of Health further cited 10 male adults who presented with a fever of unknown origin and had a symptom complex consistent with Still's disease. Interestingly, 7 of the 10 had a sore throat at the onset of their symptoms, with polyserositis associated with the fever, rash, and joint manifestations. Leukocytosis and anemia were common, but all patients had absent RF. In contradistinction to Bywaters' series, all patients had normal cervical spine radiographs, with one patient exhibiting almost complete obliteration of the intercarpal spaces in less than 2 years. Deforming arthritis developed in one patient, but the prognosis was excellent in the other nine. Others described nine females and two male adults and noted again the systemic features of the disease, with a sore throat being present at the onset. Carpometacarpal and intercarpal ankylosis, particularly involving the capitate, was apparent in 7 patients. Since the diagnosis of febrile onset JRA is made by exclusion, the characteristic spiking quotidian fever pattern, transient rash, and polymorphonuclear leukocytosis are helpful in making a positive diagnosis. Other considerations in the differential diagnosis are other systemic rheumatic diseases, granulomatous disorders, familial Mediterranean fever, and lymphoreticular malignancies.

Some of the material in the sections on *Laboratory Features* and *Immunologic Aspects* appears in similar form in Panush RS: Immunologic aspects of rheumatoid arthritis and related diseases, in Lockey RF (ed): *Allergy and Clinical Immunology.* Garden City, NY, Medical Examination Publishing Co, Inc, an Excerpta Medica company, © 1979, pp 196–199. Reprinted by permission.

BIBLIOGRAPHY

Ansell BM, Bywaters EGL: Prognosis in Still's disease. *Bull Rheum Dis* 9:189, 1959.

Ansell BM, Wood PHN: Prognosis in juvenile chronic polyarthritis. *Clin Rheum Dis* 2:397, 1976.

Bernstein B, Takahashi M, Hanson V: Cardiac involvement in juvenile rheumatoid arthritis. *J Pediatr* 85:313, 1974.

Bianco NE, Panush RS, Stillman JS, et al: Immunologic studies of juvenile rheumatoid arthritis. *Arthritis Rheum* 14:685, 1971.

Brewer EJ, Bass J, Baum J, et al: Current proposed revision of JRA criteria. *Arthritis Rheum* 20(Suppl):195, 1977.

Bujak JS, Aptekar RG, Decker JL, et al: Juvenile rheumatoid arthritis presenting in the adult as fever of unknown origin. *Medicine* 52:431, 1973.

Bywaters EGL: Still's disease in the adult. *Ann Rheum Dis* 30:121, 1971.

Calabro JJ, Holgerson WB, Sonpal GM, et al: Juvenile rheumatoid arthritis: A general review and report of 100 patients observed for 15 years. *Semin Arthritis Rheum* 5:257, 1976.

Calabro JJ, Marchesano JM: Medical management of juvenile rheumatoid arthritis. *Bull Rheum Dis* 15:378, 1965.

Carter ME: Sacroiliitis in Still's disease. *Ann Rheum Dis* 21:105, 1962.

Cassidy JT, Martel W: Juvenile rheumatoid arthritis: Clinicoradiologic correlations. *Arthritis Rheum* 20(Suppl):207, 1977.

Chylack LT, Bienfang DC, Bellows AR, et al: Ocular manifestations of juvenile rheumatoid arthritis. *Am J Ophthalmol* 79:1026, 1975.

Goel KM, Shanks RA: Follow-up study of 100 cases of juvenile rheumatoid arthritis. *Ann Rheum Dis* 33:25, 1974.

Isdale IC, Bywaters EGL: The rash of rheumatoid arthritis and Still's disease. *Q J Med* 25:377, 1956.

Lindbjerg IF: Juvenile rheumatoid arthritis. *Arch Dis Child* 39:576, 1964.

Schaller J, Beckwith B, Wedgwood RJ: Hepatic involvement in juvenile rheumatoid arthritis. *J Pediatr* 77:203, 1970.

Schaller J, Wedgwood RJ: Juvenile rheumatoid arthritis: a review. *Pediatrics* 50:940, 1972.

Stastny P, Fink CW: Different HLA-D associations in adult and juvenile rheumatoid arthritis. *J Clin Invest* 63:124, 1979.

Still GF: On a form of chronic joint disease in children. *Med Chir Trans* 80:47, 1897.

Stillman JS, Barry PE, Bell CL, et al: Clinical characteristics and classification of juvenile rheumatoid arthritis, in Jayson MIV (ed): *Still's Disease: Juvenile Chronic Polyarthritis*. London, Academic Press Inc, 1976, p 47.

13

The Spondylarthritides

Andrei Calin

In the mid-nineteenth century all forms of chronic arthritis were considered to be variants of gout. During the next decades, rheumatoid arthritis and then osteoarthritis became demarcated as separate entities. With the discovery of rheumatoid factors in 1940, a further division of inflammatory arthritis into two main groups was possible: seropositive and seronegative rheumatoid arthritis. Until the 1960s, all forms of seronegative rheumatoid arthritis were lumped together. It is now recognized that this group is heterogeneous. A small percentage of seronegative patients do indeed have rheumatoid arthritis. However, the remainder may be further subdivided into the interrelated group known as the *seronegative spondylarthritides* and a subset of patients who will become seropositive if followed up. A further group has, as yet, a seronegative inflammatory polyarthropathy of unclassified type.

SERONEGATIVE SPONDYLARTHRITIDES

As a result of meticulous clinical epidemiology, the concept of the seronegative spondylarthritides developed. This group consists of ankylosing spondylitis, Reiter's syndrome, the reactive arthritides (*Shigella, Salmonella,* and *Yersinia* arthropathy), psoriatic arthropathy, enteropathic arthropathy, juvenile chronic polyarthropathy, and possibly the rare disorders Behcet's syndrome and Whipple's disease (see Chapters 18 and 23).

The seronegative spondylarthritides are not variants of rheumatoid arthritis. Indeed, the group may be distinguished from rheumatoid arthritis on historic, racial, familial, sex, age, clinical, radiologic, pathologic, immunogenetic, and therapeutic grounds.

The characteristics of this group include: (1) pathology centered on the enthesis (i.e., the site of ligamentous insertion into bone) rather than the synovium (thus, the term *enthesopathy* is sometimes used); (2) radiologic sacroiliitis with or without ankylosing spondylitis; (3) peripheral arthropathy; (4) familial aggregation; (5) clinical interrelationships between diseases (i.e., psoriaform skin lesions, nail lesions, ocular and genitourinary inflammation, buccal, genital, and bowel ulceration, erythema nodosum, iridocyclitis, and occasionally thrombophlebitis); (6) an absence of subcutaneous nodules and (7) rheumatoid factors.

IMMUNOGENETICS: HLA B27

As mentioned above, the spondylarthropathies tend to run in families. The explanation for this recognized clinical phenomenon came in 1973 with the description of the striking association between ankylosing spondylitis and the human leukocyte antigen HLA B27. For many decades a link had been recognized between the ABO blood group system and certain disorders. Since the early 1960s there has been serologic recognition of a different antigenic system, one that results from isoantigens that are involved in cell-cell recognition.

These human leukocyte antigens now play a major role in our understanding of certain rheumatic disorders. Although there are numerous associations between the HLA system and disease, none is more striking than that between HLA B27 and the seronegative spondylarthritides. Present excitement and research activities follow not only because of the close proximity between this genetic marker and disease but also because, for the first time, this marker may be related to susceptibility to certain infective agents. For example, patients with the postdysenteric form of Reiter's syndrome (i.e., shigella) are frequently B27-positive, as are other patients with reactive arthropathy, conditions associated with specific infective agents. This link between infection and genetics will certainly help our understanding of other chronic arthritides.

The mechanism of the association between B27 and disease remains unknown, although several hypotheses exist: (1) HLA B27 may act as a receptor site for an infective agent; (2) B27 is a marker for an immune response gene that determines susceptibility to an environmental trigger; and (3) B27 may induce tolerance toward antigens with which it cross-reacts.

HLA B27 is present in about 6% of healthy whites, 3% or 4% of blacks, and less than 1% of Japanese. The prevalence of B27 in the different seronegative spondylarthritides is summarized in Table 13.1.

ANKYLOSING SPONDYLITIS

Prevalence and Epidemiology

From a clinical point of view, ankylosing spondylitis may be defined as *symptomatic sacroiliitis*. More specifically, criteria have been developed that rely on historic, clinical, and radiographic findings. Once considered a rare disease, it is now recognized that about 20% of HLA B27-positive persons develop ankylosing spondylitis. Thus, since HLA B27 is present in about 6%–8% of whites, it follows that up to 1% of persons have the disease, often remaining undiagnosed. Many of these undiagnosed but symptomatic patients have had inappropriate investigations (including myelograms), inappropriate diagnostic labels (neurosis, discogenic disease), and inappropriate management (bed rest, laminectomy).

The prevalence of ankylosing spondylitis follows the distribution of HLA B27. The disease is seen less frequently in blacks than whites, a finding related to the relative rarity of B27 in the black race (1%–4%). HLA B27 occurs in 18% of Pima and 50% of Haida Indians. Not surprisingly, ankylosing spondylitis is particularly prevalent among these and other Indian groups.

Ankylosing spondylitis may be considered a primary event or secondary to the

Table 13.1. HLA B27 and Rheumatic Disease in Whites

Group	% Positive
Healthy whites	5–14
Ankylosing spondylitis	90–100
Endemic Reiter's syndrome	70–90
Psoriasis	5–10
Psoriatic arthropathy without sacroiliitis	18–22
Psoriatic arthropathy with sacroiliitis	50–60
Seropositive juvenile rheumatoid arthritis	5–10
Juvenile chronic polyarthropathy without sacroiliitis	15–25
Juvenile chronic polyarthropathy with sacroiliitis	40–60
Inflammatory bowel disease	6
Inflammatory bowel disease with peripheral arthropathy	6
Inflammatory bowel disease with sacroiliitis	50–70
Yersinia	10
Yersinia reactive arthropathy	80
Salmonellosis	10
Salmonella reactive arthropathy	80–90
Shigellosis	10
Post-*Shigella* arthropathy (epidemic Reiter's syndrome)	80
Uveitis	40–50
Chronic balanitis	90
Rubella arthritis	6

associated spondylarthritides. Primary ankylosing spondylitis occurs most frequently toward the end of the second decade and during the third decade. Secondary spondylitic forms associated with psoriatic arthropathy, Reiter's syndrome, or inflammatory bowel disease may occur at any age.

Sex Distribution

Until recently, ankylosing spondylitis was considered to occur only rarely in women, with a sex distribution of 10 or 20 to 1 in favor of men. It is now recognized that the disease occurs more frequently than hitherto considered in women. The sex distribution may be equal or about 2 or 3 to 1 in favor of men. Until recently, women with ankylosing spondylitis were misdiagnosed as having seronegative rheumatoid arthritis. There is a natural reluctance to take pelvic radiographs in young women. Moreover, radiologists and physicians have recognized inflammatory sacroiliac disease with difficulty.

There are certain differences in the natural history of ankylosing spondylitis in men and women. Men tend to have more severe and progressive spinal disease, while women have more peripheral joint involvement. This difference probably accounts for the delay in diagnosing the condition in women.

Etiology

The cause of ankylosing spondylitis remains unknown. However, with awareness of the striking association between B27 and this disease, there is renewed interest in possible infective etiologies. For example, it is known that Reiter's syndrome is linked to shigella, yersinia, and salmonella infections. It thus remains possible that one of these or another Gram-negative organism may cause ankylosing spondylitis. Recently, there has been some enthusiasm for klebsiella as filling this role. However, it remains unknown whether one or more agents are responsible for the precipitation of ankylosing spondylitis in susceptible persons.

Clinical Features

In the same way that we recognize that rheumatoid arthritis (or better, rheumatoid disease) affects not only the joints but also extra-articular tissue, we now appreciate that ankylosing spondylitis has both skeletal and extraskeletal manifestations.

Skeletal Involvement

Spinal.   Sacroiliitis is the sine qua non of ankylosing spondylitis. Almost invariably, patients appear with back discomfort, pain, and decreased mobility. Since back pain is such a frequent occurrence and may result from nonspecific mechanical causes as well as from inflammatory spinal disease (i.e., ankylosing spondylitis), it is important to recognize features suggesting inflammatory rather than mechanical or nonspecific spinal disorders. The following characteristics may be helpful in recognizing inflammatory disease: (1) insidious onset of discomfort over days, weeks, or months rather than hours; (2) age below 40 years (especially in primary ankylosing spondylitis); (3) persistence for more than 3 months; (4) association with morning stiffness; and (5) improvement with exercise. In contrast, back pain of a mechanical nature can develop rapidly over hours, at any age, is sporadic rather than persistent, is made worse with exercise, improves with rest, and is not associated particularly with morning stiffness. Studies have shown that about 20% of persons with four or five of these features have ankylosing spondylitis.

Spinal examination may reveal muscle spasm, loss of the normal lumbar lordosis, and evidence of decreased spinal mobility. Anterior spinal flexion is measured by noting the distraction of two points, drawn 10 cm apart (Fig. 13.1*a*) on anterior flexion. Right and left lateral flexion are measured by noting the distraction of two points 20 cm apart in the midaxillary line (Fig. 13.1*b*) on contralateral flexion. In contrast to patients with nonspecific spinal disease, those with

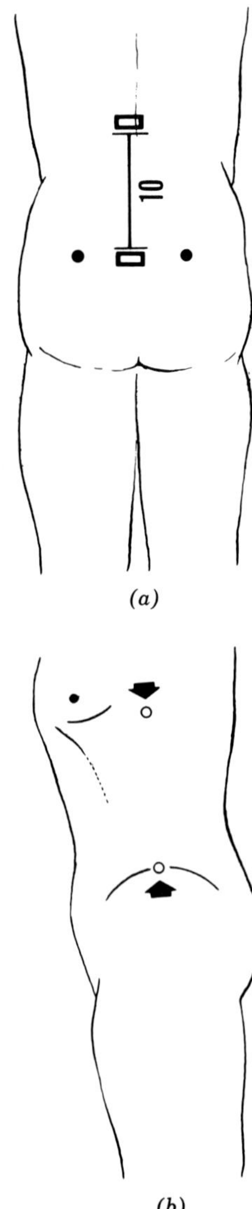

Figure 13.1. (*a*) 10-cm line drawn between two points; the lower, at the midpoint between the posterior iliac spines. (*b*) Line drawn between two arbitrary points, 20 cm apart, in the midaxillary plane.

ankylosing spondylitis have decreased mobility in the anterior and lateral planes. (Patients with the former condition may have decreased mobility in just one direction.) Since reduction in chest expansion occurs only later in the natural history of the condition, this measurement is rarely useful early on but should be performed for baseline determination.

Late spinal complications include fracture (resulting sometimes in sudden death) and a localized destructive vertebral process termed *spondylodiscitis*. This process may result from minimal trauma and is managed by rest rather than exercise, the usual treatment for active disease.

Extraspinal. Extraspinal skeletal involvement includes tenderness of enthesopathic sites (i.e., site of ligament insertion into bone). For example, the patient may have Achilles tendinitis, intercostal muscle tendinitis (the explanation for a pleuritic-like chest pain on deep inspiration), and other extraspinal problems that include peripheral joint disease, the typical dactylitis (or sausage digit), and other extra-articular findings. Peripheral joint disease occurs in up to 25% of patients with ankylosing spondylitis at some stage during the course of their disease. Typically, large joints in the lower limbs are affected. The arthropathy is often asymmetric, but an individual joint may mimic that condition seen in rheumatoid arthritis. A major problem may be hip involvement, since patients with fused spines can maintain a good degree of function, whereas bilateral hip involvement may be associated with job loss and other problems.

Extraskeletal Involvement

Every patient with ankylosing spondylitis must be questioned about the past or present existence of psoriasis, bowel disease, urethritis, and other events that may suggest one of the other secondary forms of spondylitis. Moreover, a family history should always be elicited.

Constitutional symptoms include fatigue, weight loss, and low-grade fever.

Prevalence figures for various extraspinal findings are probably lower than those published, since data result from academic centers and often hospitalized patients. Certain features may be found early or at any time in the course of the disease. For example, conjunctivitis or uveitis occurs at any time. Other manifestations such as aortic regurgitation, cord compression, upper lobe pulmonary fibrosis, and amyloid deposition occur only in the sicker patient after many years of active disease.

Rarely, patients are seen with a chronic infiltrative and fibrotic upper lobe disease that mimics tuberculosis. This fibrotic process, of unknown etiology, may result indirectly in death. The fibrotic lung may become superinfected with aspergillus, and fatal hemoptysis may follow.

Heart disease occurs primarily in those patients with more severe spondylitis. Aortic regurgitation, cardiomegaly, and persistent conduction defects are the commonest findings.

Amyloidosis is an occasional complication of ankylosing spondylitis but is rarely of clinical significance. Likewise, the kidney may demonstrate pathologic abnormalities that are of no clinical significance.

Neurologic syndromes occur rarely. The cauda equina syndrome should be considered in any patient with bowel or bladder dysfunction together with sensory and motor impairment in the buttocks and thighs and gluteal region pain.

The major features of ankylosing spondylitis are summarized and compared with those of rheumatoid arthritis in Table 13.2.

Laboratory Findings and HLA B27

The erythrocyte sedimentation rate may be elevated but can remain within normal limits in a patient with severe disease. There is often a hypochromic anemia. Tests for rheumatoid factors and antinuclear antibodies are negative.

Overreliance on HLA B27 testing should be avoided. As mentioned above, the

Table 13.2. Comparison of Ankylosing Spondylitis with Rheumatoid Arthritis

	Ankylosing Spondylitis	*Rheumatoid Arthritis*
Distribution	Racial	Worldwide
Prevalence	1%–2%	1%–2%
Positive family history	Frequent	Rare
Sex distribution	M ≧ F	F > M
Age group	Peak at 20–30 years	All ages; peak at 30–50 years
Joint involvement	Oligoarthropathy, asymmetric large joints, lower limb more than upper limb	Polyarthropathy, symmetric, small and large joints, upper and lower limb
Sacroiliac involvement	Yes	No
Spine involvement	Total (ascending)	Cervical
Nodules	No	Yes
Aortic regurgitation	Yes	No
Eyes	Conjunctivitis, uveitis	Sicca syndrome, scleritis, scleromalacia perforans
Lungs	Upper lobe pulmonary fibrosis	Pulmonary fibrosis, nodules
Rheumatoid factors	No	Yes
HLA	B27	DW4
Pathologic characteristics	Enthesopathy	Inflammatory synovitis
Radiologic characteristics	Asymmetric erosive arthropathy, new bone formation, ankylosis, sacroiliitis	Symmetric erosive arthropathy
Therapy	Indomethacin, phenylbutazone	Aspirin, gold, penicillamine

diagnosis of ankylosing spondylitis is made by radiologic evidence of sacroiliitis in a patient with back symptoms. The finding of HLA B27 does not confirm the diagnosis, since the antigen is present in 5%–10% of normal persons. Likewise, since B27 is present in only 90% of patients, its absence does not rule out the diagnosis.

Radiology

Reliance on a single anteroposterior radiograph of the pelvis is usually sufficient for discerning sacroiliitis. The radiologic grading depends on the degree of juxta-articular sclerosis, blurring of the joint margin, narrowing of the joint space, erosions, and degree of ankylosis (Figs. 13.2, 13.3).

In view of the enthesopathic nature of the disease, it is not surprising that radiologic changes occur at other sites. Typically, vertebral squaring (due to erosive disease at the corner of the vertebral body, where the annulus fibrosus infiltrates into bone), plantar spurs at the site of plantar fasciitis, calcaneal spurs at the site of Achilles tendon insertion, and other changes at sites of ligament bone contact may be seen.

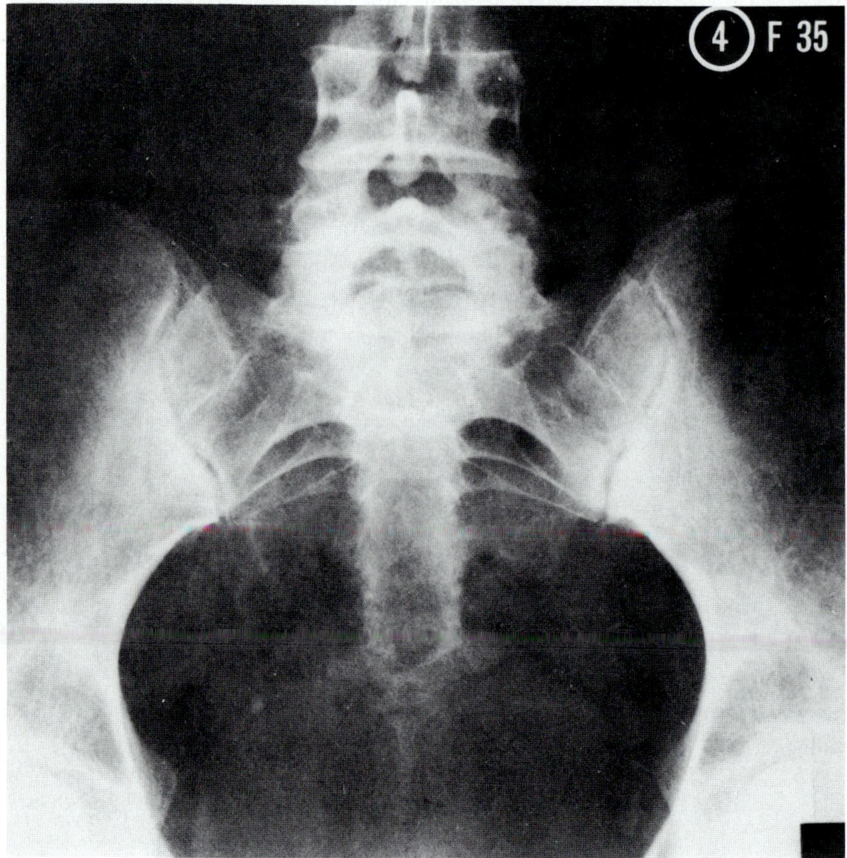

Figure 13.2. Grade II (minimal) sacroiliitis. Note blurring of the joint margin and juxta-articular sclerosis.

Syndesmophytes (new bone formation in a vertical plane, in close juxtaposition to the annulus fibrosus) must be differentiated from the horizontal osteophyte, a bony reaction to degenerative spinal disc disease. Hyperostotic lesions, seen in diffuse skeletal hyperostosis, are wax-like bony protuberances of the spine, seen predominantly in men in the seventh and later decades (Fig. 13.4*a–c*).

Extraspinal radiologic disease includes an erosive destructive arthropathy of the hip and, to a lesser extent, other joints. Radiologic features that distinguish ankylosing spondylitis from seropositive rheumatoid disease include a propensity to develop new bone formation and predominant sclerosis rather than osteoporosis and erosions (see also Chap. 5).

Natural History and Prognosis

The majority of patients with ankylosing spondylitis lead a normal life, losing little or no time from work, and are able to enjoy normal social activities. With the present awareness that ankylosing spondylitis occurs in up to 2% of the community, it is clear that only a small percentage of patients develop the typi-

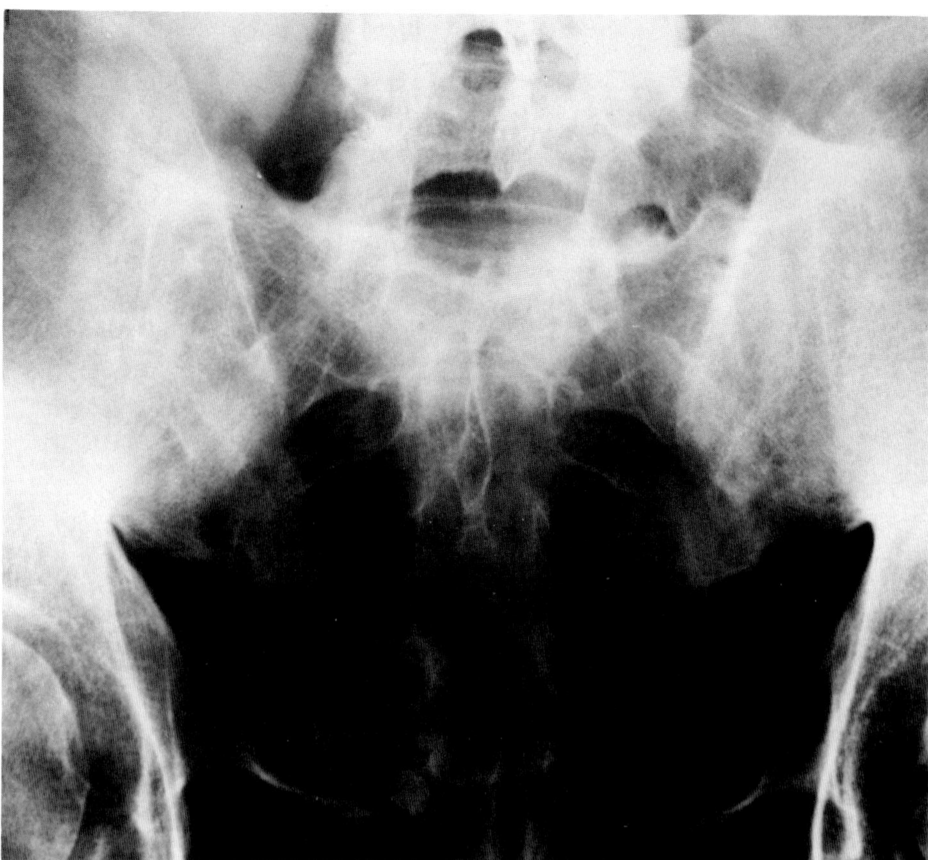

Figure 13.3. Grade IV sacroiliitis (ankylosis). Note the total loss of joint space and destruction of the joint.

cal bamboo spine. Many patients are diagnosed as having ankylosing spondylitis after many decades of minimal back pain. Clearly, there is a wide spectrum of disease activity.

Management

Ankylosing spondylitis is a gratifying condition to recognize and treat. Although it cannot be cured, it can be effectively managed. The primary objectives are to relieve pain, decrease inflammation, begin remedial strengthening exercises, and maintain good posture and function.

The patient must be encouraged to perform remedial strengthening exercises and to practice postural training. A firm mattress at night, a small pillow under the head, and attention to posture at work and at rest are all important. The best exercise regimen includes extension exercises and swimming.

By relieving inflammation, anti-inflammatory agents permit the patient to follow an adequate exercise program. Indomethacin is considered to be the drug of choice (25–50 mg tid). For those patients who are intolerant to indomethacin or

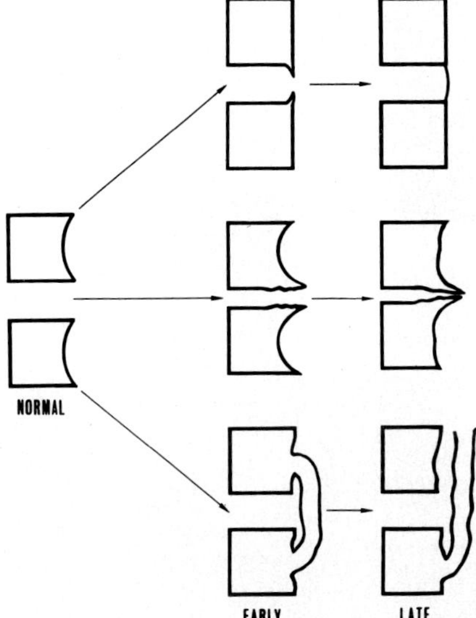

Figure 13.4. Note normal vertebral bodies on the left of the diagram. Lateral views show normal concavity. The upper section of the diagram demonstrates early vertebral loss of concavity and early new bone formation, typical of ankylosing spondylitis. The new bone occurs in the outer margin of the annulus. The middle section diagrams degenerative spinal disease with disc space narrowing associated with a horizontal plate of new bone. The bottom panel illustrates vertebral hyperostosis with a heavy paravertebral plate of new bone associated with normal disc space and vertebral contours. Progressive changes are noted on the extreme right of the diagram.

who do not demonstrate adequate efficacy, phenylbutazone may be given (100 mg tid or qid). This agent should be used cautiously in older patients and with periodic blood, urine, and liver checks. Newer nonsteroidal anti-inflammatory drugs, particularly ibuprofen or sulindac, may have a role to play in patients who do not do well with the first two. Gold, penicillamine, and the antimalarials, of value in rheumatoid disease, have not been adequately studied in ankylosing spondylitis. Radiotherapy, once considered the treatment of choice, is no longer given in view of the high risk of malignancy.

Genetic Counseling

Patients often inquire about the need to HLA-type all members of the family. At this time, patients are advised that only one in five of B27-positive subjects develop disease; since there is no cure, little more than attention to the family history is recommended to allow early diagnosis and management.

REITER'S SYNDROME

There have been dramatic advances since 1916, when Professor Hans Reiter redescribed the triad of urethritis, conjunctivitis, and arthritis that now bears his name. Reiter's syndrome provides an exciting model of a chronic rheumatic disease precipitated by a specific infection (e.g., *Shigella*) in a person with a specific genetic background (HLA B27).

Definition

Reiter's syndrome is a seronegative asymmetric arthropathy (predominantly in the lower extremity) plus one or more of: urethritis or cervicitis, dysentery, inflammatory eye disease, or mucocutaneous disease (balanitis, oral ulceration, or keratodermia). Implicit in this definition is the exclusion of primary ankylosing spondylitis, psoriatic arthropathy, or other rheumatic disease.

The concept of Reiter's syndrome as a triad of features is being replaced by a more broadly based definition. Incomplete forms are recognized, and patients may have only one or two of the typical features rather than the triad or a tetrad, pentad, or more findings. The disease may also be thought of as B27-associated reactive arthropathy. However, only 80% of patients with Reiter's syndrome are B27-positive, and therefore this concept is not totally appropriate.

Historic Review

The classic triad may follow bowel infection with shigella, salmonella, or yersinia organisms. In some parts of the world, the venereal form is considered more prevalent. Much of our understanding has followed the description by Paronen and Noer of two major classic epidemics occurring in Finland in 1944 and on board a United States naval vessel in 1962, respectively. The initial reports and follow-up data have provided important clues to the nature of the condition.

Incidence and Prevalence

The incidence and prevalence of Reiter's syndrome are difficult to assess but are almost certainly underestimated since no absolute diagnostic test exists. The illness tends to affect mobile young adults; venereal (urethritis and cervicitis), ocular, enteric, or mucosal features may be overlooked; and many patients with persistent arthropathy and relatively minimal extra-articular disease are wrongly diagnosed as having seronegative rheumatoid arthritis or psoriatic or ankylosing spondylitis.

The often-quoted sex ratio of 20 men to 1 woman may well be an exaggeration. In our own study of over 100 patients, 13% were women. It is likely that women are often misdiagnosed for the reasons mentioned above. Reiter's syndrome is most frequently seen in men during the latter part of the second and third decades. However, no age is immune.

Etiology

The relationship between genetics and the environment, as they pertain to Reiter's syndrome, is slowly becoming understood. It is hoped that within the next few years, the reasons certain organisms precipitate the disease in certain persons will become more clear. At the moment, there are only a few exciting leads to follow.

To date, it is recognized that *Chlamydia* probably causes Reiter's syndrome, and the *Shigella flexneri I* and *IIa* definitely do.

Clinical Features

Almost every system in the body may be affected by the syndrome. The prevalence of different features seen in 131 consecutive patients by the author are summarized in Table 13.3. Polyarthritis and urethritis (or cervicitis) were seen in over 90% of patients. The third most common event was back pain, often due to insertional tendinitis, in over two-thirds of patients. The patient must be examined closely to find balanitis (asymptomatic hyperkeratotic lesions on the glans penis), stomatitis, and keratodermia (psoriaform-like lesions on the soles, palms, and elsewhere), all clinically silent phenomena.

Every patient appearing with a mono- or oligoarthropathy, especially involving a lower limb joint, must be questioned about possible urethritis, balanitis, eye disease, and mouth ulcers.

In a typical patient, there is a latent period between the onset of diarrhea or urethritis and the rheumatologic syndrome. This interval may last 1 to 3 weeks. Certain features of the disorder may occur only after 20 or 30 years of disease activity. For example, aortic regurgitation and the typical spinal deformities mimicking ankylosing spondylitis occur only late in the course of the disease.

The arthritis may be acute, short-lived, and transient. However, only a fortunate patient has a self-limiting disease. For others, arthralgias, monoarthritis, polyarthritis, tendinitis, fasciitis, and spinal symptoms recur or persist. A "sausage toe" represents a typical enthesopathic lesion. Ankle and/or heel pain with or without spinal symptoms presents a major chronic problem for up to a third of patients.

Table 13.3. Characteristics at Diagnosis of 131 Consecutive Patients with Reiter's Syndrome

Feature	*Percent*
Arthritis	100
Monoarticular	4
Polyarticular	96
Urethritis/cervicitis	90
Diarrhea	18
Eye disease	63
Back pain	72
Heel pain	56
Tendinitis	52
Mucocutaneous lesions	79
Oral	27
Balanitis	46
Nails	6
Keratodermia	22

Achilles tendinitis, plantar fasciitis, and other insertional tendinitides help distinguish the arthritic component from that seen in rheumatoid arthritis.

The urethritis (or cystitis) may be a postdysenteric phenomenon (i.e., a primary feature of the disease) or a precipitating event. In the latter case, chlamydia and *Ureaplasma urealyticum* may be cultured. However, other organisms may be relevant.

Conjunctivitis, a conjunctival reaction to uveitis, or uveitis alone may occur. When mild, the symptoms and signs escape notice. The mucocutaneous manifestations mimic those seen in psoriasis (see below). However, palmar and plantar keratodermia blennorrhagica is a relatively typical event in a patient with Reiter's syndrome. The circinate balanitis is almost specific for Reiter's syndrome. Whether the ankylosing spondylitis should be considered a complication of Reiter's syndrome or a manifestation of the HLA B27 status remains unclear.

Nonspecific features include fatigue, malaise, weight loss, fever, and mental changes.

Radiologic Evaluation

Sacroiliitis, indistinguishable from that seen in ankylosing spondylitis, may occur. Sometimes asymmetric pelvic disease is noticed, and there may be spotty changes in the extrapelvic spine with sporadic syndesmophytes. Elsewhere, periostitis and other evidence of bony reaction at the site of tendon insertion into bone may be noticed. Asymmetric erosive disease of peripheral joints is occasionally seen. In contrast to rheumatoid arthritis, this change is spotty and often limited to a single small joint, often of the foot (see Chap. 5).

Laboratory Evaluation and HLA

The erythrocyte sedimentation rate may vary from 1 to 130 mm per hour. There appears to be little correlation between disease activity and this variable. Synovial fluid analysis is rarely contributory. Although synovial fluid complement levels are said to be raised in Reiter's syndrome, in contrast to depressed levels in rheumatoid disease, the physician should not have to rely on this laboratory finding to distinguish two readily separable diseases. The presence of "Reiter's cells" in the synovial fluid is no longer considered specific.

HLA B27 is of great academic interest. However, routine typing for this antigen should be unnecessary and considered an expensive test. There now seems to be little difference between HLA B27-positive and B27-negative disease. Moreover, since at least 20% of patients with classic disease are B27-negative, the test cannot be relied on too strongly. The same comments may be made for genetic counseling as for ankylosing spondylitis.

As with ankylosing spondylitis, the link between B27 and disease is less clear in nonwhites. The reason for this is unknown.

Natural History and Prognosis

Reiter's syndrome cannot be considered a benign disease. Although some patients have a self-limiting disease, as many as 25% have a persistent chronic disorder that may necessitate a change in job or loss of employment.

Management

Patients frequently have a feeling of guilt, even when the urethritis is a manifestation of the disease process rather than the precipitating event. It may be helpful to explain to the patient that the urethritis is an allergic event rather than an expression of sexual misbehavior.

The articular problems may respond to indomethacin (25–50 mg tid), phenylbutazone (100 mg tid), or one of the newer nonsteroidal agents. For those unfortunate patients whose disease progresses despite adequate anti-inflammatory therapy, azathioprine or other cytotoxic agents may be required. Corticosteroids, gold, and penicillamine appear to play no role in the management of this disease, apart from an occasional intra-articular or intralesional steroidal injection. The eye and skin lesions may require no therapy or derive no benefit from local steroid treatment.

Reiter's Syndrome versus Gonococcal Disease

The major similarities and differences between Reiter's syndrome and gonococcal arthritis are summarized in Table 13.4. In essence, Reiter's syndrome should be

Table 13.4. Comparison between Reiter's Syndrome and Gonococcal Arthropathy

	Reiter's Syndrome	Gonoccal Arthropathy
Sex distribution	M > F	M < F
Personal or family history of arthritis	+	−
Sexual activity	+	+
Fever	+	+
Urethritis	+	+
Conjunctivitis	+	−
Uveitis	+	+
Skin lesions	+	+
Balanitis	+	−
Keratodermia blennorragghica	+	−
Stomatitis	+	−
Back pain	+	−
Achilles tendinitis/fasciitis	+	−
Tenosynovitis	+	+
Migratory arthralgias	−	+
Oligoarthritis	+	+
Joint distribution	Lower > upper	Lower < upper
Synovial fluid	Inflammatory	Inflammatory
GC culture	−	+/−
HLA B27 (%)	80	5
Response to penicillin	−	+

considered the most frequent cause of an inflammatory oligoarthropathy in a young man, in contrast to gonococcal arthritis, which is much more prevalent in young women.

Reiter's Syndrome versus Psoriatic Arthropathy

The similarities and differences between Reiter's syndrome and psoriatic arthropathy are summarized in Table 13.5.

REACTIVE ARTHRITIDES

The term *reactive arthropathy* may be defined as an inflammatory arthritis related to an infective agent without microbial invasion of the synovial space. These predominantly B27-linked arthropathies follow shigella, salmonella, and yersinia infection. Shigella arthritis has been described earlier as postdysenteric Reiter's syndrome.

Reiter's syndrome (or reactive arthropathy) follows both S. enteritides and *S. typhimurium* infection. As discussed previously, about 20% of HLA B-27 positive salmonella patients will develop arthritis.

Yersinia arthritis is similar to postdysenteric Reiter's disease. Following intestinal infection with *Y. enterocolitica,* patients develop acute peripheral arthritis a few weeks later. Women are affected as frequently as men. Skin, mucous

Table 13.5. Comparison between Reiter's Syndrome and Psoriatic Arthropathy

	Reiter's Syndrome	*Psoriatic Arthropathy*
Age	20–30	Any age
Sex distribution	10 men:1 woman	3 women:2 men
Onset	Acute	Insidious
Eye disease	+	+
Skin lesions	Plantar, palmar, penile	Widespread
Relationship of arthritis to severity of skin lesions	−	+
Nail involvement	+	+
Mouth ulcers	+	−
Urethritis	+	−
Axial disease	25%	25%
Peripheral joint disease	+	+
Joint predilection	Lower limb	Upper limb
Distal interphalangeal joints	−	+
HLA	B27 (80%)	B27 (20%–50%), B13, BW17, BW38

membrane, and eye lesions are uncommon. Rarely, sacroiliitis or uveitis are seen.

PSORIATIC ARTHROPATHY

The association between psoriasis and arthritis has been recognized for several decades. Psoriatic arthropathy is considered a distinct entity. The inflammatory asymmetric oligoarthropathy appears to be enthesopathic rather than synovitic. Uveitis, sacroiliitis, and spinal disease may occur in up to 20% of cases.

Psoriasis itself is a genetically determined disease, associated with HLA B13 and BW17. HLA B27 is present in some 20% of persons with psoriatic arthropathy, and more recently, HLA BW38 has been shown to be associated with the peripheral joint disease.

Several different forms of psoriatric arthropathy are recognized, including an asymmetric oligoarthropathy, an asymmetric polyarthropathy resembling rheumatoid disease, an arthritis mutilans, psoriatic spondylitis, and psoriatic nail disease in conjunction with distal interphalangeal joint involvement. The essential differences between psoriatic arthropathy and Reiter's syndrome have been summarized in Table 13.5.

Dactylitis is a common finding in psoriatic arthropathy. Swelling of the proximal interphalangeal joint as well as the distal, together with flexor tenosynovitis, may impart a sausage shape to the digit. The distal joint involvement group has a male predominance. The deforming group, seen in about 5% of all patients with psoriatic arthropathy, may result in the classic "main en lorgnette." Whittling of bone and an associated periosteal reaction may produce a pencil-in-cup appearance.

The spondylitis associated with psoriasis is said to mimic that seen with Reiter's syndrome, in contrast to the more symmetric sacroiliitis and spondylitis seen in primary ankylosing spondylitis and inflammatory bowel disease.

Treatment includes use of indomethacin, phenylbutazone, and the other nonsteroidal anti-inflammatory drugs. These agents are more useful than aspirin. The psoriaform skin lesions should be treated as in any patient with psoriasis. The skin disease may remain clinically and pathologically indistinguishable from the keratodermia blennorrhagica seen in Reiter's syndrome.

ENTEROPATHIC ARTHROPATHY

Ulcerative colitis and regional enteritis (Crohn's disease) may be associated with arthritis. There are two rheumatic syndromes: (1) a peripheral arthropathy and (2) a seronegative spondylarthropathy. The first is a relatively mild, asymmetric involvement of the large joints associated with excerbation of the underlying intestinal inflammation and results in little deformity. This syndrome appears to be a complication of severe inflammatory bowel disease. Treatment is directed at the bowel involvement, and the arthritis remits as the bowel disease is brought under control. Thus, surgery is always successful, at least in ulcerative colitis, where the entire affected bowel can be resected. The peripheral arthropathy is considered a complication of severe disease, in contrast to the axial arthropathy

Table 13.6. Comparison of the Seronegative Spondylarthritides

	Ankylosing Spondylitis	Reiter's Disease	Psoriatic Arthropathy	Intestinal Arthropathy	Reactive Arthropathy	Juvenile Polyarthropathy
Age	20+	20+	Any age	Any age	Any age	<25
Sex	M $\geqq$ F	M $\geqq$ F	F $\geqq$ M	F = M	M = F	M $\geqq$ F
Familial aggregation	+	+	+	+	+	+
Onset	Gradual	Sudden	Variable	Peripheral joint:sudden Sacroiliac joint:gradual	Sudden	Variable
Conjunctivitis/uveitis	+/+	+++/++	+/+	+/+	+/+	+/++
Urethritis/prostatitis	−/+	+/+	−/+	+/+	+/?	−/−
Mucous membrane	−	+	−	(+)	$\pm$	−
Aortic regurgitation	+	+	?+	?	+	?
Spine	+++	+	+	$\pm$	+	$\pm$
Peripheral joints	25% Lower $\geqq$ upper	90% Lower > upper	90% Upper > lower	$\pm$ Lower > upper	90% Lower > upper	90% Upper = lower
Symmetry	+	−	−	+	$\pm$	$\pm$
Rheumatoid nodules	<1%	<1%	<1%	<1%	<1%	<1%
Rheumatoid factor	<5%	<5%	<5%	<5%	<5%	<10%
HLA B27	90%	90%	20%	5%	90%	20%
Self-limiting	−	+	$\pm$	$\pm$	$\pm$	$\pm$
Remissions	−	+	+	$\pm$	$\pm$	$\pm$

(sacroiliitis and spondylitis) that appears to be a manifestation of a similar genetic background. The latter form is considered a seronegative spondylarthropathy.

Sacroiliitis, usually bilateral, is seen, and ascending spinal changes may occur. Eye problems are common, and aortic insufficiency has been reported. This syndrome may precede the development of the intestinal disease, and in some cases two diseases may occur coincidentally in HLA B27-positive subjects. On other occasions, the articular symptoms follow the development of the intestinal inflammatory condition. About 50% of patients with inflammatory bowel disease spondylitis are B27-positive. Some 20% of patients with inflammatory bowel disease develop sacroiliitis or spondylitis.

Nonsteroidal anti-inflammatory drugs are useful but must be employed with caution because of the preexisting intestinal inflammation.

JUVENILE CHRONIC POLYARTHROPATHY

The old term *juvenile rheumatoid arthritis* is no longer appropriate. It is now apparent that children may have several forms of arthritis and that most of these forms are not analogous to adult rheumatoid arthritis. Some children have an illness quite similar to ankylosing spondylitis, albeit with more peripheral joint disease. These children, frequently boys, with HLA B27 may be considered to have spondylarthropathy. Other subsets include seropositive juvenile rheumatoid arthritis, a seronegative inflammatory oligoarthropathy, a systemic onset Still's disease that mimics infection or malignancy and other groups that are now becoming differentiated. These subsets are described in the previous chapter.

CONCLUSION

The seronegative spondylarthritides, whose clinical features are summarized in Table 13.6, form a major subsection within the field of rheumatology. The group is now undergoing extensive investigation. Appreciation of the close link between genetics and environment in these disorders will almost certainly elucidate similar problems in other branches of rheumatology.

BIBLIOGRAPHY

Bennet PH, Burch TA: *Population Studies of the Rheumatic Diseases.* Amsterdam, Excerpta Medica Foundation (Int. Long. Sev. No. 148), 1968.

Calin A: Reiter's syndrome. *Med Clin North Am* 61:365, 1977.

Calin A: HLA-B27: To type or not to type. *Ann Intern Med* 92:208, 1980.

Calin A, Fries JF: An "experimental" epidemic of Reiter's syndrome, revisited: Follow-up evidence of genetic and environmental factors. *Ann Intern Med* 84:564, 1976.

Calin A, Fries JF: *Ankylosing Spondylitis: Discussions in Patient Management.* Garden City, NY, Medical Examination Publishing Co, Inc, 1978.

Dausset J, Svejgaard A: *HLA and Disease.* Copenhagen, Munsgaard, 1977.

Good AE, Schultz JS: Reiter's syndrome following *Shigella flexneria 2a. Arthritis Rheum* 20:100, 1977.

Hill HFM, Hill AGS, Bodmer JG: Clinical diagnosis of ankylosing spondylitis in women and relation to presence of HLA B27. *Ann Rheum Dis* 35:267, 1976.

HLA-B27 and risk of ankylosing spondylitis, editorial. *Br Med J* 2:650, 1978.

Keat AC, Maini RN, Nkwazi GC, et al: Role of *Chlamydia trachomatis* and HLA B27 in sexually acquired reactive arthritis. *Br Med J* 1:605, 1978.

McDevitt HO, Engleman EG: Association between genes in the major histocompatibility complex and disease susceptibility. *Arthritis Rheum* 20:S9, 1977.

Noer HR: An experimental epidemic of Reiter's syndrome. *JAMA* 198:693, 1966.

Paronen I: Reiter's disease: A study of 344 cases observed in Finland. *Acta Med Scand* 131(Suppl 212):1, 1948.

Wright V, Moll JMH: *Seronegative Polyarthritis.* Amsterdam, North-Holland Publishing Co, 1976.

Part 4

SYSTEMIC RHEUMATIC DISEASES

14

Rheumatic Fever and Rheumatic Heart Disease

Stanford T. Shulman

The furious French blood-letter Jean-Baptiste Bouillaud is credited with recognizing the relationship of endocardial and pericardial inflammation to acute articular rheumatism, as reflected in his remarkable publications of 1836 and 1837. This chapter will present a modern view of the clinical, laboratory, pathologic, and therapeutic features of acute rheumatic fever (ARF) and rheumatic heart disease (RHD), with consideration of theories of pathogenesis.

CLINICAL FEATURES

Jones Criteria

No single clinical or laboratory finding is pathognomonic for ARF. Thus, in 1944 T. Duckett Jones established guidelines to aid in the diagnosis of ARF and to limit overdiagnosis. The need for such assistance in diagnosis related to the great overlap between manifestations of ARF and those of a number of other illnesses. The Jones criteria have been modified subsequently, most recently in 1965, primarily to reflect the importance of antecedent infection with group A beta-hemolytic streptococcus in the development of ARF. Indeed, the current Jones criteria (Table 14.1) indicate that the diagnosis of ARF requires evidence of preceding streptococcal infection. Two points are important in applying the Jones criteria: (1) the Jones criteria are not relevant to the diagnosis of chronic inactive rheumatic disease, except as applied retrospectively to data concerning an acute illness; (2) in certain circumstances ARF may be overdiagnosed even with strict application of the Jones criteria. This could occur, for example, if a patient with systemic lupus erythematosus, gonococcal arthritis, or rheumatoid arthritis, who coincidentally shows evidence of recent streptococcal infection, presents with migratory polyarthritis, fever, and an elevated sedimentation rate.

ARF primarily affects children and young adults, is uncommon below the age of 5 years, occurs occasionally in middle-aged and older adults, and has never been documented to occur after streptococcal skin infection.

Table 14.1. Jones Criteria (Revised) for Guidance in the Diagnosis of Rheumatic Fever

Major Criteria	*Minor Criteria*
Carditis	Clinical
Polyarthritis	Fever
Chorea	Arthralgia
Erythema marginatum	Previous rheumatic fever
Subcutaneous nodules	Laboratory
	Acute phase reactants:
	ESR, CRP, leukocytosis
	Prolonged P-R interval

Plus

Supporting evidence of preceding streptococcal infection (increased ASO or other streptococcal antibodies; positive throat culture for group A streptococcus; recent scarlet fever).

The presence of two major criteria, or of one major and two minor criteria, indicates a high probability of the presence of rheumatic fever if supported by evidence of a preceding streptococcal infection.

Major Manifestations of Acute Rheumatic Fever

Migratory Polyarthritis

Arthritis occurs in about 75% of ARF patients (Table 14.2). Classically, the arthritis of ARF involves large joints, particularly the knees, ankles, wrists, and elbows, rarely affecting the spine or small joints of the hands and feet. Hips are not commonly affected except in adults (vide infra). The inflamed joints and periarticular tissues are characteristically exquisitely tender, even the friction of bed clothes frequently making the patient very uncomfortable. Acutely inflamed rheumatic joints are generally hot, red, tender, and swollen. The tenderness and pain may precede the development of redness, heat, or swelling and may appear disproportionate to the objective findings. Most characteristic is the migratory nature of the arthritic involvement, so that a severely involved joint will become normal within 1–5 days without therapy, while one or more other large joints becomes inflamed. Untreated patients manifest an average of six joints involved, with the severe arthritic course lasting 1–2 weeks in the large majority of untreated patients. Monoarthritis is quite unusual unless anti-inflammatory therapy was begun very early. A dramatic response of rheumatic arthritis to even small doses of salicylates is also characteristic. Rheumatic arthritis is never deforming, with the possible exception of Jaccoud's chronic rheumatism, which is a process characterized by periarticular fibrosis, not synovitis, involving the metacarpophalangeal joints and which is of uncertain relation to ARF. Synovial fluid analysis in ARF generally shows 10,000 to 100,000 WBC/cu mm (predominantly PMNs), protein about 4 g/dl, normal glucose, and good mucin clot. Total hemolytic complement values and C3 levels in synovial fluid each average about 35% of the corresponding serum values. Arthritis is frequently the earliest manifestation of ARF and usually correlates in time with the peak in antibody titers. An inverse relationship between the severity of arthritis and the incidence of cardiac involvement has been reported.

Table 14.2. Clinical Features of Acute Rheumatic Fever

Arthritis
    75% of patients with ARF
    Migratory polyarthritis of large joints
    Spine, small joints of hands and feet rarely involved
    Dramatic response to ASA or steroids
    Nondeforming arthritis without chronicity
    Synovial fluid: 10,000–100,000 WBC/mm^3, predominantly PMNs,
       normal glucose, good mucin clot
Carditis
    50% of patients with ARF
    Endocarditis (valvulitis) almost always present
    Myocardial and pericardial involvement more variable
    Chronic valvular disease common, insufficiency early, stenosis late
    Mitral and/or aortic valve involvement almost exclusively
Chorea
    10% of patients with ARF
    Late onset with prolonged course
    Chronic neurologic sequelae rare
Subcutaneous nodules
    Rarely seen except in occasional patients with severe heart
      disease
    Extensor tendon surfaces
Erythema marginatum
    Rare
    Macular, nonpruritic rash
    On trunk or extremities

In recent years, it has been recognized that the articular manifestations of rheumatic fever in adults may be somewhat different from those observed in children. Lower extremity involvement is more common, initially including the knees and/or hips in 85% of patients. An additive polyarthritis may occur rather than a migratory form. Symmetric involvement is common, and involvement of such otherwise noncharacteristic joints as the sternoclavicular or cervical spine can be seen in adults with acute rheumatic fever. Pain seemingly out of proportion to clinical findings is frequently present in adults, as in children. A dramatic response of the symmetric large joint lower extremity arthritis to salicylates differentiates this form of arthritis from that associated with yersinia, salmonella, or shigella. It has been claimed that adult patients are more likely than children to appear with polyarthritis as their only major manifestation of rheumatic fever.

Carditis

Rheumatic carditis is characterized by active inflammation of the myocardium, pericardium, and endocardium, the term *pancarditis* referring to involvement of all three layers. Since only the endocardial manifestations of ARF result in long-term residua, they are clearly of greatest significance. The cardiac involvement during ARF varies in severity from fulminant exudative pancarditis, which can be fatal, to very mild transient cardiac involvement. Endocarditis, as manifested by one or more cardiac murmurs, is generally present whenever rheumatic carditis occurs, while pericarditis and myocarditis are much more variable. Myocarditis and/or pericarditis, in the absence of evidence of endocarditis, is rarely rheumatic in etiology. Isolated mitral, or aortic and mitral, valve disease constitutes the vast majority of cardiac murmurs in ARF. Isolated aortic and particularly right-sided valvular involvement is very unusual. Chronic RHD may develop either as a sequel to a documented attack of ARF or in the absence of a history suggesting an acute rheumatic episode and therefore presumably after a subclinical episode of ARF. When cardiac involvement occurs (50% of ARF), mitral insufficiency with or without aortic insufficiency is present early, with valvular stenosis developing only after several years or decades. In developing areas of the world, stenotic valvular lesions occur more often and develop sooner after ARF, although the reasons for this difference from the United States and Western Europe are unclear.

Chorea
Sydenham's chorea (St. Vitus' dance) is seen in about 10% of rheumatic patients and manifests as incoordination, emotional lability, decreased school performance, and facial grimacing, frequently exacerbated by stress. Symptoms may last from several weeks to a year, the mean duration being 2–3 months. A benign prognosis can be ascribed to Sydenham's chorea, since neurologic sequelae are rare. However, up to 25% of persons with chorea ultimately develop RHD because of recurrent attacks of ARF. This finding emphasizes the need for continuous rheumatic prophylaxis in such patients to prevent the development of RHD.

Subcutaneous Nodules
Firm nodules, approximately 1 cm in diameter, are rarely palpated along extensor surfaces of tendons near bony prominences in occasional patients with ARF. These patients most commonly have significant RHD.

Erythema Marginatum
Rare patients with ARF develop this macular nonpruritic rash with irregular borders on the trunk or extremities. Warming the skin can accentuate the rash.

Minor Manifestations of Acute Rheumatic Fever

These less specific criteria are either clinical (i.e., the presence of fever, arthralgia, or a previous history of rheumatic fever) or laboratory (i.e., prolongation of the P-R interval and the presence of acute phase reactants such as elevated sedimentation rate [ESR], positive C-reactive protein [CRP], or leukocytosis). Arthralgia can be used as a minor criterion only if arthritis is not used as a major criterion.

Recurrences of Rheumatic Fever

The single most important feature of ARF is its propensity to recur in persons who have had a previous attack. Osler recognized this trait and stated, "Not only does an attack not confer immunity, but predisposes the subject to the disease." While recurrences of ARF tend to mimic the manifestations of the first attack, a progressively greater percentage of rheumatic persons will manifest heart disease as the number of recurrences increases. For this reason, long-term antibiotic administration is recommended for prevention of recurrent ARF in all rheumatic persons, not just in those with cardiac disease (vide infra).

That both the severity and the incidence of ARF have decreased in the United States in recent decades is suggested by recent epidemiologic studies. However, there is evidence that high prevalence rates and severe ARF and RHD continue to exist in populations of low socioeconomic status and crowded living conditions.

LABORATORY FINDINGS

Acute Phase Reactants

As noted above, acute phase reactants are present in ARF and reflect the acute inflammatory process (Table 14.3). The ESR may be lower than expected in the presence of congestive heart failure. Acute phase reactants are so commonly present in ARF that their absence renders the diagnosis very tenuous.

Streptococcal Antibody Tests

Streptococcal antibody tests are necessary in most instances to provide the required evidence of recent infection with group A streptococcus for establishing the diagnosis of ARF. Antibodies of two kinds are produced following group A streptococcal infections, including those specific for an extracellular streptococcal product (e.g., anti-streptolysin O, anti-hyaluronidase, anti-desoxyribonuclease B [DNAase B], anti-streptokinase) and those specific for structural components of the streptococcal cell (e.g., antibodies to group A carbohydrate, peptidoglycan or mucopeptide, cell membrane, or M, T, and R proteins).

Antibodies to Extracellular Products
Most readily available antibody tests measure antibody to an extracellular product, such as the anti-streptolysin O (ASO) with its classic expression in Todd units

Table 14.3. Laboratory Features of Acute
Rheumatic Fever

Acute phase reactants
    Erythrocyte sedimentation rate
    C-reactive protein
    Leukocytosis
Streptococcal antibody tests
    Antibodies to extracellular products
        Anti-streptolysin O (ASO)
        Anti-desoxyribonuclease B (anti-DNAase B)
        Anti-hyaluronidase
        Anti-streptokinase
    Antibodies to cellular components
        Anti-A carbohydrate
        Anti-cell membrane
        Anti-M protein (and -R or -T proteins)

(the reciprocal of the highest serum dilution yielding a positive test). A recently available test, the Streptozyme, measures antibodies to five distinct extracellular products but must await further documentation of its accuracy and reliability. Antibodies to extracellular products are frequently present in elevated titer in patients with poststreptococcal sequelae but also in many who recently experienced uncomplicated streptococcal infection. While approximately the same percentage of patients in these categories have elevated titers, titers tend to be somewhat higher among rheumatics. However, there is sufficient overlap between those with ARF and those with uncomplicated infection to prevent very high antibody titers per se from being diagnostic for ARF.

Antibodies to Streptococcal Cellular Components

Antibodies to structural components of the streptococcal cell are of significance in a number of ways. Anti-M protein antibodies are the only antibodies known to confer immunity (albeit type-specific) to the streptococcus. Such immunity appears to be long-lived, having been documented up to 30 years. Anti-M, -T, and -R protein antibodies are also important in epidemiologic investigation of outbreaks of group A infections. Antibody to the group specific A carbohydrate develops after infection with group A streptococci and very frequently persists at elevated levels for a number of years in serum of patients with chronic inactive rheumatic valvular disease. Several antibodies to cellular components may have additional significance with regard to the presence of antigens in human cardiac tissue cross-reactive with streptococcal cellular constituents (see "Pathogenesis of Rheumatic Fever").

Interpretation of Antibody Tests

Two important points should be noted concerning interpretation of streptococcal tests. (1) The presence of an elevated streptococcal antibody titer may only support the diagnosis of ARF, for the recent streptococcal infection could be unrelated to the particular illness in question. This finding is most often true in children, many of whom have streptococcal impetigo (especially in summer) with a resultant elevation of several streptococcal antibody titers. This point emphasizes the importance of using the Jones criteria. (2) Only 80%–85% of patients with ARF will manifest elevated levels of any single streptococcal antibody test, while 95% or more will demonstrate elevation of at least one antibody assay if three different antibodies are sought. Because elevated antibody titers may persist only 3–6 months after streptococcal infection, they may be essentially normal in patients with isolated Sydenham's chorea, in which the period of latency between infection and rheumatic sequel may be as long as 6 months. This is in contrast to the latent period of the other major manifestations of rheumatic fever, which is usually 3 weeks.

PATHOLOGY OF RHEUMATIC FEVER

General Findings

Exudative and proliferative inflammation characterizes the pathology of ARF. Such inflammation may occur in the connective tissue of the heart, joints, vessels, and subcutaneous tissue and rarely in the lungs, pleura, and kidney. The Aschoff body, a distinctive pathologic finding of obscure significance within cardiac connective tissue, has long been considered pathognomonic of the rheumatic process. The Aschoff body consists of a perivascular collection of large mononuclear cells with basophilic cytoplasm and irregular nuclei surrounding a core of fibrinoid necrosis, with degenerated collagen fibers. The Aschoff body can be found not only during the active stage of rheumatic fever but also years later.

Specific Tissue Findings

The pathologic changes in and around acutely inflamed rheumatic joints consist of edema and exudative inflammation of the periarticular and synovial tissues. Fibrinoid degeneration and even Aschoff bodies can be seen on occasion. Chronic deforming changes do not occur.

Rheumatic subcutaneous nodules contain a central area of fibrinoid necrosis with surrounding fibroblasts and lymphocytes, closely resembling the Aschoff body.

In chorea, vascular changes in the brain have been described, including perivasculitis with mononuclear cells, petechial hemorrhage, and hyalinization of small vessels, without either Aschoff bodies or a consistent anatomic site of involvement.

Pathologic findings in RHD are present in the myocardium, pericardium, and endocardium. Myocardial lesions during ARF include varying degrees of inflammatory infiltration, often surprisingly sparse even in the presence of severe (even fatal) myocardial dysfunction. Aschoff bodies may develop, especially in the subendocardial regions of the left ventricle. Healing Aschoff bodies frequently become fibrotic intramyocardial scars, and significant myocardial fibrosis may develop. Acute rheumatic pericarditis is characterized by nondistinctive exudative inflammation of both visceral and parietal layers of pericardium with the formation of fibrinous exudate. Chronic pericardial changes that may be seen include adherence and fibrosis of the pericardial layers.

Rheumatic endocarditis affects both mural endocardium and valves, especially on the left side of the heart. Mural involvement characteristically produces MacCallum's patch, a thickened area of endocardium above the base of the posterior mitral leaflet. Valvular changes most frequently affect the mitral valve and its supporting structures, manifesting as mitral insufficiency, with aortic valvular disease next most frequent and usually in conjunction with mitral disease. Isolated rheumatic aortic disease is now considered rare. During ARF, acute inflammation and edema of the mitral valve and chordae tendinae are present with verrucae and edema of the valve edges. Dilatation of the mitral annulus often contributes to mitral insufficiency. Healing of the acutely involved valves frequently leads to fibrosis, shorening of valve leaflets and chordae, with resultant deformity. Fusion of valvular commissures and calcification may occur with time, with development of stenotic mitral and/or aortic orifices usually only after a number of years.

PATHOGENESIS OF RHEUMATIC FEVER

The pathogenesis of ARF and RHD remains obscure despite efforts by many investigators to clarify the mechanisms responsible for disease production and despite the recognition several decades ago that group A streptococcal infection is an essential antecedent. None of the numerous proposed pathogenetic theories has generated adequate supporting evidence to gain wide acceptance. That ARF develops only in a small fraction of persons after untreated streptococcal respiratory infection but fails to develop after adequately treated infection or after streptococcal skin infection must be explained.

Relation to Streptococcal Infection

The relationship of streptococcal infection to ARF was suggested by isolated nineteenth-century observations and by several epidemiologic studies in the 1930s. The serologic identification of group A streptococci by Lancefield in 1940 led to the recognition that infection with this particular streptococcus was the necessary antecedent of ARF. Further epidemiologic studies, primarily at Warren Air Force Base in the late 1940s and early 1950s, established that the attack rate of ARF was about 3% after untreated streptococcal respiratory infection in an epidemic situation. Subsequent work has established that somewhat lower attack rates prevail in nonepidemic settings.

Two additional lines of evidence confirmed the relationship between group A streptococcus and ARF. Todd's development of the ASO test in 1932 enabled immunologic documentation that persons with ARF but without a clinical history of antecedent streptococcal infection nevertheless showed evidence of recent streptococcal exposure. Additionally, the availability of sulfonamides and later penicillin led to the demonstration that recurrent attacks of ARF could be prevented by daily oral administration of antibiotics effective in the prevention of streptococcal infection. The efficacy of penicillin therapy in the prevention of a first attack of ARF was also established. From these and other studies, the necessity of treating streptococcal pharyngitis with 10 full days of antibiotic therapy has been recognized. Thus, in several ways, the link between rheumatic fever and group A streptococcal infection has been forged over a number of decades.

In recent years, it has been proposed that infection by viruses, particularly enteroviruses (Coxsackie and ECHO), may be involved in the pathogenesis of some cases of apparent RHD, either in concert with or independent of the streptococcus. However, at the present time, no direct evidence exists to implicate these agents in the pathogenesis of ARF or RHD.

Specific Pathogenetic Mechanisms

The proposed pathogenetic mechanisms for rheumatic fever generally fall into three categories: (1) persistent streptococcal infection, (2) reaction to a toxic streptococcal product or component, and (3) immunologic response to a group A streptococcal component or product. The lack of an adequate animal model for rheumatic fever has clearly contributed to the difficulty of proving pathogenetic mechanisms, resulting in a proliferation of theories.

Persistent Streptococcal Infection

The possibility that ARF represents persistent infection with group A streptococci in some form within the affected tissues has failed to attract significant supporting data. Early studies reporting the isolation of group A streptococci from rheumatic heart valves could not be confirmed. In addition, therapy with massive doses of penicillin failed to modify the activity of ARF. The persistence of L-forms derived from group A streptococci in tissues has been suggested, but the inability of tetracycline to alter ARF failed to support this concept.

Toxic Reaction

McCarty has stated, "the success of the biochemical and immunochemical studies of group A streptococci has produced a proliferation of theories of pathogenesis. In fact, even the bacteriologist without medical training has been lured into the trap of trying to relate his favorite streptococcal product to the genesis of rheumatic fever." Despite extensive investigations with streptolysin O, streptolysin S, proteinase, and DNAase B, in which toxic properties can be demonstrated, no conclusive evidence has been presented to implicate any of these or other extracellular products in the pathogenesis of ARF. Toxic effects of constituents of the streptococcal cell wall have been demonstrated, with focal cardiac lesions developing after intraperitoneal injection of sonicated cell walls into mice and arthritis after intraperitoneal injection into guinea pigs or rats. This phenomenon has been shown to be due to complexes of cell wall peptidoglycan and carbohydrate, but its relation to clinical rheumatic fever remains obscure.

Immunologic Theories

Several features support the thesis that the immune system is intimately involved in the pathogenesis of ARF: (1) the clinical similarity of this disease to certain diseases that clearly have immunopathogenetic mechanisms, (2) the presence of the latent period between streptococcal infection and ARF, and (3) the antigenicity of such a variety of streptococcal products and constituents.

The finding of higher mean streptococcal antibody levels among patients with ARF led to the hypothesis that rheumatic persons are immunologic hyper-responders. Studies employing typhoid vaccine, influenza, pneumococcal polysaccharide, and diphtheria toxoid failed to demonstrate increased responsiveness of rheumatic patients, although higher antibody levels following *Brucella abortus* vaccine were observed. Recent studies have suggested that the *quality* of antibody produced by rheumatic persons (as reflected by the finding of lower affinity of antibody to streptococcal A carbohydrate) differs from that of patients with uncomplicated streptococcal infection. Although immunoglobulin and complement have been shown to be deposited in rheumatic myocardial tissue, there is no definite evidence of classic immune complex disease. Serum complement levels are generally elevated in ARF.

Slowly accumulating evidence has suggested the possibility of an autoimmune pathogenesis of ARF. Several antigenic systems cross-reactive between group A streptococcal components and cardiac tissue have been described in the last 15 years. An immunologic relationship between human cardiac myofibrils and a streptococcal M protein-associated antigen was demonstrated. Cross-reactivity between human myocardial sarcolemmal membrane and streptococcal cell membrane was also found. Perhaps the most significant cross-reactive system reported to date is that between structural glycoprotein of bovine and human heart valves and the streptococcal cell wall A carbohydrate. This system is of particular interest because valvular involvement is clearly central to the rheumatic process and because of the finding of persistently elevated levels of antibody to the group A carbohydrate for years in sera of patients with chronic inactive RHD. These findings raise the possibility that antibody elicited by a component of the group A streptococcus and cross-reactive with a hidden valvular constituent could be involved in the pathogenesis of ARF and RHD. Definite supportive evidence for this theory, however, is still lacking.

The presence of serum antibody with reactivity to subthalamic and caudate nuclei in patients with chorea has been reported recently, further suggesting an autoimmune process. These antibodies could be adsorbed by group A but not group D streptococcal cell membranes.

Other possible mechanisms of immunopathogenesis involve T lymphocytes, cellular cytotoxicity, or antibody-dependent cellular cytotoxicity. Few data are available, although it was recently reported that migration of peripheral leukocytes from rheumatic persons was inhibited in the presence of group A streptococcal cell membrane antigens. The significance of this finding remains unclear at present.

THERAPY FOR RHEUMATIC FEVER

Acute Attacks

Treatment for ARF includes a 10-day course of penicillin or erythromycin in doses adequate to eradicate streptococcal infection (e.g., 1.2 million units of benzathine penicillin IM), as well as a course of anti-inflammatory medications (Table 14.4). Commonly used anti-inflammatory agents are salicylates and gluco-

Table 14.4. Treatment of Rheumatic Fever

Acute rheumatic fever
  Antistreptococcal therapy
    1.2×10^6 units benzathine penicillin IM *or*
    10 days oral penicillin or erythromycin
  Anti-inflammatory agents
    Aspirin: 50–100 mg/kg/day in four doses for patients without
      cardiac disease or with mild carditis *or*
    Corticosteroids: Prednisone 2 mg/kg/day in four doses for 2–4 weeks
      for patients with moderate to severe carditis
  Cardiac drugs
    Diuretic therapy as indicated
    Cautious digitalization as indicated
Chronic rheumatic disease
  Rheumatic prophylaxis to prevent recurrent acute attacks
    1.2×10^6 units LA Bicillin (benzathine) IM monthly *or*
    Sulfadiazine 500 mg po BID *or*
    Penicillin G 250 mg po BID
  Bacterial endocarditis prophylaxis (for subjects with chronic cardiac
    disease)

corticosteroids (prednisone). The available controlled studies comparing salicylates and steroids in ARF, and assessing the ultimate incidence of residual cardiac disease 1–10 years later, provide no consistent evidence that steroids prevent cardiac damage. Corticosteroids will, however, promptly decrease the acute inflammation involving cardiac, synovial, and other tissues and can be life-saving.

Patients with ARF who manifest joint symptoms without cardiac disease should be treated with salicylates administered at 50–100 mg/kg/day to maintain a blood level of 25–30 mg/dl. Salicylates should not be initiated until the diagnosis of ARF is established, for an initial period of observation to document migratory polyarthritis is most useful in establishing the diagnosis. Salicylates are generally extremely effective in producing a resolution of arthritis and should be maintained 2 weeks at full dosage and another 2–3 weeks at one-third to one-half the dosage. Patients with ARF with mild to moderate carditis (defined as lacking evidence for significant cardiomegaly or congestive heart failure) should also receive salicylates, but for a total course of 6–8 weeks. Corticosteroids (usually prednisone) are reserved for ARF patients who manifest substantial cardiac involvement, with cardiomegaly and/or congestive heart failure and/or pericarditis. Prednisone is usually administered at 2 mg/kg/day for 2–4 weeks, with the addition of salicylates as steroids are withdrawn over several weeks.

Chronic Rheumatic Disease

Rheumatic individuals require one or both of two distinct forms of prophylactic medications after the acute phase of rheumatic fever.

Rheumatic Prophylaxis

All rheumatic patients with or without cardiac involvement should receive rheumatic fever prophylaxis to prevent recurrences of ARF by the prevention of streptococcal pharyngitis. Three standard prophylactic regimens are adequate, presented in their order of preference: (1) monthly intramuscular injections of 1.2 million units of benzathine penicillin, (2) 500-mg tablets of sulfadiazine twice daily, and (3) 125–250-mg tablets of penicillin G twice daily.

The advantage of parenteral benzathine penicillin lies in the fact that one does not depend upon patient compliance; however, the injections may be painful. Strict compliance with this regimen not only prevents recurrent attacks of ARF but may allow apparent healing of cardiac lesions with a resultant disappearance of murmurs in up to 70% of patients with acute rheumatic mitral insufficiency within 7 years. The advantage of sulfadiazine over oral penicillin relates primarily to the induction of penicillin-resistant oral flora by the latter, which could subsequently predispose to an episode of bacterial endocarditis with penicillin-resistant organisms. For the rare patient allergic to both penicillin and sulfa, erythromycin has been suggested for rheumatic fever prophylaxis. A subject of some controversy is the duration of rheumatic prophylaxis. Most, including the American Heart Association, recommend lifetime prophylaxis for patients with RHD, while many physicians feel that such prophylaxis can be discontinued safely in the patient without cardiac involvement at age 21 years or 5 years after the last attack of ARF. The author recommends that lifetime prophylaxis be provided for all rheumatic individuals, since well-documented recurrences are known many years after ARF. The greatest risk for recurrences is within the first 5 years after an attack of ARF.

SBE Prophylaxis

In addition to prophylaxis designed to prevent rheumatic recurrences, patients with RHD also should receive antibiotics for the prevention of subacute bacterial endocarditis (SBE). Revised recommendations by the American Heart Association for antibiotics to precede and to follow dental extractions or procedures and genitourinary or gastrointestinal tract surgery or instrumentation have been published recently.

BIBLIOGRAPHY

Ad hoc committee to revise the Jones criteria (modified) of the Council on Rheumatic Fever and Congenital Heart Disease: *Circulation* 32:664, 1965.

Committee on Rheumatic Fever and Bacterial Endocarditis of the Council on Cardiovascular Disease on the Young of the American Heart Association: Prevention of rheumatic fever. *Circulation* 55:1, 1977.

Committee on Rheumatic Fever and Bacterial Endocarditis of the Council on Cardiovascular Disease in the Young of the American Heart Association: Prevention of bacterial endocarditis. *Circulation* 56:139A, 1977.

Denny FW Jr, Wannamaker LW, Brink WR, et al: Prevention of rheumatic fever: Treatment of the preceding streptococcal infection. *JAMA* 194:151, 1950.

Dudding BA, Ayoub EM: Persistence of streptococcal group A antibody in patients with rheumatic valvular disease. *J Exp Med* 128:1081, 1968.

Goldstein I, Halpern B, Robert L: Immunologic relationship between streptococcus A polysaccharide and the structural glycoproteins of heart valve. *Nature* 213:44, 1967.

Grahame R, Mitchell ABS, Scott JT: Chronic post-rheumatic fever (Jaccoud's) arthropathy. *Ann Rheum Dis* 29:622, 1970.

Jones TD: Diagnosis of rheumatic fever. *JAMA* 126:481, 1944.

Kaplan MH, Svec KH: Immunologic relation of streptococcal and tissue antigens. *J Exp Med* 119:651, 1964.

Lancefield RC: Specific relationship of cell composition to biological activity of hemolytic streptococci. *Harvey Lect* 36:251, 1940–1941.

Markowitz M, Gordis L: *Rheumatic Fever,* ed. 2. Philadelphia, WB Saunders Co, 1972.

McCarty M: in Wannamaker LW and Matsen JM (eds): *Streptococci* and *Streptococcal Diseases,* New York, Academic Press, Inc, 1972, p. 518.

McDanald EC, Weisman MH: Articular manifestations of rheumatic fever in adults. *Ann Int Med* 89:917, 1978.

Osler W: *The Principles and Practice of Medicine,* New York, Appleton and Co., 1892, p. 275.

Shulman ST, Ayoub EM: Qualitative and quantitative aspects of the human antibody response to streptococcal group A carbohydrate. *J Clin Invest* 54:990, 1974.

Stollerman GH: *Rheumatic Fever and Streptococcal Infection.* New York, Grune and Stratton, Inc, 1975.

Taranta A, Kleinberg E, Feinstein AR: Rheumatic fever in children and adolescents. V. Relation of the rheumatic fever recurrence rate per streptococcal infection to pre-existing clinical features of the patients. *Ann Intern Med* 60 (Suppl 5):58, 1964.

Todd EW: Antigenic streptococcal hemolysin. *J Exp Med* 55:267, 1932.

Tompkins DG, Boxerbaum B, Liebman J: Long-term prognosis of rheumatic fever patients receiving regular intramuscular benzathine penicillin. *Circulation* 45:543, 1972.

U.K. and U.S. Joint Report: The natural history of rheumatic fever and rheumatic heart disease: Cooperative clinical trial of ACTH, cortisone, and aspirin. *Circulation* 32: 457, 1965.

Wannamaker LW, Matsen JM (eds): *Streptococci and Streptococcal Diseases.* New York, Academic Press, Inc, 1972.

Zabriskie JB, Freimer EH: An immunological relationship between the group A streptococcus and mammalian muscle. *J Exp Med* 124:661, 1966.

15

Sjögren's Syndrome

Norman A. Cummings

Sjögren's syndrome is now recognized as an important and rather common symptom complex frequently associated with rheumatic diseases. This chapter will discuss the clinical aspects of this entity and emphasize the various diagnostic aids available to characterize the syndrome. A section on etiology will present some current theories of pathogenesis and delineate the concept of defining Sjögren's syndrome as part of an overall spectrum of lymphoreticular disorders. Finally, some general concepts will be given outlining principles of therapy of the various aspects of the syndrome.

Sjögren's syndrome is a clinical triad of xerophthalmia (dry eyes), xerostomia (dry mouth), and rheumatism (i.e., a rheumatic disease). In order to make the diagnosis, only two of these three findings are necessary and are in fact usually the first two mentioned. The combination of keratitis and conjunctivitis from dryness (i.e., keratoconjunctivitis sicca or KCS) and xerostomia is called the *sicca complex*. Thus if a patient appears with a sicca complex alone, and other causes can be ruled out, then criteria for the diagnosis of Sjögren's syndrome will have been satisfied.

Among patients with this triad, the rheumatic disease is rheumatoid arthritis in about one-half of the cases seen, but systemic lupus erythematosus also accounts for a large proportion of patients. In some series, more than 10% of patients with systemic lupus erythematosus will have that disease as part of Sjögren's syndrome. Other rheumatic diseases, such as progressive systemic sclerosis and polymyositis, have also been described in conjunction with the sicca complex. In addition, about 5% of patients with Sjögren's syndrome have been noted to have liver disease (usually chronic active hepatitis or primary biliary cirrhosis), and a slightly smaller proportion have fibrosing alveolitis (Table 15.1). In general, perhaps one-half to three-quarters of all patients with Sjögren's syndrome have the complete triad with one or another rheumatic disease; the remainder have sicca complex alone, sometimes referred to as the *incomplete form* of Sjögren's syndrome.

CLINICAL ASPECTS

The syndrome is usually seen in women around the age of 50 or more. It most often appears with the insidious development of the sicca complex; usually the

Table 15.1. Some Conditions Associated
with Sjögren's Syndrome

Rheumatoid arthritis
Systemic lupus erythematosus
Progressive systemic sclerosis
Polymyositis
Polyarteritis nodosa
Renal tubular acidosis
Fibrosing alveolitis
Primary biliary cirrhosis
Pancreatitis
Xerodermia
Peripheral neuritis
Cryoglobulinemia
Purpura
Pseudolymphoma
Lymphoma

patient has already had rheumatoid arthritis for several years. In only about 10% of cases of the complete syndrome will the eye and mouth findings precede the arthritis.

In the mouth, possibly because of the absence of salivary wash, rampant caries may occur. The mucosa is white and stiff, and gingivitis is not uncommon. Symptoms may vary from slight feelings of xerostomia upon awakening to almost continual distress. Common complaints may include a feeling that the mucosal surface adheres to the patient's teeth, inability of patients to wash and brush food out of their mouth after eating, necessity for alternating food with fluid in order to swallow, and inability to sleep without some oral lubricant. Dry foods, such as toast and crackers, are especially poorly tolerated.

Symptoms of lacrimal insufficiency may also be paramount. Here the patient may complain of dry feelings in the eyes, often exacerbated by breezes or smoke, a gritty sensation, other symptoms of conjunctivitis, and an inability to form tears normally when crying.

Bedside examination of these patients may reveal a normal tear film and injection from conjunctivitis or keratitis. However, a detailed ophthalmologic examination, using a slit-lamp and appropriate stain (either rose bengal or fluorescein), will often show the characteristic filamentary keratitis caused by the drying, with changes located on either side of the limbus and extending to the canthi of the eyes.

One-third to one-half of patients will experience enlargement of the salivary glands, usually the parotid, at some time during the course of their disease. Such an enlargement is either unilateral or symmetric and can be either insidious or rapid. The glands may be tender and even erythematous, and a sticky purulent discharge can sometimes be "milked" out of Stensen's duct.

In addition to dryness of the eyes and mouth, Sjögren's syndrome is not infrequently associated with signs and symptoms that may be related to dryness in other parts of the body. Thus there seems to be an increased incidence of otitis externa (probably due to cerumen impaction secondary to deficient secretion), bronchitis, vaginal dryness, and even dryness of the skin. Renal involvement is frequently noted. Most common are reports of renal tubular acidosis type I, which may be associated with interstitial nephritis and tubular atrophy, and a decrease in concentrating ability. In addition, there have been several reports of focal glomerulonephritis, immune complex glomerulonephritis with deposition of IgM and C3, and necrotizing arteritis. The association of Sjögren's syndrome with primary biliary cirrhosis, chronic active hepatitis, other forms of chronic liver disease, and fibrosing alveolitis has been mentioned. Purpura, especially of the lower extremities, can be associated with hyperglobulinemia. In addition, there seems to be an increased incidence of lymphoproliferative malignancies associated with Sjögren's syndrome; this manifestation will be discussed more fully under "Etiologic Aspects."

DIAGNOSTIC ASPECTS

Clinical Aids

In addition to characteristic signs and symptoms, a Schirmer's test is sometimes useful to document decreased tear flow. In this test, a standardized strip of filter paper is put in the lower conjunctival sac and the amount of wetting in millimeters is measured after 5 minutes. Characteristically, patients with severe xerophthalmia will have less than 5 mm of wetting for each 5-minute period, whereas many normal persons will have more than 15 mm in the same time period. However, differences may occur because of other diseases such as diabetes, malnutrition, or infection. In addition, there is a decrease in tear flow with age, so that many older persons will exhibit diminished lacrimal secretions by this test. Idiopathic xerophthalmia has also been described. Perhaps more useful than the Schirmer's test is the demonstration of filamentary keratitis in the air-exposed areas of the eye with the aid of biomicroscopic examination after staining with rose bengal.

Salivary flow rates can also be measured and are characteristically low. Measuring salivary flow is analogous to measuring tear flow; it is used as an adjunct to diagnosis. Patients with rheumatoid disease who may be mouth breathers or who have particularly fetid breath, or persons with systemic lupus erythematosus and a question of neurotic thirst, for example, are types of patients in whom salivary flow might have some value clinically. In this technique, a small double-barreled suction cup is usually put over Stensen's duct and held in place by mild suction; the patient is then stimulated by an appropriate sialogogue, such as lemon juice. The flow from the parotid is measured after 5 minutes. Normal subjects often secrete 1 ml or more of saliva in 5 minutes from each parotid gland.

Laboratory Aids

No specific laboratory abnormality is found in patients with Sjögren's syndrome. As in many other chronic inflammatory disorders, the erythrocyte sedimentation rate may be elevated, especially during times of disease activity. It is also not uncommon for patients to have some elevation in serum IgM concentration.

One interesting facet of the syndrome is the occurrence in some patients' sera of an antibody directed against the cytoplasm of normal salivary gland ducts (antisalivary duct antibody, ASDA). This antibody can be detected by an indirect immunofluorescent technique, usually using sections of normal submaxillary gland obtained from postoperative and postmortem specimens. Patients with sicca complex alone have a relatively low incidence of ASDA (10%–20%). This rate is lower even than that of patients with only rheumatoid arthritis, in whom the antibody has been detected in 30%–40% of the cases. However, patients with the complete triad of Sjögren's syndrome have positive tests for ASDA in 60%–75% of the cases.

It is also notable that the vast majority of patients with Sjögren's syndrome, either complete or incomplete, have rheumatoid factor in their serum. Thus this IgM anti-IgG antibody, usually detected by latex fixation or bentonite flocculation, is found in over 90% of patients with Sjögren's syndrome. Cryoglobulinemia has been noted frequently, usually of the mixed type, representing IgM rheumatoid factor reacting with the patient's IgG.

Other signs of disordered immunity have also been described. Thus more than 50% of sera from patients with sicca complex have precipitating antibodies to a soluble nuclear antigen extracted from lymphoid cells referred to as SS A, and SS B, or Ha, whereas only 5%–10% of sera from patients with rheumatoid arthritis and sicca complex contain such antibodies. In addition, there may be impaired cellular immunity, reflected by decreased responsiveness of peripheral blood lymphocytes to phytohemagglutinin, especially in those patients with the complete triad.

HLA-B8 antigen was increased in populations with sicca syndrome alone but decreased in patients with Sjögren's syndrome and rheumatoid arthritis. Similarly, these populations displayed frequencies of B-cell alloantigens, especially DW-3, different from normals and from one another.

Radiologic Aids

Secretory sialography has been used to assess the degree of involvement of the major salivary glands in Sjögren's syndrome. Various patterns of sialectasia, that is, ectasia of the ducts, have been described. They include punctate, globular, and cavitary changes. The disadvantages of these techniques are that the procedure can be quite painful for the patient and can itself result in parotitis. In addition, the findings are relatively late and not necessarily specific for Sjögren's syndrome.

Salivary gland scintigraphy is essentially a technetium 99^m scan of the salivary glands, which is safe and objective. In this technique, scintiphotographs are taken periodically for the first hour after injection, so that a dynamic, rather than a routine static, oral view is obtained. The scans are classified according to how rapidly the isotope is taken up, how actively it is concentrated by the glands, and how promptly it is secreted into the oral cavity. These scans have been shown to correlate well with clinical symptoms of xerostomia, salivary flow rates, and findings in late disease on secretory sialography. They do not correlate with ASDA or histology.

Biopsy Aids

The pathologic basis of glandular disorder in Sjögren's syndrome seems to be a lymphoid infiltrative process. It has been found that the ubiquitous minor salivary glands of the lower lip or palate are involved in this same process that had previously been seen in the major salivary glands. Therefore a simple lower lip or palate biopsy, performed under local anesthesia, can supply ample material for histologic classification without the risk of facial nerve injury or parotitis that parotid biopsy may carry.

A normal biopsy from the lip of a control subject will usually reveal acinar tissue as well as ducts from accessory salivary glands. Slight or 1+ infiltration of the connective tissue between acini and ducts may occasionally be seen; the infiltrates are usually made up of plasma cells or lymphocytes. More suspicious and characteristic of Sjögren's syndrome would be a 2+ biopsy, which denotes multiple aggregates of round cells. With a 3+ labial biopsy, generalized lymphocytic infiltration as well as atrophy of acinar tissue may be seen. In addition to infiltration and atrophy, biopsies sometimes show extensive acinar destruction, with round cell infiltrates replacing lobular architecture (4+). Additional classification is sometimes found useful by quantitating the number of lymphoid aggregates (of 50 or more lymphoid cells) in a given area of the lip biopsy slide, to give a "focus score."

A close inspection of normal salivary ducts will reveal two types of cells: the epithelial cell lining the duct lumen, and the so-called myoepithelial cell in the periphery of the duct. Ductal proliferation is a characteristic of Sjögren's syndrome and, in particular, proliferation of the myoepithelial cells has been noted. In some cases, the round cell infiltrate has essentially replaced lobular architecture and obliterated almost all the acinar tissue. At the same time, the myoepithelial cells have proliferated to such an extent that the duct lumen is essentially closed, and the circular remnants of these ductal structures are seen to be almost swimming in a sea of lymphocytes. These are referred to as *epimyoepithelial islands* and are pathognomonic for the diagnosis of Sjögren's syndrome. However, they are seen only in a biopsy of major salivary glands, and not from the lip or palate. They are not constant, but they will rule out other possible causes of salivary gland infiltration, including tuberculosis, sarcoidosis, and lymphoma.

Available diagnostic aids (Table 15.2) are relatively nonspecific for Sjögren's syndrome. Therefore diagnosis is usually approached by detecting a constellation of such findings within the appropriate clinical setting. In one such diagnostic approach, a focus score of greater than one in a labial salivary gland biopsy was present in over 95% of patients. This finding is borne out by other experience, so that demonstration of characteristic involvement of minor salivary glands by lip biopsy is a wise and necessary technique to use when the diagnosis of Sjögren's syndrome is being seriously considered. Other rheumatic diseases were also present frequently (a possible bias in the study), but KCS was found in only about half of the patients.

In general, it is best to view the entire patient, using the laboratory findings mentioned above as indices to gauge the probability of diagnosis and the dynamic salivary gland scans to document the extent of involvement. It should be emphasized that a rheumatic disease may not be present; rheumatoid factor is usually

Table 15.2. Diagnostic Aids in Sjögren's Syndrome

Clinical
    Characteristic history
    Findings of xerostomia, xerophthalmia, rheumatic disease
    Diminished tear flow (Schirmer test)
    Keratoconjunctivitis sicca (rose bengal; fluorescein)
    Diminished salivary flow (Lashley cup)
Laboratory
    Signs of inflammation
    Hyperglobulinemia
    Rheumatoid factor
    ASDA
    Anti-SS A, B
    Other "autoimmune" findings (ANA, antithyroid antibodies)
Radiologic
    Secretory sialography
    Salivary gland scintigraphy
    Signs of accompanying arthropathy, if present
Pathologic
    Lymphoproliferation
        Glandular—e.g., labial biopsy
        Extraglandular (see text)

present, ASDA is nonspecific, KCS is detected in only some, and a positive labial salivary gland biopsy is the single most frequent finding in Sjögren's syndrome. Table 15.3 lists some other causes of salivary gland enlargement, some of which (as noted) may be associated directly or indirectly with arthritis.

ETIOLOGIC ASPECTS

The lymphocytes and plasma cells that infiltrate the salivary glands are functionally active; both B cells and T cells have been identified in such infiltrates. Furthermore, such cells locally synthesize IgG and especially IgM to a considerable extent. In some cases these lymphocytes synthesize monoclonal immunoglobulins, sometimes of the same chain type as that found in the patient's sera when Waldenström's macroglobulinemia coexisted. Because such lymphocytes show increased IgM synthesis, and because of the high incidence of rheumatoid factor in Sjögren's syndrome, the antibody activity of this IgM was investigated. The results indeed showed active and local synthesis of rheumatoid factor in many patients with Sjögren's syndrome. This finding has not been the case with the majority of patients with rheumatoid arthritis alone (whether or not rheumatoid factor was present in the peripheral circulation) or with other rheumatic diseases.

What has emerged is the concept that Sjögren's syndrome appears as a clinical spectrum of lymphoproliferative disease from benign to malignant (Table 15.4). The benign portion of the spectrum is the typical syndrome discussed here, whereas in the malignant portion are Waldenström's macroglobulinemia, reticu-

Table 15.3. Conditions Associated with
Salivary Gland Enlargement

Infections[a]
(Viral, bacterial, fungal)
Hypersensitivity reactions
(Especially iodides, propylthiouracil,
isoproterenol, and phenylbutazone[a])
Diabetes mellitus
Pregnancy
Malnutrition
Chronic liver disease[a]
Ductal obstruction
Chronic inflammation, stones
Sarcoidosis[a]
Neoplasms[a]
Sjögren's syndrome[a]

[a] May be associated with arthritis.

Table 15.4. Lymphoproliferative Spectrum of Sjögren's Syndrome

	Benign	*Intermediate*	*Malignant*
Entity	Sicca complex	Pseudolymphoma	Lymphomas
Site of involvement	Glandular	Extraglandular	Extraglandular
Some possible manifestations	Xerostomia	Interstitial nephritis	Malignant progression
	Xerophthalmia	Renal tubular acidosis	
	Parotidomegaly	Fibrosing alveolitis	
	Xerodermia	Purpura	
	Pancreatitis	Cryoglobulinemia Lymphadenopathy	
	Hyperglobulinemia	$\uparrow$ or $\downarrow$ IgM	
	Rheumatoid factor	$\downarrow$ Rheumatoid factor	
	ASDA (see text)	$\downarrow$ ASDA	
Pathology	Glandular lymphoproliferation	Benign extraglandular proliferation	Malignant extraglandular proliferation
	Acinar atrophy		Lymphoma
			Waldenström's macroglobulinemia
Course	Benign	May progress or regress	Malignant

lum cell sarcoma, and various lymphomas. An intermediate or middle portion of the spectrum has been called *pseudolymphoma,* which denotes a condition of extraglandular proliferation and signs and symptoms depending on the organ and site of involvement. According to this concept, such a lymphoproliferative spectrum, progressing from glandular infiltration through pseudolymphoma and developing into malignant lymphoproliferation, is an expression of the basic disease process in Sjögren's syndrome. Indeed, the incidence of lymphoid malignancy has been shown to be far in excess of that expected in the non-Sjögren's population.

The characteristics, then, of pseudolymphoma would be those of extraglandular lymphoproliferation in which the cells would not meet pathologic criteria for classification as malignant. In such cases, the signs and symptoms depend upon the site or organ involved. Thus renal tubular acidosis and/or defects in concentrating ability may be associated with interstitial nephritis. Lymphadenopathy, sometimes of frightening proportions, may also be a manifestation of pseudolymphoma. Interstitial pneumonitis, dramatic elevations of serum IgM, purpura, cryoglobulinemia, perhaps pancreatitis, and involvement of the liver with "autoimmune liver disease" may all be signs of pseudolymphoma.

Clinically, patients have been noted to progress from common Sjögren's syndrome through pseudolymphoma and then to regress under certain conditions to the "garden variety" syndrome, or to progress to frank lymphoma or reticulum cell sarcoma. In some patients, ASDA has been negative or turns negative during the progression to pseudolymphoma; rheumatoid factor similarly has been absent or found in decreased titers, and serum IgM concentration may be low. All of these are atypical findings in benign Sjögren's syndrome. However, in some patients with pseudolymphoma, serum IgM levels may be very elevated, and a few of these have subsequently progressed to Waldenström's disease. In others, a fall in serum IgM concentration and a disappearance of serum rheumatoid factor was associated with progression of the pseudolymphoma to frankly malignant lymphoma.

In up to 50% of the specimens examined, virus-like particles have been found in the tissues of patients with sicca complex but not in those from patients with Sjögren's syndrome and rheumatoid arthritis. These particles have been myxoma-like in nature, and occurred in the rough endoplasmic reticulum of endothelial and sometimes glomerular cells. The presence of these clues to viral infection, and the signs of abnormal immunity discussed above, have led some investigators to postulate that Sjögren's syndrome is a dysfunction of the exocrine gland apparatus due to autoimmune activity. This activity may be based upon a response to an infectious agent in genetically susceptible persons. These persons respond with abnormal activation of B cell and subsets of T cell populations, with resultant characteristic round cell infiltration of the target organs. Further immunologic imbalance in certain of these patients may then lead to more generalized malignant degeneration of such infiltrates.

THERAPEUTIC ASPECTS

It is now the general consensus that the rheumatoid arthritis that may be part of the complete Sjögren's triad is not treated differently from that of rheumatoid disease alone. Thus administration of gold, for example, is no longer thought to be associated with a high risk of toxic reactions in patients with Sjögren's syndrome.

Treatment of xerophthalmia usually focuses on supplementation with artificial tears, commonly containing methylcellulose. More serious dryness of the eyes may sometimes necessitate the use of protective soft contact lenses. Some groups have used cauterization of the main lacrimal ducts in order to divert the small amount of lacrimal flow available to a wider area of the conjunctival sac.

Xerostomia, when severe, has been most refractory to therapy. The patient must be cautioned against the use of hard candies to stimulate salivary flow, as this practice may accelerate the already serious dental problems. Often frequent small sips of water can relieve the mouth dryness; it has been found empirically that cool and alkaline mouthwashes may be more effective in ameliorating the sensation of oral dryness than warm acid solutions. In addition, some prefer to use a lubricating substance, such as methylcellulose, in the mouthwash. At times, noncarbohydrate-bearing flavoring may help somewhat to stimulate salivary flow. Introduction of a fluoride gel into the mouthwash is often recommended. In addition, it is noted, but not documented by controlled studies, that supplements of zinc sulfate (for example, 50 mg qd) may decrease some of the unpleasantness associated with dry mouth, although they do not seem actually to increase salivary flow. Finally, vigorous programs of oral hygiene and continuing dental care must be strictly maintained to limit the severity of side effects of the xerostomia on dental health.

Parotid gland enlargement is treated conservatively, if possible; analgesics, nonsteroidal anti-inflammatory drugs (which the patient may be receiving anyway), and appropriate measures to rule out infection, stone, or unrelated causes may suffice. Excision of the salivary gland should not be carried out; however, at times, fear of lymphomatous progression may dictate the need for direct parotid gland biopsy. For very active inflammation, systemic corticosteroids will sometimes be necessary.

In general, the treatment of pseudolymphoma involves balancing the possibility of target organ damage against potential risk from corticosteroids or immunosuppressive agents. Dramatic lymphadenopathy, renal disease, alveolitis, pneumonitis, purpura, macroglobulinemia, pancreatitis, liver disease, the development of cryoglobulins, negative or disappearing antisalivary duct antibody, and the absence or disappearance of rheumatoid factor are all danger signs that the Sjögren's syndrome may be progressing along the postulated spectrum toward pseudolymphoma or beyond. In such cases, because the disease is immunopathic and involved with abnormal lymphoproliferation, it seems reasonable to consider the use of those drugs.

For example, prednisone has been shown to be associated with amelioration of aggregates of lymphocytes and plasma cells in the interstitial pneumonia associated with the pseudolymphoma of Sjögren's syndrome. Similarly, cyclophosphamide use has been associated with decrease in parotid swelling, decrease in previously elevated serum IgM concentration, increase in salivary flow rate, decrease in synthesis of IgM by lymphocytes infiltrating the lips, and even occasionally with improvement of the grade of involvement documented by lip biopsy.

Therefore, although so-called uncomplicated Sjögren's syndrome may be a rela-

16

Systemic Lupus Erythematosus and Related Disorders: Clinical Aspects

John B. Winfield

Robert J. Quinet

SYSTEMIC LUPUS ERYTHEMATOSUS

Systemic lupus erythematosus (SLE) is a chronic, multisystem disorder typically affecting young women and characterized serologically by the presence of multiple autoantibodies, particularly antinuclear antibodies (ANA). Major organ systems involved include skin, joints, kidneys, serosal membranes, and the central nervous system. Estimates of prevalence in the general population range from 0.001% to 0.05%. There is general agreement that SLE is much more common than previously appreciated and that the majority of patients exhibit a relatively benign course without inevitable progression to major target organ injury.

The sex ratio is approximately 9 females: 1 male except at the extremes of age, where there is only a slight female predominance. The peak period of onset is the twenties and thirties. A genetic component has been clearly defined, with greatly increased incidence among first-degree relatives of patients with SLE.

Diagnostic Approach

Diagnosis in a given patient requires familiarity with the common clinical manifestations and their modes of presentation, the demonstration of certain immunologic abnormalities (e.g., ANAs), and the exclusion of other entities resembling SLE. Precise diagnostic classification often is not possible after a single evaluation, but generally it is not difficult when patients are followed over time. The relative incidence of the most common clinical features is shown in Table 16.1. Among these manifestations, arthralgia/arthritis and mucocutaneous inflammation are most common, with an overall incidence of approximately 90%. The absence of both of these features is distinctly unusual in SLE. Glomerulonephritis is extremely common but, contrary to popular opinion, is often mild and non-progressive. Recurrent pleuritis and/or pericarditis is present in the majority of

Table 16.1. Clinical Features of SLE

Common
  Arthralgia[a]
  Arthritis
  Fever and constitutional symptoms[a]
  Mucocutaneous involvement[a]
  Nephritis
  Pleuritis[a] and pericarditis
  Pulmonary function test abnormalities
  Libman-Sacks endocarditis (at autopsy)
  Lymphadenopathy
  Neuropsychiatric disease
  Anemia
  Leukopenia[a]
Uncommon
  Hepatomegaly
  Splenomegaly
  Retinopathy
  Abdominal pain
  Myalgia
  Aseptic necrosis of bone
  Raynaud's phenomenon
  Sjögren's syndrome
  Chronic lupus pneumonitis
  Thrombocytopenia
  Hemolytic anemia
  Lupus anticoagulant
Rare
  Cardiac valvular disease (clinically significant)
  Myocarditis (clinically apparent)
  Acute lupus pneumonitis
  Bowel hemorrhage or necrosis
  Ascites

[a] Frequent presenting manifestations.

patients. Patients with active SLE exhibit prominent constitutional symptoms including malaise, mild weight loss, and fever. With the exception of leukopenia and mild anemia, other features occur less frequently and are helpful in diagnosis only if present.

Insidious onset of polyarthritis or polyarthralgias is the single most common initial manifestation of SLE (50%–60%). Patients present with mucocutaneous involvement less frequently (20%). Other modes of initial presentation are distinctly uncommon: glomerulonephritis (0%–6%), fever (4%–5%), neuropsychiatric disease (3%–4%), pleuropericarditis (0%–5%), thrombocytopenic purpura (2%–4%), hemolytic anemia (2%–4%), and Raynaud's phenomenon (0%–3%). When only one system is involved, for example, arthralgia, it may remain the sole system for years before the development of other manifestations. Thus the multisystem nature of SLE may become apparent only after prolonged follow-up and observation.

Given a patient with signs and symptoms consistent with SLE, the diagnostic effort next should be directed at documenting certain immunologic abnormalities that are almost universally present. These include hypergammaglobulinemia; the presence of ANAs, often in high titer; and hypocomplementemia. A positive immunofluorescence assay for ANA in a high titer suggests a diagnosis of SLE. The demonstration of anti–double-stranded DNA or anti-Sm antibodies is confirmatory. Immunofluorescent staining for immunoglobulin or complement along the dermal-epidermal junction of a biopsy specimen from uninvolved skin also is quite specific for SLE. Laboratory assessment of SLE is discussed more fully in a later section.

The disorders most commonly confused with SLE diagnostically are listed in Table 16.2. Rheumatoid arthritis (RA) in its early stages may be indistinguishable from SLE both clinically and serologically. While it is easy to distinguish classic RA (rheumatoid factor-positive, marginal erosions, and rheumatoid nodules) from SLE (nonerosive arthritis or arthralgia and the presence of glomerulonephritis), the differentiation of SLE from seronegative arthritis is often difficult when constitutional symptoms and articular complaints dominate the clinical picture. Diagnostic difficulty also arises in patients with "overlap" syndromes with features of scleroderma, dermatomyositis, and RA. Precise characterization of serologic abnormalities often is extremely helpful in such cases. Both the entity known as mixed connective tissue disease (MCTD) and drug-induced lupus share many features with idiopathic SLE and will be discussed in subsequent sections. "Lupoid" hepatitis, although characterized by the presence of a positive lupus erythematosus (LE) preparation and other SLE-like serologic abnormalities, is a subset of chronic active hepatitis and completely distinct from SLE. Primary

Table 16.2. Disorders Clinically
Resembling SLE

Rheumatoid arthritis
Polyarteritis nodosa (vasculitides)
Polymyositis/dermatomyositis
Rheumatic fever
Scleroderma
Sarcoidosis
Lymphoma
Chronic active hepatitis (lupoid hepatitis)
Drug-induced lupus
Mixed connective tissue disease
Adult Still's disease
Relapsing polychondritis
Weber-Christian disease
Mixed cryoglobulinemia
Other malignancies
Whipple's disease
Periodic syndromes

Table 16.3. Preliminary Criteria for SLE[a]

Facial erythema

Discoid lupus

Raynaud's phenomenon

Alopecia

Photosensitivity

Oral or nasopharyngeal ulceration

Arthritis without deformity in $\geq$ 1 peripheral joint

LE cells

Chronic false-positive serologic test for syphilis

Profuse proteinuria

Pleuritis or pericarditis

Psychosis or convusions

Cellular casts

Hemolytic anemia, leukopenia, thrombocytopenia

[a] The presence of four or more criteria serially or simultaneously indicates a diagnosis of SLE with 90% sensitivity and 98%–99% specificity.

liver involvement in SLE is highly unusual, and when evidence for liver dysfunction is present, it is usually simply a transaminitis secondary to salicylate therapy.

Perhaps the most common question asked the rheumatology consultant is, "The lab just turned up a positive ANA test result on my patient; does she have lupus?" Although it is true that a positive ANA test result is virtually a sine qua non for the diagnosis of SLE, the converse does not obtain. An ANA positive in low titer is ubiquitous in clinical medicine, occurring in patients with common viral infections, cancer, Hashimoto's thyroiditis and other autoimmune endocrine syndromes, a variety of other rheumatic diseases, and in a significant proportion of the normal elderly population.

The preliminary criteria of the American Rheumatism Association for classification as SLE are shown in Table 16.3. These criteria were derived to distinguish unequivocal SLE from classic or definite RA or nonrheumatic disease and were meant to classify populations of patients in a uniform fashion for the purpose of clinical investigation. These criteria were not intended for diagnosis in individual patients and should not be applied in this way. For the practitioner, the criteria are most useful as a guide to direct questioning to some of the multisystem problems present in SLE.

Clinical Manifestations

Constitutional Symptoms

Fatigue and malaise are present in the majority of patients both initially and chronically, often despite improvement in other clinical symptoms. Fever secondary to SLE may follow any pattern. When present, it demands a compulsive search for superimposed infection, especially in the presence of shaking chills, polymorphonuclear leukocytosis, and in patients receiving corticosteroid or other immunosuppressive therapy. Weight loss and anorexia may be severe and, together with malaise and fever, constitute excellent indices of systemic disease activity.

Joint Involvement

Symmetric arthralgia or polyarthritis, usually accompanied by morning stiffness and affecting the proximal interphalangeal joints, metacarpal phalangeal joints, wrists, and knees, is the most common initial and recurrent clinical manifestation. The polyarthritis generally is migratory or transient but may be persistent. Physical findings often are minimal, but objective evidence for tenosynovitis, frank synovial effusion, and periarticular inflammation may be seen. Synovial analysis is helpful only to exclude infection in the unusual patient with prominent arthritis in an asymmetric distribution. Synovial fluid findings are either normal or only mildly inflammatory (Chap. 3). True erosions are never seen radiographically. Nevertheless, deforming arthropathy (ulnar deviation, swan neck, or boutonniere deformities) may occur in approximately 5% of patients, presumably due to long-standing, recurring synovitis.

The major orthopedic problem in SLE is aseptic (avascular) necrosis, which occurs in the hips of at least 5% of patients. The early symptoms are nonspecific and usually consist of pain in the groin or buttock, often radiating to the anterior thigh or knee. Aseptic necrosis of the femoral head is best recognized, but it is not generally appreciated that many patients also develop aseptic necrosis in multiple joints in addition to the hip, including the shoulders, wrists, and ankles. X-rays are not helpful in diagnosis during the first several months of symptoms, although bone-seeking polyphosphate radionuclide-labeled tracers may reveal increased or decreased uptake in the femoral head as early as 7–10 days after onset. Radiographic changes are described and illustrated in Figures 5.20*a* and 5.20*b*. Although the development of aseptic necrosis is highly correlated with antecedent corticosteroid therapy, the basis for this association is unclear. Early lesions may respond to analgesic or nonsteroidal anti-inflammatory agents and limitation of weight bearing. Core (medullary) decompression shows promise for halting disease progression. Total joint replacement is usually required for advanced lesions.

Mucocutaneous Manifestations

The classic cutaneous finding is a fixed, finely scaling erythematous malar rash, but in practice this sign is encountered infrequently. The "butterfly" distribution reflects photosensitivity with sun exposure. Physical examination reveals erythema, slightly raised and sharply defined borders, follicular plugging, telangiectasia and, in older lesions, atrophy and scarring. A nonspecific, diffuse erythematous rash also occurs frequently. Skin rash often recurs in association with other systemic manifestations such as fever, malaise, weight loss, alopecia, pleurisy, and arthritis. Manifestations of dermal vasculitis, which occurs in 20%–30% of patients, include periungual erythema, nail-fold infarcts, and livedo reticularis. Dermal vasculitis may progress to ischemic skin ulceration. Other cutaneous features include periungual telangiectasia, purpura/petechiae (generally related to thrombocytopenia, qualitative platelet dysfunction, or corticosteroid therapy), angioedema, urticaria, vesicobullous lesions, subcutaneous nodules, erythema nodosum, and erythema multiforme. A small minority of patients develop acute and chronic inflammation of subcutaneous fat (lupus profundus).

Discoid lupus is a distinctive skin lesion characterized by red-violaceous papules or plaques with elevated "active" borders and scaly, pale centers with adherent scales and wide follicles filled with keratinous debris. As the lesions advance, atrophy and scarring appear in the center and the active peripheral region extends outward. Typical distributions are the malar region, ears and scalp, forearms, hands, and less frequently the trunk. Discoid lupus may be considered a chronic, cutaneous form of SLE; with prolonged follow-up, multisystem disease often develops.

Hair loss develops in approximately 25% of patients and tends to be recurrent. Alopecia generally is associated with other manifestations of systemic disease activity. Because scarring changes usually are absent, remission is accompanied by complete hair regrowth.

Oral ulcerations most commonly are located on the central-posterior hard palate, but also occasionally on the gingiva or buccal mucosa. Early lesions present as small, erythematous, slightly elevated lesions and are painless. These lesions progress to form typical shallow ulcerations that, if large, are painful. Similar lesions in the nasopharynx may progress to nasal septal perforation. Oral and nasopharyngeal ulcerations are an important index of systemic disease activity. Large, painful ulcerations may be treated with viscous Xylocaine and/or local corticosteroids. Healing occurs without residua.

Patients with photosensitivity may develop exacerbation of cutaneous and systemic symptoms after exposure to excessive sunlight. This exacerbation is due to ultraviolet irradiation and accounts for the higher incidence of cutaneous lupus in the spring and summer months.

Renal Disease

Clinically evident nephritis eventually develops in 50%–75% of patients and is presenting features in 5%–8%. In the majority of patients, renal disease is clinically silent. Its detection requires performance of a complete urinalysis on a freshly voided urine sample, and serum BUN and creatinine determinations as a routine during each follow-up visit. Symptomatic renal disease, for example, nephrotic syndrome with edema/anasarca, hypertensive encephalopathy associated with rapidly progressive glomerulonephritis, and frank uremia are unusual modes of presentation; they generally occur as late manifestations in a minority of patients. Findings upon urinalysis include hematuria, leukocyturia, cylindruria, and proteinuria. Microhematuria usually is mild. An RBC greater than 200/hpf implies menstrual contamination, urinary tract infection, or some other cause of capillary bleeding, for example, thrombocytopenia, vasculitis, or drug effect (cyclophosphamide). Leukocyturia generally indicates urinary tract infection, but sterile pyuria may occur during an exacerbation of lupus nephritis, often associated with WBC casts. Detection of significant proteinuria by qualitative tests should be followed by quantitative determinations on a 24-hour urine collection. More than 200–500 mg of protein excreted every 24 hours is a reliable index of lupus nephritis. Proteinuria in excess of 2–3 g/24 hr is associated with an increased risk of decline in renal function; this finding thus is of prognostic significance. Proteinuria is less satisfactory as a guide to therapeutic response, however, because it often persists long after clinical remission has been achieved.

Renal function is best assessed by serial determinations of serum creatinine. Calculation of creatinine clearance provides more quantitative data but suffers in an outpatient setting from inadequate 24-hour urine collection. Increases in serum creatinine that steadily progress over months to years are associated with greatly increased risk of end-stage renal failure. More acute declines in glomerular filtration during exacerbations of nephritis, even to the point of frank uremia, may reverse completely and do not necessarily imply irreversible loss of function.

Because renal injury in SLE is related pathogenetically to the deposition of DNA–anti-DNA complexes along the glomerular basement membrane, serial complement and anti-DS DNA determinations provide useful information both diagnostically and as a guide to therapy. With many patients, however, correlation of these serologic indices with active nephritis is imprecise. Indeed, certain patients may exhibit hypocomplementemia and increased anti-DS DNA antibody levels for many months without any evidence of overt nephritis. It is for this reason that serologic assessment should be adjunctive, not definitive, in regard to initiation of therapy or estimation of prognosis. On the other hand, the clinician may predict with some confidence a stable or improved course for glomerulonephritis when anti-DS DNA antibodies are absent and the complement level is normal.

Study of tissue obtained at renal biopsy by light, immunofluorescence, and electron microscopic techniques has provided an enormous amount of useful information concerning the nature of glomerulonephritis in SLE. The most widely accepted classification is based upon the light microscopic histologic appearance and includes five relatively distinct patterns: mesangial, focal-proliferative glomerulonephritis, diffuse proliferative glomerulonephritis, membranous glomerulonephritis, and glomerular sclerosis. Immunofluorescence studies, enabling rough quantitation and localization of IgG and C3 deposits, contribute additional useful information. With electron microscopy, electron-dense immune complex deposits can be more precisely localized to the subepithelial or subendothelial regions of the glomerular tuft.

For the clinician, the purposes of renal biopsy are to estimate prognosis, aid in establishing the diagnosis of SLE in questionable cases, and provide information with regard to choice of therapy. For example, a decision to institute therapy specifically directed at glomerulonephritis, and the vigor with which a chosen regimen is pursued, require information concerning the activity or inactivity of the renal lesion and, if active, whether the lesion is mild or severe. Although the issue is controversial, most would agree that renal biopsy alone frequently fails to provide such specific information in an individual patient. Present knowledge about the prognostic and therapeutic implications of the various histologic subtypes is obscured by selection bias in performing renal biopsies, noncomparative histologic criteria from study to study, and variable and uncontrolled treatment regimens. Transformations from one histologic category to another may sometimes occur when one performs serial biopsies on an individual patient, for example, membranous glomerulonephritis → diffuse proliferative glomerulonephritis. Perhaps the major limitation of renal biopsy is that by necessity it provides information at only a single point in the patient's illness and thus fails to reflect the tempo and evolution over time. Therefore, the wise clinician judiciously chooses patients on whom to perform a biopsy and integrates the biopsy findings with those obtained from serologic, urinary, and other clinical data in making an assessment of the patient's renal status.

Mesangial Glomerulonephritis. All patients with SLE have at least minor histologic or immunopathologic evidence of renal injury when a biopsy is performed. The earliest lesion is in the mesangium. The glomeruli are either normal or exhibit mild mesangial hypercellularity by light microscopy. Immunofluorescence studies show deposits of IgG and C3. It has been recognized that the mesangial lesion may progress to focal proliferative or diffuse proliferative glomerulonephritis. There is little correlation between the presence or absence of clinical evidence for renal disease in patients with mesangial deposits, although it is unusual for this lesion to be associated with marked proteinuria or abnormal renal function.

Focal Proliferative Glomerulonephritis. Focal proliferative glomerulonephritis is characterized by segmental proliferation and minor necrosis of tufts in less than half of the glomeruli. There is minimal glomerular sclerosis and epithelial crescent formation. Granular deposits of IgG and C3 are found in the mesangium and scattered in limited fashion along the glomerular basement membrane. Electron-dense deposits also are limited primarily to the mesangium. Their presence subendothelially may indicate a progression toward more diffuse disease. Clinically, patients with focal proliferative glomerulonephritis exhibit minor urinary abnormalities, and only occasionally renal insufficiency and/or nephrotic syndrome. Many patients with this lesion follow an indolent, nonprogressive course. However, because focal proliferative glomerulonephritis and diffuse proliferative glomerulonephritis are in a continuum, the potential for progressive disease exists.

Diffuse Proliferative Glomerulonephritis. Diffuse proliferative glomerulonephritis is the most common histologic pattern encountered in most series. All or most glomeruli exhibit global cellular proliferation. Necrosis and crescent formation are prominent. Many glomeruli are sclerotic. IgG, C3, and IgM generally are deposited in large amounts diffusely throughout the glomerulus. Large subendothelial deposits may be seen with electron microscopy and correspond to the classic "wire loop" lesions seen by light microscopy. As a group, patients with biopsies showing the diffuse proliferative histologic pattern and extensive deposits of immunoglobulin and complement have heavy proteinuria and are at increased risk for progressive renal failure. The appearance of edema and acellular necrosis of arterioles and intralobular arteries may herald the onset of rapidly progressive glomerulonephritis. Even advanced diffuse proliferative lesions may be transformed into the mesangial pattern after clinical remission.

Glomerular Sclerosis. Occasional patients, usually with a nephrotic syndrome and evidence of renal insufficiency, may exhibit only glomerular sclerosis on biopsy. It is unclear whether the antecedent immunopathology in such patients is long-term but relatively mild nephritis, or whether the sclerotic glomeruli are the healed residua of an episode of severe nephritis. Patients with inactive renal lesions obviously do not require therapy.

Membranous Glomerulonephritis.   Approximately 10% of patients are found to have membranous glomerulonephritis, which histologically and clinically is virtually identical to the idiopathic lesion seen in non-SLE patients. Light microscopy reveals uniform thickening of the capillary wall with minimal or no cellular proliferation. Immunoglobulin is deposited in a diffuse, finely granular pattern subepithelially in the glomerular capillary wall. Renal function usually remains stable. Very marked proteinuria with nephrotic syndrome is a key feature. In contrast to diffuse proliferative glomerulonephritis, which is associated with cryoglobulinemia, hypocomplementemia, and high levels of anti-DS DNA antibodies, serologic findings in patients with membranous glomerulonephritis generally may be normal or minimally abnormal. Renal vein thrombosis may complicate membranous glomerulonephritis.

Tubulointerstitial Nephritis.   An uncommon but increasingly recognized renal lesion in SLE is tubulointerstitial nephritis. Granular peritubular deposits of IgG and C3 are associated with interstitial inflammation and fibrosis, tubular atrophy, and thickening and reduplication of tubular basement membranes. Patients with predominant tubulointerstitial disease are characterized clinically by impaired excretion of potassium and acid. Proteinuria may be entirely absent.

Pulmonuary Manifestations

The most common pulmonary manifestations of SLE are pleuritis (30%–50% of patients) and asymptomatic pulmonary function test abnormalities. Pleuritis is typically recurrent and may be associated with pericarditis or other systemic manifestations of active disease. Physical examination reveals an inconstant pleural friction rub, elevated and relatively immobile diaphragms, and dry, end-expiratory basilar rales that presumably reflect basilar atelectasis secondary to splinted respiration. Chest radiographs show diaphragmatic elevation, a pleural effusion that is usually small, and plate-like atelectasis at the involved base. Pleuritis without a visible pleural reaction or effusion may be seen occasionally. Patients with a nephrotic syndrome may develop large, asymptomatic pleural effusions as part of generalized anasarca. Pleural fluid obtained at thoracentesis typically is a straw-colored exudate containing several thousand leukocytes, predominantly mononuclear. Pleural fluid glucose is normal. LE cells, ANAs, and depressed serum complement components may be seen. Complement levels are lower in SLE pleural effusions than in those associated with malignancy, but the degree of overlap among these conditions is such that complement levels seldom provide definitive information diagnostically.

A surprisingly large number of patients without symptoms of pulmonary disease are found to have mild pulmonary function abnormalities indicative of restrictive lung disease and decreased diffusion capacity. Although they are rarely progressive, careful questioning of such patients often will elicit symptoms of mild breathlessness.

Pulmonary infiltrates, erroneously termed *lupus pneumonitis,* usually are secondary to complications of SLE, for example, uremic pulmonary edema, superimposed infection, or patchy basilar atelectasis due to painful pleuritis. Concurrent infection is the most common cause of a radiographic infiltrate in SLE, particularly in the absence of associated pleural disease. Uremic pulmonary edema is characterized radiographically by vascular and interstitial congestion with fluffy alveolar infiltrates in the perihilar and lower lobe regions. Associated cardiomegaly and/or pleural effusion frequently are present.

True lupus pneumonitis does occur as a primary manifestation of SLE but should always be a diagnosis of exclusion. Acute pneumonitis is rare, occurring in less than 5% of patients. It is characterized by dyspnea, fever without pleuritis, nonproductive cough, and occasionally hemoptysis. The patient presents with tachypnea and may be cyanotic. A chest x-ray reveals diffuse, patchy infiltrates with a predilection for basilar areas. Lung biopsy is often required to exclude definitively opportunistic infection. The lung histology is nonspecific, revealing hyaline membranes, interstitial edema, and alveolitis. In certain patients with acute lupus pneumonitis, major pulmonary hemorrhage dominates the clinical picture. A sudden decrease in hematocrit is often a clue to the etiology of the diffuse infiltrates. Such patients often progress to respiratory failure, and the outcome frequently is fatal. At postmortem examination, there is evidence of severe intra-alveolar hemorrhage with immunopathologic and ultrastructural evidence of immune complex formation in alveolar septae, large blood vessels, and bronchioles. Chronic lupus pneumonitis is indistinguishable from idiopathic pulmonary fibrosis (fibrosing alveolitis), and it is unclear whether pulmonary fibrosis is a specific manifestation of SLE. Occasional patients develop pulmonary arterial hypertension that frequently progresses to cor pulmonale and death. In such patients, vasculitis involving pulmonary arterioles, arteries, and veins is a prominent finding pathologically.

Cardiac Manifestations

Pericarditis, myocarditis, and endocarditis may occur singly or in combination. Coronary vasculitis and, more recently, accelerated coronary atherosclerosis have been described. Arterial hypertension, which often precedes the onset of clinically significant renal disease, is prevalent and undoubtedly contributes to cardiac and renal compromise. Symptomatic pericarditis is the most common cardiac manifestation, occurring in 20%–50% of patients during the course of their illness, often in association with pleuritis and other manifestations of systemic disease activity. The relative incidence of pericardial inflammation in echocardiographic surveys of unselected patients and at postmortem examination is much higher, which indicates that pericarditis is relatively asymptomatic in many patients. A pericardial rub is heard in only 10%–30% of patients. Physical examination should include careful measurement of pulsus paradoxus and a search for Kussmaul's sign. An electrocardiogram usually reveals tall T waves and elevated ST segments acutely. It is of interest that similar electrocardiogram changes may be found in asymptomatic patients. Although infectious pericarditis complicating SLE has been reported, in practice pericarditis nearly always is a primary manifestation. Pericardiocentesis or anterior pericardiectomy is reserved for those patients not responding rapidly to therapy or exhibiting persistent hemodynamic compromise. Progression to cardiac tamponade occurs but is highly unusual. Constrictive pericarditis has been reported as well. Pericardial fluid resembles other "third-space" fluids in SLE.

Clinical diagnosis and assessment of lupus myocarditis are difficult. Frequently it is not possible to distinguish between myocarditis and other etiologies of congestive heart failure, for example, fluid retention secondary to renal disease or corticosteroid therapy, arterial hypertension, and chronic anemia or pleural pulmonary disease. In the absence of obvious secondary etiologies, cardiomegaly and the presence of gallop rhythm correlate reasonably well with histopathologic evidence of myocarditis. Other clinical findings that may be helpful in assessment are softened S1, resting tachycardia without fever, and conduction abnormalities on the electrocardiogram. Use of echocardiographic and gated blood pool scanning techniques hold promise for more definitive evaluation of myocarditis in future studies. Based upon catheterization data, preliminary evidence suggests that definite myocardial dysfunction is relatively common in unselected patients. At autopsy, histologic evidence of myocarditis is found less frequently than in patients examined in the precorticosteroid era. Findings include small collections of lymphocytes and plasma cells in the interstitium, focal scars, and fibrosis.

Libman-Sacks endocarditis historically is the classic cardiac lesion in SLE. Verrucae usually are located on the ventricular aspect of the posterior mitral leaflet, ventricular mural endocardium, chordae, and papillary muscles. The aortic valve is less commonly involved, and the right heart rarely. Active lesions consist of small clumps of fibrin deposited on leaflets that may exhibit focal areas of necrosis and lymphocyte and plasmocyte infiltrations. With healing, dense, vascularized scar tissue with secondary dystrophic calcification develops. Libman-Sacks endocarditis almost never results in hemodynamically significant valvular dysfunction. For the most part, the verrucae are below the resolution of echocardiography. It is distinctly unusual for these verrucae to dislodge and embolize. Thus, the vast majority of heart murmurs in SLE are unrelated to verrucus endocarditis. The most common murmur is an innocent, mid-systolic ejection type related to fever, anemia, or tachycardia. Pathologic murmurs suggest coincidental rheumatic heart disease of infectious endocarditis.

Although there are well-documented case reports of autopsy-proven myocardial infarction secondary to coronary vasculitis in SLE, atherosclerosis appears to be a much more frequent cause of ischemic heart disease. It is possible that after initial immunologic injury to the coronary endothelium, arterial hypertension and prolonged corticosteroid therapy lead to accelerated atherosclerosis.

Gastrointestinal Manifestations

Recurrent abdominal pain develops in the majority of patients with SLE. Frequently it is difficult to distinguish whether the abdominal symptoms are a primary manifestation of SLE or are secondary. This problem is particularly vexing in patients receiving corticosteroids, as many of the usually reliable signs of intra-abdominal catastrophe may be masked. It is good to remember that appendicitis, ruptured ectopic pregnancy, cholecystitis, and other common etiologies of significant abdominal pain are no less common in SLE than in the population at large. Patients with SLE are at increased risk for peptic ulcer disease due to the combined administration of nonsteroidal anti-inflammatory agents and corticosteroids.

Several clinical syndromes peculiar to SLE are encountered sufficiently frequently to merit special mention. The first is a syndrome mimicking an acute surgical abdomen. The patient presents with abdominal pain that is nonspecific but often crampy or colicky. Examination reveals distension, guarding, and rebound tenderness but absence of true rigidity. Bowel sounds often are surprisingly normal but may be hypoactive or absent. Ascites may or may not be present. The result of rectal examination is unremarkable. Such symptoms frequently recur in an individual patient. Short of laparotomy, it is exceedingly difficult to distinguish this clinical picture from perforated viscus or bowel obstruction. Confidence in the diagnosis is enhanced somewhat by the occurrence of this syndrome in the setting of active SLE. Serial radiographic examinations to detect pneumoperitoneum generally reveal only ileus. Other radiographic findings include mucosal changes, particularly in the jejunum, with narrowing of the lumen, effacement of mucosal folds, thumb printing, and spasticity similar to that seen with infarcted bowel. Diagnostic paracentesis should be considered to exclude infectious peritonitis or free perforation. Selective mesenteric arteriography occasionally is helpful in documenting vasculitis or a site of bleeding. The precise indication for and timing of surgical intervention require the most experienced judgment. Surgery in patients with active SLE is hazardous, often leading to further deterioration. In the absence of septicemia, evidence of gastric or duodenal ulceration, urinary tract infection, or the diffuse pain suggestive of impending small bowel infarction, most rheumatologists would offer a trial of corticosteroids. Exploratory surgery should be strongly considered if, after 24–48 hours of this therapy, there has been no improvement. The role of laparoscopy in this situation has not been defined clearly but holds promise. It is important to remember that this syndrome, which may be due either to abdominal serositis or to vasculitis, generally is reversible without surgical intervention.

Bacterial peritonitis, either spontaneous or secondary to ruptured viscus, also presents as an acute surgical abdomen. A diagnostic paracentesis should be done even in the absence of demonstrable ascites. Both gram-positive and gram-negative bacteria have been implicated and generally can be cultured from blood and peritoneal fluid.

Other gastrointestinal manifestations of SLE include ascites, protein-losing enteropathy, and aspirin-induced hepatotoxicity. Ascites generally is secondary to nephrotic syndrome but may be a manifestation of true serositis. The ascitic fluid usually is an exudate containing moderate numbers of lymphocytes. Protein-losing enteropathy has been well documented in several patients by measuring ^{51}Cr-labeled albumin in the stool. Protein loss may be of sufficient magnitude to result in severe hypoalbuminemia and ansarca.

Significant liver involvement is not a primary manifestation of SLE. Although minimal liver function test abnormalities occasionally may be seen, significant elevation of liver enzymes more often is secondary to dose-related salicylate-induced hepatotoxicity. Such patients may exhibit many of the symptoms of acute viral hepatitis. The prognosis generally is good, with rapid return of biochemical evidence of liver dysfunction to normal upon discontinuation of salicylates. *Lupoid hepatitis* is a misnomer. It refers to a subset of chronic active hepatitis with prominent ANAs completely distinct from SLE.

Neuropsychiatric Manifestations

The diagnostic classification of neuropsychiatric manifestations of SLE is exceedingly difficult and challenging. Problems include the frequent occurrence of subtle or transient symptoms or signs; difficulty in distinguishing SLE and non-SLE etiologic relationships; and the absence of discriminative diagnostic laboratory tests to identify SLE-related neuropsychiatric disease. The best overall estimate of the incidence of neuropsychiatric disease in SLE is that it is common. If one discounts secondary brain dysfunction in chronically ill patients or patients with severe extracentral nervous system systemic activity, recent data suggest that central nervous system (CNS) disease tends to appear relatively early during the course of SLE. It is distinctly uncommon for patients to appear with neuropsychiatric disease as the sole or initial manifestation of SLE, however. There appears to be no clear age, sex, or race predilection for neuropsychiatric disease, nor have associations of neuropsychiatric manifestations with specific extra-CNS findings been definitively identified.

Psychiatric disease and seizures, which are frequently associated with each other, are most common. Psychotic behavior often suggests schizophrenia and is marked by visual and auditory hallucinations and paranoid ideation. Careful examination generally reveals the presence of organicity with disorientation, disturbance of consciousness, confusion, and focal neurologic signs. Functional psychoses also occur, both acute and chronic. Functional psychoses and neurotic disorders are difficult to ascribe to SLE per se and usually are secondary to premorbid personality, reaction to illness, or corticosteroid therapy. Grand mal seizures are most common, although any type may occur transiently or recurrently.

Cranial nerve disorders also are frequent and may occur singly or in combination with very complex symptoms. Particularly common are abnormalities of extraocular and pupillary movement, facial weakness, tinnitus and vertigo, and palatal weakness. Blindness and homonymous hemianopic defects occur. These conditions are generally central in origin, and defects in vision are infrequently related to retinal changes at the present time.

Overt paralysis or paresis is encountered infrequently, although transient pyramidal tract signs are commonly elicited. Occasional patients develop hemiplegia due to large vessel occlusion or transverse myelopathy.

Infrequent neurologic manifestations include peripheral neuropathies, cerebellar dysfunction, scotomata, pseudotumor, chorea, and aseptic meningitis. Peripheral neuropathies may be sensory, sensorimotor, or pure motor.

Pathologic findings at autopsy generally provide little information correlative with clinical findings during life. Not infrequently, the brain will be completely normal in patients with severe, diffuse organic dysfunction. The most common abnormality is disseminated areas of focal encephalomalacia. Fibrinoid degeneration and vascular occlusion have been described, but vasculitis is not a prominent finding in most patients. Other findings may include large or small intercerebral hemorrhages and micro-infarcts. When present, the latter often correlate well with clinical findings. For example, cranial neuropathies are frequently associated with brain stem micro-infarcts; seizures have been related to micro-infarcts in the cerebral cortex. The finding of cerebral abscesses or viral inclusion bodies, totally occult during life, is distressingly common.

Laboratory neurologic investigation in the assessment of the patient with SLE and neuropsychiatric manifestations usually is helpful only in a negative sense. The electroencephalogram is abnormal in the majority of patients, but the findings are nonspecific and not directly correlated with the clinical findings. Brain scan and computerized axial tomography are usually normal. Cerebral arteriography generally reveals large vessel occlusion in patients with hemiparesis. Lumbar puncture yields abnormal findings in only a minority of patients. The cerebral spinal fluid (CSF) pressure is normal. Mild increase in CSF protein, slight pleocytosis that is generally mononuclear, and decreased CSF sugar are seen occasionally. Determination of C4 levels in the CSF has not proved to be useful.

In most patients, there is no clear correlation between neuropsychiatric manifestations and extrasystemic disease activity or serologic abnormalities. While an elevated erythrocyte sedimentation rate, anemia, lymphopenia, increased anti-DS DNA antibody levels, and hypocomplementemia in the serum may be present in patients with neuropsychiatric disease, these laboratory indices are usually associated with extra-CNS systemic illness, and not with brain dysfunction. Indeed, a very common presentation for a neuropsychiatric illness is its development in a patient whose illness by other clinical and laboratory measures would be considered to be in remission. Thus, the main task for the clinician in assessing the patient with neuropsychiatric illness is to exclude non-SLE related etiologies.

The course of an individual episode of neuropsychiatric disease cannot be predicted by the manifestations. The great majority of patients recover, either completely or partially. CNS disease is an uncommon primary cause of death, even in patients dying with neuropsychiatric manifestations. Life-table analysis indicates that the long-term survival of patients with neuropsychiatric disease is not less than that of persons without neuropsychiatric manifestations.

Hematologic Manifestations

Anemia develops in 50%–75% of patients. The usual hematologic picture is that of anemia of chronic disease, that is, normochromic/normocytic smear, depressed plasma iron and decreased total iron-binding capacity, and normal bone marrow findings and adequate iron stores. The presence and degree of anemia parallel SLE activity, both clinically and serologically. It has been suggested that severe anemia has prognostic significance, particularly with regard to renal disease. Therapy directed at the anemia per se is ineffective. The anemia resolves with remission of overall disease activity.

Overt hemolytic anemia is distinctly uncommon, occurring in less than 10% of patients. The clinical features and course of hemolytic anemia in SLE are similar to those of idiopathic acquired autoimmune hemolytic anemia. Indeed, an appreciable number of patients presenting with idiopathic hemolytic anemia subsequently develop SLE. A positive direct Coombs' test may be present frequently in the absence of significant hemolysis. A warm-reactive IgG antibody, generally of the IgG_{1-3} subclasses, as well as C3 or C4, is usually detected by direct Coombs' test when there is active hemolytic disease. During periods of quiescent hemolysis, complement alone may be observed in the direct Coombs' test. IgM antibodies and cold agglutinins are only occasionally responsible for hemolytic anemia.

Anemia secondary to a variety of non-SLE-related etiologies also occurs and includes iron deficiency, renal disease, and reactions to drugs. Gastrointestinal blood loss due to salicylate or other nonsteroidal anti-inflammatory drugs or prednisone may be particularly troublesome.

Leukopenia is a frequent hematologic manifestation and is a particularly useful laboratory index of SLE disease activity. Rarely does the total white blood count fall below 2,000/cu mm, however; in such cases, immunosuppressive therapy is usually a major contributing factor. Although the absolute numbers of granulocytes and lymphocytes are generally decreased together, a relative lymphopenia is most prominent. The basis for granulocytopenia has not been clarified fully. Present concepts include action of antipolymorphonuclear antibodies, decreased marrow mobilization, and central bone marrow suppression of granulopoiesis. In addition, there are qualitative functional abnormalities of granulocytes that may be relevant in regard to altered host defense against microbial organisms.

Lymphopenia is strongly correlated with the presence of cold-reactive IgM anti-lymphocyte antibodies. Although the absolute number of lymphocyte subpopulations defined by surface markers is decreased in lymphopenic patients, T cells are disproportionately decreased even in patients without lymphopenia. These unusual lymphocyte subpopulation abnormalities may be of fundamental significance and will be discussed further in the subsequent chapter. Lymphopenia in active SLE is paralleled by skin test anergy and decreased lymphocyte proliferative responses to mitogens and antigens in a variety of in vitro assays. Most of these functional lymphocyte abnormalities return toward normal during remission.

Less than 20% of patients develop thrombocytopenia, although when present, thrombocytopenia may be the most prominent feature of SLE. Thrombocytopenia is due to IgG antiplatelet antibodies that mediate peripheral destruction. Platelet survival is decreased and bone marrow megakaryocytes are increased in number. It is of interest that even in patients without thrombocytopenia, both the number and size of bone marrow megakaryocytes are increased, indicating the presence of a compensated immune thrombolytic state. Rarely is thrombocytopenia due to decreased thrombocyte production. Qualitative platelet defects have been described in relationship to a serum inhibitor of thrombocyte aggregation with effects similar to those of aspirin, that is, decreased collagen-, ADP-, and epinephrine-induced aggregation. This qualitative platelet defect is associated with purpura but not with increased bleeding tendencies.

From 5% to 10% of patients with SLE exhibit a lupus anticoagulant. The lupus anticoagulant has been found to be an autoantibiody directed against the platelet phospholipid portion of the prothrombin activator complex. Its effect is to inhibit the conversion of prothrombin to thrombin. The lupus anticoagulant is not specific for SLE, occurring in drug-induced lupus, polyarteritis nodosa, chronic active hepatitis, Laennec's cirrhosis, and certain carcinomas and lymphoproliferative malignancies. Coagulation test results suggesting the presence of the lupus anticoagulant are an increased activated partial thromboplastin time that remains increased when the patient's plasma is mixed with an equal volume of normal plasma. The prothrombin time is normal or only slightly increased, and the thrombin time is normal. The thromboplastin generation test is normal using normal plasma substrate and abnormal using the patient's plasma as substrate.

The great majority of patients with circulating lupus anticoagulant do not have increased bleeding tendencies and may undergo major surgery without risk of increased postoperative bleeding. Patients who are at risk for clinically significant bleeding generally have in addition to the lupus anticoagulant, marked thrombocytopenia, uremia, or an associated deficiency of factor II activity. The cause of the decreased factor II activity is unknown, but its presence may be suspected if the prothrombin time is increased. In such patients, a specific assay for factor II should be done before surgery. Approximately 50% of patients with the lupus anticoagulant have associated thrombocytopenia. Sporadic reports of inhibitors to factors XII, IX, and VIII have appeared, but these are quite rare in SLE.

Muscle Involvement

Recurrent proximal myalgias, characterized by tenderness, minimal or absent weakness, and normal or modest elevation in muscle enzymes develop in approximately one-third of patients. Profound proximal muscle weakness may occur in patients with "overlap" features of polymyositis but is quite rare. Other causes of proximal muscle weakness frequently encountered are chloroquine neuromyopathy and corticosteroid myopathy.

Initial evaluation focuses on whether myalgia or weakness is the primary problem. Myalgias usually are transient and respond rapidly to anti-inflammatory drugs. If true proximal muscle weakness is present, the medication history should be reviewed. If the patient has been receiving hydroxychloroquine, this drug should be discontinued. It may be difficult to distinguish corticosteroid myopathy from myositis. If muscle enzymes are significantly elevated, corticosteroid myopathy is unlikely to be the sole cause of weakness. Electromyographic (EMG) findings in corticosteroid myopathy are "myopathic" and in myositis "irritative" or "neuromyopathic." If muscle enzyme changes and the EMG suggest myositis, a muscle biopsy should be obtained in the region most abnormal on EMG. Any of the biopsy findings of polymyositis may be seen in SLE (including muscle necrosis, regeneration, mononuclear interstitial infiltration, and vasculitis), but generally changes are milder, with true necrosis occurring rarely and vasculitis also uncommon. With a diagnosis of primary myositis, corticosteroid therapy should be initiated or increased in dosage (60 mg/day), as in polymyositis. If corticosteroid myopathy is suspected, or if the data concerning this differential diagnosis are equivocal, corticosteroid therapy should be tapered or changed to an alternate-day regimen. Improved muscle strength confirms the diagnosis of corticosteroid myopathy.

Ocular Manifestations

Retinopathy occurs in 10%–25% of patients but rarely leads to visual impairment. Ophthalmologic examination reveals cotton-wool spots identical to those seen in hypertensive or diabetic retinopathy. Their appearance is that of fluffy white oval or circular lesions adjacent to vessels, occasionally associated with superficial flame-shaped or preretinal hemorrhages. Both retinal vasculitis and arterial hypertension are thought to contribute to the lesions. The cotton-wool spots are of no prognostic value but may aid in the initial diagnostic evaluation. Uveitis and scleritis are not primary manifestations of SLE.

Xerophthalmia and xerostomia (dry eyes, dry mouth) are relatively uncommon in SLE and, when present, are associated with two of the new antinuclear antibodies, anti–SS-A and anti–SS-B, in serum. Salivary and lacrimal gland enlargement also occurs occasionally. If Sjögren's syndrome is suspected, a Schirmer's test should be done; if it is positive, the patient should have a slit-lamp examination with rose bengal staining to detect interstitial keratitis. For symptomatic patients, methyl cellulose eye drops are prescribed.

Lymphadenopathy

Lymphadenopathy develops in 30%–40% of patients, with the largest nodes occurring in the axillary and anterior cervical chains. Lymphadenopathy correlates poorly with disease activity and may persist indefinitely. Findings in biopsy specimens are nonspecific. Routine biopsy is unnecessary in a patient with well-documented SLE. As in Sjögren's syndrome, there may be a spectrum of lymphoproliferation ranging from that associated with autoimmune disease to immunoblastic lymphadenopathy to lymphoma. For this reason, a disproportionately or progressively enlarging lymph node requires a biopsy.

Splenomegaly

Splenomegaly is detectable on physical examination only during active disease. There is a weak negative correlation between splenomegaly and hemoglobin level, but true hypersplenism is rare. When removed in patients with corticosteroid-resistant immune cytopenias, the histopathologic examination reveals congestion, scattered infarcts, prominent follicles, and "onion skin" thickening of splenic arterioles. Splenectomized patients are particularly susceptible to pneumococcal and *Hemophilus influenzae* sepsis.

Raynaud's Phenomenon

The incidence of Raynaud's phenomenon in SLE is approximately 30%. It may be the presenting feature. Typically, cold exposure or emotion induce a tri-color change with initial pallor, progressing to cyanosis upon continued cold exposure and rebound hyperemic erythema upon rewarming. Raynaud's phenomenon in SLE is less severe and disabling than that in progressive systemic sclerosis and infrequently progresses to digital skin ulceration.

Laboratory Assessment

Initial laboratory assessment should be directed at confirming the clinical impression of a diagnosis of SLE, gauging the extent of SLE disease activity, and defining major organ system involvement. An adequate laboratory evaluation may be accomplished using the assays and procedures listed in Table 16.4. A diagnosis of SLE is supported by the presence of serum ANA in a high titer (e.g., greater than 1 : 256), although ANA titers in this range may be seen in certain other disorders, including drug-induced lupus, RA, juvenile RA, MCTD, scleroderma, Sjögren's syndrome, and "lupoid" hepatitis (Table 4.4). ANA in lower titer, while still supportive of a diagnosis of SLE, is much less specific for this entity.

Many clinical laboratories will report patterns of antinuclear fluorescence in addition to titer. A homogeneous ANA indicates the presence of antibodies to deoxyribonucleoprotein (DNP). Large amounts of anti-DNP in serum are responsible for the LE cell phenomenon. A speckled ANA usually indicates the

Table 16.4. Laboratory Evaluation of SLE

ANA (titer, fluorescence pattern)
Anti-DS DNA
Anti-Sm
CH50 (C3, C4)
Cryoglobulin determination
Rheumatoid factor
IgG, IgM, IgA quantitation
Erythrocyte sedimentation rate
Complete blood count
Urinalysis/24-hr TUP
BUN and serum creatinine
(Skin biopsy for D-E junction Ig staining)

presence of an antibody to one of the acidic nuclear glycoproteins, Sm, or nuclear ribonucleoprotein (nRNP). Anti-Sm is virtually diagnostic of SLE. Anti-nRNP, when present in extremely high titers, that is, greater than 1 : 100,000, is associated with but not diagnostic for the syndrome known as MCTD. Immunofluorescent staining of nucleoli is seen primarily in patients with scleroderma. Immunofluorescent staining of the periphery of the nucleus (rim or shaggy pattern) may reflect the presence of antibody to DS DNA ,Table 4.3).

Because anti-DS DNA antibody is so intimately involved with the pathogenesis of organ-system injury in SLE and because its presence is virtually restricted to patients with this disease, an assay for anti-DS DNA antibody should be included in the initial evaluation of patients suspected of having SLE. A wide variety of assays are currently available, some in commercial kit form: radioimmunoassays based upon ammonium sulfate precipitation of antibody bound to radiolabeled DNA; assays in which antibody bound to DNA is retained on millipore filters; hemagglutination; immunodiffusion; and indirect immunofluorescent assays. All of these techniques may provide quantitative, reproducible measurements. Confusion and difficulty arise, however, if special care is not taken in the laboratory to ensure that the DNA used in these assays is truly DS. DNA is a fragile molecule and easily becomes unraveled, exposing antigenic determinants that react with anti-sDNA (single-stranded) antibody. As anti-sDNA antibody is not at all specific for SLE and correlates relatively poorly with SLE disease activity, the clinician must be certain that the laboratory is really measuring anti-DS DNA antibody. Several recent advances have made this task easier. Certain radioimmunoassays use a synthetic DS DNA, known as dAdT, which can exist only in DS form. Another approach has been to perform indirect immunofluorescence using the hemoflagellate *Crithidia luciliae,* which has a microscopically visible kinetoplast containing DS DNA.

A serum complement determination should be performed in the initial evaluation of patients suspected of having SLE. Most useful is the measurement of total hemolytic complement activity (CH50). A decrease indicates that complement is being consumed in vivo by the presence of immune complexes or, in occasional patients, the presence of a genetically determined complement component deficiency. In the absence of a genetic complement deficiency, depressed CH50 is an extremely sensitive index of ongoing tissue injury, particularly glomerulonephritis. In addition to this functional assay, it may be desirable to obtain immunochemical measurements of the individual components C3 and C4. Decreased C4 levels indicate activation of the classic complement pathway; decreased C3 levels may indicate activation of either the classic or alternate pathways.

Cryoglobulins in SLE have been classified immunochemically as type III. They contain various complement components, polyclonal IgM rheumatoid factor, and polyclonal IgG. Although often detectable in only trace quantities, cryoglobulins reflect the presence of circulating immune complexes, especially DNA–anti-DNA. In combination with hypocomplementemia, cryoglobulinemia is highly correlated with clinically significant active glomerulonephritis.

Other laboratory studies useful in initial assessment include measurement of the erythrocyte sedimentation rate; a complete blood count, including platelet count; urinalysis; and rheumatoid factor assay. If available, additional diagnostic precision may be provided by immunodiffusion or hemagglutination assays for anti-Sm and anti-nRNP. The LE preparation has been superseded by antinuclear fluorescence assays. Skin biopsy to detect dermal-epidermal immunoglobulin and C3 deposition infrequently is required for diagnosis.

A patient who is ill usually manifests mild to moderate anemia, relative lymphopenia, elevation of the Westergren sedimentation rate, hypocomplementemia, cryoglobulinemia, and increased anti-DS DNA antibody levels. In remission, all of those indices return toward normal. In the individual patient, these laboratory indices often do not correlate precisely with the physician's clinical assessment of the patient's disease status, however. For example, certain patients have marked hypocomplementemia for many months without significant symptoms or organ system deterioration. Similarly, an increased anti-DNA antibody level may precede by months or even years overt evidence of glomerulonephritis. Such observations argue strongly for treating the patient and not the laboratory tests. Nevertheless, if the results from clinical evaluation and laboratory evaluation agree with the physician's assessment that a patient is ill, laboratory studies become very useful in monitoring the response to therapy and the adequacy of remission.

As a general rule, it is advisable to obtain as a minimum the following laboratory studies at each patient visit: complete blood cell count; erythrocyte sedimentation rate; either C3, C4, or CH50; urinalysis; BUN; serum creatinine; and anti-DS DNA antibody determination. Special studies are included depending upon the clinical manifestations, that is, a 24-hour total urinary protein determination in a patient with glomerulonephritis. Other studies, including ANA, rheumatoid factor, quantitative immunoglobulin levels, anti-sDNA antibody determination, and assay for the newer ANAs are not required routinely. Assessment of laboratory values should never replace the physician's careful interview and examination of the patient. A patient who is doing well looks well; a patient who is ill generally exhibits specific, identifiable signs and symptoms.

Course of Illness and Choice of Therapy

Course of Illness
The natural history of SLE is highly variable but nevertheless frequently follows several well-recognized patterns in individual patients. Disease often remains mild

for many years without severe exacerbations. Such patients with benign SLE are essentially asymptomatic or exhibit only arthralgia or mild constitutional symptoms. Management requires periodic reassessment to exclude the development of major organ system involvement and intermittent therapy with nonsteroidal anti-inflammatory agents or low-dosage prednisone (less than 20 mg/day). The fulminant, persistently active course culminating in early death described in the older literature is extremely uncommon today. Patients with rapidly progressive SLE often fail to achieve remission despite vigorous immunosuppressive therapy.

Most patients with SLE exhibit fluctuations in disease activity characterized by moderate to severe constitutional symptoms, frequently prominent serologic abnormalities, and clinically evident major organ system injury. Disease activity in patients with recurrently active SLE typically is maximal during the first several years after diagnosis. Subsequently, there is gradual improvement, usually without new major organ system involvement and accompanied by complete or partial resolution of the earlier manifestations. Although exacerbations and remissions may recur for many years, the tempo is one of milder exacerbations and longer remissions. Such patients are often difficult to treat, however. The problem here lies not with therapeutic induction of remission but rather with avoiding overtreatment.

The prognosis for SLE is on the whole good. The 5-year survival in all series published since 1970 is greater than 90%. At 10 years, survival is 80%–90%. Thus, the physician can present an optimistic picture to the patient and his/her family, at least in terms of mortality. Survival in SLE has been improving in linear fashion since 1930. There is no single factor that can account for such improvement. A number of developments, or combinations thereof, are likely responsible. These include improvement in general medical supportive care, earlier diagnosis, detection of milder cases, and the development of antibiotics, diuretics, and antihypertensive medications. The widespread use of hemodialysis and renal homotransplantation has dramatically improved the outlook for the small group of patients who progress to end-stage renal disease. The degree to which corticosteroid therapy has improved survival is controversial, although most rheumatologists would agree about the importance of corticosteroids in very ill patients or patients with persistently active disease. Additional benefit from more potent immunosuppressive agents, such as azathioprine and cyclophosphamide, remains unestablished. The best evidence would appear to indicate that any positive effects of such drugs are largely negated by increased mortality due to infections and other complications of therapy.

Major causes of death in SLE include infection, renal failure and its complications, and, in patients dying later in the course of their illness, ischemic heart disease. This accelerated atherosclerosis has been correlated with prolonged corticosteroid use. Death due to uremia or to CNS disease occurs much less frequently than previously. Recently, an increase in malignancy-related deaths has been noted, but it is unclear whether this pattern merely reflects better survival into older age.

Patients on no or low-dose corticosteroids have higher rates of bacterial infection relative to control patient groups. The frequency of infections, especially those due to opportunistic organisms, rises dramatically with high-dose corticosteroid therapy. The risk for infection also is higher for patients with an active renal sediment or nephrotic syndrome, but probably not for patients with other manifestations of clinically active SLE, for example, hypocomplementemia or leukopenia. The most common major infection is bacterial pneumonia. Failure to culture the usual pathogens or to respond to broad-spectrum antibiotics requires urgent consideration of tuberculosis, nocardiosis, *Pneumocystis carinii,* and histoplasmosis. Septicemia may occur suddenly and often without a definite source. Blood cultures should be obtained routinely in febrile patients. Meningitis also occurs. India ink smear of CSF and cryptococcal antigen studies of CSF should be obtained routinely, because meningitis from this organism occurs with unusual frequency in SLE. Other less common major infections include spontaneous or secondary bacterial peritonitis, septic arthritis, disseminated candidiasis, and disseminated aspergillosis. A wide variety of mild infections occurs with extremely high frequency: urinary tract infections, oral and vaginal candidiasis, bacterial cellulitis and skin abscesses, sinusitis, and so on. Herpes zoster is particularly common in patients receiving cytotoxic agents but has a benign prognosis even in the unusual event of dissemination.

Choice of Therapy

Glomerulonephritis.   The traditional therapeutic approach with glomerulonephritis is to use the renal histopathologic and immunopathologic findings as a guide. Mesangial and focal proliferative glomerulonephritis in the absence of compromised renal function do not require specific therapy. Most rheumatologists would institute moderate to high prednisone therapy for membranous and diffuse proliferative glomerulonephritis. The practice of automatically instituting high-dose corticosteroid therapy for 6 months at the first appearance of a nephritic sediment is not justified, however. A wiser course is first to document the presence of significant nephritis and, if present, to begin a trial of 40–60 mg of prednisone/day orally using the urinary sediment, 24-hour urine protein determinations, serum creatinine, serum complement, and anti-DS DNA levels as guides to therapy in consultation with an experienced rheumatologist or nephrologist. Prednisone should be tapered as clinical and serologic indices improve, for example, clearing of nephritic sediment and rise in serum complement. The objective is to decrease the prednisone to a low-dosage range (10–20 mg/day) as rapidly as possible as the glomerulonephritis improves. Prednisone therapy should not be initiated on an alternate-day schedule. Alternate-day prednisone is effective only as a tapering maneuver or to maintain an established regimen.

It should be remembered that with the general availability of renal hemodialysis and renal homotransplantation, development of uremia is no longer necessarily a terminal event. In such patients, it may be safer to make a judgment that the glomerulonephritis is nonresponsive to prednisone and to decrease or discontinue this medication. Data from the few well-performed, double-blind control trials of cyclophosphamide and/or azathioprine alone or in combination with corticosteroids have failed to support the efficacy of these agents in diffuse proliferative glomerulonephritis. Therapy with immunostimulatory drugs, for example, levamisole, remains experimental. Plasmapheresis is a promising new approach, but its use should be restricted to controlled trials in order to establish better the indications and effectiveness.

Central Nervous System Disease. Neither consensus nor controlled-prospective studies are available to guide the choice of therapy in CNS disease. Until better data are available, it appears reasonable to administer prednisone in moderate dosage for patients not receiving it at the onset of their neuropsychiatric disease and to increase the dosage in those already receiving prednisone. Administration of massive doses of prednisone is not justified. Good evidence indicates the absence of improved therapeutic efficacy and greatly increased risk for serious infectious complications. Few data are available concerning the use of cytotoxic agents or plasmapheresis, although the latter approach deserves investigation because of its lack of toxicity. Anticonvulsant medications and cytotropic drugs should be used according to standard indications.

Cutaneous Manifestations. A generally conservative approach should be used. Precautionary measures include avoidance of excessive sun exposure and liberal use of sunscreens containing 5% para-aminobenzoic acid. Mild lesions usually respond to local corticosteroid creams and ointments in progressively greater strength. More severe lesions may require intralesional or local corticosteroids under plastic wraps. Hydroxychloroquine is effective in many patients with chronic discoid lesions. Oral corticosteroids or cytotoxic agents should be avoided. An exception here is the occasional patient with widespread, disfiguring discoid lesions refractory to other modes of therapy.

The response of acute lupus pneumonitis to corticosteroids usually is dramatic, with a rapid return to normal of temperature and respiratory rate and clearing of pulmonary infiltrates. The benefit of corticosteroid therapy in chronic lupus pneumonitis is less clear. A reasonable approach is to discourage smoking, exclude reversible airway obstruction, and reserve corticosteroids in a brief trial for severe functional limitation. Although data in SLE are lacking, therapy with cytotoxic agents has not been shown to be effective in other types of fibrosing alveolitis. Pleuritis and pleural effusion respond to low-dosage (10–30 mg qd) prednisone or nonsteroidal anti-inflammatory agents. Therapy for pericarditis is similar to that for pleuritis.

Arthritis. Arthritis usually is well controlled with salicylate or other nonsteroidal anti-inflammatory medications. Corticosteroids generally should not be used as a primary therapy for arthritis in the absence of significant extra-articular systemic disease.

Hematologic Manifestations. Anemia of chronic disease and leukopenia reflect active SLE and resolve with the remission of systemic disease. The recommended regimen for hemolytic anemia is 60 mg qd of prednisone for 3–4 weeks followed by rapid tapering of the dosage if there is a positive response. Corticosteroids suppress hemolysis primarily by inhibition of erythrocyte sequestration. If the hemolytic anemia is unresponsive to corticosteroids, splenectomy may be considered.

High-dose corticosteroid therapy is indicated as the initial therapy for significant thrombocytopenia. Failure to respond may require subsequent splenectomy. Little information is available concerning the role of nonsteroidal and immunosuppressive agents. Vincristine may be used as short-term therapy in life-threatening situations. The utility of vincristine for prolonged use has not been established. The presence of a lupus anticoagulant generally does not require corticosteroid therapy.

Raynaud's Phenomenon.   Therapy for Raynaud's phenomenon includes discontinuation of tobacco products, careful attention to hand care, and central and peripheral warming. In patients with severe, persistent symptoms, guanethidine is a useful agent. Alternative medications include reserpine, tolazoline, phenoxybenzamine, and alpha-methyl-dopa. Sympathectomy is of little value. Medications that exacerbate peripheral vasoconstriction, for example, beta blockers, methysergide, and ergotamine, should be avoided.

SLE and Pregnancy.   Approximately 50% of patients will have no change in disease activity during or after pregnancy. SLE will flare up in one-third of patients, most commonly during the first 8 weeks postpartum or during the first trimester. Corticosteroids may be used in pregnancy with little risk to the fetus, although rare cases of neonatal adrenal insufficiency have been noted. Aspirin is also relatively safe but may cause prolonged gestation. Therapeutic abortion may precipitate a flareup or further exacerbate already established disease activity. It is recommended that high-dose corticosteroid therapy be administered before, during, and after therapeutic abortion. Spontaneous abortion and prematurity occur more frequently in SLE than in the general population. Perinatal infant mortality is normal. Toxemia is appreciably increased. Contraception, preferably with intrauterine devices, is advised for patients with active SLE.

DRUG-INDUCED LUPUS

The diagnosis of drug-induced lupus should be suspected in patients exhibiting features of idiopathic SLE who are receiving certain drugs. Diagnosis is confirmed by complete or partial resolution of all symptoms after withdrawal of the drug. Certain clinical and serologic features, including positive ANA, the presence of anti-SS DNA antibodies but the absence of anti-DS DNA, the absence of hypocomplementemia, the absence of nephritis or neurologic dysfunction, and the development of a symptom complex in an atypical patient (e.g., an elderly man) are supportive diagnostic features. Table 16.5 lists the drugs most fre-

Table 16.5. Drugs Implicated
in Drug-induced Lupus

Procainamide
Hydralazine
Chlorpromazine
Alpha-methyl-dopa
Diphenylhydantoin
Trimethadione
Isoniazid

quently incriminated in this syndrome. The vast majority of patients with drug-induced lupus have received either procainamide or hydralazine. The majority of patients receiving 1–2 g/day of procainamide will develop a positive ANA. Symptomatic illness generally does not appear until a total dose of more than 500 mg has been taken. Patients developing procainamide-induced lupus are generally middle-aged or elderly men who have received this medication for arrhythmias in association with ischemic heart disease. Hydralazine-induced lupus is seen primarily in younger women with arterial hypertension. The risk of symptomatic illness increases markedly with dosages greater than 400 mg/day but may occur with dosages as little as 75 mg/day for 1 month. Most patients have received more than 100 mg of hydralazine. The ANA becomes positive 3–20 months after initiation of hydralazine therapy, with the onset of symptoms 3–6 months later. Ultimately, perhaps 50%–60% will develop a positive ANA. Individuals with a "slow acetylator" phenotype are at particular risk for developing ANA positivity and earlier symptoms with both hydralazine and procainamide and require less total drug exposure. The other group of drugs particularly associated with development of an SLE-like illness are antiseizure medications, especially diphenylhydantoin and trimethadione. Such patients present special problems in diagnosis because seizures are a frequent central nervous system manifestation of idiopathic SLE. A minority of patients receiving alpha-methyl-dopa, chlorpromazine, or isoniazid will develop a positive ANA, but symptomatic illness is rare. Isolated case reports suggest the possibility that SLE may develop after treatment with an enormous number of other medications, but in virtually all cases a true association has not been established.

The symptoms and signs of hydralazine and procainamide-induced lupus are similar in both type and relative frequency to those in idiopathic SLE. Virtually all patients have arthralgia or nondeforming arthritis. Other prominent manifestations include fever, pleuritis, and pericarditis. Anemia, lymphadenopathy, and splenomegaly occur infrequently. Although patients with hydralazine-induced lupus not infrequently have renal disease, this disease is not a feature of the lupus syndrome. The laboratory features of drug-induced lupus are summarized in Table 16.6. Features distinguishing drug-induced lupus from SLE are normal white blood count, hematocrit and platelet count, and absence of anti-DS DNA and anti-Sm.

Drug-induced lupus is generally a benign illness that resolves promptly after withdrawal of the inciting medication. Occasional patients may require therapy with nonsteroidal anti-inflammatory drugs or low to moderate doses of prednisone for weeks to months, however. Rarely, serious complications may develop, for example, cardiac tamponade, constrictive pericarditis, or pulmonary fibrosis, which progress despite discontinuation of the drug. The real medical importance of drug-induced lupus is the diagnostic confusion presented by individual patients. For example, a patient with known cardiac disease who presents with the acute onset of chest pain due to procainamide lupus-related pericarditis or pleuritis may be diagnosed as acute myocardial infarction or pulmonary embolism. In occasional instances, it may be impossible to distinguish hydralazine-induced lupus from idiopathic SLE. Certain authorities suggest that patients who develop hydralazine-induced lupus have a preexisting "lupus diathesis" that is unmasked by hydralazine. Such patients may have ANA positivity before receiving hydral-

Table 16.6. Laboratory Findings in
Drug-induced Lupus Contrasted to Those
in SLE

	Drug-induced Lupus	*SLE*
ESR	↑	↑
Serum Ig	↑	↑
WBC	Normal	↓
HCT	Normal	↓
Platelets	Normal	↓
ANA	Positive	Positive
CH50	Normal	↓
RF	+	+
Anti-DS DNA	−	+
Anti-S DNA	+	+
Anti-DS RNA	(+)	+
Anti-nRNP	(+)	+
Anti-Sm	−	+
Antihistone	+	+

azine and continue with smoldering rheumatic complaints for years after discontinuation of this drug. The mechanisms by which certain drugs induce an SLE-like illness are unknown.

MIXED CONNECTIVE TISSUE DISEASE

The original concept of MCTD developed in 1975 was that of a syndrome encompassing clinical features of SLE, progressive systemic sclerosis, and polymyositis. In the initial descriptions, there was a low incidence of renal disease and a generally favorable prognosis. Many of the clinical manifestations were responsive to corticosteroids. Serologically, patients with MCTD were characterized by a high titer of antibody to extractable nuclear antigen (ENA), which through its sensitivity to ribonuclease has been characterized as anti-nRNP. In subsequent years, there has been considerable debate as to whether MCTD is a distinct clinical entity or simply one of the classic rheumatologic disorders, that is, SLE, RA, scleroderma, or dermatomyositis with overlap features. Certain authorities consider MCTD to be basically progressive systemic sclerosis with features of other connective tissue disorders. Others would classify MCTD as SLE or RA with atypical serologic or clinical features.

Regardless of whether MCTD is a distinct clinical entity, there is general agreement that patients classified as such share a number of common features. Eighty percent of patients are women, with a peak incidence in the 20–40 age group. Virtually all patients have arthralgias, and approximately two-thirds have frank arthritis that is generally nondeforming but occasionally indistinguishable from that of RA, with erosions and rheumatoid nodules. Hands frequently are swollen, with sausage fingers and telangiectasias. Over time, the hands become scleroderma-like, although necrotic ulcers are rare. Occasional patients exhibit a violaceous rash over the eyelids and erythematous changes over the small joints of the hands, findings typical of dermatomyositis. Raynaud's phenomenon is present in the vast majority of patients. A minority have an SLE-like rash and may exhibit dermal-epidermal immunoglobulin deposits on skin biopsy. Esophageal motility dysfunction, with dilatation of the distal two-thirds of the esophagus and absent peristalsis. Although usually asymptomatic, patients may develop severe dysphagia as well as progressive involvement of the duodenum and the colon, which have both the clinical and histopathologic features of progressive systemic sclerosis. The majority of patients have myalgias or overt myositis with proximal muscle tenderness and weakness, and elevated CPK and aldolase levels. EMG and muscle biopsy findings are similar to those in polymyositis. Pericarditis is the most frequent cardiac manifestation. Pulmonary disease is also common, although generally not detectable unless careful radiographic and pulmonary function studies are performed. The major features that occur in approximately 70% of patients include diffuse interstitial infiltrates, decreased diffusing capacity, and occasionally decreased lung volume.

The prognosis for patients with MCTD generally is good. In initial descriptions, this prognosis was related to the absence of serious major organ system involvement. However, as patients have been followed up for longer periods, it has become apparent that certain patients develop serious manifestations. Renal disease that is clinically and immunopathologically identical to that of SLE occurs in a small minority of patients. Several deaths from typical scleroderma kidney have occurred as well. Pulmonary disease may lead to severe exertional dyspnea or pulmonary hypertension and rarely dominates the clinical picture. Neurologic manifestations are infrequent in MCTD. The most common manifestation is trigeminal neuralgia, but transverse myelitis, seizures, aseptic meningitis, and cerebral infarction have been reported. These features are indistinguishable from those in SLE. Other features of SLE sometimes seen in MCTD include lymphadenopathy, splenomegaly, fever and other general systemic manifestations, serositis, and leukopenia.

With the exception of high-titer anti-nRNP, the laboratory features of MCTD are not specific for this entity. Moderate anemia and leukopenia are frequent, and an occasional patient may develop autoimmune hemolytic anemia and thrombocytopenia similar to that in SLE. Rheumatoid factor is positive in approximately 50% of patients. Antibodies to DS DNA, LE cells, and hypocomplementemia are unusual. Hypergammaglobulinemia is generally present.

Initial therapy in MCTD generally consists of the administration of prednisone in a dosage of 40–60 mg/day. The therapeutic response is often prompt, particularly for SLE and polymyositis features. However, advanced scleroderma-like changes in the skin, serious neurologic dysfunction, and gastrointestinal motility disturbances may persist or progress. Follow-up data concerning the eventual outcome of patients initially classified as MCTD is incomplete at the present time. It would appear that very few patients die. Those who do die from manifestations of advanced scleroderma or SLE-like glomerulonephritis. The clinical picture in many patients continues to evolve and often acquires characteristics of classic progressive systemic sclerosis, and less frequently SLE or RA.

BIBLIOGRAPHY

Baldwin DS, Gluck NC, Lowenstein J, et al: Lupus nephritis: Clinical courses related to morphologic forms and their transitions. *Am J Med* 62:12, 1977.

Budman DR, Steinberg AG: Hematologic aspects of systemic lupus erythematosus. *Ann Intern Med* 86:220, 1977.

Bulkley BH, Roberts WC: The heart in systemic lupus erythmatosus and the changes induced in it by corticosteroid therapy: A study of 36 necropsy patients. *Am J Med* 58:243, 1975.

Discussion of gastrointestinal involvement in SLE: Case records of the Massachusetts General Hospital (Case 47–1976). *N Engl J Med* 295:1187, 1976; and case records of the Massachusetts General Hospital (Case 25–1978). *N Engl J Med* 298:1463, 1978.

Estes D, Christian CL: The natural history of systemic lupus erythematosus by prospective analysis. *Medicine (Baltimore)* 50:85, 1971.

Fauci AS, Dale DC, Balow JE: Glucocorticosteroid therapy: Mechanisms of action and clinical considerations. *Ann Intern Med* 84:304, 1976.

Fries JF, Holman HR: Systemic lupus erythematosus: A clinical analysis, in Smith LH (ed): *Major Problems in Internal Medicine,* vol. 6. Philadelphia, WB Saunders Co, 1975.

Ginzler EM, Kaplan D: Adrenocorticosteroids in lupus nephritis. *Trans Proc* 7:109, 1975.

Harvey AM, Shulman LE, Tumulty PA, et al: Systemic lupus erythematosus: Review of the literature and clinical analysis of 138 cases. *Medicine (Baltimore)* 33:291, 1954.

Hejtmancik MR, Wright JC, Quint R, et al: The cardiovascular manifestations of systemic lupus erythematosus. *Am Heart J* 68:119, 1964.

Holgate ST, Glass DN, Haslam P, et al: Respiratory involvement in systemic lupus erythematosus. *Clin Exp Immunol* 24:385, 1976.

Johnson RT, Richardson EP: The neurological manifestations of systemic lupus erythematosus: A clinical-pathological study of 24 cases and review of the literature. *Medicine (Baltimore)* 47:337, 1968.

Karsh J, Klippel JH, Balow JE, et al: Mortality in lupus nephritis. *Arthritis Rheum* 22:764, 1979.

Labowitz R, Schumacher HR: Articular manifestations of systemic lupus erythematosus. *Ann Intern Med* 74:911, 1971.

Matthay RA, Schwarz, MI, Petty TL, et al: Pulmonary manifestations of systemic lupus erythematosus: Review of 12 cases of acute lupus pneumonitis. *Medicine (Baltimore)* 54:397, 1975.

Prystowsky SD, Herndon JH Jr, Gilliam JN: Chronic cutaneous lupus erythematosus (DLE). *Medicine* 55:183, 1976.

Reichlin M: Problems in differentiating SLE from mixed connective-tissue disease. *N Engl J Med* 295:1194, 1976.

Wagner L: Immunosuppressive agents in lupus nephritis: A critical analysis. *Medicine* 55:239, 1976.

17

Systemic Lupus Erythematosus: Immunologic Aspects

John B. Winfield

In the preceding chapter, systemic lupus erythematosus (SLE) was described clinically as a multisystem disorder. In this chapter, SLE will be considered as a multifaceted entity reflecting the interplay of immunologic, genetic, biochemical, hormonal, and, possibly, virologic factors. While immunologic abnormalities have been the major focus for investigation so far, it is not at all clear that a strictly immunologic defect is most basic or pivotal. The development of high levels of unusual autoantibodies and their participation in immune complex-mediated tissue injury may be paramount in regard to clinical disease expression, but these are clearly secondary phenomena. None of the multiple immune system regulatory deficiencies that have been described have yet been shown to be truly primary. Recognition that SLE is in part a genetic disease obviously is a key recent development. This fact is particularly true in view of the identification of SLE-associated alleles in that region of the major histocompatibility complex most involved with regulation of the immune response. Also of potential importance are recent observations that both male and female patients with SLE may have subtle endocrinologic abnormalities leading to a relatively estrogenic state. The hormonal milieu has many incompletely defined effects on the immune system. The search for factors in the environment that might cause SLE, either directly or through interaction with host factors, has yielded intriguing but largely inconclusive information thus far. Thus, while an enormous amount of information has been accumulated concerning the basic nature of SLE, full understanding has not been achieved. In essence, the many isolated observations have not yet been related to each other in a way that provides a truly comprehensive picture accounting for all elements of the disease.

ETIOLOGIC CONSIDERATIONS

Genetic Factors

Several lines of evidence indicate that SLE is, in part, a genetic disease. The prevalence of SLE in first-degree relatives of patients with SLE is 1.5%, which is

both consanguineous and nonconsanguineous, for autoantibodies. The rationale here is that while consanguineous relatives might be expected to have certain autoantibodies as markers of a genetic predisposition to this disease, the presence of such markers in nonconsanguineous relatives would imply horizontal transmission of an infectious agent. Indeed, certain data indicate that antilymphocyte autoantibodies and ANAs are present in a high proportion of spouses of patients with SLE. These studies are of great interest, but their significance is unclear at the present time because the findings have not been generally reproducible.

IMMUNOLOGIC ABNORMALITIES IN SLE

Overview

The most prominent humoral immunologic abnormalities in SLE are hypergammaglobulinemia, the development of multiple autoantibodies, and hypocomplementemia. Humoral hyperresponsiveness is not generalized to all antigens, however. Although titers of antibodies to B blood group substances may be extremely high, immunization with other antigens, including A blood group antigens and influenza vaccines, results in an immune response no different from that of control populations. Associated with hypergammaglobulinemia in patients with active disease is evidence for endogenous B-cell activation. B cells freshly placed in culture spontaneously proliferate and secrete an exaggerated amount of IgG for a short period. Perhaps because of this in vivo activation, B cells from patients with SLE cannot be stimulated normally with pokeweed mitogen to become further activated.

Patients with active SLE generally exhibit cutaneous anergy to antigens such as purified protein derivative (PPD), candida, and mumps. In vitro stimulation of T cells from such patients with soluble antigens and mitogens, including concanavalin A and phytohemagglutinin, is abnormally low. As a rule, most of these humoral and cellular immunologic abnormalities reverse almost completely during periods of remission. Thus while mild hypergammaglobulinemia and low-level ANA positivity may persist indefinitely, a patient with SLE in prolonged remission and not receiving therapy may be essentially normal when assessed by routine immunologic assays.

The bases for these interesting immunologic abnormalities are the subject of intense investigation, conjecture, and controversy. While expectations for more complete understanding of the fundamental mechanisms involved are high, at the present time concepts are largely speculative and based upon phenomenologic data interpreted in the context of postulates derived from experimentation in mice. It is clear, however, that the final common pathway resulting in humoral abnormalities, for example, anti-DS (double stranded) DNA or anti-Sm antibody production, involve genetic, hormonal, immunologic, and possibly physical or virologic factors. Current thinking is moving away from unifying concepts applicable to all patients with SLE. Indeed, it is likely that SLE is not a single disease, but rather a limited number of closely related but nevertheless distinct illnesses with different genetic, immunologic, and pathogenetic bases. For example, patients with SLE and homozygous C2 deficiency are characterized clinically by an unusual rash, absent or low-level anti-DS DNA antibodies, and relatively mild glomerulonephritis. A second SLE subset might be defined serologically by the presence of anti-Sm antibodies as the sole or dominant autoantibody present, and clinically by indolent, nonprogressive glomerulonephritis. Further impetus to the concept that SLE might not be a single disease entity has been provided by studies in several strains of mice that develop an SLE-like disease. Experimental evidence strongly indicates that, while anti-DNA antibodies and glomerulonephritis may be characteristic of all, the underlying immunologic abnormalities and pathogenetic mechanisms differ markedly.

Having raised the issue that SLE may not be a single disease entity, in fairness we must discuss a number of immunologic features shared generally by patients given this diagnosis. T cells are decreased both in absolute numbers and in relative proportions in the peripheral blood of patients, particularly during periods of active disease. Several lines of evidence indicate that a functionally important subpopulation of T cells may be particularly involved in this regard. Although the nature of this minor T-cell subset has not been characterized fully, it appears to have surface receptors for the Fc region of IgG and the T cell differentiation antigen, T5, and the functional capacity to suppress humoral and cellular immune responses. Studies demonstrating this missing or decreased T-cell subpopulation are in good agreement, with data indicating that nonspecific suppressor T-cell function induced in vitro by convanavalin A is abnormally low in active SLE. It is debatable, however, whether the major defect in SLE responsible for hypergammaglobulinemia and autoantibody formation will be so simple as a deficiency of a single cell type.

It is unknown whether the T-cell abnormalities in SLE represent a primary defect or are secondary to the effects of circulating immune complexes or anti-lymphocyte antibodies. Antilymphocyte antibodies in SLE have been shown to react with specific lymphocyte subpopulations and to effect their removal from the circulation either by direct complement-mediated cell lysis or by opsonization with phagocytosis. Because the immunologic abnormalities in SLE are largely reversible, the hypothesis that antilymphocyte antibodies might deplete a suppressor T-cell subset either during or preceding periods of active disease is an attractive one. The increase in the level of antilymphocyte antibodies during active disease and decrease during periods of remission is consistent with such a mechanism.

Lessons learned from the study of New Zealand and other strains of mice that develop an illness similar to human SLE are instructive and caution us against viewing the situation in humans too simplistically. For years, research efforts in the murine lupus model were concentrated on the study of New Zealand Black (NZB) mice and F_1 hybrid offspring of New Zealand Black × New Zealand White parents. The latter develop anti-DS DNA antibodies, anti–T-cell antibodies, and progressive glomerulonephritis leading to early death, a clinical picture similar to that of human SLE. Initial experiments suggested that the fundamental defect was a loss of suppressor T cells with consequent abnormal immune regulation. Mechanisms postulated to be responsible for the loss of suppressor T cells, and for which there is some experimental support, include an abnormal thymus gland with decreased thymic hormone and depletion of suppressor T cells by anti–T-cell antibody. As understanding of the different types of mechanisms involved in regulation of the immune response in mice became more sophisticated, it became apparent that the abnormal immune regulation in New Zealand mice was much more complex. For example, conventional suppressor T cells bearing the Lyt 2,3$^+$ surface antigens were found to be increased rather than decreased in NZB mice, and under the proper experimental conditions, suppressor cell function was hypernormal rather than deficient. At the present time, more elaborate mechanisms, involving deficiency of a different type of T cell functionally important in a negative feedback loop suppressing the immune response, are receiving experimental support.

More recent studies of murine lupus have been expanded to involve a number of strains other than New Zealand mice. Certain investigators believe that there are different immunoregulatory defects in each or these autoimmune mouse strains. Others are unable to define any consistent immunoregulatory abnormalities and question whether a deficient suppressor cell function exists at all. Resolution of the many apparently contradictory findings in murine lupus probably must await further clarification of the normal immune response in the mouse. With this background, however, it is apparent that the situation in human SLE will probably be much more complex than the currently available experimental data would lead us to expect. It is impossible to determine whether the primary problem in human SLE lies with defective genetic control of immune responses, deficient suppressor T-cell function, abnormal macrophage function, an intrinsic B-cell defect, a deficient host response to an exogenous infectious agent, an inherited enzyme deficiency, or a combination of such elements. It is entirely possible that completely different factors, or combinations of factors, may be operant in individual patients.

Autoantibodies

An increasingly complex array of autoantibodies to host constituents has been described in SLE. Antibodies to DS DNA and to Sm, a nuclear glycoprotein, are virtually specific for this disease and have proven to be of great usefulness diagnostically. While certain of the autoantibodies undoubtedly represent phenomena of no etiologic or pathogenetic significance, a surprisingly large number have been implicated directly in the natural history of SLE. Strong evidence supports the involvement of anti-DNA and, to a lesser extent, antibodies to certain nuclear glycoproteins in immune complex tissue injury, particularly glomerulonephritis. While likely in certain cases, the contribution of other autoantibodies to circulating immune complex systems has not been fully resolved. Autoantibodies to leukocytes, platelets, erythrocytes, and clotting factors are all relevant pathogenetically through direct antigen-antibody interaction. Antilymphocyte antibodies, through depletion of circulating lymphocytes or lymphocyte surface receptor blockade, may also be broadly related to abnormalities of both humoral and cellular immune responses that are characteristic of this disease.

Anti-DNA Antibodies

Operationally, there are two main types of anti-DNA antibodies in SLE, those reactive with native (n) or double-stranded DNA (DS DNA) and those reactive only with single-stranded or denatured DNA (sDNA). Anti-sDNA binds purine and pyrimidine bases or short oligonucleotide sequences thereof. Anti-nDNA binds to deoxyribose-phosphate situated externally on the double helix.

Anti-sDNA antibodies are found in SLE but also in rheumatoid arthritis and many other connective tissue and autoimmune diseases. Anti-DS DNA antibodies are highly specific for SLE and represent a primary diagnostic marker of this disease. Much confusion concerning the diagnostic specificity of anti-DS DNA antibodies for SLE persists, however, because of technical difficulties in assay procedures. DNA is an extremely fragile molecule, and even slightly denatured DS DNA will react with anti-sDNA in many of the sensitive assays currently in use clinically. This problem has been largely resolved by the introduction of newer assays, for example, the *Crithidia luciliae* immunofluorescent assay and radioimmunoassays using highly purified or synthetic DS DNA.

The origin of anti-DS DNA antibodies is not known, although both experimental and clinical observations have identified several modes by which these antibodies might arise. It is likely that genetic factors are implicated, perhaps involving immune response genes. Candidates for the DNA immunogen in humans include a viral or bacterial DNA source, endogenous DNA largely denatured by ultraviolet radiation exposure of the skin (sunburn), or endogenous DNA altered antigenically by complex formation with drugs. In experimental animals, anti-DNA antibodies have been induced by hyperimmunization with bacteria and with bacterial lipopolysaccharide.

Anti-DNA antibody is primarily of the IgG class, particularly in patients with ongoing tissue injury. IgM anti-DS DNA antibodies are less common and do not appear to be directly related to the pathogenesis of SLE. Very recent evidence suggests that anti-DS DNA antibodies may vary considerably in their avidity for DNA, that is, in the strength with which they bind DNA, and that antibodies of high avidity may be those most likely to form DNA–anti-DNA complexes injurious to the kidney.

The DNA–anti-DNA immune complex system is predominantly involved in the pathogenesis of glomerulonephritis. Initial information in this regard came in the late 1950s from immunofluorescent studies of kidney biopsy sections from patients with SLE that identified immunoglobulin in deposits along the glomerular basement membrane. Subsequent investigations localized complement components and DNA in a distribution similar to that of immunoglobulin in kidney. A fundamental advance was provided by the observation that immunoglobulin eluted from isolated glomeruli from cadaver kidneys contained anti-DNA antibody and that anti-DNA activity was specifically concentrated in such eluates relative to the serum level. Much useful information has come from longitudinal studies of patients during the course of their illness. Increased levels of anti-DS DNA and, to a lesser extent, of anti-sDNA are found in patients with active glomerulonephritis. If patients are followed up very closely, and if the amount of anti-DS DNA antibody is quantitated precisely, the serum level of anti-DS DNA often falls slightly just before the appearance of clinically evident nephritis. This fall presumably reflects the binding of anti-DNA with DNA to form immune complexes that deposit along the glomerular basement membrane. The hypocomplementemia characteristic of active nephritis in SLE closely parallels the associated elevation of anti-DNA antibodies, elevated serum levels of anti-DS DNA, and immune complexes. Free DNA and anti-DNA antibodies have been shown to alternate with each other in the serum of patients followed up for long periods in a manner entirely analogous to the serum sickness model so well studied in rabbits.

Although there is no doubt that immune complexes of DNA and anti-DNA represent the most important mechanism leading to glomerular injury, a question has arisen concerning whether this type of complex forms in the circulation and is deposited in the kidney secondarily, or whether DNA binds initially to collagen-like material in the glomerular basement membrane through charge effects, with secondary binding of DNA antibodies. Some evidence exists to support each of these possible mechanisms, and it is likely that both may be operant.

A role of DNA–anti-DNA immune complexes in other types of tissue injury in SLE, while likely, has been much less well defined. Immunofluorescence studies of uninvolved skin frequently reveal immunoglobulin and complement deposited along the dermal-epidermal (D-E) junction (lupus band test). It is thought that this immunoglobulin staining at the D-E junction reflects the deposition of DNA–anti-DNA complexes, but this issue has not been fully clarified. Bright staining at the D-E junction for IgG correlates with hypocomplementemia, increased anti-nDNA antibodies, and progressive glomerulonephritis. Whether this phenomenon will prove to be of general applicability and thus a useful tool for the assessment of patients has not yet been fully determined. It is likely that DNA–anti-DNA complexes contribute to skin injury and vasculitis, at least in certain patients, but this remains to be proven. There is no solid evidence to support a role for DNA–anti-DNA complexes in most types of SLE pulmonary disease or in diffuse central nervous system (CNS) dysfunction.

Deoxyribonucleoprotein Antibodies

Antibodies to deoxyribonucleoprotein (DNP) are primarily responsible for the lupus erythematosus (LE) cell phenomenon and give a diffuse pattern of antinuclear immunofluorescence. Anti-DNP antibodies react with a complex of histone and DNA, and both of these moieties are required for full antigenicity. With complement-fixation techniques or radioimmunoassays using radiolabeled soluble DNP, the presence of anti-DNP is largely restricted to SLE. The level of anti-DNP exhibits the same association with active glomerulonephritis as anti-DNA, which raises the possibility that antibody to DNP may also contribute to immune complex-mediated renal injury.

Special immunofluorescent approaches recently have indicated that antibody to histones may be much more prevalent in patients with rheumatoid arthritis and other non-SLE disorders than previously thought. Antihistones appear to be particularly prominent ANAs in drug-induced lupus and in rheumatoid arthritis. It is of interest that in rheumatoid arthritis many such ANAs may actually represent rheumatoid factors (anti-IgG antibodies) that cross-react with histones, a phenomenon not observed in SLE.

Antibodies to RNA and RNA-Protein Antigens

A large number of antibodies to RNA and complex RNA-protein antigens have been described. Antiribosomal antibodies are present in approximately 70% of patients with active SLE and have been detected less frequently in rheumatoid arthritis and chronic active hepatitis. Two major types of antibodies have been defined: antiribosomal ribonucleoprotein and antiribosomal RNA. The level of antiribosomal antibodies correlates with that of anti-sDNA, suggesting the possibility that the immunogen for both may arise secondary to tissue breakdown.

Many different types of RNA antibodies have been detected in SLE sera, including those directed to high-molecular-weight RNA, low-molecular-weight RNA (transfer RNA), and isolated nuclear RNA. In addition, antibodies to synthetic DS RNA and sRNA exist. RNA antibodies have attracted great interest because it has been thought that they might reflect a causal link between an RNA-containing virus and SLE. Despite a great amount of investigation, such an association has not been established, however.

The best studied RNA-protein antibody is antinuclear ribonucleoprotein (nRNP). This antibody is directed to both the RNA and nuclear protein components, and antigenicity is destroyed by ribonuclease. Together with anti-Sm and anti–SS-B, anti-nRNP is one of the major antinuclear antibodies that gives a speckled ANA pattern. Anti-nRNP is present in approximately 30% of patients with SLE, 20% of patients with scleroderma, and rarely in patients with rheumatoid arthritis. Extremely high titers are characteristic of mixed connective tissue disease (MCTD). Saline extracts of nuclear homogenates contain nRNP and a number of other nuclear antigens (ENAs). In qualitative (immunodiffusion) or semiquantitative (hemagglutination) assays for antibodies to ENA, the presence of anti-nRNP is established by loss of reactivity after digestion of the ENA with ribonuclease. The level of anti-nRNP varies little with changes in disease activity and has not been firmly related to immune complex-mediated tissue injury.

Antibodies to Nonnucleic Acid, Nonhistone, Nuclear Protein Antigens
Autoantibodies to a complex group of nuclear proteins have been identified through immunodiffusion analysis. A common denominator for this group of antigens is that they are extractable with buffered saline from homegenates of nuclei and are not destroyed by either deoxyribonuclease or ribonuclease. The number of such antigens identified by reactivity with SLE sera is increasing continuously, but their significance pathogenetically or as etiologic clues remains obscure. Nomenclature is very confusing, being derived in most cases from the name of the patient in whom antibody of a given specificity was first described, for example, Sm (*Smith*). Anti-Sm was the first to be discovered. It is distinguished from anti-nRNP in hemagglutination assays using ENA-coated erythrocytes by its resistance to ribonuclease digestion. Antibody to Sm is highly specific for SLE, and its presence generally is a reliable marker of this disease. Approximately 50% of patients with active SLE exhibit anti-Sm in their sera. The exact role of anti-Sm in the pathogenesis of SLE is unclear.

Anti–SS-A and anti–SS-B are two more recently described ANAs detectable in immunodiffusion assays using ENA. Both are found in only a minority of patients with SLE. The major disease association of anti–SS-A and anti–SS-B is with sicca complex.

Autoantibodies to Cytoplasmic Constituents
In addition to ribosomes, a variety of autoantibodies to cytoplasmic organelles and soluble antigens have been described including lysosomes, mitochondria,

and certain soluble glycoproteins. Antigens in the last category include Ro and La. Ro and La are found predominantly in SLE and Sjögren's syndrome. It has recently been shown that Ro is immunologically identical to the nuclear antigen SS-A and La to SS-B. It is of interest that anti-La is frequently found in patients who have typical clinical features of SLE but lack ANAs detectable by conventional immunofluorescent techniques (ANA-negative lupus). Antimitochondrial antibodies in SLE are similar to those in primary biliary cirrhosis but are present in low titer. Because of their reactivity with cardiolipin, antimitochondrial antibodies give rise to false-positive serologic tests for syphilis.

Antibodies to Lymphocyte Surface Antigens

Antilymphocyte antibodies are found in the serum of most patients with SLE. The most common type is of the IgM class and is easily detected by complement-dependent cytotoxcity assays performed at low temperatures or by immunofluorescence techniques. IgM antibodies react with a number of different cell surface antigens, including those specific for B cells and T cells, as well as antigens shared with other cell types, including monocytes, erythrocytes, and brain cells. IgG antibodies appear to be much less frequent and are more difficult to characterize and study.

Antilymphocyte antibodies have been of special interest because of experimental data suggesting an important role in the development of other immunologic abnormalities. The level of IgM antilymphocyte antibodies correlates with disease activity and has been associated with lymphopenia in sick patients. This lymphopenia may involve all circulating lymphocytes or possibly functionally important lymphocyte subsets. Although many issues remain to be clarified, certain data suggest that antilymphocyte antibodies may deplete suppressor T cells specifically. Thus, antilymphocyte antibodies might contribute to the perpetuation of disordered immune regulation.

The origin of antilymphocyte antibodies is unclear. It is certain, however, that nonspecific stimuli such as vaccination with killed bacterial vaccines or infection with a variety of common infectious diseases may lead to their development. Antilymphocyte antibodies usually are reactive with the patient's own lymphocytes, but an SLE-specific surface antigen target has not been identified. Several fascinating, albeit controversial, studies suggest that nonconsanguineous spouses of patients with SLE frequently have antilymphocyte antibodies of the same type found in SLE. This finding has been taken as evidence for horizontal transmission of a viral agent as possibly etiologic in SLE.

Lymphocyte antibodies are thought to contribute to a number of the functional immunologic abnormalities of SLE lymphocytes. Serum from patients with SLE frequently has suppressive effects upon lymphocyte responses in various in vitro immune assays. In certain instances, the suppressive effects have been related to activity of antilymphocyte antibodies. For example, antilymphocyte antibodies can block the proliferation of lymphocytes in mixed lymphocyte cultures and in cultures in which lymphocytes are stimulated by soluble protein antigens or lectins such as phytohemagglutinin and concanavalin A. The mechanism by which antilymphocyte antibodies suppress these different types of immune responses is thought to be either the stripping or the blockade of surface receptors.

Antigranulocyte Antibodies

Antibodies of the IgG class have been found in occasional patients to bind to polymorphonuclear leukocytes. Such antibodies have the capacity to opsonize neutrophils for ingestion by other neutrophils. The association of such antibodies with severe polymorphonuclear leukocyte depletion, which is unusual in SLE, suggests that neutropenia may be mediated by antigranulocyte antibodies. Thus, the mechanism for neutropenia in SLE may be similar to that in certain patients with Felty's syndrome and idiopathic neutropenia.

Antibrain Antibodies

Considerable interest recently has been stimulated by the demonstration of antibodies to neuroblastoma cell surface antigens in patients with active CNS dysfunction. These "antibrain" antibodies are of several types. IgG antibodies that cross-react poorly with lymphocyte and other non-CNS surface antigens are increased in titer in patients with active-diffuse CNS dysfunction. This class of antibodies is not found in patients without CNS disease. IgM antibodies appear to be directed at surface antigens present on neuronal cells, lymphocytes, and erythrocytes. Antibodies of this type do not appear to be particularly associated with CNS disease. Although it is possible that antibrain antibodies may be causally related to neuropsychiatric illness, for example, by interfering with synaptic transmission, this connection has not yet been established.

Immune Complexes

A pathogenetic role for circulating immune complexes was initially defined in the "one shot" serum sickness model. Here the onset of glomerulonephritis is closely associated with the appearance of soluble immune complexes in the circulation, hypocomplementemia, and deposition of immune complexes in the kidney. This model led to the development of SLE as the prototype of immune complex deposition disease in humans. In addition to inducing inflammation, immune complexes may function as regulators of cellular and humoral immunity through their capacity to interact with receptors for the Fc fragment of IgG and complement (see also Chaps. 7 and 8).

There are three main ways in which immune complexes may be formed. First, antibody can react with soluble antigens in the circulation. Second, antibody can react with fixed antigens on the surfaces of cells. Third, antibody can react with antigens released into interstitial fluids, for example, the Arthus reaction. A number of variables control the formation of immune complexes, their fate, and their biological properties vis-à-vis tissue injury. Among these variables are the immunoglobulin class of the antibody, its avidity (strength of interaction with antigen), and the capacity of the resultant complex to fix complement. The ratio of antigen to antibody also is important. Very small complexes containing one or two antigen molecules per antibody molecule tend to circulate for long periods without tissue deposition. Larger complexes are cleared rapidly from the circulation, largely by the reticuloendothelial system. Perhaps the most important factor affecting the pathogenicity of complexes is the duration with which antigen is released into the circulation. In this situation, continuing immune complex formation occurs (chronic serum sickness) that has many of the features of progressive glomerulonephritis in SLE.

A major effect of immune complex formation is activation of the complement system (Chap. 8). Activation of the classic complement pathway is initiated primarily by interaction of immune complexes with Clq. Alternative complement pathway activation involves C3 directly, bypassing C1, C4, and C2. Activation of the complement system by immune complexes is accompanied by a number of biologic effects. Immune complexes and bound complement components attached to complement receptors on neutrophils and macrophages (immune adherence) may trigger phagocytosis and the release of biologically active substances. Chemotaxis of leukocytes is stimulated by C5a and other activation products. Vasoactive amines are released after binding of C3a and C5a to mast cells and basophils. Complement-dependent lysis of cells is mediated by attachment of antibody to cell surface antigens through formation of the C5–9 terminal attack sequence. The pathogenetic effects of immune complexes deposited in tissue, for example, along the glomerular basement membrane in the kidney or in blood vessel walls, are largely a consequence of complement activation. An increase in vascular permeability is in part mediated by C3a and C5a anaphylatoxins. An influx of inflammatory cells is dependent upon immune adherence and chemotactic stimuli.

Certain complement-independent mechanisms also are involved in immune complex-related tissue inflammation. These mechanisms include release of platelet-activating factors from basophils, with subsequent aggregation and release of vasoactive amines from platelets. This release of vasoactive amines contributes to increased vascular permeability, which in turn is a major prerequisite for immune complex deposition. The importance of this mechanism for tissue injury is underscored by experiments showing that depletion of platelets prevents immune complex disease in animals. A major end result of the interplay of all of these factors is phagocytosis by macrophages and neutrophils of immune complexes, with the subsequent release of hydrolytic enzymes from lysosomes that then effect tissue injury.

Because many types of tissue injury in SLE are related causally to immune complex formation, a variety of techniques for immune complex detection and quantitation in serum and other biologic fluids have been developed (Chap. 4). Most useful have been methods based upon physical characteristics of immune complexes, for example, increased molecular size or decreased solubility at low temperatures (cryoglobulins), or upon biologic characteristics involving fixation to complement components or attachment to complement receptors on cell surfaces. An example of the latter approach is the Raji technique, in which immune complexes are quantitated on the basis of their binding to C3 receptors on the surface of the Raji B cell tissue culture line. Binding of immune complexes to Clq is the basis for a number of quantitative radioimmunoassays. An additional series of quantitative assays are based upon the binding of immune complexes to monoclonal IgM rheumatoid factor. In all, there are more than 30 different tests for measuring immune complexes. Each test is subject to artifacts of various types. In addition, it has become apparent that different types of immune complexes in various diseases are best measured with specific assay methods. Thus, tests for measuring immune complexes in rheumatoid arthritis may not be suitable for determining immune complexes in SLE.

In SLE, immunoglobulin has been detected by immunofluorescence techniques in the kidney, at the D-E junction in the skin, in venules and small arterioles in patients with necrotizing vasculitis, in the choroid plexi, and in the lung. Analysis of immunoglobulin eluted from glomeruli of patients with glomerulonephritis and immunoglobulin contained in cryoprecipitates from serum suggests that the major antibody in immune complexes in SLE is anti-DNA antibody. Immune complex assays based upon C1q binding have been particularly useful in SLE and indicate that increased levels of circulating immune complexes are associated with hypocomplementemia in patients with active nephritis. The Raji cell assay also has proven useful in this regard.

The exact role of quantitative immune complex determinations in the management of patients with SLE has not been completely defined. There is evidence that immune complexes disappear with remission and that elevated immune complex levels may be the first indication of a flareup in activity. A major problem has been the lack of a precise correlation between immune complex measurements and clinical indices of disease activity in individual patients. Indeed, at the present time, assessment of anti-DS DNA antibody and serum complement levels appears to offer as much, if not more, useful information than quantitative immune complex assays.

BIBLIOGRAPHY

Eichmann K: Expression and function of idiotypes on lymphocytes. *Adv Immunol* 26: 195, 1978.

Gibofsky A, Winchester RJ, Patarroyo M, et al: Disease associations of the Ia-like human alloantigens: Contrasting patterns in rheumatoid arthritis and systemic lupus erythematosus. *J Exp Med* 148:1728, 1978.

Koffler D, Agnello V, Kunkel HG: Polynucleotide immune complexes in serum and glomeruli of patients with systemic lupus erythematosus. *Am J Pathol* 74:109, 1974.

Kunkel HG: The immunologic approach to SLE. *Arthritis Rheum* 20:S139, 1977.

Markenson JA, Phillips PE: Current comment: Type C viruses and systemic lupus erythematosus. *Arthritis Rheum* 21:266, 1978.

Ross GD: Identification of human lymphocyte subpopulations by surface marker analysis. *Blood* 53:799, 1979.

Symposium on Immune Regulation. *Fed Proc* 38:2051, 1979.

Tan EM: Immunospecificities of antinuclear antibodies. *Arthritis Rheum* 20:S187, 1977.

Winchester RJ (ed): Proceedings of the ARA conference on new directions for research in systemic lupus erythematosus. *Arthritis Rheum* 21(suppl):S1, 1978.

18

Vasculitis

John S. Sergent

VASCULITIS

Vasculitis syndromes represent a bewildering area of medicine, especially upon first being encountered by a medical student or young physician. The problem is so confusing that many students of medicine simply lump all of the types of vasculitis together into the convenient term *polyarteritis nodosa* and make no further attempt to appreciate the various syndromes involved. Others, perhaps more immunologically oriented, tend to assume that all manifestations of all immune-mediated diseases are due to vasculitis and fall into the trap of overinterpreting clinical data based on experimental techniques. Finally, a large group of students and house officers conclude that the vasculitis syndromes are so rare and represent such a subspecialized area of medicine that they are of no concern to the average physician. It is the intent of this chapter to demonstrate that clinical vasculitis syndromes are (1) common, (2) clinically important, and (3) understandable.

The term *necrotizing vasculitis* is suggested as a generic term to apply to all situations in which widespread necrotizing vasculitis is a predominant clinical feature. Some diseases with prominent vascular manifestations are generally excluded from this category. These diseases include Buerger's disease and scleroderma, in which vessels are obliterated but necrosis and inflammation are rare.

Incidence

Table 18.1 shows the types of vasculitis seen at Vanderbilt University and the Nashville Veterans Administration Hospital over a 3-year period. These are both referral hospitals, with approximately 1,100 medical beds combined. Necrotizing vasculitis associated with rheumatic diseases accounted for the largest proportion of these patients. However, a variety of other syndromes were seen, including three cases of hepatitis B-associated vasculitis, six cases of Wegener's granulomatosus, and a variety of others. Eight of these patients died. The long-term morbidity in the remainder includes blindness, chronic hemodialysis, severe hypertension, and crippling residual neuropathy.

Of special importance is the incidence of vasculitis in this medical center. Although these figures may represent a somewhat higher incidence than is seen in the average community hospital, clinically important generalized necrotizing

Table 18.1. Generalized Vasculitis at Vanderbilt Medical Center during a 3-year Period

Rheumatic diseases		18
Rheumatoid arthritis	8	
Systemic lupus erythematosus	8	
Dermatomyositis	1	
Mixed connective tissue disease	1	
Henoch-Schönlein purpura		5
Wegener's granulomatosis		6
Essential cryoglobulinemia		4
Giant cell (cranial) arteritis		3
Hepatitis B vasculitis		3
Takayasu's arteritis		2
Behçet's disease		2
Serous otitis		1
Idiopathic polyarteritis nodosa		1
Total		45

vasculitis is not rare at all. Approximately one new patient with vasculitis has been seen every 3½ weeks by the rheumatology unit in these hospitals.

History

The term *periateritis nodosa* was first used to describe a young man who died of a mysterious disease characterized by fever, cough, renal disease, muscle weakness, peripheral neuritis, and abdominal pain. The postmortem examination demonstrated widespread inflammation in nodular lesions along the course of major arteries; thus the term *periarteritis nodosa*. The first understanding of the problem emerged in the 1930s, when necrotizing vasculitis was noted in patients treated with sulfonamides or with horse serum. Shortly thereafter, several investigators injected serum into experimental animals to induce experimental serum sickness. The animals became ill with fever, glomerulonephritis, and arthritis; microscopic study revealed necrotizing vasculitis in various organs. Thus was born the immunologic study of necrotizing vasculitis.

Clinical Appearance of Vasculitis

Since the target organs are the blood vessels, the clinical appearance depends on the part of the body affected by the vasculitis and also on the type of vessel involved, that is, large artery, small arteriole, or vein. However, a number of clinical features are frequently seen in most types of vasculitis and deserve emphasis.

Fever

Fever and other systemic signs, such as weight loss and night sweats, occur in the vast majority of patients with necrotizing vasculitis. Patients with vasculitis limited entirely to the skin, such as peripheral ulcers in rheumatoid arthritis and some forms of idiopathic cutaneous vasculitis, may lack prominent constitutional symptoms.

Joint Pain

Pain in and around joints is also seen in virtually all patients, although frank arthritis as a manifestation of vasculitis is much less common.

Skin Lesions

A variety of skin lesions may be associated with necrotizing vasculitis. Certain forms of vasculitis, such as rheumatoid arthritis, almost invariably have skin involvement. However, in other syndromes, involvement of the skin may be uncommon or rare. The lesions seen probably depend on the size of vessels predominantly involved in the vasculitic process. Thus petechiae and purpura, such as seen in Henoch-Schönlein purpura, probably represent injury to arterioles and capillaries. Tender nodular lesions are seen in the involvement of larger vessels, such as medium-sized arteries and veins. Gangrene of fingertips, toes, and other areas usually implies involvement of small arteries. Frank necrosis with ulceration usually accompanies a localized venulitis.

Abdominal Pain

Various types of abdominal pain may be seen in patients with vasculitis. The most frequent is cramping postprandial pain, suggestive of ischemic bowel disease. However, infarction of bowel, gallbladder, and kidney may all appear with pain. Many patients complain of vague, nondescript abdominal pains with no clear localization or relationship to meals or bowel movements. In most large series of patients with vasculitis, some will be diagnosed at exploratory laparotomy.

Renal Disease

Renal disease has occurred in about half of our patients as an important apparent manifestation of vasculitis. Almost by definition, it is seen uniformly in Wegener's granulomatosis and in the vasculitis accompanying systemic lupus erythematosus. However, it has been extraordinarily rare in rheumatoid vasculitis and certain other syndromes. Renal disease due to vasculitis usually appears as hypertension, mild to moderate azotemia, and mild proteinuria. A nephrotic syndrome is very unusual. The urine sediment is usually not very impressive, although hematuria may be prominent.

Other Manifestations

Severe headaches are the rule in patients with giant cell arteritis, whether due to temporal arteritis or aortic arch arteritis. Episcleritis of the type seen in rheumatoid arthritis occurs in a small percentage of patients, as do nondescript chest pain and mild pleurisy. A variety of central nervous system manifestations, including strokes, seizures, and dementia, may also be prominent apparent manifestations.

Pathology

The pathology of necrotizing vasculitis varies depending on the age of the lesion and the location. Active lesions in medium-sized vessels are usually accompanied by necrosis of the vessel wall associated with intense eosinophilic staining of the wall, known as *fibrinoid necrosis*. The surrounding inflammatory infiltrate in active lesions contains many polymorphonuclear leukocytes and eosinophils. As the lesion ages, the active fibrinoid necrosis is usually absorbed and the infiltrate around the vessel becomes predominantly mononuclear (lymphocytes and plasma cells). The vascular channel may be completely obliterated by a thrombus, but there is often intense endothelial proliferation with a remnant of a small vessel remaining.

Although some forms of vasculitis, such as that accompanying hepatitis B antigenemia, have been associated with prominent depositions of immunoglobulins and complement, this is by no means the rule. In spite of the evidence demonstrating that vasculitis can be caused by circulating immune complexes, one must not assume that immune complex deposition is the only mechanism of inducing vasculitis. In fact, some forms of vasculitis, especially Wegener's granulomatosis and idiopathic polyarteritis nodosa, are striking for their paucity of immunologic findings.

Diagnosis of Vasculitis

There are a number of clinical situations in which the possibility of a generalized necrotizing vasculitis should be considered. Certain patients have preexisting diseases that raise one's index of suspicion—for example, a patient with longstanding rheumatoid arthritis who suddenly develops peripheral neuropathy, or a patient with preexisting asthma and eosinophilia. In patients with no preexisting disease, any two or three of the clinical manifestations listed above should suggest the possibility of a generalized vasculitis. Some clinical features have more significance than others. Thus, mononeuritis multiplex and various skin lesions such as digital gangrene tend to be highly specific, while abdominal pain and hypertension are not.

When a vasculitis is suspected, a number of studies are available and help confirm the diagnosis. First, certain serologic studies, such as a search for cryoglobulins, hepatitis B surface antigen, and a serum complement determination, are called for in virtually all cases. The only two definitive ways of further confirming a diagnosis of vasculitis are arteriography and biopsy. Arteriography can be highly specific, if positive. In certain cases, such as aortic arch arteritis, the arteriogram may be the only diagnostic study performed. Many radiologists have described the characteristic widespread aneurysms seen throughout the mesenteric circulation in patients with various types of necrotizing vasculitis (Fig. 5.25), so that a mesenteric arteriogram is occasionally performed as a diagnostic procedure. Often, the arteriogram is done as an evaluation for another disease, and the demonstration of vasculitis is a surprise to both the clinician and the radiologist.

If one decides to perform a biopsy, the decision regarding location is always of major concern. Although a number of early studies showed that certain organs, such as the testis, have a high incidence of involvement in patients with vasculitis, it has not been our policy to do a biopsy on the testis. We have demonstrated vasculitis in occasional patients as a result of renal biopsy performed for evaluation of azotemia and an abnormal urinalysis. In addition, occasional patients have the diagnosis made by biopsy of suspicious skin lesions, such as tender erythematous nodules or early necrotic lesions. However, by far the commonest way to establish a diagnosis is by biopsy of muscle and/or nerve. Although the lesions may be focal and scattered, "blind" biopsy of the deltoid or quadriceps muscle is frequently diagnostic. The gastrocnemius muscle is often chosen because a biopsy can be done of the sural nerve at the same time. In patients with mononeuritis, this procedure will improve the chance of a positive biopsy. In diseases such as temporal arteritis and Wegener's granulomatosis, the diagnosis is established by biopsy of the lesion itself.

Classification

Through the years, there have been many attempts to classify patients with necrotizing vasculitis. None of these attempts has been entirely successful. The first classification attempt, by Zeek, was based primarily on the pathologic appearance of the vasculitis. Although this classification was extremely helpful in identifying certain pathologic features that tended to accompany particular clinical syndromes, it was unsuitable for many patients. Another classification was based on the presence or absence of lung disease, since it was observed that patients with pulmonary disease tended to have a high incidence of granulomatous lesions, eosinophils, and preexisting asthma, whereas those without lung involvement had none of these features. Through the years, many modifications have been offered.

Table 18.2 gives an updated and useful classification of the vasculitis syndromes. This categorization (1) deals with clinical rather than pathologic manifestations, (2) recognizes that some forms of vasculitis (secondary) are superimposed on preexisting disease syndromes (3) emphasizes certain causes of vasculitis that should be sought (cryoglobulins and hepatitis B antigen), and (4) denotes that some syndromes (temporal arteritis and Wegener's granulomatosis) are well defined and deserve a distinct classification.

Table 18.2. Classification of Vasculitis

Diseases characterized by necrotizing vasculitis	
Giant cell (cranial) arteritis	Henoch-Schönlein purpura
Wegener's granulomatosis	Churg-Strauss vasculitis
Aortic arch arteritis	Classic polyarteritis nodosa
Diseases sometimes complicated by vasculitis	
Rheumatic diseases	Respiratory diseases
Rheumatoid arthritis	Loeffler's syndrome
Systemic lupus erythematosus	Asthma
Dermatomyositis	Serous otitis media
Rheumatic fever	Hypersensitivity
Mixed connective tissue disease	Serum sickness
Infectious diseases	Drug allergy
Hepatitis B	Amphetamines
Streptococcal infections	Cryoglobulinemia
Bacterial endocarditis	Others
	Ulcerative colitis
	Dermal vasculitis
	Cogan's syndrome

PRIMARY VASCULITIS

Classic Polyarteritis Nodosa

Classic polyarteritis nodosa is rare, accounting for less than 5% of all cases of generalized necrotizing vasculitis seen on general medical services. For many years the terms *polyarteritis nodosa* and *generalized vasculitis* were used synonymously, so that many patients in older series would probably be reclassified today. (Table 18.3).

To be classified according to this system as polyarteritis nodosa, the following criteria must be met: (1) there must be no underlying chronic infectious or rheumatic disease; (2) prominent pulmonary involvement must not be present; (3) the basic vascular lesion must involve medium-sized and large vessels; (4) there must be no conspicuous immunologic abnormalities, such as prominent cryoglobulinemia; (5) there must be no clear-cut relationship to drug hypersensitivity. With these considerations, polyarteritis nodosa will be rare and reasonably well defined.

Historical

The disease first called *periarteritis nodosa* over 100 years ago was a vasculitis involving primarily large vessels, especially at their bifurcations. It was because of the large nodular lesions at these bifurcations that the term *periarteritis nodosa* was used.

Clinical Features

The disease is about twice as prevalent in men as in women. Most patients are relatively young—that is, about half are in their teens or twenties. The illness usually begins abruptly, with high fever, constitutional symptoms, and sudden de-

Table 18.3. Primary Vasculitis Syndromes

Disease	Predominant Age and Sex Affected	Typical Onset	Vessels Affected	Predominant Distribution
Polyarteritis nodosa	Young men	Often abrupt	Medium-sized arteries	Renal, mesenteric, peripheral
Wegener's granulomatosis	Middle-aged men	Gradual	Small arteries	Upper and lower respiratory tract, renal
Henoch-Schönlein purpura	Children of both sexes	Abrupt	Small veins and arteries	Skin, renal, mesenteric
Aortic arch arteritis	Young oriental women	Gradual	Large arteries	Arteries arising from aortic arch
Giant cell (cranial) arteritis	Elderly of both sexes	Abrupt	Medium-sized arteries	Cranial
Churg-Strauss arteritis	Middle-aged of both sexes	Gradual	Small arteries	Lung, peripheral

velopment of arterial occlusion. Especially prominent presenting manifestations
are renal disease and neurologic complaints.

Renal Disease.   In the majority of patients (c. 75%), hematuria, mild to moderate proteinuria, hypertension, and azotemia are the only findings of renal disease.
Rarely, spontaneous rupture of the kidney may be the initial manifestation of
the illness. A frank nephrotic syndrome is rare. Renal biopsy usually shows little
or no glomerulonephritis with prominent vasculitis in the arterioles.

Neurologic Disease.   Neurologic symptoms occur in nearly 80% of patients. Although major central nervous system manifestations may dominate the picture,
much more common is the sudden development of mononeuritis multiplex.

Other Features.   Since virtually any organ system may be involved secondary to
vascular ischemia, the clinical features are protean. Gastrointestinal symptoms
(c. 30%) are pain, nausea, vomiting, anorexia, diarrhea, ulceration, perforation,
hemorrhage, or infarction secondary to vascular involvement. The liver (c. 50%),
spleen (c. 35%), pancreas (c. 40%), or gallbladder, depending on affected vessels,
may also be involved. In about 35%–50% of patients, cardiac changes are found—
coronary arteritis, involvement of the endocardium, myocardium, or pericardium—
or manifestations secondary to renal hypertension. Musculoskeletal symptoms occur in 30%–60% of patients as myositis, atrophy, or nonerosive synovitis. Skin
involvement is found in 25%–50% of patients and consists of nodules, purpura,
urticaria, bullae, necrotic ulcers, subcutaneous hemorrhages, or livedo reticularis.
Ovaries, testes, epididymis, bladder, adrenals, or other organs can also be affected.

Laboratory Data

Anemia is usually secondary (blood loss, renal disease). Leukocytosis, with polymorphonuclear response, is frequent. Urinalysis often reveals hematuria, proteinuria, or casts. Results of other studies may be abnormal depending on clinical
involvement—electrocardiogram, electroencephalogram, liver function studies, and
muscle enzymes. Idiopathic polyarteritis nodosa is notable for the paucity of immunologic findings; striking abnormalities usually indicate another disease. Virtually all patients have an elevated erythrocyte sedimentation rate; a normal
value might suggest an alternative diagnosis (e.g., Buerger's disease).

The following test results are usually normal and if abnormal suggest an alternative diagnosis: (1) rheumatoid factor, (2) antinuclear antibody, (3) hepatitis B
antigen and antibody, and (4) cryoglobulins. In addition, the serum complement
level is usually normal or even mildly elevated.

Pathologic Changes

The process affects medium and small muscular arteries. Lesions are segmental
and frequently found at bifurcations of vessels. Lesions at different stages of inflammatory change or healing may occur together. The characteristic histologic
change is fibrinoid necrosis. Polymorphonuclear cells disrupt the internal elastic
lamina and infiltrate the intima, media, and adventitia. Plasma and mononuclear
cells with healing and fibrosis may be found at later stages. Intimal proliferation

may cause vascular occlusion. Inflammation can lead to aneurysm formation, rupture, or dissection.

Course and Prognosis

Untreated multisystem disease usually progresses to death within one year. Death is due to renal disease in the majority of patients. Other causes are cardiac, gastrointestinal, or cerebrovascular. In contrast to 5-year survival of 10%–13% for untreated patients, estimates for steroid-treated patients are nearly 50% for 5-year survival. Recent observations of patients treated aggressively with cytotoxic agents have been dramatic, as in Wegener's granulomatosis (see below).

Management

As with virtually all of the vasculitides, the therapy for polyarteritis nodosa is empiric. Generally high-dosage (e.g., 1 mg/kg/day prednisone) corticosteroids are begun, but no adequately controlled studies exist. Cytotoxic drugs, especially cyclophosphamide, are also popular; again, controlled studies are lacking.

A widespread practice is to initiate therapy with corticosteroids and to add cytotoxic drugs only if the disease progresses despite corticosteroids. Occasionally, cytotoxic drugs are advised for their "steroid sparing" effect, when the disease is controlled with high-dose steroid therapy but flares as the steroids are reduced. Finally, in occasional very rapidly progressive disease, both cytotoxic drugs and steroids are used from the beginning.

Adequate attention must be paid to management of the varied problems these patients often have, including hypertension, renal failure, congestive heart failure, and complicating bacterial infections.

The decision on the timing of withdrawal of drug therapy is always difficult. Generally, one likes to establish the following clinical situation before beginning drug withdrawal: (1) no further clinical progression of disease; (2) stable laboratory tests, especially renal function and urinalysis; (4) improvement or return to normal in indices of chronic inflammation, especially erythrocyte sedimentation rate and hematocrit.

When reduction of drugs is undertaken, corticosteroids are withdrawn gradually, usually at the rate of 5 mg qd of prednisone every week or two. If there are any clinical or laboratory signs of disease flareup as the corticosteroids are reduced, the dose is increased and one usually waits another 6–12 weeks before attempting to withdraw the drugs again.

Immunology

No genetic factors have been clearly identified among patients with polyarteritis nodosa. Tissue typing has not yet been reported in series of patients. Particularly because it has been thought that polyarteritis nodosa may be a chronic form of serum sickness, possible environmental influences have been sought. Patients have been reported with illnesses resembling polyarteritis nodosa after drug ingestion or, rarely, infections.

In animals, arteritis occurs spontaneously in New Zealand black/white F_1 hybrid mice and Aleutian mink and can be induced by other means. The most comprehensive and pertinent studies have been those of immune-complex-induced serum sickness in animals. If rabbits are injected daily with heterologous serum proteins, some become tolerant of antigen and others form nonprecipitating antibody and eliminate antigen. Another group forms nonprecipitating antibody, clears antigen slowly, and develops a chronic serum sickness type of immune-complex-deposition disease. These latter animals develop chronic glomerulonephritis but not systemic arteritis. It is not known why arteritis is absent. Animals show proteinuria, azotemia, elevated cholesterol, glomerular capillary thickening, endothelial cell proliferation and swelling, and crescent formation. Granular deposition of immune complexes and complement has been shown by immunofluorescent and electron microscopic techniques.

If animals are given a large single injection of foreign protein (antigen), antibodies to antigen are made; circulating antigen-antibody complexes form in antigen excess and may cause an acute serum sickness type of immune-complex-deposition disease. These animals develop an arteritis with lesions in arteries (coronary, pulmonary), glomeruli, joints, and heart. Acute serum sickness is also characterized by deposition of antigen, antibody, and complement. Histologically, the lesion shows endothelial cell proliferation, polymorphonuclear infiltration, and fibrinoid necrosis. Phagocytosis of immune complexes occurs rapidly so that the complexes are often difficult to detect in the experimental disease (and presumably in human disease). Serum complement levels in these animals are reduced.

Mechanisms by which immune complexes deposit and produce tissue injury are reviewed in Chapters 7 and 8. These mechanisms are relevant not only to polyarteritis nodosa but to other rheumatic diseases, particularly rheumatoid arthritis and systemic lupus erythematosus. Many factors enter into the fate of complexes—quantity, size, solubility, antigen-antibody ratio, antigen sites per molecule, and type and class of antibody. It appears that large complexes (potentially injurious) are cleared more rapidly than small ones by the reticuloendothelial system. When the reticuloendothelial system is saturated, complexes localize elsewhere. Several experiments have indicated that it is large (19 S) complexes that deposit along filtering membranes. Their deposition is aided by hydrodynamic forces and local increases in vascular permeability. It is thought that antigen in complexes interacts with basophils or mast cells containing immunoglobulin (Ig) E on their surface. These cells at a particular site release a soluble mediator, platelet-activating factor. This factor activates platelets to release vasoactive amines that increase vascular permeability and influence complex deposition. Complement may not be needed for selective deposition of complexes. Once deposited, complexes activate the classic complement pathway and, through complement-derived chemotactic factors and increased immune adherence, recruit polymorphonuclear cells to the site of inflammation. Tissue injury results from complement-mediated mechanisms and release of neutrophil constituents, thus leading to digestion of vessel walls.

How closely this model applies to polyarteritis nodosa is uncertain. Autoantibodies (antinuclear antibodies, rheumatoid factor) are uncommon in human disease. Some patients with polyarteritis nodosa had elevated IgE levels. Other patients had IgG cytotoxic to leukocytes or kidney cells. Serum complement levels are inconsistently decreased; they are often normal or increased. Circulating cryoglobulins are demonstrable in some patients and immune complexes in many. Immunofluorescent studies demonstrate Ig, complement, and fibrinogen. An association between hepatitis B surface antigen (HBsAg) and polyarteritis nodosa occurs (see below). Studies of some of these patients indicated the presence of circulating HBsAg-anti-HbsAg and Clq precipitins (immune complexes), as well as immunofluorescent localization of HbsAg, Ig, and complement to vessel walls or glomeruli. Hepatitis-associated antigen has not been found in patients with other rheumatic disorders.

Thus, insofar as human polyarteritis nodosa resembles experimental acute serum sickness in rabbits, the pathogenesis appears to be immune complex formation and deposition in vessels, with resultant complement- and neutrophil-mediated inflammation. Evidence suggests that the vasculitis may result from an immunologic reaction to a virus in some patients. The etiology for most other patients with polyarteritis nodosa, aside from rare drug hypersensitivity, remains unknown.

Wegener's Granulomatosis

Wegener's granulomatosis has been recognized for about 40 years. It consists of necrotizing granulomatous vasculitis in the respiratory tract and glomerulonephritis. In most cases there is evidence of a widespread and generalized vasculitis as well.

Clinical Features

Although the disease may occur at any age and in either sex, approximately 60% are men and the peak age of onset is the fourth or fifth decade. Many of the patients have a history of a relentless and progressive sinusitis that does not respond to antibiotics or surgical therapy. Virtually all patients have nonspecific systemic symptoms such as fever, weight loss, and malaise. Multiple pulmonary infiltrates, hemoptysis, and evidence of active glomerulonephritis may develop abruptly. At this stage, many patients will also have skin lesions and other manifestations of generalized vasculitis.

The sinusitis is often very destructive and may erode the floor of the orbit and maxilla. Chest x-ray shows multiple infiltrates, some of which may change rapidly.

Diagnosis

With the classic triad of necrotizing upper respiratory tract lesions, pulmonary infiltrates, and glomerulonephritis, the diagnosis is usually established by demonstrating necrotizing granulomatous arteritis on a biopsy of either the upper respiratory tract lesions or a pulmonary nodule. Occasionally, especially in the sinuses or nasal septum, the biopsy may show only intense granulomatous inflammation with necrosis. In these cases, a repeat biopsy is indicated.

Biopsy of the kidney in these patients shows a segmental necrotizing glomerulonephritis. In rare cases, granulomatous inflammation may be seen in the interstitium around the glomeruli. Immunofluorescence studies usually show minimal if any immunoglobulin or complement deposition. Electron microscopy shows only scattered immune deposits.

Differential Diagnosis. In patients with hemoptysis and glomerulonephritis, the differential diagnosis is usually between Wegener's granulomatosis and Goodpasture's syndrome. The definitive differentiation of these two entities can be made by renal biopsy. Goodpasture's syndrome shows a linear, smooth deposition of immunoglobulins along the glomerular basement membrane. The light microscopic appearance is that of rapidly progressive glomerulonephritis with diffuse involvement of all glomeruli and early crescent formation. Sinusitis and other upper respiratory tract lesions are not seen in Goodpasture's syndrome. These patients also do not have a generalized vasculitis. Other conditions that frequently enter into the differential diagnosis include poststreptococcal glomerulonephritis, pulmonary emboli, embolic renal disease, and other causes of vasculitis.

Laboratory Data

Laboratory findings may include anemia, leukocytosis, elevated erythrocyte sedimentation rate, eosinophilia, hyperglobulinemia, x-ray abnormalities appropriate to organ involvement, and renal function abnormalities.

Course and Management

It was previously reported that all patients with this disease had a relentless downhill course and died within several months. Adrenal corticosteroids prolonged life somewhat but did not result in complete remission. A variety of alkylating and cytotoxic drugs, including nitrogen mustard, azathioprine, chlorambucil, and cyclophosphamide, resulted in prolonged survival and some apparent cures. Of these drugs, the experience of Fauci and his co-workers with cyclophosphamide is by far the greatest, and this is now regarded as the standard drug for therapy of this condition.

The recommended dosage is 1–2 mg/kg/day, with adjustments to maintain the total white blood count above 3,000/cu mm. Higher doses for a short period have been used in occasional very ill patients. The dose is gradually increased until a clinical response is seen. The response can be measured in various ways, including pulmonary infiltrates, urinalysis, erythrocyte sedimentation rate, and the subjective impression of well-being. Most seriously ill patients are simultaneously placed on corticosteroids in large doses for 2–4 weeks. The corticosteroids are gradually reduced over a period of several weeks.

These patients are often very ill. Careful attention to other problems, including renal failure, cardiac disease, pulmonary disease, and hypertension, often makes the difference between survival and death.

Once the disease is under control, the patient is maintained on cyclophosphamide for 1–2 years, after which the drug is gradually withdrawn. Fauci and his co-workers have described a gradual loss of bone marrow reserve in these patients, so that the dose of cyclophosphamide occasionally must be gradually decreased over this period. Using this approach, approximately 60% of all patients with Wegener's granulomatosis survive 2 years, and most of the 2-year survivors appear to remain well indefinitely. Patients with significant renal insufficiency, such as serum creatinine above 3 or 4 mg%, usually do poorly. Also, other patients simply cannot tolerate cytotoxic drugs in therapeutic doses and succumb to a relentless progression of disease.

Immunology and Pathogenesis

The etiology and pathogenesis of Wegener's granulomatosis are not known, although the disease has some immunologic abnormalities. It has been speculated that Wegener's granulomatosis is caused by hypersensitivity to an unknown antigen. Patients were found to have elevated IgA, secretory IgA, and C3 levels before treatment. Rheumatoid factor is commonly detected. Circulating immune complexes or cryoglobulins are often found. Tissue immunofluorescence has revealed glomerular Ig and complement. Cutaneous anergy occurs inconstantly. Impaired in vitro lymphocyte responsiveness is noted in some patients. Cyclophosphamide-treated patients showed suppressed antigen responsiveness in vitro, monocytopenia, depressed responses to new antigens, and reduction of IgA levels to normal. Although it is not known how immunologic events participate in the pathogenesis of Wegener's granulomatosis, it appears that theropeutic alterations of immune responses are associated with disease remission.

Henoch-Schönlein Purpura

Henoch-Schönlein purpura, also known as *anaphylactoid purpura,* is a condition primarily of children in which three organ systems are characteristically involved—the skin, gastrointestinal tract, and kidneys.

Clinical Features

The skin lesion (c. 100% of patients) is a purpuric macule present over the buttocks and lower extremities. The typical lesion progresses from an erythematous raised papule approximately 5–10 mm in diameter to a dusky purple flat lesion over a period of about 24 hours. The lesions usually occur in crops so that most of the anterior surfaces of the lower extremities will be covered with these lesions over a fairly short period. To a lesser extent, they may also be found on the trunk and the arms.

The gastrointestinal manifestations (c. 50% of patients) of the disease are due to hemorrhage in the wall of the small intestine from focal areas of vasculitis. This hemorrhage may then cause sudden gastrointestinal bleeding or abdominal colic or may be the leading point of an intussusception.

The renal disease of these children appears as hematuria with mild to moderate proteinuria. Biopsy of the kidney reveals a glomerulonephritis of variable severity. In the majority of cases, a focal glomerulonephritis is noted, although diffuse proliferative lesions may be seen. Occasional patients may have diffuse proliferative lesions with crescent formation.

The child frequently has a prodrome consisting of malaise and influenza-like symptoms, which may last for several days before the development of purpura. The onset is usually abrupt, with the rapid development of purpura and often abdominal colic. About half the patients have guaiac-positive stools, although gross gastrointestinal bleeding is less common. Renal disease is generally present from the onset if it is going to develop. Over half of the cases have gross hematuria.

Course

Although this condition was previously thought benign and self-limiting, as many as 20% of children eventually develop renal insufficiency. In adults, that figure may be as high as 40%. Most of those who do poorly have recurrent attacks, each of which results in progressively greater destruction of renal tissue.

Laboratory Data

Except for those mentioned above, laboratory studies are normal. Pathologic changes are those of small vessel angiitis, with a pleomorphic cellular response with a preponderance of neutrophils.

Management

No studies have clearly demonstrated the benefit of any form of therapy in these patients. In patients with abdominal pain or gastrointestinal bleeding, the gastrointestinal tract should be rested, using nasogastric suction and parenteral alimentation. Corticosteroids and cytotoxic drugs are occasionally used in progressive and severe disease, but the benefits, if any, are marginal. Fortunately, in children, the majority of acute attacks resolve.

Immunology and Pathogenesis

Many patients have histories of antecedent viral or bacterial (streptococcal) infections. Hypersensitivity to drugs or food has similarly been implicated, although not rigorously proved. Immunologic studies of patients showed generally normal serum complement levels; normal or elevated antistreptolysin-O titers; occasional cryoglobulinemia; variable immunofluorescent localization of IgG, IgA, C3, or properdin in glomeruli; and less constant localization of immunoreactants in skin. Rare cases of Henoch-Schönlein purpura have been reported in patients with hereditary deficiencies of certain complement components. Thus, a typical clinical syndrome associated with the absence of hemolytic complement activity should alert one to this possibility.

Aortic Arch Arteritis

Aortic arch arteritis (Takayasu's arteritis) is a very rare condition in the United States, although it is common in the Orient. It affects the main arteries as they arise from the aortic arch and, to a lesser extent, the abdominal aorta.

Clinical Features

The typical patient is a young oriental woman with the onset of malaise, low-grade fever, and claudication in the arms. Visual problems, including transient blindness, and severe recurrent migraine-type headaches are common. Since other branches of the aorta may also be involved, patients have been reported with intestinal ischemia and severe hypertension due to involvement of the mesenteric and renal arteries.

This disease is often called *pulseless disease*. The diagnosis should be suspected when a striking difference between the blood pressures in the arms is noted by the examiner. In some patients, the pulses cannot be demonstrated in the upper extremities. Other clinical manifestations include aortic insufficiency, prolonged fever of unknown origin, transient ischemic attacks, and Raynaud's phenomenon.

Pathology

The lesions consist of an intense granulomatous vasculitis involving large arteries, often associated with intimal proliferation and thrombosis of the vessel itself. Immunofluorescence studies have been scanty, but immunoglobulins and complement are not prominent in lesions.

Laboratory Data

Except for an elevated erythrocyte sedimentation rate and mild anemia, most laboratory test results are normal. The results of immunologic studies, such as rheumatoid factor, antinuclear antibodies, complement, and cryoglobulins, are normal.

Diagnosis

The diagnosis is usually confirmed by arteriography, which reveals variable stenosis and aneurysmal dilatation in many of the vessels arising from the aortic arch and the abdominal aorta. Occasional patients will appear with enlargement of arteries, especially the carotid. Biopsy will show giant cell arteritis.

Course and Therapy

The natural history of the disease, especially outside of the Orient, is unclear. Most patients have a progressive and deteriorating course, with occasional acute flareup of clinical symptoms. Corticosteroid therapy has been used for about 30 years, with many instances of transient or sustained improvement. However, no controlled studies are available, and it is unclear whether these drugs actually prolong survival or not. Certainly, adequate control of blood pressure and other general measures are essential in therapy.

Giant Cell (Cranial) Arteritis

Clinical Features

Giant cell arteritis is a spectacular disease in its most characteristic appearance. It occurs primarily in persons over the age of 50, with the peak age of onset at about 65. The onset is often abrupt, although many patients may have had insidious symptoms for weeks or even months before seeking medical care. The symptoms can be divided into two groups: constitutional and those related directly to the cranial arteritis. The constitutional symptoms generally are known as *polymyalgia rheumatica*. This syndrome occurs in at least two-thirds of the patients with giant cell arteritis. It consists of severe aching and stiffness in the large proximal muscles, especially around the shoulder and pelvic girdles. Most patients are disabled by the pain and stiffness. In fact, it is common to see patients who are unable to roll over in bed. Some patients may have mild synovitis. Many of them have a low-grade fever.

The cranial arteritis itself appears in a fairly characteristic way. Headache is the rule, occurring in up to 90% of the patients. The typical patient complains of an excruciating headache that may vary in severity but never clears completely. The onset of the headache may be abrupt and frequently begins at night. It is due to inflammatory arteritis in the cranial arteries and is often localized over the temporal arteries. Thus, many people termed this entity *temporal arteritis*. Occipital arteries are also commonly involved; patients may have areas of tenderness located elsewhere on the scalp.

Cranial arteritis may include visual problems, such as transient or permanent blindness, with or without any predisposing visual symptoms, diplopia, and blurred vision. Additional symptoms of cranial arteritis include claudication of the jaw with chewing, and occasional claudication of the tongue as well.

A very small percentage of patients may have evidence of arteritis in arteries other than those in the head. These patients may appear with claudication in the upper and/or lower extremities, mesenteric vasculitis, or similar evidence of widespread vasculitis. However, this condition is rare. Physical examination of patients with temporal arteritis is often remarkable for the paucity of abnormalities. Careful palpation of the scalp may reveal localized areas of tenderness. In some patients the temporal arteries themselves will be found to be enlarged, firm, and pulseless. However, severe giant cell arteritis may be found in patients with absolutely asymptomatic temporal arteries.

In spite of the severe symptoms relating to the proximal musculature in at least two-thirds of the patients, muscle examination may reveal tenderness only to deep palpation. Strength is usually normal except for poor compliance because of pain. No atrophy is evident, and results of electrodiagnostic studies are normal. Although synovitis has been reported by scan and other techniques, it is rarely notable on physical examination.

In those patients with eye involvement, funduscopic examination may show blanching of the disc, hemorrhages, and occasional exudates.

Laboratory Data

A striking elevation of the erythrocyte sedimentation rate is the only consistent laboratory abnormality in this disease. As a general rule, the diagnosis should not be made unless the sedimentation rate (Westergren) is greater than 50 mm/hr. In many cases, the sedimentation rate is 100 mm/hr or greater.

External carotid arteriography has been used to help define areas of likely vasculitis. Although this technique is still sometimes employed, the difficulties in differentiating atherosclerotic from vasculitic lesions have made it of only occasional benefit, and it has not been widely accepted.

A variety of nonspecific laboratory abnormalities have also been reported in recent years. These include mild anemia, thrombocytosis, mildly abnormal liver function tests, and occasional evidence of mild inflammation on synovial fluid analysis.

Pathology

Involved arteries typically show a characteristic arteritis that consists of intimal thickening, thrombosis, and focal granulomatous arteritis with giant cells, lymphocytes, histiocytes, and a background of plasma cells and eosinophils. The internal elastic membrane is usually disrupted.

Course

The natural history of this disease is probably not fully appreciated, since it has been shown that as many as 15% or 20% of patients with polymyalgia rheumatica and giant cell arteritis may simply have different manifestations of the same disease.

In those patients with clinical and biopsy-proven cranial arteritis, however, it is known that the incidence of involvement of intracranial arteries, especially the ophthalmic, may be as high as 10%. This condition usually appears early in the course of the disease and is often sudden and permanent. Other evidence of intracranial disease, including transient ischemic attacks, strokes, seizures, and organic brain syndromes, has been reported.

Management

Because of the fear of blindness and other major intracranial complications, therapy for patients with established giant cell arteritis should be instituted immediately. Most observers use relatively high dosages of corticosteroids, in the range of 60 mg/day of prednisone. A recent study showed that alternate-day prednisone was not adequate to control this disease and that a divided daily dose was preferable to a single morning dose. This regimen is usually maintained for the first 6 to 12 weeks of the disease. When the erythrocyte sedimentation rate returns to normal, the prednisone dose is gradually converted to a single daily dose and its level is then reduced gradually. Although it was formerly believed that cranial arteritis was universally a self-limited illness in which all patients could be weaned from their steroids within a few months, it has been seen recently that most patients require at least small doses of corticosteroids for more than 1 year. These patients are often exquisitely sensitive to slight changes in their steroid doses, especially when the dosage level is below 15 mg/day. For that reason, when the dosage has been reduced to approximately this level, further reductions are made cautiously—2.5 mg/day decrements every 2 to 4 weeks.

The erythrocyte sedimentation rate should be followed carefully during this period. Cranial arteritis is one of the few rheumatic diseases in which there is compelling reason to treat even if the only abnormality is a laboratory one. Therefore, if the erythrocyte sedimentation rate abruptly rises, serious consideration should be given to raising the steroid dosage again, regardless of whether or not the patient is symptomatic.

Appropriate therapy for patients with polymyalgia rheumatica without proven arteritis is controversial. This syndrome is common; at least as many patients appear at rheumatology clinics with polymyalgia rheumatica as with typical cranial arteritis. It is known that some patients without symptoms referable to cranial arteritis will have arteritis on biopsy. Also, it is known that the arteritis is not uniform in distribution, so that a negative biopsy result does not rule out arteritis. However, due to the toxicity of high-dose corticosteroids in the older age group, it is common clinical practice to treat polymyalgia rheumatica, in the absence of clinical or pathologic arteritis, with low dosages of prednisone, for example, 5–15 mg/day, or even with nonsteroidal anti-inflammatory drugs alone. These patients require careful and frequent observation, but most do well and do not develop overt arteritis.

Immunologic Studies

Test results for rheumatoid factor, antinuclear antibody, serum complement, and immunoglobulin levels have been normal or only mildly abnormal in virtually all patients studied. Results of immunofluorescent studies of temporal arteries have usually been normal or have shown weak staining with antisera to immunoglobulins. More promising were early reports of enhanced cell-mediated immunity directed against vascular antigens, although recent work showed no significant differences when comparing patients with giant cell arteritis to those with either rheumatoid arthritis or to normal control subjects. The etiology and pathogenesis of giant cell arteritis are unknown. There have been reports of familial polymyalgia rheumatica and of increased incidence of HL-A8, HL-A10, and HL-A16 in patients. Increased contact of polymyalgia rheumatica patients with parakeets, the presence of anti-HBSAg antibody in patients, normal viral antibody study findings, and deposition of Ig and C3 were also reported.

Allergic Granulomatous Arteritis

Allergic granulomatous arteritis, also known as *Churg-Strauss vasculitis,* is often considered a variant of either Wegener's granulomatosus or typical polyarteritis nodosa.

Clinical Features
These patients are usually middle-aged or older and have a history of asthma or other chronic lung disease. Patients may become abruptly ill, with dyspnea, worsening asthma, and other symptoms of generalized vasculitis including hypertension, renal failure, neuropathy, and various skin lesions.

Laboratory Data
Over half of these patients have peripheral eosinophilia, but otherwise the laboratory data are identical to those found in other forms of vasculitis. Chest x-ray frequently shows fleeting pulmonary infiltrates, some of which may cavitate.

Pathology
The lesions on biopsy may vary from well-formed granulomas to simply a focal necrotizing vasculitis. In the lung, granuloma formation is most prominent. It usually consists of striking eosinophilia around areas of necrotizing granulomatous vasculitis. Peripheral biopsies have a lower incidence of granuloma formation and may simply show a focal necrotizing vasculitis. However, cases have been reported in which typical granulomas were present in a generalized distribution.

Prognosis, Course, and Treatment
Approximately half of the patients with this syndrome die of complications of their vasculitis. No specific treatment is known. High-dose corticosteroids, with or without cytotoxic drugs, are usually employed as for polyarteritis nodosa or Wegener's granulomatosis.

Immunology
There are no characteristic immunologic abnormalities. The erythrocyte sedimentation rate is uniformly elevated, and immunoglobulins are usually increased. Serum complement levels are normal, and results of few immunofluorescent studies have been reported.

SECONDARY VASCULITIS

Many patients with generalized vasculitis have an underlying diagnosis (Table 18.2); the vasculitis is simply one of a variety of complications of another illness. Unlike most of the primary syndromes, the secondary vasculitides are usually accompanied by striking evidence of immunologic abnormalities.

Rheumatoid Vasculitis

Clinical Features

Clinical rheumatoid vasculitis appears in two ways. By far the most common, occurring in up to several percent of hospitalized patients with rheumatoid arthritis, is a low-grade vasculitis that includes insidious onset of skin ulcers, stocking-glove peripheral sensory neuropathy, and small infarcts in and around the nail folds and finger pulp areas. Biopsy shows low-grade vasculitis involving small blood vessels, especially venules.

Much less common, but much more severe, is a syndrome identical to polyarteritis nodosa. These patients, many of whom have recently been on high-dose corticosteroid therapy, may have the abrupt onset of mononeuritis multiplex, with or without other evidence of vasculitis. Unlike polyarteritis nodosa, involvement of the renal arteries is rare. However, involvement of other viscera, especially the mesenteric arteries, may be seen and may be life-threatening.

In these patients, biopsy of muscle may show segmental necrotizing arteritis as in polyarteritis nodosa (Chap. 10).

Laboratory Data

Laboratory studies during episodes of fulminant rheumatoid vasculitis reveal hypocomplementemia in over one half of patients and mixed cryoglobulins in most of them. These patients with vasculitis virtually all have rheumatoid factor, usually in high titer. It has been shown that these patients are more apt to have low-molecular-weight IgM rheumatoid factor and a high level of circulating immune complexes. Also, 7S IgM avidly fixes early complement components and may thereby generate significant amounts of complement-derived fragments with potent vasoactive properties. Eosinophilia in varying degrees has also been reported in an increased percentage of patients with rheumatoid vasculitis.

Course

The prognosis for patients with generalized rheumatoid vasculitis is poor. Death, either as a result of visceral involvement or due to severe inanition, occurs in approximately one-half of patients within 5 years.

Management

Patients with skin ulcers and nail fold infarcts probably should not be treated in a vigorous manner. Local measures may suffice for the skin ulcers, which are the most painful and debilitating aspect of this form of vasculitis. These measures include careful debridement, whirlpool baths, wet-to-dry dressings, and topical adsorbents. The wounds are kept as clean as possible, and occasional surgical excision is required. For patients who have poor formation of granulation tissue, especially with painful ulcers, topical oxygen therapy applied by using a plastic "oxygen boot" is often successful. When good granulation tissue appears, skin grafting is often required to heal these ulcers. If an ulcer has developed over a bony prominence, such as a malleolus, a cast or other immobilizing device to limit trauma to the skin is recommended.

Therapy for fulminant generalized vasculitis is more aggressive, including high doses of corticosteroids, with the recognition that rapid reduction of corticosteroids may actually induce rheumatoid vasculitis. Cytotoxic agents, as for polyarteritis nodosa, are also used in some patients.

Other Rheumatic Diseases

Systemic Lupus Erythematosus

Systemic lupus erythematosus (SLE), although characterized pathologically by inflammation in small blood vessels all over the body, is not accompanied by clinically important generalized arteritis in most patients. However, perhaps 5% of patients with SLE will develop a fulminant vasculitis characterized by mononeuritis multiplex, skin ulcers, gangrene, and visceral involvement, especially of the colon. This complication often arises abruptly and is usually seen in patients who do not have severe glomerulonephritis. Biopsy of muscle and other tissues may show a large vessel arteritis identical to polyarteritis nodosa (Chap. 16).

Dermatomyositis

Childhood dermatomyositis is occasionally complicated by a vasculitis that is primarily limited to the intestinal tract, although involvement of the eye, skin, and other tissues has been reported (Chap. 19).

Sjögren's Syndrome

Sjögren's syndrome may be associated with non-thrombocytopenic purpura, although clinically important vasculitis is rare. Patients with purpura typically have hypergammaglobulinemia involving all Ig classes, and occasionally mixed cryoglobulins will be found. Rarely, purpura may be a manifestation of the hyperviscosity syndrome, usually seen in persons with large amounts of IgG rheumatoid factor.

Cryoglobulinemia

Cryoglobulins are abnormal immunoglobulins that undergo precipitation at low temperatures and redissolve when warmed (Chap. 4). They may occur secondary to other disease processes or be idiopathic (essential). They are described as monoclonal or polyclonal (mixed). Monoclonal cryoglobulins occur most frequently with lymphoproliferative disorders (myeloma, macroglobulinemia, lymphocytic leukemia, lymphosarcoma) and less commonly without an underlying disorder. Mixed cryoglobulins are frequently associated with other immunologic or rheumatic diseases, infectious diseases (subacute bacterial endocarditis, syphilis, leprosy, toxoplasmosis, mononucleosis, cytomegalovirus), skin disorders, lymphoproliferative disorders, and chronic disease (ulcerative colitis, liver disease, sarcoid) or are idiopathic. Secondary cryoglobulinemia is discussed with the appropriate primary disease. Essential cryoglobulinemia, usually mixed, can give rise to a small-vessel vasculitis and is considered a distinct entity (Table 4.6).

Clinical symptoms may include Raynaud's phenomenon, acrocyanosis, livedo reticularis, peripheral numbness or paresthesia, vascular occlusion, infarct, digital ulceration, lower-extremity purpura, leg ulcers, hyperviscosity syndrome, urticaria, arthralgia/arthritis, or glomerulonephritis. Laboratory studies demonstrate rouleaux formation, a rapid erythrocyte sedimentation rate, cryoprecipitation, abnormalities on protein and immunoelectrophoresis, and low serum complement. Pathologic changes consist of small vessel vasculitis. Immunofluorescent studies show deposition of Ig and complement.

The cryoglobulins in essential cryoglobulinemias, and associated with rheumatic disease in general, are almost always mixed. The majority of these patients probably have a chronic infection as the stimulus for their mixed cryoglobulinemia. Over half of the originally described patients had either hepatitis B antigen or antibody. Cryoglobulins may be IgM anti-IgG:IgG, monoclonal IgG anti-IgG: polyclonal IgG, or IgA:IgG and may contain C3 or DNA. The mechanisms of cryoprecipitation are unclear but appear related to molecular physicochemical factors and protein-water interaction, pH, ionic strength, temperature, charge, conformation, and state of hydration. The stimulus (or loss of regulatory function) leading to the production of these abnormal immunoglobulins in this group of patients is not known. They are presumably analogues of circulating immune complexes with a propensity to cause small-vessel lesions.

Treatment of this disorder has consisted of cold avoidance, corticosteroids, immunosuppressive agents, penicillamine, splenectomy, plasmapheresis, and hydroxychloroquine and has been variably successful.

Hepatitis B Vasculitis

Hepatitis B-associated vasculitis, first described in 1970, has accounted for 30%–40% of the cases of idiopathic necrotizing vasculitis in some series. This association indicates that (1) a common infectious agent can cause a chronic rheumatic disease, (2) the host response may be the determining factor in the clinical syndrome seen, and (3) hepatitis B vasculitis is a chronic immune-complex-mediated disease.

Epidemiology
The epidemiology of hepatitis B vasculitis parallels that of hepatitis B itself. The disease is seen with increased frequency in drug users, homosexuals, and chronic dialysis patients.

Clinical Features
Patients with hepatitis B vasculitis have symptoms resembling those of most other types of generalized vasculitis. Fever, arthralgias, weight loss, and mononeuritis multiplex are seen in nearly all patients, and abdominal pain, central nervous system disease, and skin lesions are common.

Course
The relationship between the vasculitis and the liver illness is unpredictable (Fig. 18.1). Patients were seen who had preexisting chronic active hepatitis, who were asymptomatic carriers, and who had apparently recovered from acute hepatitis B. One patient clearly had vasculitis as the initial manifestation of hepatitis B infection, followed several months later by typical hepatitis.

Management
Therapy has consisted of corticosteroids and sometimes cytotoxic drugs, in a manner similar to that of polyarteritis nodosa treatment. Approximately 30%–40% of

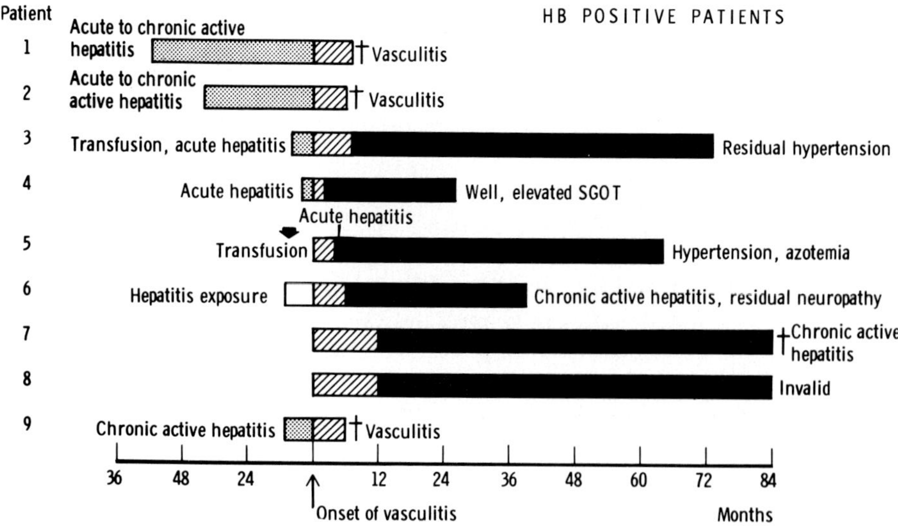

Figure 18.1. Summary of the course of hepatitis B-positive patients with vasculitis. Lightly stippled bars indicate known antecedent liver disease. Diagonally hatched bars indicate the periods of clinically active vasculitis. Dark stippled bars indicate the duration of follow-up after recovery from vasculitis. Dagger denotes death. (Reprinted with permission from Sergent JS et al: Vasculitis with hepatitis B. *Medicine* 55:12, 1976)

the patients have died of their vasculitis. Among the survivors, hepatitis B vasculitis has been found to be a "one-shot" illness that runs its course in 6–12 months. After this time, if the patients can be weaned from the drugs, recurrences are rare. This is true despite the fact that all patients have remained chronically antigen or antibody positive. Residual morbidity, including hypertension, neuropathy, and chronic active hepatitis, is high.

Hypersensitivity Angiitis

Hypersensitivity angiitis is distinguished by an involvement of small arteries, arterioles, and venules. Pathologic changes consist of fibrinoid necrosis with pleomorphic cellular infiltration, neutrophil predominance, prominent eosinophils, and lesions at similar stages of evolution. Hypersensitivity angiitis has also been termed *leukocytoclastic angiitis* or *small-vessel vasculitis*.

Human acute serum sickness is similar to that in the animal model discussed previously. It was originally described when antisera produced in animals were frequently administered to treat human diseases. The same process can follow certain drug hypersensitivities. Approximately 1–2 weeks after exposure (1–3 days in previously sensitized persons), symptoms occur. These are fever, urticaria, arthralgias, arthritis, myalgias, adenopathy, or vasculitis of other organs (uncommonly). Laboratory features are leukocytosis, eosinophilia, elevated erythrocyte sedimentation rate, and low complement values. The syndrome is self-limited. Treatment is symptomatic. It has recently been shown that treatment with antihistamines (cyproheptadine or hydroxyzine) reduced the incidence of symptoms of patients given equine diphtheria antitoxin, which suggests that complex deposition was inhibited. Mechanisms of acute hypersensitivity or serum sickness in humans are thought to be those outlined in animal models. Occasional patients with drug hypersensitivities and serum sickness symptoms have manifested lymphocyte sensitivity to the drugs, as assayed in vitro by transformation or mediator production.

Behçet's Disease

Behçet's disease is a multisystem disease of unknown cause. It is suggested that this diagnosis be made if certain criteria are met: three major or two major and two minor. Major criteria are (usually) oral ulceration, genital ulceration, ocular changes, or skin disease. Minor criteria are gastrointestinal, central nervous system, articular, or cardiovascular involvement or a positive family history. The true incidence and epidemiology of Behçet's disease are not known.

Behçet's disease occurs most commonly in the Middle East and Japan and in men more often than in women. Familial incidence has been recognized, and an association with HL-A5 has been reported. Etiologic studies have been inconclusive.

Clinical manifestations are diverse. They include mucosal (recurrent oral ulcers resembling aphthous stomatitis, scanty lingual fungiform papillae), ulcerative genital lesions, cutaneous lesions, and ocular, gastrointestinal, cardiovascular, neurologic, and other manifestations (pulmonary infiltrates, myalgias, fever, constitutional symptoms, epididymitis, orchitis, malignant lymphoma, and adenopathy).

Laboratory findings include elevated acute phase reactants, elevated erythrocyte sedimentation rate, anemia, polyclonal hypergammaglobulinemia, negative antinuclear antibody, negative rheumatoid factor, occasional positive cryoglobulins, occasional eosinophilia, normal complement levels, normal blood coagulation test results, positive anticytoplasmic antibodies, and variably impaired cell-mediated immunity.

Roentgenographic changes are not pathognomonic. Pathologic changes reveal vasculitis that may be necrotizing, endothelial swelling, vascular occlusion, fibrinoid deposition, and mononuclear inflammatory cell infiltration.

The natural history is variable, with spontaneous remissions and exacerbations. Morbidity from major organ system disease can occur. Without consistent success or controlled observations, many therapeutic approaches have been tried: topical and systemic steroids, immunosuppressives, blood transfusions, fibrinolytic drugs, and transfer factor.

The pathogenesis is unknown. Behçet's disease bears a resemblance to other systemic rheumatic diseases, vasculitis, mucocutaneous syndromes, and periodic syndromes, but its relationship to them is uncertain.

Erythema Nodosum

Erythema nodosum is manifested by painful, inflamed subcutaneous nodules frequently accompanied by arthritis and associated with underlying disease. The tender, slightly raised red nodules appear suddenly, usually over anterior tibia, and heal within 3–6 weeks. Young women are most frequently affected. Constitutional symptoms with fever are common. Articular symptoms occur in nearly three-fourths of patients with synovitis or the knees, ankles, or small joints. Erythema nodosum has been associated with sarcoidosis, tuberculosis, streptococcal infection, inflammatory bowel disease, lymphogranuloma venereum, fungal infections, leprosy, cat-scratch disease, trichophyton, Behçet's disease, other infections, and drugs, or it may be idiopathic.

Laboratory tests reveal acute inflammation and reflect the underlying abnormality.

Pathologic changes are probably those of tissue inflammation rather than vasculitis. They include panniculitis in lower dermal and subcutaneous tissue; polymorphonuclear and later round cell infiltration; endothelial proliferation; and inconstant thrombosis, arteriolitis, or venulitis.

Erythema nodosum usually resolves within a few months. Recurrence or persistence is usually the result of persistent underlying disease or unrecognized drug ingestion. Treatment is conservative and consists of leg elevation and analgesic anti-inflammatory drugs. Colchicine has been effective in some patients. Corticosteroids are effective but not usually recommended for a self-limited process.

Immunologic studies are incomplete. Immunoglobulin or complement levels have been raised in occasional patients. Tissue immunofluorescence has inconstantly demonstrated Ig or complement.

Weber-Christian Disease (Nodular Panniculitis)

Weber-Christian disease is an uncommon syndrome characterized by recurrent febrile nodular panniculitis. Nodules are usually subcutaneous on the trunk and extremities but can occur and cause symptoms elsewhere—mesentery, marrow, pericardium, or other internal organs. Pathologic changes include edema, fat necrosis, and mononuclear cellular infiltrate, and possibly also vasculitis. Treatment generally consists of anti-inflammatory drugs, systemic steroids, and immunosuppressives. Recent studies have found low-molecular-weight (7S) IgM; circulating complexes of 7S IgM:IgG; and reduced serum C1, C4, and C2 during disease activity. These data suggest that systemic Weber-Christian disease may be immune-complex-mediated.

Cutaneous Vasculitis and Arthritis

A syndrome of recurrent maculopapular erythematous or urticarial skin eruptions, angioedema, synovitis, and glomerulonephritis has been reported. Histologic studies demonstrated a leukocytoclastic angiitis of cutaneous vessels. Patients had recurrent episodes and had been treated with salicylates, indomethacin, hydroxyzine, antimalarials, steroids, azathioprine, cyclophosphamide, or chlorambucil. Immunologic studies revealed negative rheumatoid factor; positive antinuclear antibodies in some patients, but usually negative anti-DNA; trace cryoglobulins; low serum complement (CH50, C1, C4, C2, C3, factor B; usually normal C1 inhibitor), circulating immune complexes in some patients; and vascular deposition of IgM, IgA, and complement in some. This syndrome therefore appeared to be immune-complex-mediated.

Polyarthritis with Intestinal Bypass

Polyarthritis, usually mild and nondeforming, has been recognized in some patients who have undergone jejunocolostomies for obesity. Treatment consists of salicylates and oral corticosteroids if needed. Restoration of normal bowel anatomy can lead to resolution of symptoms. Cryoproteins were identified containing Ig, C, and antibody to colonic bacteria. These observations suggest that absorbed intestinal bacterial antigens may evoke immune complex formation with classic and alternative complement pathway activation.

Portions of the material in immunology of polyarteritis nodosa, immunology and pathogenesis of Wegener's granulomatosis, immunology and pathogenesis of Henoch-Schönlein purpura, immunologic studies of giant cell arteritis, cryoglobulinemia, hypersensitivity angiitis, Behçets disease, erythema nodosum, Weber-Christian disease, cutaneous vasculitis and arthritis, and polyarthritis with intestinal bypass appear in similar form in Panush RS: Immunologic aspects of vasculitis in Lockey RF (ed): *Allergy and Clinical Immunology*. Garden City, NY, Medical Examination Publishing Co, Inc, an Excerpta Medica company, © 1979, pp 244–247, 249–255. Reprinted by permission.

BIBLIOGRAPHY

Blomgren SE: Erythema nodosum. *Semin Arthritis Rheum* 4:1, 1975.

Brouet JC, Clauvel JP, Danon F, et al: Biologic and clinical significance of cryoglobluins: A report of 86 cases. *Am J Med* 57:775, 1974.

Caldwell JR, Cusamano C, Ludwig F: Circulating 7S IgM immune complexes and low serum complement in a patient with systemic Weber-Christian disease. *Clin Res* 22:416A, 1974.

Chajek T, Fainara M: Behçet's disease: Report of 41 cases and a review of the literature. *Medicine* 54:179, 1979.

Christian CL, Sergent JS: Vasculitis syndromes: Clinical and experimental models. *Am J Med* 61:385, 1976.

Cochrane CG, Koffler D: Immune complex disease in experimental animals and man. *Adv Immunol* 16:185, 1973.

Fauci AS, Haynes BF, Katz P: The spectrum of vasculitis: Clinical, pathological, immunological, and therapeutic considerations. *Ann Intern Med* 89:167, 1977.

Fauci AS, Katz P, Haynes BD, et al: Cyclophosphamide therapy of severe systemic necrotizing vasculitis. *N Engl J Med* 301:235, 1979.

Fauci AS, Wolff SM: Wegener's granulomatosis: Studies in eighteen patients and a review of the literature. *Medicine* 52:535, 1973.

Hunder GG, Sheps SG, Allen GL, et al: Daily and alternate-day corticosteroid regimens in treatment of giant cell arteritis: Comparison in a prospective study. *Ann Intern Med* 82:613, 1975.

Levo Y, Gorevic PD, Kassab et al: Mixed cryoglobulinemia—an immune complex disease often associated with hepatitis B virus infection. *Trans Assoc Am Physicians* 90:167, 1977.

McDuffie FC, Sams WM, Maldonado JE, et al: Hypocomplementemia with cutaneous vasculitis and arthritis. *Mayo Clin Proc* 48:340, 1973.

Mowrey RH, Lundberg EA: The clinical manifestations of essential polyangiitis (periarteritis nodosa) with emphasis on the hepatic manifestations. *Ann Intern Med* 40: 1145, 1954.

Sergent JS, Lockshin MD, Christian CL, et al: Vasculitis with hepatitis B antigenemia: Long-term observations in nine patients. *Medicine* 55:1, 1976.

Theofilopoulos AN, Burtonboy G, Lo Spalluto J, et al: IgG rheumatoid factor and low molecular weight IgM: An association with vasculitis. *Arthritis Rheum* 17:272, 1974.

Zeek PM: Periarteritis nodosa and other forms of necrotizing angiitis. *N Engl J Med* 248:764, 1953.

19
Polymyositis and Dermatomyositis

Norman L. Gottlieb

Robert G. Gray

Polymyositis (PM) is an inflammatory muscle disease characterized by symmetric weakness of the proximal extremities and neck. Other systems (e.g., pulmonary, cardiac, gastrointestinal) may be involved (Table 19.1). When accompanied by typical inflammatory cutaneous lesions, the disorder is termed *dermatomyositis (DM)*, a clinical entity first described by Unverricht nearly a century ago. Myopathies of PM and DM are clinically and histologically indistinguishable, and aberrant cellular immunity (vide infra) has been documented in both disorders. However, the more intimate relation of DM with malignancy, and the higher frequency of DM in the pediatric population, suggest that different precipitating events may be present.

CLASSIFICATION

Several classifications of inflammatory myopathy have been proposed. One widely used categorization (Table 19.2) emphasizes the variable clinical expression, prognosis, and disease associations of idiopathic myositis. Acute myolysis, characterized by noninflammatory muscle cell necrosis, elevated serum muscle enzymes, and myoglobinuria, previously was classified as a type of PM, although it occurred rarely. Currently, rhabdomyolysis is known to encompass a heterogeneous group of disorders that include crush injuries, alcohol-induced myolysis, McArdle's syndrome, primary metabolic myopathies, sea snake envenomation, and others.

PREVALENCE

Estimates of the prevalence of PM/DM in European and American populations vary from 0.1% to 0.6%. PM is the most common primary adult myopathy but is observed in childhood less frequently than muscular dystrophy, from which it must be differentiated. Several new cases of PM/DM generally are encountered

Table 19.1. Clinical Features of Polymyositis/Dermatomyositis

Muscle	Weakness
	Symmetric proximal extremity
	Anterior neck flexor
	Pharyngeal
	Pain and/or tenderness
	Atrophy (in advanced disease)
Skin	Heliotrope lids and periorbital edema
	Erythematous eruption on face, neck, trunk
	Gottron's papules
	Cuticular hyperkeratosis, periungual erythema
	Calcinosis (predominantly childhood DM)
Articular	Arthralgias
	Mild inflammatory polyarthritis
Gastrointestinal	Esophageal and small bowel hypomotility
	Malabsorption
Pulmonary	Inflammatory infiltrates
	Fibrosing alveolitis
Cardiac	Atrial arrythmias
	Conduction disturbances
	Rarely, frank myocardiopathy, pericarditis
Vascular	Raynaud's phenomenon
	Necrotizing vasculitis of gut, skin, subcutaneous
	tissues, vasa nervorum (childhood DM)

each year on the medical services of large hospitals, and the age-adjusted incidence is five cases per mission per year in the United States. These disorders may develop at any age but are diagnosed most frequently in the fifth and sixth decades. The age distribution is bimodal, 20% of cases occurring under the age of 15 years. In common with systemic lupus erythematosus (SLE) and scleroderma (PSS), these conditions exhibit a female predominance (2 : 1) and an apparent racial predilection for blacks.

Table 19.2. Classification of Idiopathic Inflammatory Myositis

Type	*Name*
I	Polymyositis in adults
II	Typical dermatomyositis
III	Inflammatory myositis associated with malignancy
IV	Childhood myositis
V	Myositis associated with the overlap syndromes

SOURCE: From Pearson and Bohan (1977).

CLINICAL FEATURES

Symmetric proximal muscle weakness is present ultimately in all cases of PM/DM, with rare exception. It is the initial disease manifestation in 50%. Disease onset generally is insidious, evolving over weeks to months; occasionally it is fulminant. Pelvic girdle weakness usually precedes upper limb involvement, and early complaints are difficulty in arising from a chair or squatting position and in stair climbing. Upper extremity myositis is heralded by an increasing difficulty in maintaining the arms overhead, as in hair combing. Weakness of the neck musculature is characterized by loss of the ability to elevate the head from a pillow or to maintain the head in a fixed position against resistance. The "tripod" sign, wherein both upper extremities are used by the patient for support while in a sitting position, should alert the clinician to weakness of the trunk muscles. Posterior pharyngeal muscle involvement may produce a pseudobulbar palsy; dysphagia and dysphonia with nasal twang may develop. Dysphagia with nasal regurgitation generally portends a poor prognosis, leading to aspiration pneumonia and reflecting extensive myositis. Chest wall and diaphragmatic muscle weakness cause restrictive pulmonary dysfunction that, in severe cases, may terminate in respiratory failure. Myalgias, muscle tenderness, muscle atrophy, and myoedema frequently are present but usually are overshadowed by loss of muscle strength.

Dermatitis develops in nearly half of all cases of inflammatory myositis. Generally it accompanies or occurs shortly after the onset of muscle involvement. However, skin eruptions may precede other disease features by months or, rarely, years. Typical, widespread DM cutaneous lesions occasionally are seen with only minimal myositis (amyopathic DM). Periorbital and facial edema are frequent findings; a heliotrope or lilac discoloration or suffusion of the upper eyelids, considered pathognomonic for DM, occurs less often. Dusky erythematous eruptions of the face (especially in a malar distribution), "V" of the neck, upper torso, shoulders, and arms are typical (Fig. 19.1). Red, raised, scaly or smooth patches (Gottron's papules) over the knuckles, elbows, knees and, less often, medial malleoli are characteristic of DM but are found only in 10% of cases (Fig. 19.2). Linear bands of erythema over the dorsum of the hands, and periungual or fingerpad erythema, are observed commonly. Figure 19.3 shows the hand of a DM patient with biopsy-proven leukocytoclastic angiitis. Bedside nail-fold capillaroscopy, using immersion oil and an ophthalmoscope set at 40+ diopters, often demonstrates capillary dilatation and tortuosity. Such periungual vascular changes at times may be discerned by careful clinical examination, even without the aid of instrumentation (Fig. 19.4). Similar capillary abnormalities may be seen in mixed connective tissue disease (MCTD) and SLE. Periungual vascular distortion, often with focal "drop-out," is a regular and prominent feature of PSS. Thick, rough, hyperkeratotic cuticles are observed frequently, even in the absence of periungual erythema or telangiectasia. Atypical skin lesions, including extensive sclerodermatous induration, widespread dermal atrophy, and eczematoid eruptions, are seen uncommonly. Subcutaneous calcinosis is limited almost exclusively to pediatric DM, generally as a late finding (Fig. 19.5). In some long-standing "burned-out" cases with minimal or no active myositis, widespread

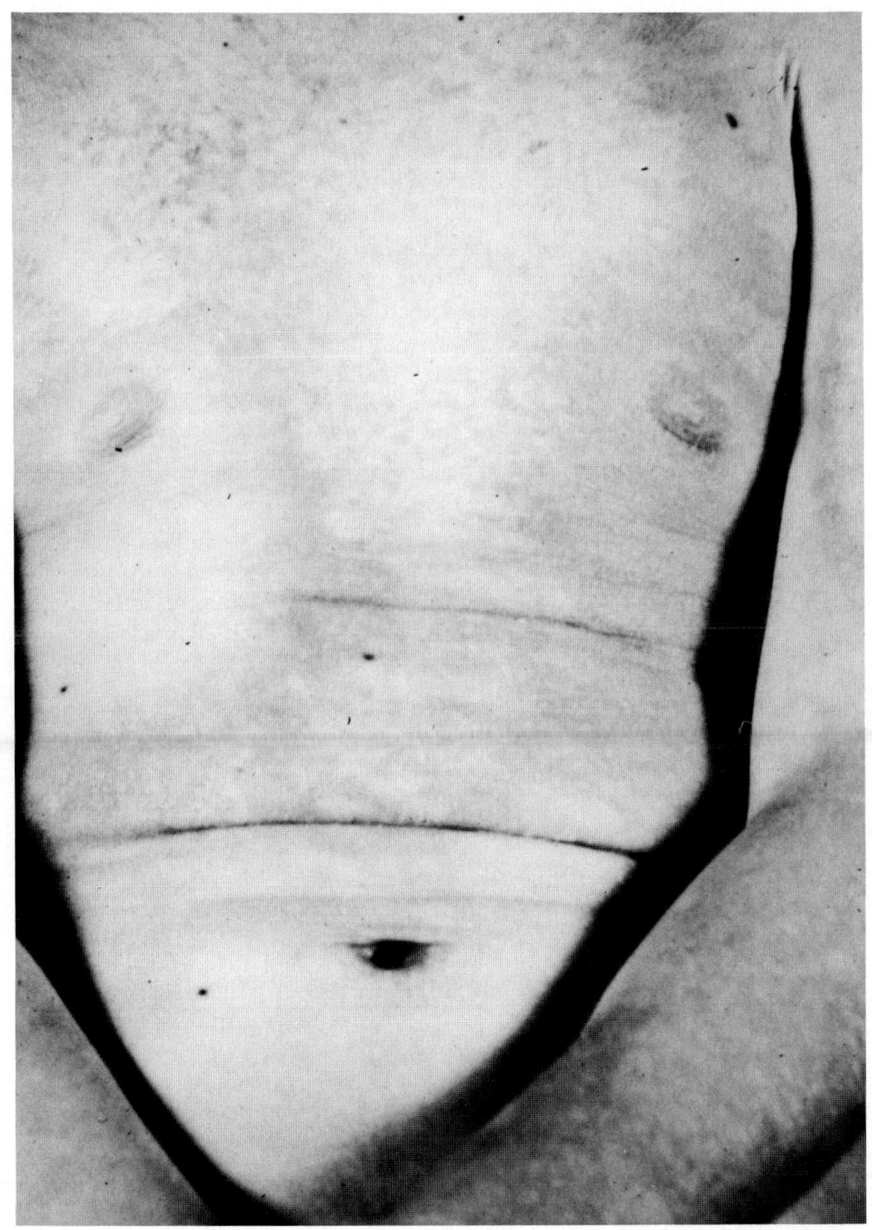

Figure 19.1. Poikiloderma of the anterior chest wall and upper extremities with areas of hypopigmentation, hyperpigmentation, and erythema.

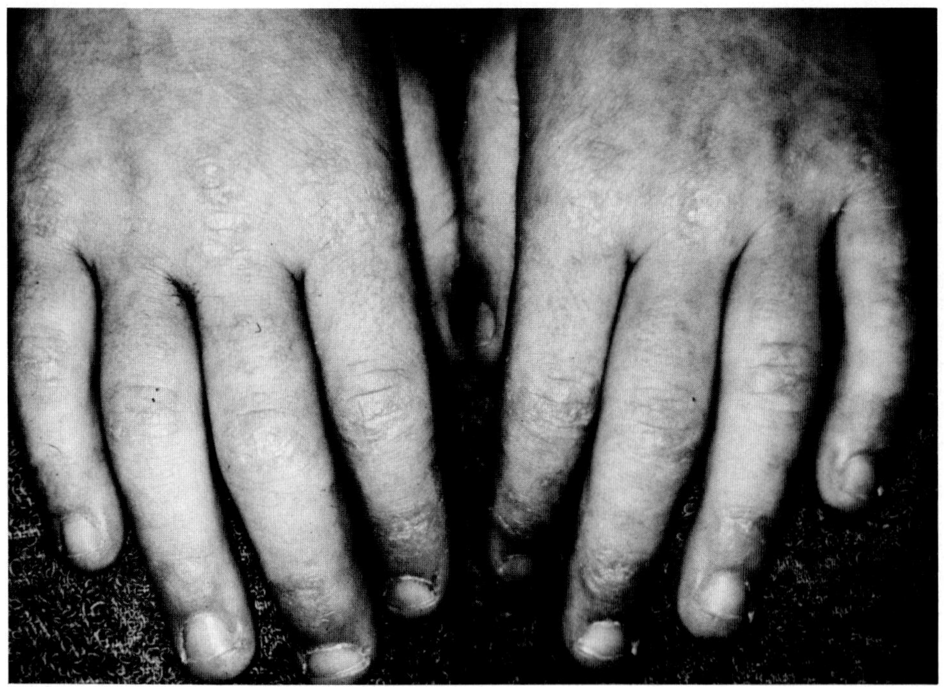

Figure 19.2. Gottron's papules developed over most of the metacarpophalangeal and interphalangeal joints simultaneously with the onset of myopathy.

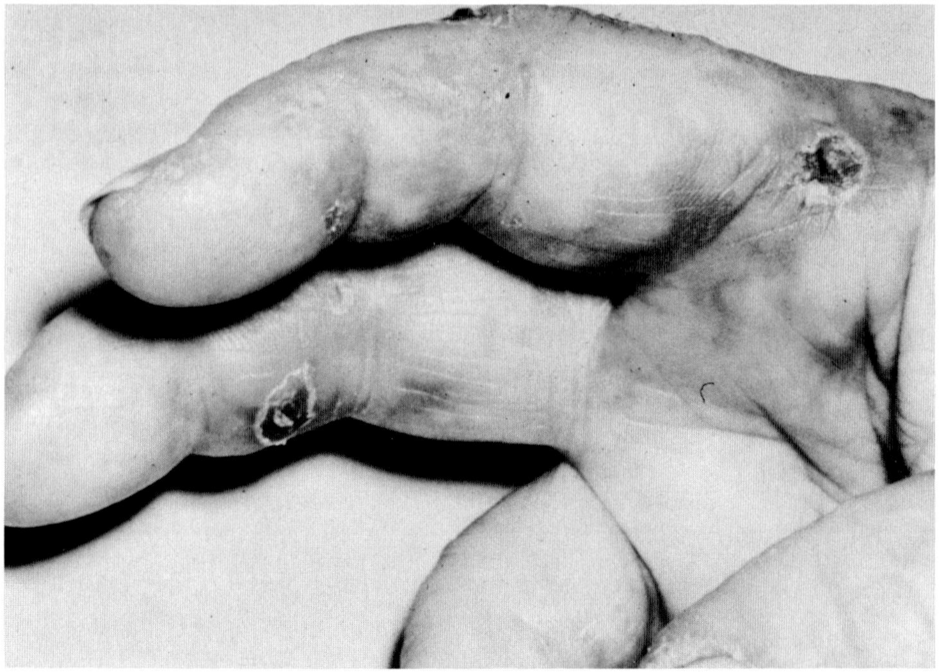

Figure 19.3. Vasculitic lesions developed on the digits, palms, and forearms of a woman with DM.

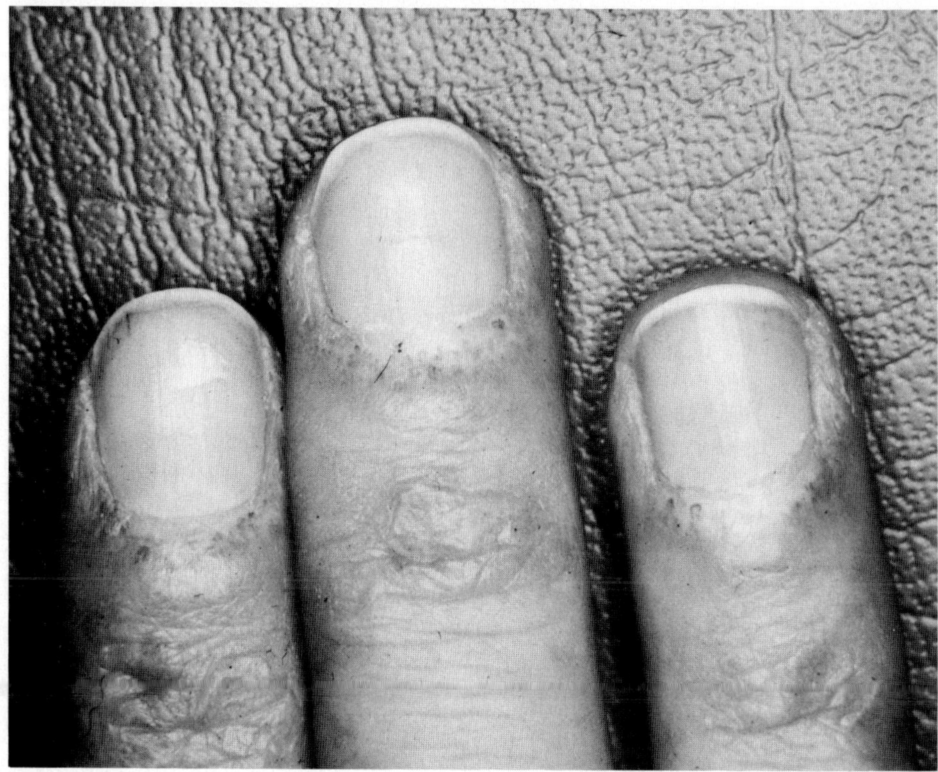

Figure 19.4. Prominent vascular dilatation and tortuosity of the proximal nail fold, and thickened, hyperkeratotic cuticles are evident. Note the Gottron's papules over the distal interphalangeal joints.

sheets of subcutaneous calcinosis (calcinosis universalis) may be a disabling aspect of DM, contributing to progressive joint contractures and immobilization.

Arthralgias occur in the majority of cases, and a nondeforming, often transient polyarthritis having a predilection for the knees and small joints, is found in 25%–35% of patients. Articular disease may precede dermal and muscle involvement by more than a year and be confused with rheumatoid arthritis (RA). The absence of subchondral erosions, mildly inflammatory synovial fluid (WBC < 5,000/cu mm), and the usual absence of serum rheumatoid factor serve as helpful distinguishing features. Infrequently, independent criteria for both RA and PM coexist, representing a true overlap syndrome.

Recently, a distinct syndrome, consisting of extreme lateral instability of the thumb interphalangeal joint ("floppy thumb" sign), periosteal and synovial calcification, and erosive arthritis of hand interphalangeal joints with sparing of other articulations, was reported. Raynaud's phenomenon frequently accompanied these findings, but serum rheumatoid factor generally was absent.

Raynaud's phenomenon is present in a third of PM/DM patients. Vascular changes generally are mild and unassociated with the distal digital ulcerations and pitted scars characteristic of PSS.

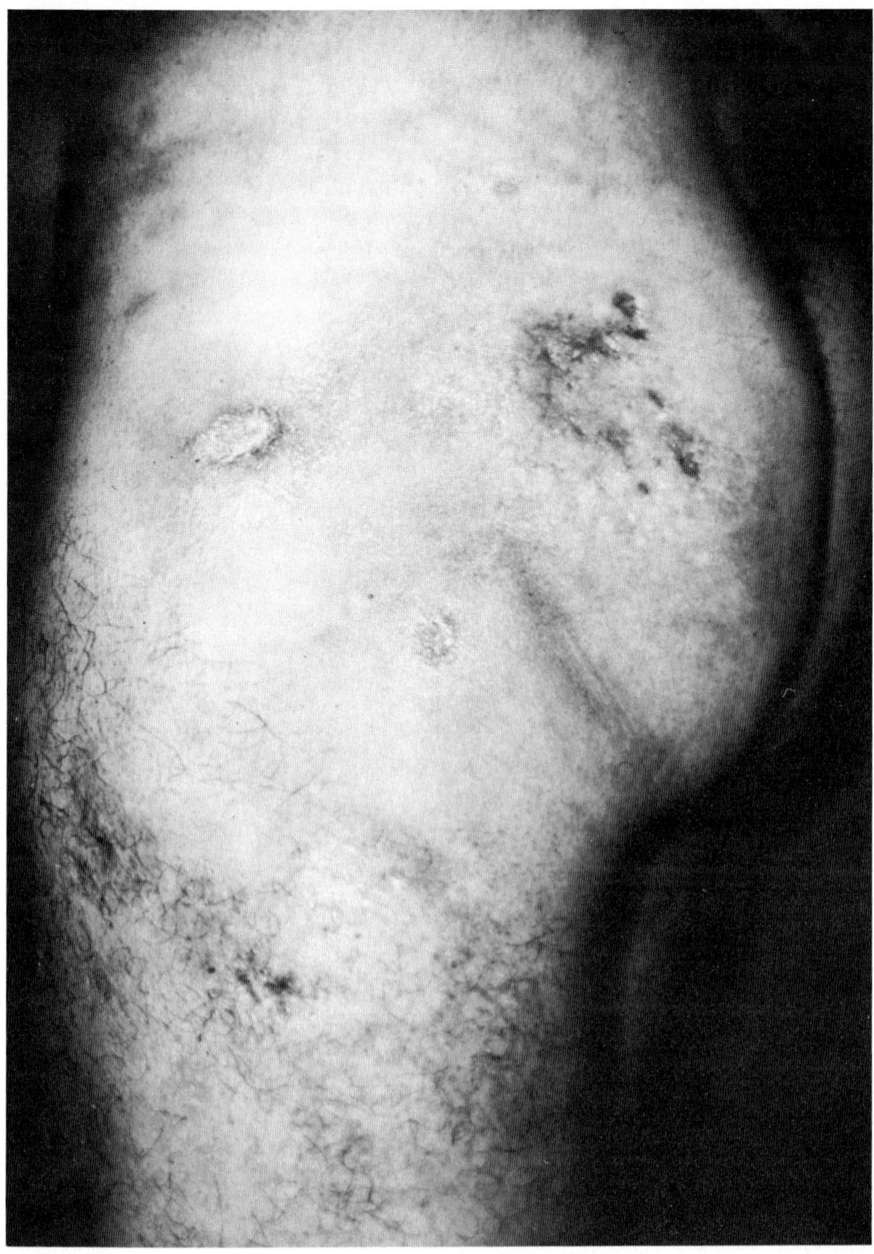

Figure 19.5. Subcutaneous calcinosis, ulceration, and poikiloderma are present on the buttocks and adjacent areas.

Heart involvement occurs more often in PM/DM than hitherto appreciated. Electrocardiographic abnormalities are detected in 30% of cases; nonspecific ST-T wave changes, atrial arrhythmias, and conduction disturbances (notably, left anterior hemiblock) are found most frequently. Left ventricular dysfunction, established by noninvasive systolic time interval measurements, is evident in the majority of patients with abnormal electrocardiographic findings. Clinically apparent pericarditis, cardiomyopathy, or congestive heart failure are unusual sequelae, however. Pathologic cardiac findings generally are limited to sparse interstitial fibrosis and mononuclear cell infiltration.

Intrinsic pulmonary disease consists of acute, sterile inflammatory infiltrates or chronic fibrosing alveolitis. Differentiation clinically, or pathologically by open lung biopsy, is important, as the former condition is corticosteroid-responsive. An empiric trial of corticosteroids (e.g., prednisone 40–60 mg daily in divided doses) may be justified in equivocal cases when infectious etiologies have been excluded and lung biopsy is inadvisable.

Lower esophageal and small intestinal hypomotility may be indistinguishable from sclerodermatous involvement of the gastrointestinal tract. Dysphagia, esophageal reflux with stricture formation, and malabsorption secondary to intestinal stasis with bacterial overgrowth may result. In juvenile onset PM/DM, marked oral and pharyngeal mucosal erythema may be noted. Mesenteric and small-vessel bowel vasculitis is a unique feature of childhood DM that presents as abdominal pain and often leads to fatal hemorrhage, ulceration, perforation, or infarction of bowel.

ASSOCIATION WITH MALIGNANCY

An association between inflammatory myositis, especially DM, and malignancy is well supported in the literature. The prevalence of cancer in PM/DM patients ranges from an overall estimate of 15% to a maximum of 71% in men over 40 years of age. The heterogeneity of myositis populations, the occasional failure to distinguish PM from carcinomatous myopathy, the varied or unspecified diagnostic criteria for PM, and the lack of large, controlled studies are responsible for the continuing controversy concerning the statistical relationship between PM/DM and malignancy. In an extensive literature review, it was observed that patients with both DM and malignancy were older than the general DM population but younger than the general cancer population; a predilection for women was seen. Both conditions generally become manifest within one year of each other, and in some cases myositis activity correlates with the extent and activity of the underlying malignancy. The relative frequency of specific tumors associated with DM differs from that of the general population in that ovarian and gastric carcinomas are overrepresented and colorectal carcinoma is seen less often than anticipated. Based on the current wealth of clinical data, a malignancy evaluation appears warranted in PM/DM patients over the age of 40, especially if clinical or laboratory findings suggest the presence of underlying tumor. Childhood myositis, in contrast to adult cases, rarely is associated with malignancy, although concomitant PM/DM and acute leukemia or non-Hodgkin's lymphoma have been reported.

LABORATORY FINDINGS

Muscle-derived serum enzymes almost invariably are elevated in PM/DM (Table 19.3). Creatine phosphokinase (CPK), aldolase, serum glutamic oxaloacetic transaminase (SGOT), and lactic dehydrogenase (LDH) generally parallel one another, although serial CPK and aldolase determinations probably are the most sensitive and specific enzymes for measuring myositis activity. Only skeletal and cardiac muscle and the central nervous system contain significant quantities of CPK; therefore, serum levels are not affected by hepatic disease or hemolysis, which may spuriously elevate other enzymes. However, CPK elevations may follow intramuscular injections, strenous physical exertion, trauma, brain infarction, excessive alcohol intake, certain drugs, and other muscle disorders.

Serum enzyme activity generally declines several weeks before clinical improvement. Similarly, enzyme levels may rise 3–6 weeks before muscle weakness is evident. Serum enzymes may be normal in greatly advanced cases because fibrous connective tissue has replaced muscle mass.

Two alternative methods for assessing myositis activity have been advocated recently. One is calculation of the urinary clearance ratio of creatine/creatine + creatinine. An elevated ratio (> 0.4) reflects muscle injury with increased creatine release and excretion. The second is measuring serum myoglobin content by radioimmunoassay. These sensitive tests may allow earlier diagnosis and prediction of relapse in certain patients.

The Westergren erythrocyte sedimentation rate (ESR) is moderately elevated (usually less than 50 mm/hr) in about half of the patients. Alpha-2 globulins, gammaglobulins, and other acute-phase reactants also may be increased, reflecting a systemic inflammatory process. A mild neutrophilic leukocytosis is present commonly; anemia is unusual in the absence of associated malignancy or treatment complications. Antinuclear antibody, usually in low titer and displaying a homogeneous or speckled immunofluorescent pattern, is found in less than 15% of cases. A highly specific antibody directed against a nuclear acidic (nonhistone) antigen (PM-1) has been noted in 50% of a small series of myositis patients. Serum rheumatoid factor is detected in half of the cases, whether or not articular

Table 19.3. Laboratory Features of Polymyositis/Dermatomyositis

Characteristics of myositis	Elevated serum muscle enzyme (CPK, aldolase, SGOT, LDH)
	Elevated serum myoglobin (radioimmunoassay)
	Creatinuria (urinary clearance ratio of creatine/creatine + creatinine > 0.4)
Acute phase reactants	Elevated Westergren sedimentation rate
	Elevated alpha-1 and gammaglobulins
Autoantibodies	ANA, low titer (usually homogeneous or speckled) in less than 15% of patients
	Rheumatoid factor (latex fixation) in 50% of patients
	Antibodies to a nuclear acidic antigen (PM-1)

disease exists. Serum complement levels generally are normal, even with severe disease.

ELECTROMYOGRAPHY

Electromyographic (EMG) abnormalities in PM/DM are nonspecific and suggest a mixed neuromyopathic process. Myositis causes random degeneration of myofibrils within each motor unit; a total reduction of motor units per se, characteristic of a pure neuropathy, is absent. During voluntary muscle contraction the EMG wave form is of short duration, reduced amplitude, and disintegrated (polyphasia). Abnormal muscle irritability accounts for salvos of high frequency and repetitive potentials ("pseudomyotonic" discharges) elicited by mechanical stimulation of affected muscle.

The primary inflammatory process may extend to terminal nerve fibers, producing denervation of adjacent muscle fibers. Spontaneous fibrillation (sawtooth) potentials, and positive sharp waves, characteristic of denervation, are evident at rest and after mechanical stimulation. The typical EMG changes associated with myositis may be fully or partially present and uncommonly are absent; furthermore, EMG interpretation is subject to observer experience and bias.

PATHOLOGY

Muscle biopsy is recommended in most, if not all, suspected cases of PM. A clinically affected proximal muscle (e.g., quadriceps femoris or deltoid) without significant wasting, contralateral from one showing EMG abnormalities, is selected. An open excisional biopsy is preferred to a closed needle biopsy.

The histologic hallmark of myositis is muscle cell degeneration and regeneration (Fig. 19.6). Degeneration is shown by variation in the size of contiguous muscle fibers, frank myofibrillar necrosis or vacuolar change, and macrophage ingestion of necrotic cell particles. Regenerating fibers are identified by enhanced basophilia, enlarged sarcolemma, and the presence of large, hyperchromatic nuclei lying centrally within sarcoplasm.

Perivascular and interstitial round cell infiltration is a common but not invariable finding; inflammatory changes may be lacking in otherwise typical cases. Interstitial fibrosis is usual in advanced disease. An angiitis characterized by nonreactive fibrinoid change in the media of large muscular arteries may be found in childhood PM.

No single histopathologic feature is pathognomonic of PM, although the collective presence of typical features, interpreted in light of clinical findings, is highly suggestive. Histochemical staining may differentiate lower motor neuron disease (predominantly type II fiber atrophy) and myotonic dystrophy (predominantly type I fiber atrophy) from PM (random types I and II fiber atrophy). Local trauma may produce changes indistinguishable from those of PM, emphasizing the importance of appropriate biopsy site selection. Focal variation of muscle fiber size, and occasionally nuclear centralization, may be seen in muscular dystrophy; significant inflammatory change, however, is rare. RA and other disorders

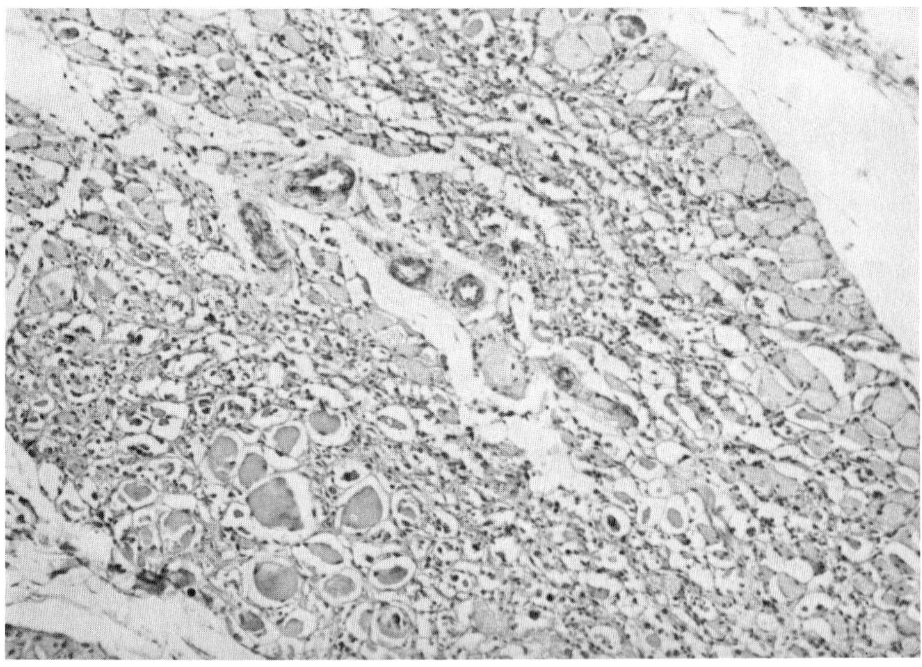

Figure 19.6. Cross-section of skeletal muscle ($\times$400) showing extensive lymphocytic infiltation, muscle fiber atrophy, and degeneration.

may be associated with mononuclear cell infiltrates interspersed between muscle bundles. Infrequently, muscle histologic findings in PM are normal due to sampling error, mandating repeat biopsy.

The skin lesions of DM are nonspecific histologically, and skin biopsy is of little diagnostic value. However, dermal biopsy is a relatively benign technique and may exclude other conditions at times confused with DM, such as SLE. Usual findings in DM include epidermal atrophy, basal cell degeneration, vascular dilatation, dermal lymphocytic infiltration, and mucinous (glycosaminoglycan) deposits in involved and uninvolved skin in 30% of cases.

IMMUNOLOGIC FEATURES

The evidence that PM/DM are immune-mediated is less convincing than for other rheumatic disorders, such as RA and SLE. Nonetheless, a number of immunologic aberrations have been observed.

Aberrant cellular immunity has been implicated in the pathogenesis of myositis. Lymphocytes from PM patients demonstrate blastogenic transformation, increased synthesis of nucleic acids, and the release of lymphokines (e.g., migration inhibition factor, lymphotoxin) when exposed to muscle antigens. In addition, peripheral lymphocytes from patients with myositis show in vitro cytotoxicity against fetal and neonatal rat muscle in tissue culture. Thus, circulating sensitized T cells in PM patients may be transformed by exposure to muscle tissue and exert a lymphokine-mediated effect. Corticosteroids and immunosuppressive agents appear to protect target muscle cells from the detrimental actions of liberated lymphokines and reduce the capacity of T cells to react abnormally to autologous muscle.

Attempts to identify antibodies to a variety of muscle antigens, using gel diffusion, tanned RBC agglutination, and immunofluorescent techniques, generally have proved unrewarding. Autoantibodies to muscle have been detected in a minority of PM/DM patients and occasionally are present in other disorders. Circulating autoantibody to purified skeletal muscle myoglobin was recently identified by a passive hemagglutination method in 71% of 31 PM patients. The prevalence and titer of antimyoglobin antibody were significantly higher than in other myopathic and rheumatic diseases. These promising findings await confirmation.

Immune complex-induced vascular injury may occur in some patients with childhood DM. Circulating immune complexes, as determined by Raji cell assay and C1q binding, are present in some cases. Endothelial damage and thrombi in muscle vessels, and vascular deposits of IgG, IgM, and C3, have been described in both childhood and adult disease. However, such deposits correlate poorly with sites of muscle inflammation and are not specific for PM/DM.

A few patients with defects in humoral immunity, such as congenital and acquired agammaglobulinemia and congenital C2 deficiency, have developed PM/DM. Such associations are of uncertain significance and may be fortuitous.

PATHOGENESIS

The pathogenesis of PM/DM is undefined. Aberrant cellular and, possibly, humoral immunity may be important etiologic factors. Infection is a possible precipitating event; intranuclear and cytoplasmic inclusions in muscle cells and tubuloreticular cytoplasmic inclusions in endothelial cells of muscle and skin blood vessels have been seen in some PM/DM patients using electron microscopy. These aggregates closely resemble those produced by myxovirus or picornavirus infection. Attempts at virus isolation have been unrewarding, however, and virus-like inclusion particles have been observed in other rheumatic disorders. An increased prevalence and high titers of anti-toxoplasma antibodies have been reported in PM patients, but *T. gondii* has not been isolated, and anti-toxoplasma treatment has not affected the disease course.

DIFFERENTIAL DIAGNOSIS

Polymyositis should be considered whenever proximal muscle weakness is present and is confirmed by the presence of elevated serum muscle enzyme levels, EMG abnormalities, and muscle pathology. Distinctive skin lesions are an extremely valuable diagnostic feature of DM. Criteria have been proposed that provide useful guidelines for patient evaluation (Table 19.4); a thorough workup is essential for accurate classification of muscle disorders (Table 19.5).

Primary muscle diseases must be differentiated from neurogenic conditions that

Table 19.4. Proposed Diagnostic Criteria for Polymyositis/Dermatomyositis

---

Symmetric proximal muscle and anterior neck flexor weakness
Characteristic muscle histologic changes
    Muscle fiber necrosis (types I and II fibers) with phagocytosis
    Muscle fiber regeneration with basophilia, large central nuclei, and variation in fiber size
    Mononuclear cellular infiltration, perivascular and interstitial
Elevation of serum muscle enzymes
Characteristic EMG changes
    Myopathic changes: short, small polyphasic potentials
    Denervation changes: fibrillation potentials, positive sharp waves
    Muscle irritability: salvos of high-frequency repetitive discharges
Characteristic dermal lesions
    Heliotrope rash and periorbital edema
    Erythematous eruption of face, neck, or upper torso
    Gottron's papules (virtually pathognomonic)
PM: no rash; 4 criteria = definite; 3 criteria = probable; 2 criteria = possible.
DM: rash plus 3 criteria = definite; plus 2 criteria = probable; plus 1 criterion = possible.

SOURCE: Adapted from Bohan A, Peter JB (1975).

frequently cause secondary changes in muscle function and structure. Peripheral neuropathy due to diabetes mellitus, chronic alcoholism, nutritional deficiency, or carcinomatosis may cause a secondary myopathy. Other neurologic disorders, such as multiple sclerosis, Guillan-Barre syndrome, myasthenia gravis, spinal stenosis, myelitis, and nerve root entrapment syndromes may at times be erroneously diagnosed as primary myopathic conditions. Careful neurologic history and examination, coupled with EMG and nerve conduction studies, usually delineate appropriately the primary organ system affected.

Muscular dystrophy may be associated with elevated creatine phosphokinase

Table 19.5. Diagnostic Considerations in Patients with Muscle Weakness and Elevated Serum Muscle Enzymes

---

Polymyositis/dermatomyositis
Other rheumatic disorders (e.g., RA, SLE, PSS, MCTD)
Muscular dystrophies (Duchenne's pelvifemoral, limb-girdle, facioscapulohumeral)
Alcoholic myopathy
Metabolic myopathies (e.g., hypothyroidism, McArdle's syndrome)
Drugs: penicillamine, chloroquine, hydroxychloroquine, clofibrate, corticosteroids
Infections: trichinosis, viral myositides (including hepatitis B), toxoplasmosis, trypanosomiasis, schistosomiasis, tuberculosis, mycoses, syphilis
Noninfectious granulomatous disorders: sarcoidosis, Crohn's disease, idiopathic
Central nervous system insults (e.g., stroke)
Miscellaneous: heat stroke, strenuous muscle exertion

Table 19.6. Differentiation between Muscular Dystrophy (MD) and Polymyositis/Dermatomyositis (PM/DM)

	MD	*PM/DM*
Onset	Insidious; < 40 yrs[a]	Acute-subacute; any age
Family history	+	−
Rash	−	±
Muscle weakness		
Limb-girdle	±	+
Facial	±	−
Distal extremity	±	−
Elevated serum CPK	±	+
Electromyography	Myopathy	Myopathy Denervation Irritability
Muscle pathology		
Degeneration	+	+
Regeneration	±	+
Inflammatory infiltrate	−	+

[a] Distal muscular dystrophy onset in midlife.

(CPK) levels and muscle biopsy findings similar to those of PM. However, dystrophic myopathies generally are familial, usually are manifest clinically before the fourth decade of life, evolve insidiously over several years, prominently involve the cervical and cranial musculature, and follow an unremitting course (Table 19.6). Other rheumatic features, such as arthralgias and Raynaud's phenomenon, are absent.

Endocrinologic disorders may be confused with PM. A noninflammatory myopathy with increased serum CPK occasionally in the initial manifestation of myxedema; therefore, thyroid function should be measured in all patients with proximal muscle weakness. Thyrotoxicosis, hyperparathyroidism, and other chronic hypercalcemic states may produce proximal muscle weakness, occasionally as an early feature of the disorder. Muscle enzyme concentrations are usually normal, and other findings often make the underlying condition apparent clinically.

Numerous drugs have been incriminated in myopathic syndromes. Penicillamine may produce a myositis clinically and histologically indistinguishable from idiopathic PM. Clofibrate, chloroquine, hydroxychloroquine, and corticosteroids may cause a proximal myopathy, occasionally with modest enzyme elevations. Muscle biopsy in the case of antimalarials and corticosteroids shows a vacuolar myopathy similar to that observed in SLE. Corticosteroid myopathy generally affects the pelvic girdle before the shoulder girdle and spares the pharyngeal musculature. Steroid myopathy may develop with as little as 10 mg of prednisone daily but is more common with the fluorinated compounds (e.g., triamcinolone); resolution rapidly follows termination of therapy, but improvement may follow reduction of the dose.

Polymyalgia rheumatica, a syndrome of shoulder and pelvic girdle myalgias and stiffness, may simulate PM. This affliction of the elderly is associated with an elevated erythrocyte sedimentation rate (> 50 mm/hr) and at times anemia, low-grade fever, hepatic involvement, and giant cell arteritis. However, muscle weakness is lacking and muscle enzymes, EMG, and muscle biopsy are normal.

Inflammatory myositis may be a prominent feature of other rheumatic disorders, including SLE, RA, PSS ("sclerodermatomyositis"), and MCTD. The last syndrome is defined by high titers ($> 1 : 1000$) of antibodies directed against the ribonucleoprotein component of extractable nuclear antigen (ENA), in association with one or more of the following clinical features: Raynaud's phenomenon, hand edema, sclerodactyly, arthralgias, serositis, fever, and a low incidence of renal disease. Weakness and muscle atrophy may develop, occasionally associated with myalgia. Frequently, myositis is evident histologically, even in the absence of symptoms.

Trichinosis may produce severe myalgias and moderate muscle weakness, with slight elevations of serum enzymes. The precipitous onset, generalized muscle involvement, and dietary history suggest the correct diagnosis. Serologic studies (trichinella antibodies, eosinophilia, normal ESR) and demonstration of parasitic infestation in muscle biopsy specimens are confirmatory.

A generalized granulomatous myositis may accompany sarcoidosis, Crohn's disease, and various infectious processes such as tuberculosis, mycoses, syphilis, and toxoplasmosis. Clinical features and muscle biopsy usually establish the appropriate diagnosis. Idiopathic giant cell polymyositis, characterized by a predilection for women, generalized skeletal muscle granulomata, serum muscle enzyme elevation, and giant cell myocarditis, may mimic PM. This syndrome frequently is preceded by thymoma and myasthenia gravis and may be associated with lymphocytic infiltration of the thyroid gland and refractory mucocutaneous candidiasis. The aforementioned abnormalities suggest a primary defect in cellular immunity. Atheromatous microemboli, carcinomatous thromboembolism, and emboli from a left atrial myxoma may produce muscle (especially calf) pain and elevations of serum muscle enzymes, simulating a primary inflammatory myositis.

PROGNOSIS

Life-table survivorship studies of treated PM patients indicate a relatively high mortality early in the disease, with a 2-year cumulative survival rate (CSR) of 72%. A less dramatic decline in survival is observed subsequently; the 5-year CSR is 54%. Childhood myositis has a more benign course, the 7-year CSR being 90%. Pneumonitis, usually attributable to aspiration due to pharyngeal muscle involvement, is the most dire prognostic sign. Underlying malignancy and advanced age at disease onset adversely affect the outcome. Dysphagia, extensive dermatitis, and profound muscle weakness are thought to worsen the prognosis, although definitive studies are lacking. Spontaneous remissions are not well documented in adult PM/DM but are in childhood disease. Early treatment, before the development of muscle atrophy, generally improves the prognosis.

Epidemiologic studies, comparing heterogeneous myositis populations from the precorticosteroid and postcorticosteroid eras, suggest a decline in mortality. Prospective, controlled trials supporting the generally accepted view that corticosteroids improve survival are unavailable. One report detected no difference in mortality between two small age-matched groups of adult PM patients, whether steroid-treated or not. A retrospective study showed no significant difference in survival between PM patients treated with high-dose (> 20 mg prednisone) or low-dose corticosteroids (< 10 mg prednisone). The mortality exceeded the anticipated death rate in both groups. Nevertheless, most clinicians agree that corticosteroids improve the quality if not the quantity of life in this disorder.

TREATMENT

Corticosteroids are the agents of choice in the management of PM/DM. Divided dosages of prednisone (40–100 mg/day) generally are preferred; fluorinated preparations (e.g., triamcinolone) are avoided, as they convey the greatest risk of steroid myopathy. A concomitant antacid regimen is recommended, and a potassium supplement frequently is required. After clinical improvement and return of serum enzymes toward normal, corticosteroids are gradually tapered off to a maintenance level of 10–15 mg prednisone daily. Reduction in dose is made slowly, with the patient's clinical status and serum muscle enzyme levels monitored frequently to reduce the risk of disease exacerbation. Corticosteroids may be administered as a single daily dose, and some patients achieve adequate control on an alternate-day regimen. Termination of corticosteroids ultimately is possible in many cases of childhood disease; adults usually require long-term maintenance therapy. Anecdotal experience suggests that steroid resistance is more common in the presence of underlying malignancy than when tumor is absent.

Immunosuppressive treatment often proves beneficial for patients who fail to improve on high-dose corticosteroids or who develop serious steroid-related adverse effects, although controlled studies are not available. Combined prednisone and intravenous methotrexate (10–15 mg initially, gradually increasing to 30–50 mg/day, given at 5–7-day intervals) brought improvement in 77% and had a "steroid-sparing" effect in patients unresponsive to moderate–high-dose prednisone alone. Methotrexate toxicity was minor and included stomatitis, gastrointestinal upset, skin rash, purpura, and fever. Hepatotoxicity was not evident clinically or by laboratory values after an average of 1 year's therapy and a mean cumulative dose of 1 g methotrexate.

Azathioprine (1.5–2.0 mg/kg/day initially, adjusted to maintain mild leukopenia) was given to patients treated primarily with high-dose prednisone who suffered myositis relapse whenever steroids were reduced or who developed significant steroid complications. Disease control and reduction of steroid dose without disease exacerbation was achieved in the majority. Other immunosuppressive agents, such as cyclophosphamide and chlorambucil, reportedly are beneficial in PM/DM.

Correct positioning and passive range of motion exercises are mandatory to prevent flexion contractures. Active range of motion and muscle-strengthening exercises are instituted as the myositis is controlled. Precautions against pulmonary aspiration are essential in patients with pharyngeal muscle involvement.

BIBLIOGRAPHY

Barnes BE: Dermatomyositis and malignancy: A review of the literature. *Ann Intern Med* 84:68, 1976.

Benson MD, Aldo MA: Azathioprine therapy in polymyositis. *Arch Intern Med* 132:547, 1973.

Bohan A, Peter JB: Polymyositis and dermatomyositis. *N Engl J Med* 292:344 and 403, 1975.

Bohan A, Peter JB, Bowman RL, et al: A computer-assisted analysis of 153 patients with polymyositis and dermatomyositis. *Medicine* 56:255, 1977.

Bunch TW, O'Duffy JD, McLeod RA: Deforming arthritis of the hands in polymyositis. *Arthritis Rheum* 19:243, 1976.

Dawkins RL, Mastaglia FL: Cell-mediated cytotoxicity to muscle in polymyositis. *N Engl J Med* 288:434, 1973.

Haas DC: Treatment of polymyositis with immunosuppressive drugs. *Neurology (Minneapolis)* 23:55, 1973.

LeConant P, Texier L: Histologic lesions of muscles in dermatomyositis: Differentiation from related musculocutaneous syndromes. *Br J Dermatol* 69:299, 1957.

Maricq HR, Spencer-Green G, LeRoy EC: Skin capillary abnormalities as indicators of organ involvement in scleroderma (systemic sclerosis), Raynaud's syndrome, and polymyositis. *Am J Med* 61:862, 1976.

Metzger AL, Bohan A, Goldberg LS, et al: Polymyositis and dermatomyositis: Combined methotrexate and corticosteroid therapy. *Ann Intern Med* 81:182, 1974.

Medsger TA Jr, Dawson WN Jr, Masi AT: The epidemiology of polymyositis. *Am J Med* 48:715, 1970.

Medsger TA Jr, Robinson H, Masi AT: Factors affecting survivorship in polymyositis: A life-table study of 124 patients. *Arthritis Rheum* 14:249, 1971.

Pearson CM, Bohan A: The spectrum of polymyositis and dermatomyositis. *Med Clin North Am* 61:439, 1977.

Rose AL: Childhood polymyositis: A follow-up study with special reference to treatment with corticosteroids. *Am J Dis Child* 127:518, 1974.

Schwarz MI, Matthay RA, Sahn SA, et al: Interstitial lung disease in polymyositis and dermatomyositis: Analysis of six cases and review of the literature. *Medicine* 55:89, 1976.

Sharratt GP, Danta G, Carson PHM: Cardiac abnormality in polymyositis. *Ann Rheum Dis* 36:575, 1977.

Talbott J: Acute dermatomyositis—polymyositis and malignancy. *Semin Arthritis Rheum* 6:305, 1977.

Winkelmann RK, Mulder DW, Lambert FM, et al: Course of dermatomyositis-polymyositis: Comparison of untreated and cortisone-treated patients. *Mayo Clin Proc* 43:545, 1968.

20

Progressive Systemic Sclerosis and Associated Disorders

Thomas A. Medsger, Jr.

CLASSIFICATION

The term *scleroderma* means hardening and/or thickening of the skin, which may occur in a variety of conditions including both systemic disorders and those limited to the integument. Classifications of sclerodermatous cutaneous changes emphasize this generalized-localized distinction (Table 20.1).

Progressive systemic sclerosis (PSS), which affects both skin and internal organs, is considered one of the diffuse rheumatic diseases. Features shared with the other recognized conditions in this group include (1) overlap of clinical features, (2) a tendency to affect blood vessels as a common target organ, and (3) a variety of common serologic and cellular immune abnormalities. Thus, immunologic mechanisms are believed to play an important role in pathogenesis.

Some authors have considered PSS to be a homogeneous spectrum of disease, although several patient subgroups have been identified according to the extent of cutaneous involvement (diffuse versus restricted) and the presence or absence of clinical features of other rheumatic diseases. Individuals with diffuse (generalized) skin thickening (both the distal and proximal extremities and trunk) tend to have a more rapidly progressive illness, a higher frequency of renal and cardiac involvement, and a poor survival rate. In contrast, those with the CREST syndrome variant (*c*alcinosis, *R*aynaud's phenomenon, *e*sophageal hypomotility, *s*clerodactyly, and *t*elangiectasia) appear to have a more limited and relatively benign course without renal or cardiac sequelae, but instead have a tendency to develop, after many years, distinctive visceral complications including "primary" pulmonary hypertension, intestinal malabsorption, and/or several autoimmune disorders including primary biliary cirrhosis, Sjögren's syndrome, and Hashimoto's thyroiditis.

A third group of PSS patients is that having typical extremity scleroderma changes associated with manifestations of other connective tissue diseases, the so-called *overlap* syndromes. The best described such entity is mixed connective tis-

Table 20.1. Classification of Scleroderma

Progressive systemic sclerosis (PSS)
 With diffuse or generalized involvement of skin (scleroderma affecting the trunk, face, proximal and distal extremities); tendency to relatively early appearance of visceral disease (esophagus, intestine, lung, heart, kidney)
 With limited or restricted involvement of skin, often confined to the fingers and face; prominence of calcinosis, Raynaud's phenomenon, esophageal dysfunction, sclerodactyly, and telangiectasia (CREST syndrome); prolonged delay in the appearance of distinctive internal manifestations (including severe pulmonary arterial hypertension and biliary cirrhosis)
 In overlap with other connective tissue diseases, including rheumatoid arthritis, systemic lupus erythematosus, polymyositis-dermatomyositis (e.g., mixed connective tissue disease)
Eosinophilic fasciitis
Localized forms of scleroderma
 Morphea: single or multiple plaques, occasionally generalized
 Linear scleroderma, with or without melorheostosis
Drug-induced scleroderma-like conditions
 Polyvinyl chloride disease
 Bleomycin-induced fibrosis

SOURCE: Adapted from Rodnan (1979).

sue disease (MCTD), with shared features of PSS, sytemic lupus erythematosus (SLE), and polymyositis.

Finally, a number of sclerodermatous conditions may occur without visceral manifestations, including eosinophilic fasciitis, localized forms of skin thickening (morphea) and linear localized scleroderma, and several drug-induced scleroderma-like conditions.

PROGRESSIVE SYSTEMIC SCLEROSIS

Epidemiology

Although no formal criteria for PSS exist, classification criteria have been developed utilizing a multicenter study and three comparison groups (SLE, polymyositis-dermatomyositis [PM-DM], and Raynaud's phenomenon alone). A single *major criterion,* sclerodermatous skin proximal to the digits (hands, forearms, face, neck, thorax, or abdomen), identified 239 of 264 (91%) clinically diagnosed definite PSS patients. At least two or three *minor criteria*—(1) sclerodactyly (sclerodermatous skin change limited to the digits), (2) digital pitting scars, or (3) bilateral basilar pulmonary fibrosis on chest roentgenogram—brought the number of patients satisfying these criteria to 97% compared with only 10 of 413 (3%) of the comparison patients. Unfortunately, "overlap" patients could not be adequately separated from PSS patients in this study. These criteria will help to establish the reliability of series of PSS cases reported in the literature but are not intended as diagnostic criteria for the individual case.

Estimates from epidemiologic studies suggest that the annual incidence of PSS is 5–10 new patients diagnosed per million population at risk. PSS is thus far less frequent than rheumatoid arthritis (RA) (500 per million annually) and SLE (75 per million annually) and approximately as common as PM-DM. Women are more often affected than men; the overall female : male ratio is 3 : 1 but, as with SLE and RA, is considerably higher during the childbearing years. PSS is unusual during childhood and is uncommon in men under age 30. Blacks, especially black women, have a higher incidence than whites, but this difference is minimal compared with the dramatic racial differences observed in SLE. U.S. national mortality statistics, based on death certificate reporting, have confirmed these incidence figures.

PSS may be more frequent in underground miners (gold, coal) or others occupationally exposed to silica dust. A scleroderma-like illness has been described in workers exposed to unfinished plastics in the manufacture of polyvinyl chloride. Serum antinuclear antibodies have been found in over half of the first-degree relatives of patients with PSS, and chromosomal abnormalities appear to be more common in PSS patients. A number of convincing case reports of familial PSS have been recently published. Although one such report noted a common HLA A and B locus haplotype, overall no tissue-typing abnormalities in PSS patients have been confirmed.

Initial Symptoms

In most cases, the initial complaint is either Raynaud's phenomenon, symmetric painless edema, or gradual thickening of the skin of the distal extremities, particularly the fingers and hands. Rheumatic symptoms, most commonly arthralgias and stiffness of the finger joints and knees, may be an early feature, often with objective polyarthritis or tenosynovitis (carpal tunnel syndrome). In the remaining patients, myositis, dysphagia, or heartburn are the presenting problems. Rarely, some typical visceral finding, such as malabsorption, may long antedate the development of cutaneous changes.

Organ Involvement

The involvement of various organ systems in PSS is described below. Certain clinical and laboratory abnormalities are more meaningful than others, and these findings are listed in Table 20.2 as a guide to the evaluation of such patients.

Skin

In our experience, approximately one-half of patients have diffuse scleroderma and the remainder have more limited (restricted) cutaneous changes. The latter group has, classically, sclerodermatous changes limited to the fingers (sclerodactyly) and other features of the CREST syndrome. In either case, the skin of the fingers is affected first, often with tight swelling ("sausage fingers"). These puffy fingers may persist indefinitely or evolve to a more indurative, "hidebound" phase. Diffuse involvement of skin tends to occur in the setting of antecedent Raynaud's phenomenon of short duration and results in rapid progression (within months) of skin changes to the more proximal portions of the extremities (forearms, arms, thighs) and subsequently to the trunk (chest, abdomen, back). These skin changes

Table 20.2. Evaluation of Organ Systems in Patients with Proven or Suspected Progressive Systemic Sclerosis

	History	Physical Examination	Laboratory Evaluation	
			Helpful	Not Generally Helpful
Skin		Thickening, especially of digits and distal extremities		Skin biopsy
		Hyperpigmentation		
		Telangiectases (periungual, fingers, palms, face, lips)		
		Calcinosis (fingers, elbows, knees)	Roentgenograms	
Raynaud's phenomenon	Triphasic change, especially blanching distal to PIP joints	Digital pitting scars, ulcers, or gangrene	Provocative test if history and PE inconclusive	Arteriogram
Joints	AM stiffness	Swelling, synovial thickening, and/or effusion	Synovial fluid analysis	Roentgenograms
Skeletal muscle	Proximal weakness	Proximal weakness	EMG, CPK and aldolase, biopsy	SGOT, LDH
Gastrointestinal tract Esophagus	Lower dysphagia, heartburn, regurgitation		Cine esophagram (especially in prone or supine position) or esophageal manometric study	Unspecified UGI series
Small bowel	Postprandial bloating, diarrhea	Abdominal distension, hypertympany, diminished bowel sounds	Small bowel series, 72-hr total fecal fat excretion while on 100 g fat diet, D-xylose excretion test, duodenal culture (aerobic and anaerobic)	Small bowel biopsy

Colon	Constipation		Barium enema	Proctosigmoidoscopy
Lung	Dyspnea	Dry or "velcro" bibasilar rales, pleural friction rub, increased P2	Chest roentgenogram, pulmonary function tests (including vital capacity, $DLco$, and pO_2), pulmonary arterial pressure determination via right-sided cardiac catheterization	Lung scan, lung biopsy
Heart	Dyspnea, orthopnea, peripheral edema	Signs of left-sided congestive heart failure	Chest roentgenograms, EKG, echocardiogram, right-sided cardiac catheterization	Coronary arteriogram
Kidney	Headache, visual disturbance, seizures	Malignant hypertension, grade III–IV hyptertensive retinopathy	Urinalysis, serum creatinine, plasma renin, renal arteriogram or biopsy	IVP, retrograde pyelography, 24-hour urine protein
Immunologic				
Sjögren's syndrome	Scratchy eyes, dry mouth	Glossitis, salivary gland enlargement	Schirmer test, slit lamp examination, lip biopsy	
Hashimoto's thyroiditis	Symptoms of hypothyroidism	Goiter	T_4, TSH, serum antithyroid antibodies	
Biliary cirrhosis	Jaundice, pruritis	Jaundice	Serum alkaline phosphatase, antimitochondrial antibody titer, liver biopsy	
General			ANA titer, ANA fluorescence pattern, anti-ENA (before and after RNase)	CBC, ESR, platelet count, LE cell preparation, rheumatoid factor, anti-DNA, serum protein electrophoresis, serum complement

are accompanied, or occasionally preceded, by impressive hyperpigmentation, often stippled with a regular pattern of hypopigmentation (salt-and-pepper appearance).

When underlying structures are involved, flexion contractures develop, and skin overlying bony prominences becomes taut, shiny, and extremely vulnerable to breakdown. Painful ulcerations often result, become secondarily infected, especially with staphylococci, and are notoriously difficult to heal.

Facial tightness leads to loss of normal skin folds and the characteristic "pinched" facies. Should the patient survive a number of years, this skin thickening usually recedes somewhat, leaving the integument thin and atrophic with prominent, grossly visible linear telangiectatic vessels.

In contrast, the CREST syndrome most often evolves from pure Raynaud's phenomenon to Raynaud's plus sclerodactyly over a period of years or even decades. Telangiectases, consisting of dilated capillary loops and postcapillary venules, appear late in the course especially on the fingers, nail folds, face, and lips and tend to be punctate rather than linear. In long-standing CREST syndrome, roentgenograms of the hands, elbows, or knees disclose subcutaneous deposits of calcium salts. Calcinosis may also appear as palpable nodules, which

Table 20.3. Comparison of Organ System Involvements in PSS According to Extent and Location of Sclerodermatous Skin Change

	Diffuse Scleroderma	*CREST Syndrome*
Skin	Generalized (trunk, face, proximal and distal extremities)	Restricted (fingers, face); occasionally hands, forearms; rarely absent (PSS sine scleroderma)
Raynaud's phenomenon	95%	98%
Joints/tendons		
Arthralgias	75%	50%
Arthritis	40%	20%
Tendon friction rubs,	60%	Rare
contractures	75%	40%
Muscle (myopathy)	15%	$< 5\%$
Gastrointestinal tract		
Esophageal dysmotility	70%	70%
Malabsorption	10%	15%
Lung		
Pulmonary fibrosis	40%	40%
Pulmonary hypertension	Rare	10%
Heart		
Pericarditis	5%	5%
Congestive failure	10%	Rare
Kidney		
Malignant hypertension with renal failure	25%	Rare

may erode through skin and drain "gritty" calcific material. Although a clear-cut distinction between these two ends of the spectrum is not always possible, this separation is useful because of the somewhat different natural history likely to ensue (Table 20.3).

During the active indurative phase, skin biopsies show a striking increase in collagen in the dermis, which on electron microscopy appears to have an excess of thin, beaded, "early" extracellular forms of the collagen fibril resembling embryonic skin collagen. Although not common, variably large accumulations of T lymphocytes have been identified in interstitial areas (Fig. 20.1). Later in the course of PSS, the skin tends to be strikingly atrophic and acellular histologically.

Raynaud's Phenomenon

Paroxysmal vasospasm in the fingers (and less often in the toes) is present in over 95% of patients with PSS. The most reliable historic point is homogeneous blanching of the digits distal to the proximal interphalangeal (PIP) joints associated with numbness and pain on exposure to cold or during periods of emotional stress. Cyanosis and intense erythema on rewarming are also common. Although such phenomena are normal physiologic responses to cold and may be familial, most investigators feel that Raynaud's phenomenon in PSS is attributable primarily to structural changes within blood vessel (arteriolar) walls, notably vessel wall and intimal thickening with resultant luminal narrowing (Fig. 20.2). Mor-

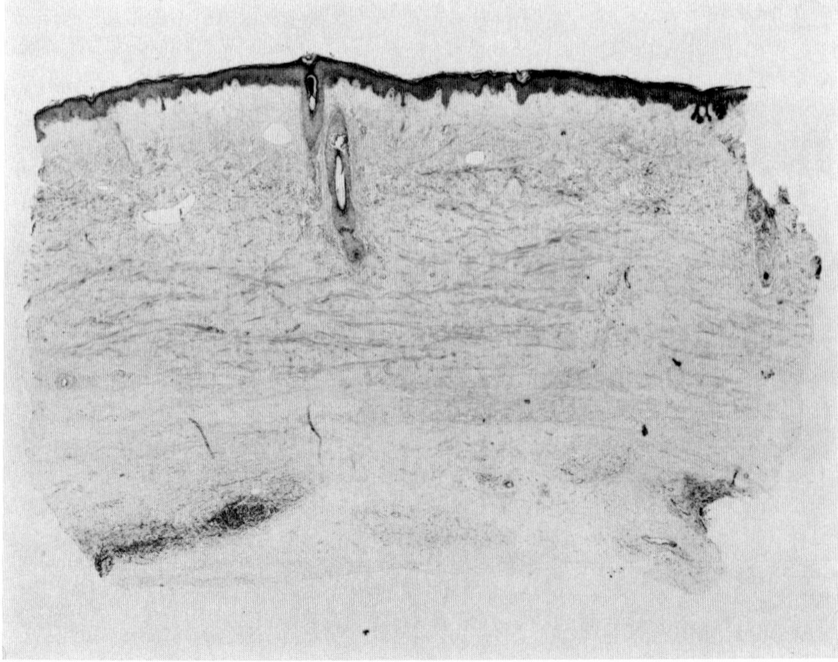

Figure 20.1. Photomicrograph of forearm skin biopsy from a 53-year-old woman with diffuse scleroderma showing marked dermal thickening and collections of lymphocytes in the deeper layers of the dermis (×18).

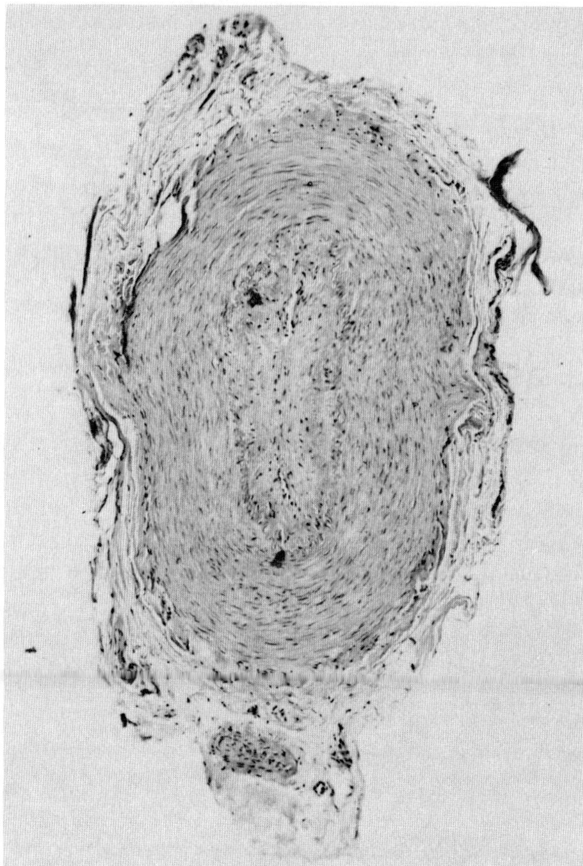

Figure 20.2. Cross-section photomicrograph of a digital artery taken at postmortem from a 58-year-old woman with scleroderma kidney. Note the marked thickening of the intima with nearly complete occlusion of the lumen and adventitial fibrosis ($\times$75).

phologic evidence for this conclusion is found in arteriographic studies, histologic and electronmicroscopic findings, and capillary microscopy.

Occlusion of a sizeable digital vessel may result in digital tip infarction; lesions may take the form of hard, painful digital tip sores with subsequent tissue loss (pitting), ulcerations, or frank gangrene. Tissue loss is the end result, and progressive reduction in digital tip soft tissue and bone (distal phalangeal tufts) occurs. Such complications are more frequent in CREST syndrome than in diffuse scleroderma. In contrast to atherosclerosis, major pulses are normal to palpation, and the fingers are affected far more commonly than the toes.

Joints and Tendons

Symmetric arthralgias of finger joints, wrists, elbows, knees, and ankles are common, but palpable synovial thickening is unusual. Synovial fluid is generally scant, with low white blood cell counts ($<$ 3,000/cu mm). Synovial biopsy in such instances has revealed predominantly fibrosis with minimal inflammation. Although juxta-articular osteoporosis is common, there is little tendency to joint space narrowing or erosion.

Tendon sheaths are also affected by PSS, becoming thickened and adherent to surrounding structures. A leathery friction rub is often palpable over wrist, ankle, and knee tendons. This physical finding is attributable to fibrinous deposits in tenosynovium and overlying fascia. It is nearly specific for diffuse PSS and rarely, if ever, occurs in the CREST variant. Carpal tunnel syndrome may result from such involvement of the wrist flexor tendons. Due to the combined effects of skin, tendon, and articular involvement, alarmingly rapid contractures may develop, particularly affecting the fingers.

Skeletal Muscle

Muscle atrophy is common in PSS, especially in diffuse scleroderma when severe cutaneous and articular involvement causes contractures and marked limitation of motion. A proximal myopathy is also encountered, but this complication is usually less dramatic and incapacitating than typical PM. The degree of muscle weakness is less, serum enzyme elevations are less, and biopsies tend to show more interstitial fibrosis than myofibril degeneration or chronic inflammatory cell infiltration. Most often, this subtle myopathy does not progress rapidly, even without therapy.

Gastrointestinal Tract

Esophageal dysfunction is the most common visceral manifestation of PSS, occurring in at least 70% of patients. The most prominent symptoms are lower dysphagia (retrosternal "sticking" of solids), retrosternal burning due to reflux esophagitis, and postprandial (especially nocturnal) regurgitation. Persistent esophagitis may result in stricture formation, forced reduction in oral intake, and marked weight loss. This problem is particularly common in patients with CREST syndrome.

Cinefluoroscopic or manometric studies usually show diminished or absent peristaltic activity in the distal two-thirds of the esophagus, even in persons without symptoms. Decreased lower esophageal sphincter tone accounts for reflux of gastric contents. Histologic changes show lymphocytic infiltration in submucosal areas as well as atrophy and fibrous replacement of the muscularis but normal myenteric plexuses of Auerbach. Thickening of blood vessel walls and intimal proliferation in small arterioles may contribute to the dysfunction via ischemia.

Small and large intestinal involvement may dominate the picture, especially in CREST syndrome patients, causing postprandial fullness and severe bloating, vomiting, crampy abdominal pain, episodic diarrhea, and constipation. Roentgenographic studies show markedly diminished activity (hypomotility) and dilatation (Fig. 20.3). Such hypomotility favors the overgrowth of intestinal microorganisms in usually sterile areas (duodenum, upper jejunum), leading to excessive bile salt deconjugation (hydrolysis), impaired micelle formation, and interference with absorption simulating a "blind-loop" syndrome. Patchy atrophy of the muscularis layer, particularly in the colon, may result in the formation of wide-mouthed sacculations (diverticulae) on the antemesenteric border. Although seldom the cause of symptoms except possibly constipation, these sacculations may rarely perforate or produce obstruction after becoming impacted with fecal

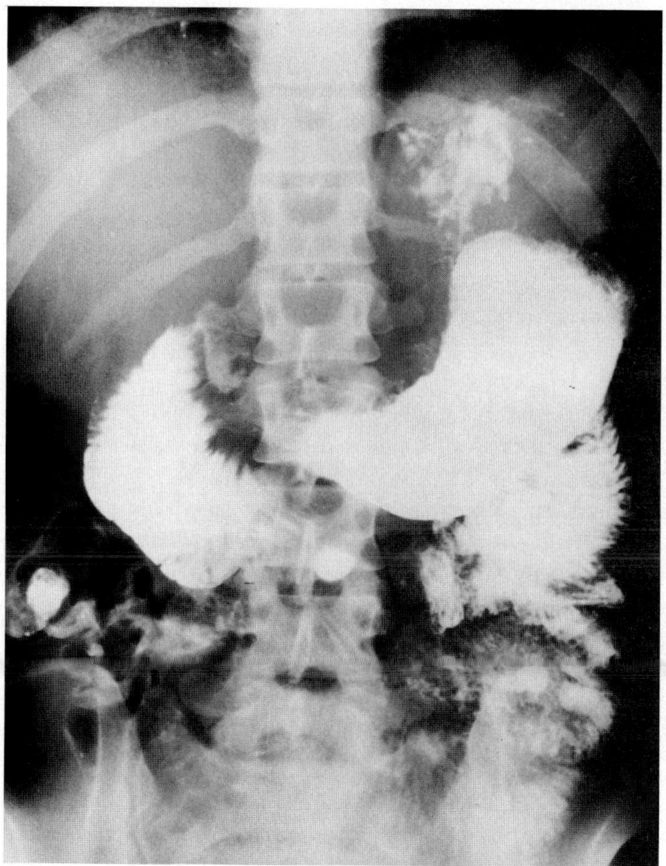

Figure 20.3. Roentgenogram of the upper gastrointestinal tract showing marked duodenal dilatation in a 33-year-old woman with Raynaud's phenomenon, digital pitting scars, and polymyositis (PSS sine scleroderma).

matter. The pathologic findings are similar to those described above for the esophagus, with prominent atrophy and fibrosis.

Primary disease of intestinal tract solid organs is distinctly unusual in patients with classic diffuse scleroderma, although biliary cirrhosis has been described in a number of women with CREST syndrome who have pruritis, jaundice, intrahepatic cholestasis, and serum antimitochondrial antibodies.

Lungs

Pulmonary involvement is a frequent clinical feature of PSS and is a nearly universal pathologic finding at postmortem examination, chiefly interstitial and alveolar fibrosis. Patients often complain of exertional dyspnea, and dry fibrotic "velcro" rales are heard on auscultation. The earliest detectable physiologic evidence of impaired gas exchange is a low diffusing capacity for carbon monoxide. Subsequently, chest roentgenograms show bilateral basilar interstitial fibrosis (40%), occasionally with "honeycombing." In many cases, a restrictive ventilatory defect (decreased vital capacity) can be shown on pulmonary function studies, chiefly due to peribronchial fibrosis. Despite these alterations, chronic respiratory insufficiency is rare, although superimposed bacterial infections may prove fatal.

Although pulmonary hypertension may be superimposed on such fibrosis, it is usually mild and only slowly progressive. In contrast, a modest proportion (10%) of CREST patients, frequently without significant pulmonary fibrosis, develop severe "primary" pulmonary hypertension. This complication, often appearing after several decades of benign CREST syndrome, is progressive and almost uniformly fatal over a 2- to 3-year follow-up period. The pulmonary vascular lesions may be dramatic, with marked muscularis hypertrophy, bland intimal proliferation and deposition of mucopolysaccharide-like material, internal elastic membrane fragmentation, and luminal obliteration.

Pleural fibrosis is a common autopsy finding, but symptomatic pleurisy and/or effusion is somewhat unusual. Alveolar (or bronchiolar cell) carcinoma is now an accepted late sequel of PSS, especially in CREST patients with long-standing alveolar fibrosis.

Heart

Cardiac involvement may be either primary or secondary to pulmonary or renal PSS. Primary processes include pericarditis and myocardial fibrotic infiltration. Although acute pericarditis is rare, fibrous pericardial adhesions are encountered in over 60% of autopsies, implying subclinical disease. Echocardiographic studies are now beginning to assist in the evaluation of the natural history of such asymptomatic processes. Primary myocardiopathy, the most common clinically recognizable form of PSS cardiac involvement, occurs in less than 10% of patients and almost exclusively in the diffuse variant. In these cases, slowly progressive cardiomegaly and congestive heart failure develop, the latter often refractory to standard therapy. Arrhythmias, including complete heart block, and electrocardiographic abnormalities (particularly conduction disturbances) are common. Autopsy studies suggest that the functional disturbances in life are contributed to by both conduction system fibrosis and fibrosis of working myocardium. Ischemia and Raynaud's phenomenon may play a role, as evidenced by extensive thickening of small coronary vessels and "contraction band" necrosis of myocardium.

Secondary changes in the heart may result from the abrupt onset of malignant hypertension and/or fluid retention secondatry to renal insufficiency in "scleroderma kidney." In this situation, congestive heart failure and pulmonary edema occur with a normal-size heart. With control of fluid overload and hypertension, the heart again functions normally. Another secondary problem is the right-sided cardiac failure that may accompany the types of pulmonary PSS described above.

Kidney

Renal involvement is frequent in PSS and usually takes the form of highly malignant arterial hypertension. The typical setting is diffuse, progressive cutaneous thickening of less than 4 years' duration. Hypertension onset is usually abrupt and dramatic, associated with severe headache, visual disturbances, grade IV retinopathy, seizures, and acute congestive heart failure. Rarely, the arterial blood pressure has remained normal, but the rule is significant hypertension with marked hyperreninemia. At this early stage, urinalysis usually shows 1–3+ protein and 5–20 red blood cells per high-power field. At the outset, or within several days or weeks, azotemia is obvious and becomes rapidly progressive, often terminating in anuria. Almost without exception, untreated patients succumb to renal or cardiac failure or to subarachnoid hemorrhage within days or a few weeks. Nearly half of the deaths attributed to scleroderma occur as the result of this serious complication. The diagnosis is easily made clinically but can be confirmed by attenuation of vasculature on renal arteriogram or biopsy showing intimal hyperplasia, mucopolysaccharide deposition, fibrinoid necrosis, and peri-adventitial fibrosis in intralobular and smaller-size arteries (Fig. 20.4). Immunoglobulins, especially IgM, and complement components have been identified in these lesions, although not in impressive amounts.

Other

Sedimentation rate elevation is not dramatic in PSS, and anemia is uncommon. Leukopenia, autoimmune hemolytic anemia, and thrombocytopenia are likewise unusual, and their occurrence should raise the suspicion of an overlap syndrome. Trigeminal sensory neuropathy has been described, although a number of af-

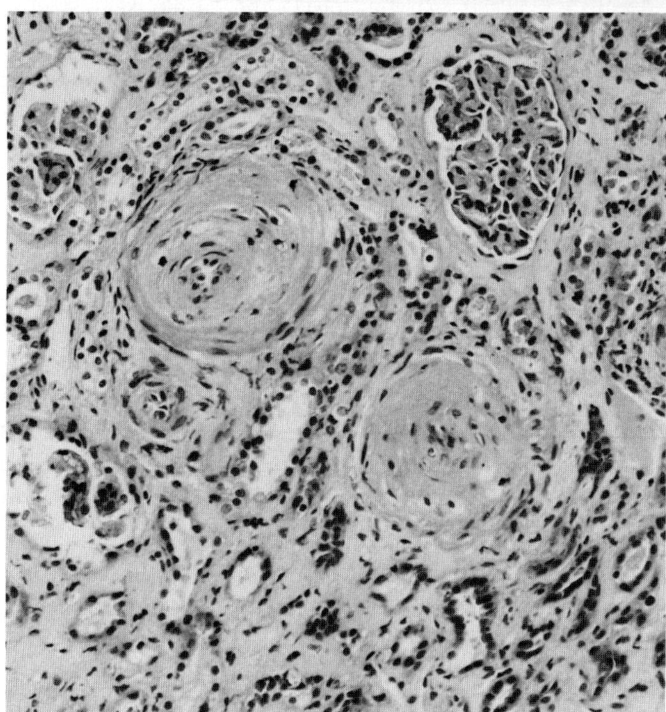

Figure 20.4. Photomicrograph of a kidney biopsy from a 46-year-old woman with severe renal involvement. Note the subintimal proliferation and fibrinoid change in the arterial walls and periarterial fibrosis (×185).

fected persons appear to have polymyositis and also Sjögren's syndrome. The central nervous system is rarely, if ever, affected primarily. When the sicca complex is present (estimated minimum 20% among PSS patients), minor salivary gland periglandular fibrosis is a more frequent histopathologic finding than lymphocytic infiltration. Even in the absence of Sjögren's syndrome, oral hygiene tends to be a problem for PSS patients. Two contributing factors are decreased oral aperture, making dental work technically difficult, and a tendency to resorption of the periodontal membrane, leading to loosening of permanent teeth.

Course of Disease

The natural history of PSS is extremely variable. Early in the disease, it is difficult to judge the prognosis with respect to either death or disability. There may be some spontaneous improvement in skin thickening and the severity of Raynaud's phenomenon. However, visceral involvement tends to be progressive, even in the presence of stable or improving cutaneous scleroderma.

The most important determinants of ultimate survival appear to be the involvement of certain internal organs, especially the kidney, heart, and lung (Fig. 20.5). Since diffuse skin involvement correlates with cardiac and renal PSS, it is also a poor prognostic sign. In contrast, CREST patients show improved survival since the above mentioned potentially fatal sequelae of CREST appear late in the disease course. Anemia and sedimentation rate elevation are also associated with

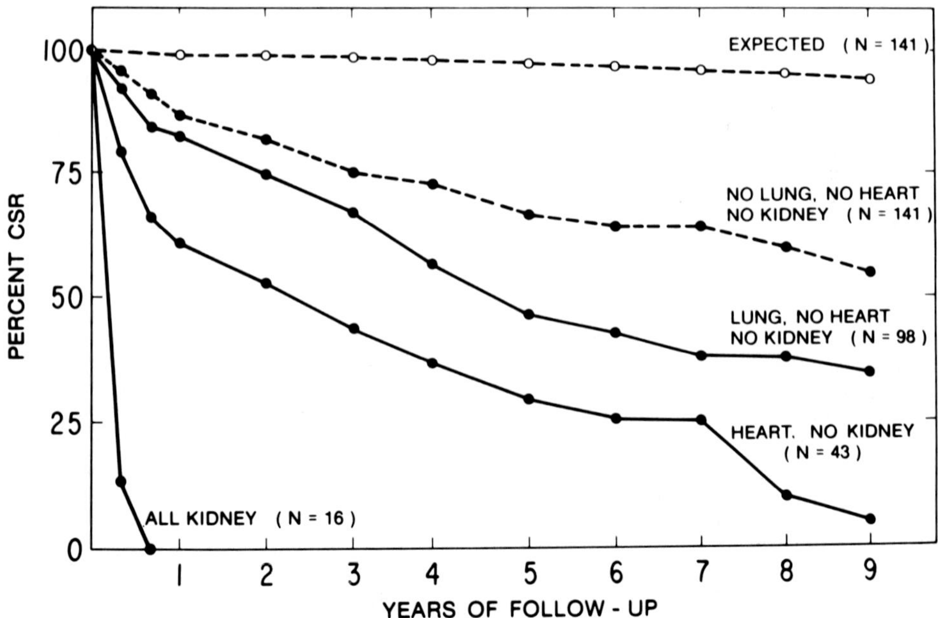

Figure 20.5. Cumulative survival rate (CSR) in 309 patients from Memphis and Pittsburgh with progressive systemic sclerosis according to involvement of internal organs at the time of first hospital diagnosis. (Adapted with permission of the author and publisher from Medsger TA, Masi AT, Rodnan GP, et al: *Ann Intern Med* 75:373, 1971.)

reduced survival, but no single pathophysiologic process is suggested by these nonspecific abnormalities.

The prognosis with respect to disability is most often related to contractures of upper extremity joints, particularly hands in diffuse PSS, and digital ischemia, which is more prominent in CREST patients.

Etiology and Pathogenesis

Collagen Metabolism

There is now convincing evidence from a variety of sources that fibrosis of the skin and internal organs in PSS is the result of overproduction of collagen. Absolute increases in the collagen content of skin biopsy plugs of uniform diameter have been reported, and electron microscopic studies show PSS skin fibroblasts to be very active in fibrilogenesis. Dermal fibroblasts from PSS patients, especially cells derived from the lower dermis, grown in tissue culture, produce abnormally large quantities of collagenase-sensitive protein. The factors that regulate collagen production and degradation are still unknown.

Immunologic Abnormalities

Both clinical and pathologic similarities, particularly a tendency to affect blood vessels, have tended to link PSS with the other connective tissue diseases. In addition, impressive collections of lymphocytes and plasma cells have occasionally been detected, especially in the skin and gastrointestinal tract.

Approximately one-third of patients with PSS have polyclonal hypergammaglobulinemia, and the same proportion demonstrate positive serum test results for rheumatoid factor. Antinuclear antibodies, usually in low titer, have been found in the sera of nearly 90% of persons with PSS and are usually of the fine or large speckled patterns, but are occasionally nucleolar. These antibodies have no apparent clinical associations or significance. Several new serum antibody systems have been reported in PSS patients, including anti-Scl 70 and anticentromere antibodies, the latter being particularly frequent among CREST patients. These findings have not yet been confirmed. Antibodies to nuclear ribonucleoprotein (anti-RNP) are present in nearly 20% of PSS patients, but in amounts far less than are commonly reported in cases of MCTD. Antibodies directed against native DNA or Sm antigen are absent or conspicuously unusual in PSS.

Peripheral blood lymphocytes from PSS patients have shown a variety of abnormal responses indicating cell-mediated hypersensitivity. When cultured in the presence of human skin collagen, these cells produce soluble factors chemotactic for monocytes and human dermal fibroblasts and a macrophage migration inhibition factor. The lymphocytes of patients with PSS and diffuse scleroderma (but not CREST syndrome) are stimulated to produce macrophage migration inhibition factor by skin extracts of both normal and sclerodermatous skin. Coupled with the independent observations that lymphokines are capable of localizing human dermal fibroblasts and of increasing collagen production by embryonic lung fibroblasts, these observations suggest that immunologic mechanisms may be implicated in the genesis of the fibrotic lesions of PSS.

Treatment

General

Management of the patient with PSS requires, first, the establishment of a good relationship between patient and physician. It is essential to discuss the variable nature of PSS and to differentiate between the diffuse and CREST forms and their prognostic implications. Detailed instruction using diagrams of the skin, blood vessels, and esophagus, for example, and a rational approach to each problem posed by the patient help to establish the needed rapport.

A number of factors make the evaluation of potential therapeutic agents extremely difficult. These factors include the variable and slowly progressive course, the lack of easily quantitated indices of improvement (or deterioration), especially of viscera, the difficulty in judging changes in skin thickening objectively, and the influence of psychophysiologic factors on many subjective symptoms.

In considering the pathogenetic events cited above, three theoretical sites of drug action are possible (Fig. 20.6). Beneficial results might be gained from (1) suppressing the appearance and/or function of lymphocytes distributed in affected tissues, (2) blockade of overactive fibroblasts, and (3) enhanced solubilization and/or metabolism of the excessive extracellular collagen.

The influence of corticosteroids on both cutaneous and visceral PSS has been disappointing, although they are effective for certain specific problems such as active proliferative synovitis, acute pericarditis, myositis, and some other features of MCTD. Patients with MCTD often respond dramatically to small doses of corticosteroids (e.g., 10 mg prednisone daily) and may even show some regression of cutaneous changes. Potassium para-aminobenzoate (Potaba) and dimethyl sulfoxide (DMSO) have been used but evidence for their benefit is unconvincing.

Recent attention has focused on *d*-penicillamine, a compound known to interfere with the intermolecular cross linking of collagen. In one study, 25 of 34 patients were stated to be improved on an average daily dosage of 1,000 mg given

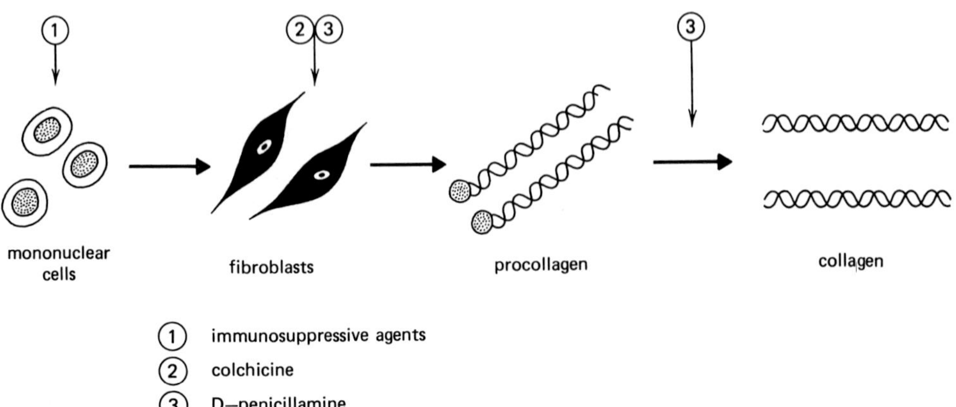

Figure 20.6. Proposed location of drug action in the skin of patients with progressive systemic sclerosis (adapted from a drawing with permission of Gerald P. Rodnan, M.D.)

for a mean of 2.3 years. Since serious side effects may ensue and experience with this drug in PSS is limited, it should be considered chiefly for patients with rapidly progressive diffuse skin involvement.

The use of colchicine has also been advocated on the basis of its preventing collagen accumulation by inhibiting the conversion of procollagen to collagen, possibly through interference with microtubule-mediated intracellular transport, or perhaps via stimulation of collagenase production. No confirmatory studies have supported the initial enthusiasm for this agent in treating patients with PSS.

For reasons cited above, the participation of immune mechanisms in PSS pathogenesis has kindled interest in the use of immunosuppressive agents. The literature in this regard is still meager and largely anecdotal, but the use of such drugs also has been considered in persons with rapidly progressive disease who appear destined to develop disabling contractures or life-threatening internal organ involvement.

Supporting Measures

A commonsense approach to Raynaud's phenomenon should be suggested, including dressing warmly and avoiding unnecessary or prolonged cold exposure and cigarettes if possible. Vasodilating drugs have proved disappointing, although some patients appear to improve on reserpine given in 0.25–0.50 mg dosages daily or methyldopa in doses of 500–1,000 mg daily. Intra-arterial reserpine (1 mg into the brachial artery) has had variable results; some patients report sustained improvement lasting several months or more. Intermittent cervical sympathetic blockade may help to diminish pain and increase circulation to digital infarctive lesions. Surgical thoracic sympathectomy usually results in only transient relief of vasospasm and appears to have no significant influence on the course of cutaneous or visceral sclerosis. Some voluntary control over vasospasm can be achieved using biofeedback training.

Uninfected painful digital tip infarcts are best left alone and dry to demarcate by autoamputation. Pain and minor trauma may be minimized by the use of a protective and immobilizing finger cast that patients may be taught to make themselves, and adequate oral analgesics should be used. Surgical intervention is rarely required, and then only for drainage or debridement of secondarily infected nonviable tissue. Open finger ulcers should be kept clean and fibrinous exudate removed several times daily after soaking in half-strength hydrogen peroxide. Although local pain may be relieved by topical antibiotic and corticosteroid ointments, these compounds do not aid healing.

Excessive skin dryness and pruritis may be relieved by the use of special lotions, soaps, and bath oils rubbed thoroughly into the thickened areas. Household detergents should be avoided. Patients with diffuse scleroderma are unable to dispense heat adequately and are predisposed to heat stroke after excessive sun exposure. Subcutaneous calcinosis cannot be dissolved by chelating agents. Surgical removal of these deposits is often complicated by persistent draining fistulous tracts that become secondarily infected.

Joint pain and tenosynovitis often respond adequately to the use of salicylate or nonsteroidal anti-inflammatory agents. Corticosteroids are seldom required for arthritis, but some physicians prefer to use them during the acute puffy and painful hand stages. Some improvement in joint mobility may be achieved by an active exercise program. We teach our patients stretching exercises to improve motion in upper extremity joints, especially the hands.

Patients with dysphagia for solid foods must learn to masticate completely and to avoid tough meat and dry bread. Reflux esophagitis can usually be minimized by the routine use of antacids and elevation of the head of the bed. In resistant cases, cimetidine has proved efficacious. The development of esophageal stricture may require periodic dilatation. Successful excision of strictures and correction of gastroesophageal reflux by gastroplasty have been reported. Direct stimulation of gastrointestinal smooth musculature by metaclopromide has been reported to increase lower esophageal sphincter tone and increase peristaltic activity. When malabsorption syndrome results from small intestinal involvement, the use of broad-spectrum antibiotics reduces bacterial overgrowth and often dramatically improves symptoms. Ideally, the proper choice is made after duodenal intubation for aerobic and anaerobic cultures. We have used intermittent (2–3-week) courses of tetracycline or ampiçillin, followed by rest periods of 1–2 weeks.

No primary therapy is available for pulmonary fibrosis. Prompt antibiotic administration is necessary in the event of superimposed bacterial pneumonia. The treatment of congestive heart failure due to PSS is difficult because of a poor response to digitalis, digitalis toxicity, and arrhythmias related to the conducting system and myocardial fibrosis. A greater reliance is placed on diuretics in this situation. Acute pericarditis and inflammatory myositis are two clear-cut indications for the use of corticosteroids.

Several advances have been made in the treatment of patients with malignant hypertension and renal failure due to "scleroderma kidney." Very aggressive antihypertensive therapy appears to decelerate the progression of azotemia and in some cases may abort the process completely. Agents directed against the hyperreninemia, such as propranolol, appear to be useful, and a recently used group of inhibitors of angiotension-converting enzyme is promising. Such inhibitors might conceivably be effective in modifying the usually ingravescent course of pulmonary hypertension in PSS. Prompt bilateral nephrectomy should be performed if hypertension cannot be controlled medically. Many patients have now been carried successfully on hemodialysis, although vascular access has been limited due to scleroderma involvement of vessels and poor flow through fistulae. Several successful renal transplants have been performed, but scleroderma changes have been detected in one donor kidney on subsequent biopsy.

SCLERODERMA VARIANTS

Eosinophilic Fasciitis

Eosinophilic fasciitis is a recently recognized scleroderma variant in which skin, subcutis, and deep fascia are inflamed and markedly thickened. This disorder appears to be more frequent in men. Its onset is often after a period of unusually vigorous physical activity. The most common initial symptoms are tightness, swelling, and pain in the hands, forearms, and upper arms, followed by induration and thickening, especially of the subcutis. Later, these tissues become irregularly contracted and grossly dimpled. Marked limitation of motion of the hands and feet may occur. Typical carpal tunnel syndrome is present in up to one-third of patients. Characteristically, the digits are spared cutaneous thickening in this process, although they may be affected by significant contractures due to more proximal tendinous entrapment. Skin of the trunk may also be affected, but facial involvement is uncommon. In addition, Raynaud's phenomenon and other visceral features of PSS are absent. Laboratory clues to the diagnosis include prominent peripheral eosinophilia and often hypergammaglobulinemia (IgG). Tissue specimens are most appropriately evaluated by deep en bloc biopsies that include skin, subcutaneous tissue, fascia, and muscle (Fig. 20.7). Early in the course of the disease, the deep fascia and lower subcutis are edematous and infiltrated with chronic inflammatory cells and eosinophils. Dermis and interstitial areas of underlying muscle are also affected. As the illness progresses, these structures become intensely sclerotic. Deposits of immunoglobulin (especially IgG) and complement (C3) have been identified in some specimens, suggesting the contribution of humoral immune mechanisms in pathogenesis. Although the natural history of eosinophilic fasciitis is not known, preliminary reports suggest that the disease

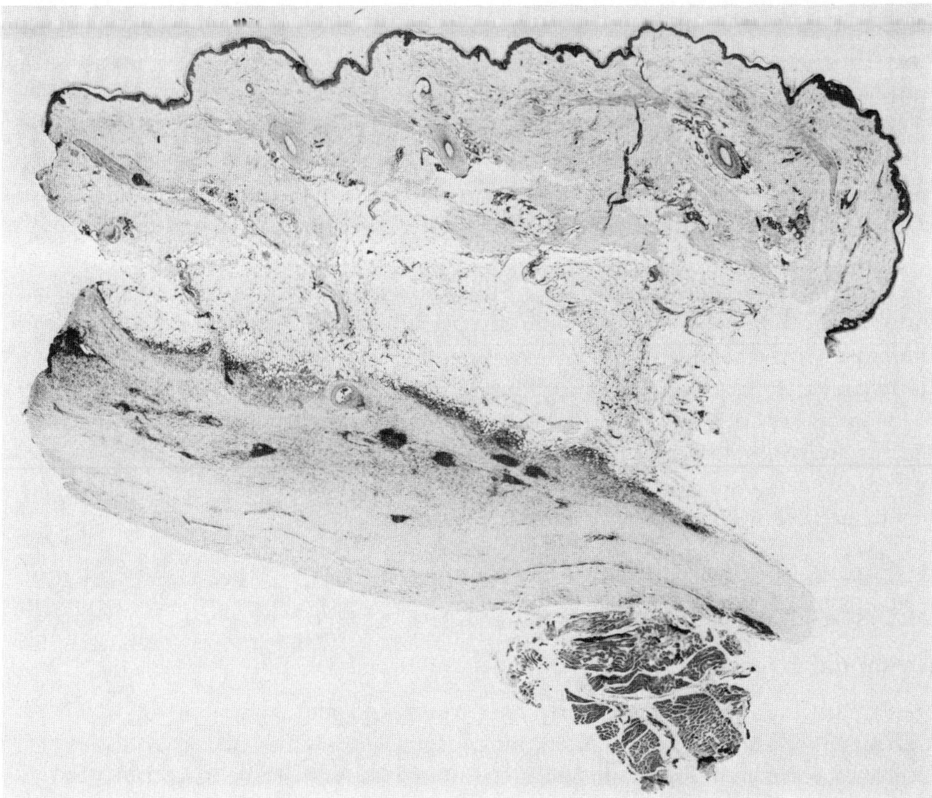

Figure 20.7. Low-power magnification of en bloc leg biopsy from a 35-year-old woman with eosinophilic fasciitis. Note the dramatic thickening of the deep fascia and collections of inflammatory cells in this area (×9.5).

is most often self-limited, undergoing spontaneous remission usually over a period of several years. Corticosteroid therapy in low dosage (prednisone 10 mg per day or less) often results in marked symptomatic improvement and suppression of eosinophilia but does not necessarily alter the long-term course. Several of our patients have had disease exacerbations in new anatomic distributions years after the first onset; these flareups became quiescent after short courses of corticosteroid therapy.

Morphea

Morphea is a form of scleroderma that appears as localized patches or plaques of skin thickening. These lesions begin with erythematous or violaceous discoloration and progress to firm, yellowish areas of induration of widely variable diameter. With time, there may be considerable softening of these areas with cutaneous atrophy. The process is limited to the skin and subcutis. It seldom involves an extensive area of the integument. Histologically, a chronic inflammatory cell reaction is present, usually more pronounced than that encountered in PSS.

Linear Scleroderma

Linear scleroderma consists of a band or streak of sclerosis that usually appears in an upper or lower extremity or on the scalp (en coup de sabre). Children are most frequently affected. In this circumstance, intense fibrosis and inflammation occur in the dermis and subcutis, as in morphea, but most often they extend to include underlying fascia and muscle. Resulting contractures may seriously impair joint mobility (usually knees, elbows, or fingers). Adjacent bone may also be involved in this process, resulting in a linear hyperostosis termed *melorheostosis*. A number of patients with linear scleroderma have developed a rheumatoid arthritis-like nonerosive polyarthritis, chiefly affecting the small joints of the hands. Some of these persons also have serologic abnormalities (antinuclear antibodies, antibodies to single-stranded DNA, and rheumatoid factor) and peripheral eosinophilia, raising the possibility that immune mechanisms are involved.

BIBLIOGRAPHY

Alarcón-Segovia D: Progressive systemic sclerosis: Management. IV. Colchicine, in Rodnan GP (ed): *Clinics in Rheumatic Diseases*. London, WB Saunders Co, Ltd, 1979, p 294.

Barnes EL, Rodnan GP, Medsger TA Jr, et al: Eosinophilic fasciitis: A pathologic study of twenty cases. *Am J Pathol* 96:493, 1979.

Bulkley BH: Progressive systemic sclerosis: Cardiac involvement, in Rodnan GP (ed): *Clinics in Rheumatic Diseases*. London, WB Saunders Co, Ltd, 1979, p 131.

Cannon PJ, Hassar M, Case DB, et al: The relationship of hypertension and renal failure in scleroderma (progressive systemic sclerosis) to structural and functional abnormalities of the renal cortical circulation. *Medicine* 53:1, 1974.

Clements PJ, Furst DE, Campion DS, et al: Muscle disease in progressive systemic sclerosis: Diagnostic and therapeutic considerations. *Arthritis Rheum* 21:62, 1978.

D'Angelo WA: Progressive systemic sclerosis: Management. I. Introduction and general commentary, in Rodnan GP (ed): *Clinics in Rheumatic Diseases.* London, WB Saunders Co, Ltd, 1979, p 263.

Guttadauria M, Ellman H, Kaplan D: Progressive systemic sclerosis: Pulmonary involvement, in Rodnan GP (ed): *Clinics in Rheumatic Diseases.* London, WB Saunders Co, Ltd, 1979, p 151.

Jayson MIV, Weiss JB: Progressive systemic sclerosis: Metabolism of connective tissue, in Rodnan GP (ed): *Clinics in Rheumatic Diseases.* London, WB Saunders Co, Ltd, 1979, p 185.

Kondo H, Rabin BS, Rodnan GP: Cutaneous antigen-stimulating lymphokine production by lymphocytes of patients with progressive systemic sclerosis (scleroderma). *J Clin Invest* 58:1388, 1976.

LeRoy EC: Increased collagen synthesis by scleroderma skin fibroblasts in vitro: A possible defect in the regulation or activation of the scleroderma fibroblast. *J Clin Invest* 54:880, 1974.

Maricq HR, LeRoy EC: Progressive systemic sclerosis: Disorders of the microcirculation, in Rodnan GP (ed): *Clinics in Rheumatic Diseases.* London, WB Saunders Co, Ltd, 1979, p 81.

Masi AT, Medsger TA Jr, Rodnan GP, et al: Methods and preliminary results of the scleroderma criteria cooperative study of the American Rheumatism Association, in Rodnan GP (ed): *Clinics in Rheumatic Diseases.* London, WB Saunders Co, Ltd, 1979, p 27.

Medsger TA Jr, Masi AT: Epidemiology of progressive systemic sclerosis, in Rodnan GP (ed): *Clinics in Rheumatic Diseases.* London, WB Saunders Co, Ltd, 1979, p 15.

Medsger TA Jr, Masi AT, Rodnan GP, et al: Survival with systemic sclerosis (scleroderma): A life-table analysis of clinical and demographic factors in 309 patients. *Ann Intern Med* 75:369, 1971.

Myers AR: Progressive systemic sclerosis: Gastrointestinal involvement, in Rodnan GP (ed): *Clinics in Rheumatic Diseases.* London, WB Saunders Co, Ltd, 1979, p 115.

Nassonova VA, Ivanova MM: Progressive systemic sclerosis: Management. II. D-penicillamine, in Rodnan GP (ed): *Clinics in Rheumatic Diseases.* London, WB Saunders Co, Ltd, 1979, p 277.

Rodnan GP: Progressive systemic sclerosis, in McCarty DJ Jr (ed): *Arthritis and Allied Conditions.* Philadelphia, Lea & Febiger, 1979, p 762.

Rodnan GP: Progressive systemic sclerosis: Clinical features and pathogenesis of cutaneous involvement (scleroderma), in Rodnan GP (ed): *Clinics in Rheumatic Diseases.* London, WB Saunders Co, Ltd, 1979, p 49.

Rothfield NF, Rodnan GP: Serum antinuclear antibodies in progressive systemic sclerosis (scleroderma). *Arthritis Rheum* 11:607, 1968.

Salerni R, Rodnan GP, Leon DF, et al: Pulmonary hypertension in the CREST syndrome variant of progressive systemic sclerosis (scleroderma). *Ann Intern Med* 80:394, 1977.

Steigerwald JC: Progressive systemic sclerosis: Management. III. Immunosuppressive agents, in Rodnan GP (ed): *Clinics in Rheumatic Diseases.* London, WB Saunders Co, Ltd, 1979, p 289.

21
Infections of Bones and Joints

Martha L. Lee

J. Douglas Lee

An appreciation of bone and joint infections is important in the evaluation of rheumatologic patients. Infection may mimic or complicate certain rheumatologic diseases and must be identified so that correct therapy is promptly initiated. The penalty for belated diagnosis and treatment may be loss of joint function and even of life.

Bone and joint infections occur by three major routes: direct inoculation, extension from a contiguous infectious focus, or hematogenous spread. Direct inoculation of virulent organisms into a bone or joint occurs most commonly in the extremities, particularly the feet. At risk are persons who work barefoot and those who operate high-speed equipment that may implant foreign bodies into the extremities. Sensory deficits, as in diabetic neuropathy, also predispose to infection. Contiguous spread is characteristically seen adjacent to mucous membranes of the head or chest, as with infection due to actinomycosis and from infected ulcers in neuropathic feet.

Clinically significant bacteremias often involve organisms considered to be of primary virulence, such as *Staphylococcus aureus, Streptococcus pyogenes, S. pneumoniae,* and *Neisseria gonorrheae.* In children under the age of 6, *Hemophilus influenzae* must also be included. Bacteremias involving these organisms frequently cause metastatic bone and joint infections, whereas *N. meningitidis* and Gram-negative organisms commonly cause bacteremias but less often result in metastatic orthopedic infection.

The probability that any bacteremia will cause metastatic infection is modified by host factors. Local mechanical tissue damage such as occurs in rheumatoid arthritis, at fracture sites, or at the site of bone infarcts from sickle cell anemia and other hemoglobinopathies increases the susceptibility to infection. For reasons not well understood, osteoarthritis does not appear to increase the probability of developing septic arthritis in the setting of bacteremia. Defects in host resistance as seen in diabetes, cirrhosis, corticosteroid therapy, cytotoxic therapy, leukemias, and lymphomas increase susceptibility, particularly to Gram-negative rods and other unusual organisms. Patients with rheumatoid arthritis seem more prone to develop septic arthritis, especially with *S. aureus*.

SEPTIC ARTHRITIS

Definition

Pyarthrosis is any inflammatory condition involving a joint caused by a replicating microorganism.

Etiology

Organisms that cause septic arthritis are outlined in Table 21.1.

Clinical Picture

The patient with septic arthritis is usually indistinguishable from one with crystal-induced synovitis. The onset is acute and involvement is generally pauci-articular. Large joint rather than small joint involvement, as is seen with gout, is usual. Joint pain is extreme, and pseudoparalysis due to pain in the affected extremity may be seen in children and infants. Local redness, heat, and swelling are usually present. A fever is noted in 90% of patients. In the absence of antipyretic use, recurrent rigors may indicate bacteremia. The presence of other foci of infection, particularly in the skin, respiratory or genitourinary tracts, increases the probability of infectious etiology.

Laboratory Data

Most patients with septic arthritis exhibit leukocytosis with a left shift in the differential white count and an elevated erythrocyte sedimentation rate (ESR). Examination of the synovial fluid usually reveals a polymorphonuclear pleocytosis

Table 21.1. Septic Arthritis

Organism	Overall Frequency[a]	Comment
Neisseria gonorrheae	~ 20%	Most common cause of septic arthritis in young adults
Staphylococcus aureus	~ 41%	
Streptococci	~ 16%	Group B streptococcus very common in neonates
Streptococcus pneumoniae	~ 6%	
Hemophilus influenzae	~ 5%	Very common in children less than 6 years of age
Gram-negative organisms	~ 12%	Compromised hosts

[a] Figures depend on the ratio of pediatric and adult patients in each series, decade of series, and type of patient population.

of greater than 85% with an elevated protein level, decreased glucose, and poor mucin clot. Positive Gram stain is diagnostic. Cultures are positive in most cases, although arthritis due to *N. gonorrheae* is often culture-negative and the diagnosis must be made on a clinical basis. Granulomatous arthritides generally require synovial biopsy for culture and for histopathologic diagnosis. Comparison of synovial fluid findings in different rheumatic conditions, including septic arthritis, is shown in Table 3.1.

Radiology

X-rays are initially normal with the exception of soft tissue swelling and, in some cases, evidence of synovial effusion. After 10 to 14 days, periarticular osteoporosis and joint space narrowing due to cartilage loss may occur. With chronicity, subchondral erosions, reactive sclerosis, and even bony ankylosis may be seen.

Diagnosis

A diagnosis is made by examination of the joint fluid, which should be carried out immediately if the diagnosis of septic arthritis is considered. No acute pauci-articular arthritis should be treated without joint aspiration, and the fluid should be studied as outlined in Table 3.1. A culture must be done in all cases. Counter-immunoelectrophoresis, if available, may give an immediate specific diagnosis.

Therapy

Therapy should be instituted as soon as synovial fluid from each affected joint has been examined. Therapy is bimodal, including both antibiotics and drainage of the joint. The initial choice of antibiotic therapy is based on the Gram stain. Gram-negative stains in children, generally denote *H. influenzae, N. meningitidis, S. pneumoniae,* or *S. pyogenes.* These microorganisms are usually all ampicillin sensitive, although an increasing number of Hemophilus are ampicillin resistant. *S. aureus* is usually Gram-positive and should be treated with nafcillin or oxacillin intravenously in high doses. If the stain is Gram-negative, if the patient has other Gram-negative infections as a possible source, and if the patient has a serious underlying disease, Gram-negative coverage should be added, such as tobramycin intravenously or intramuscularly, adjusted for renal function. In the neonate, Gram-negative and group B streptococcal infections are most common and may require initial treatment with ampicillin and tobramycin (Table 21.2).

The duration of therapy must be individualized for each patient and depends on age, organism, clinical response, site of infection, the presence of other infection, and the presence of underlying disease. The length of parenteral therapy ranges from as little as 2 weeks in children and in adults with gonococcal arthritis to 6 weeks in staphylococcal infections and most adult infections. A total of at least 6 weeks of treatment (intravenous followed by oral therapy) is generally recommended in adults. The adequacy of oral treatment should be demonstrated by measurement of serum antibiotic levels. A peak serum bactericidal level of 1 : 8 is adequate.

Table 21.2. Antibiotic Choices: Initial Therapy

Organism	*Drug*
Neisseria gonorrheae	Penicillin 6–10 million units a day IV adult
Staphylococcus aureus	Oxacillin or nafcillin 150 mg/kg/day IV
Streptococcus	Penicillin 8–10 million units/day
Hemophilus influenzae	Cefamandole 150 mg/kg/day
Gram-negative organisms	Tobramycin and cefazolin adjusted for renal function and weight
Negative gram stain	
Age 0–3 months	Ampicillin 150 mg/kg/day and tobramycin
3 months to 5 years	Cefamandole 100–150 mg/kg/day
> 5 years	Nafcillin 150 mg/kg/day
Compromised host Nosocomial infection	Tobramycin and cefazolin adjusted for renal function

Joint drainage is universally recommended. Indications for surgical drainage versus repeated needle aspiration are debated. Gonococcal arthritis rarely requires open drainage. As a minimum, all joints should be aspirated on a daily basis or more frequently whenever there is detectable fluid present. This regimen may require aspiration several times a day during the first few days of therapy. A septic hip joint should be drained surgically because repeated needling is difficult and the hip capsule is not distensible. The blood supply of the femoral head may thus be easily compromised, leading to aseptic necrosis of the femoral head. Joints that are responding poorly to repeated aspiration, especially if the fluid remains purulent, should be opened surgically and irrigated. However, there is no universal agreement regarding when the decision to drain surgically should be made.

Physical therapy plays an important role in treatment. Splinting during the acute phase reduces pain. As soon as pain permits, which is usually after 2 or 3 days of therapy, physical therapy, beginning with range-of-motion exercises and progressing to weight bearing as tolerated, is important to restore joint function.

Prognosis

The prognosis is dependent on early recognition and treatment, the site of infection, and the organism type. Infections not treated within 7 days have a much higher incidence of permanent joint damage and disability. Infection of the hip joint has a particularly bad prognosis, apparently because of the difficulty with diagnosis and the tenuous blood supply of the femoral head. Infections in other weight-bearing joints, particularly the knee and ankle, commonly result in some usually mild disability. Infections with Gram-negative bacilli often result in joint damage, presumably because these patients tend to be elderly, often have other joint disease, have underlying illnesses, and Gram-negative bacteria are more difficult to treat. *N. gonorrheae,* however, rarely causes significant long-term dysfunction.

GONOCOCCAL ARTHRITIS

Gonococcal arthritis is the most common infectious arthropathy in adults and can be distinguished from other pyogenic arthritides. It is more common in women than men and at times of menses or pregnancy. The organism usually enters through the genitourinary tract or, less often, the oral or rectal mucosa.

The clinical spectrum of disseminated gonococcal infection includes cutaneous lesions, pharyngitis, urethritis, hepatitis, meningitis, endocarditis, myocarditis, or conjunctivitis. During the septicemic phase of illness, patients have fever, chills, tenosynovitis, or a fleeting polyarthralgias arthritis. Other patients have or develop persistently inflamed "septic" joints. Not all patients fall clearly into categories of septicemic (hematogenous) or septic joint (localized) gonococcal arthritis. Synovial fluid cultures are positive in about 50% of patients thought to have gonococcal arthritis and are more often found in septic joints. Although it has been speculated that certain symptoms of gonococcal arthritis could be the result of hypersensitivity mechanisms rather than of direct bacterial invasion, neither immune complexes nor serum or synovial fluid hypocomplementemia have been consistently found in patients with disseminated infection. Persons deficient in C6, C7, or C8 are at increased risk of developing one or more episodes of neisseria infection. Hemolytic complement studies are indicated in subjects with recurrent bacteremia. Disseminated gonococcal infection is treated with aqueous penicillin G 10 million units intravenously daily until improvement, followed by ampicillin 0.5 g qid, to complete 7 days of treatment. Alternatives include: ampicillin 3.5 g or amoxicillin 3 g po, each with probenecid 1 g, followed by 0.5 g antibiotic quid for 7 days; tetracycline or erythromycin 0.5 g po qid for 7 days; or spectinomycin 2 g intramuscularly for 3 days.

OSTEOMYELITIS

Definition

Osteomyelitis is any inflammatory process within the substance of bone caused by replicating microorganisms.

Etiology

Organisms causing bone infection are similar to those causing joint infections and are outlined in Table 21.3. The organism varies with the site of infection.

Table 21.3. Organisms Causing Osteomyelitis

Organism	Frequency[a]	Comment
Staphylococcus aureus	70%+	
Streptococcus	10%	Group A streptococci, *S. pneumoniae* Group B streptococcus in neonates
Gram-negative organisms	20%	*Hemophilus influenzae* in children; any Gram-negative rod in adults or compromised hosts

[a] Figures depend on patient population, age, and years covered by any series.

For example, polymicrobial infections are seen most commonly in the feet, where puncture wounds and neurotropic soft tissue infections are the major causes of osteomyelitis.

Clinical Picture

Over 90% of patients with bone infection have an acute or subacute illness characterized by local pain, swelling, and tenderness, with variable degrees of fever. In children, infections typically occur in the metaphysis of the bone, and 70% involve the lower extremity, either the tibia or femur. In patients less than 3 years of age having femoral infection, 70% also have septic arthritis of the hip joint. It is this group that usually has pseudoparalysis. In adults, long bones are usually not involved, and the forms of osteomyelitis in adults are described below.

Laboratory Data

Most patients exhibit a leukocytosis and elevated ESR. In subacute cases, anemia may also be present. Blood cultures may be positive in children but are rarely positive in adults.

Radiology

Except for the presence of soft tissue swelling, x-rays of the involved bone are normal for the first 10–14 days. At about 2 weeks, a periosteal reaction may be seen and may be associated with decreased density of the bone and lytic defects within the bone. As more time passes, sequestra or foci of necrotic tissue within the bone may be seen.

Diagnosis

Early diagnosis depends on a high index of suspicion. The presence of an inflammatory process over the metaphysis of a long bone in a child with fever is osteomyelitis until proven otherwise. This diagnosis is not altered by the presence of a negative x-ray. In this situation, culture of blood and periosteal aspirate should be obtained. If adequate material is present, Gram stain often will give an immediate diagnosis. If radiographic abnormality is present, surgical drainage of the area to obtain material for culture should be undertaken. In atypic cases, bone scans using either gallium 67 (and/or technetium 99) labeled compounds may be useful in demonstrating the presence of a bony lesion before x-rays are abnormal (Figs. 21.1–21.3). In this situation, tomograms also may be helpful. Scans are particularly useful in the feet when there is a history of puncture wound and when the diagnosis of osteomyelitis may be difficult to make. Scans may also be useful in differentiating bone from joint infection. In the presence of chronic osteomyelitis, relapse may be evident on scan at a time when the diagnosis is difficult to make radiographically (Figs. 21.4, 21.5).

Therapy

The first line of therapy is antibiotics parenterally in high doses for 6–8 weeks. Initial therapy with oxacillin or nafcillin should be instituted immediately after

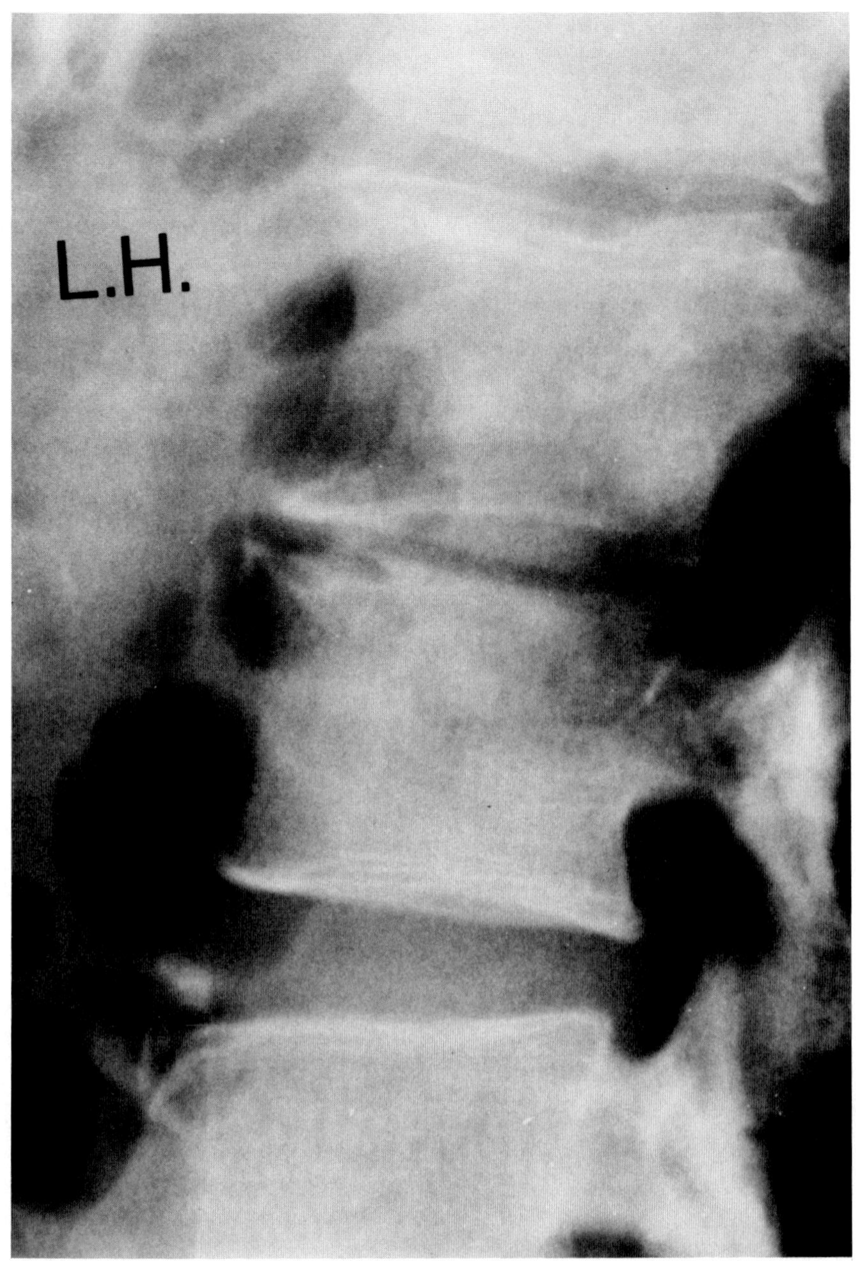

Figure 21.1. Nondiagnostic lateral spine in a patient with back pain.

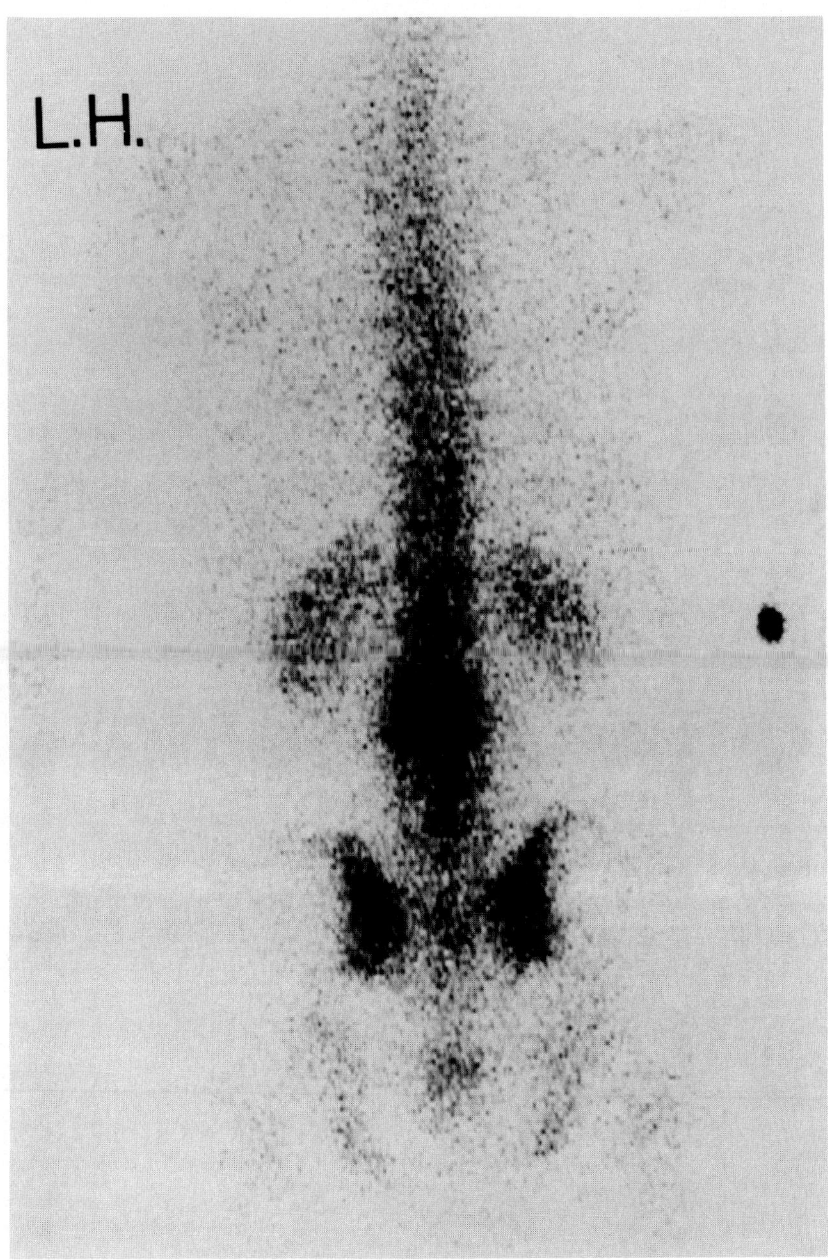

Figure 21.2. Bone scan showing increased uptake reflecting osteomyelitis.

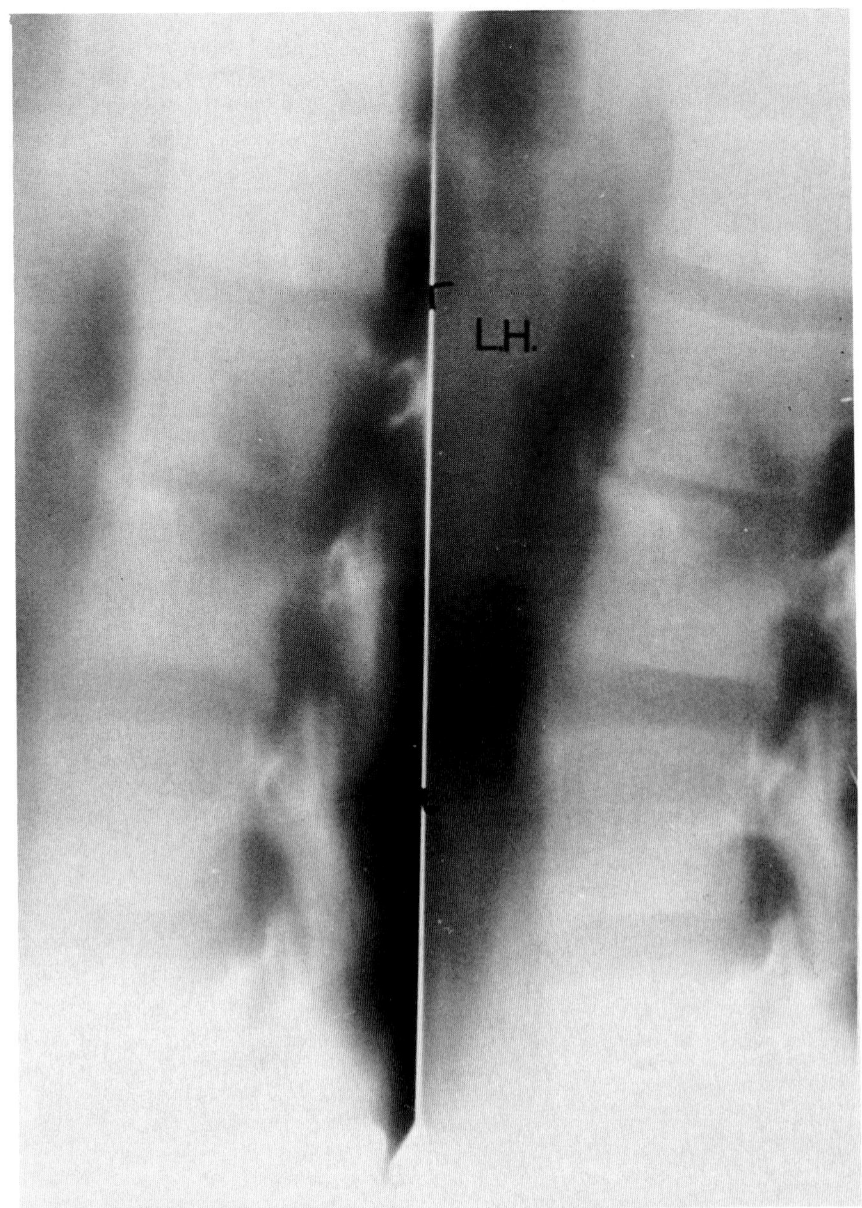

Figure 21.3. Tomograms of the same patient showing bone destruction.

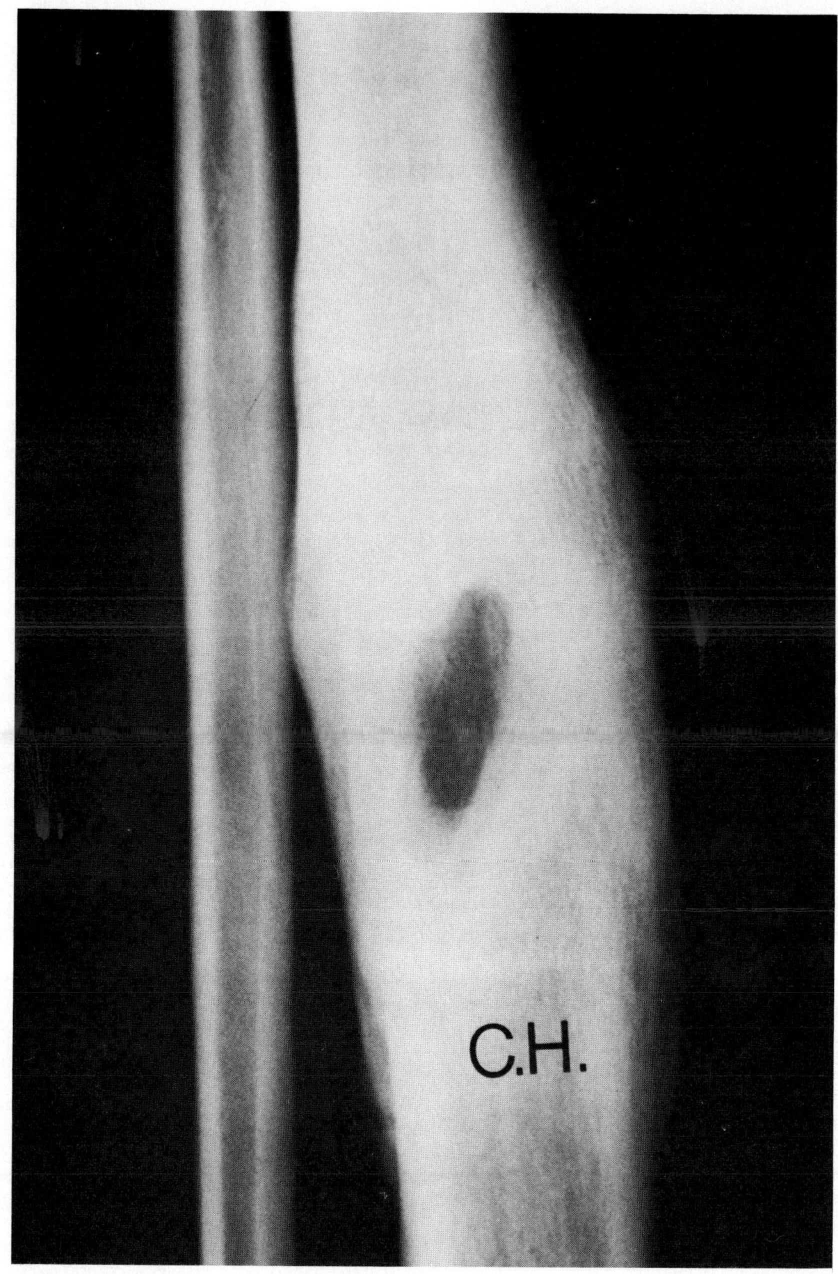

Figure 21.4. Radiographically stable tibial lesion.

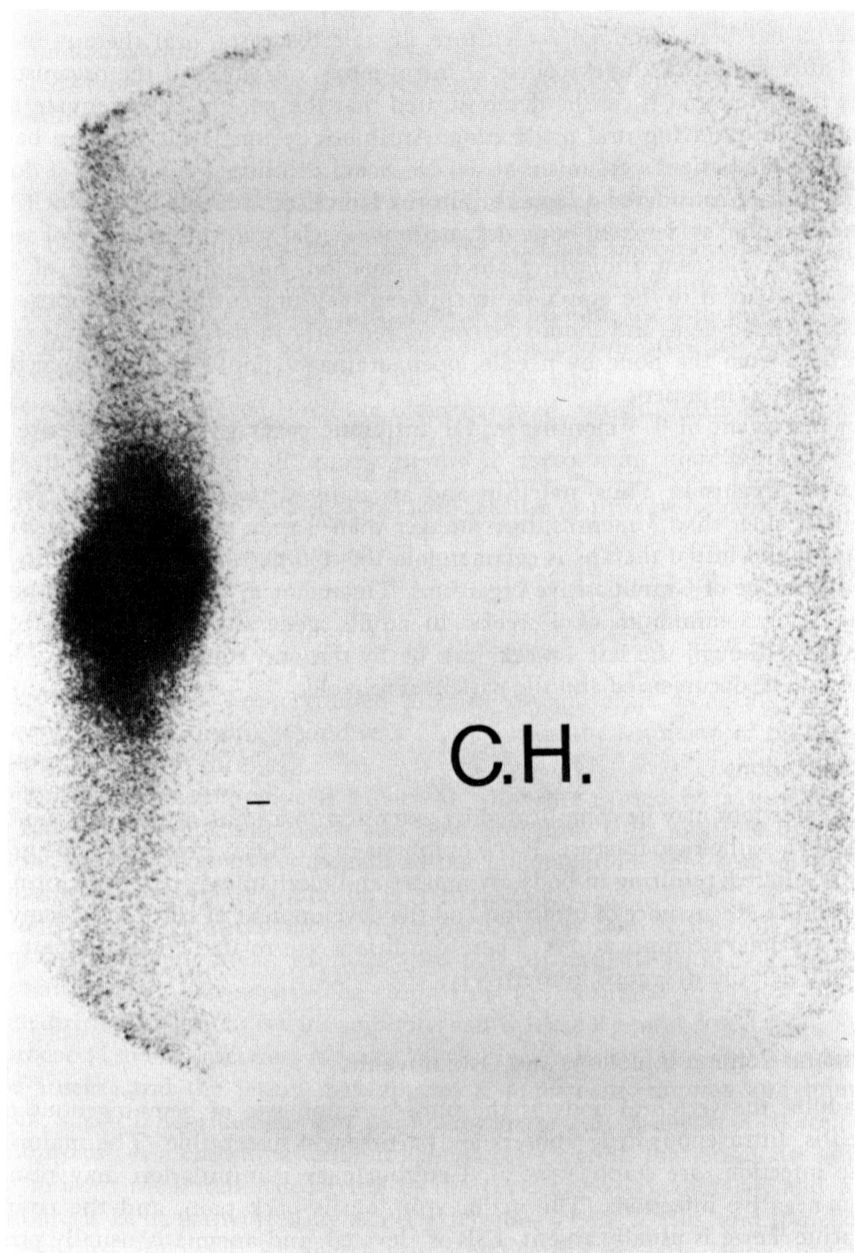

Figure 21.5. Bone scan showing increased uptake indicating osteomyelitis, later proven at surgery.

Sporotrichosis is an inoculation-acquired disease of the skin and lymphatics in an extremity. Arthritis, tenosynovitis, and osteomyelitis of the infected limb may be seen rarely. The combination of nodular lymphangitis and osteomyelitis or subacute septic arthritis is virtually diagnostic. The treatment consists of amphotericin B.

TUBERCULOUS OSTEOMYELITIS AND ARTHRITIS

Tuberculous osteomyelitis and arthritis appear clinically as manifestations of reactivation tuberculosis. When bone and joint involvement is the apparent manifestation, the majority of patients do have evidence of active disease elsewhere. The disease is usually low grade and of insidious onset. Arthritis is usually monoarticular. Knees, wrists, ankles, hips, and elbows are most frequently involved. Osteomyelitis most commonly involves lumbar vertebrae (Pott's disease). The diagnosis requires biopsy with acid-fast stains and culture. The culture of synovial fluid is rarely useful. Treatment of tuberculous bone and joint infections require a minimum of two drugs for 1 year (isoniazid and ethambutol), followed by a single drug for an additional year (isoniazid). This regimen may be altered depending upon the extent of disease, resistance of the organism, and clinical response.

SYPHILITIC INFECTIONS

Secondary syphilis may cause bone pain and tenderness, with x-ray evidence of periostitis. Treatment is as for other forms of secondary syphilis. Infants born with congenital syphilis frequently manifest periostitis on x-ray. In late syphilis, osteomyelitis and gummatous disease of bone may be seen.

LYME ARTHRITIS

Lyme arthritis was first recognized in Connecticut as a seasonal, usually self-limited illness characterized by brief recurrent episodes of asymmetric large joint oligoarthritis. There is strong epidemiologic evidence for transmission of a causative agent by the tick vector *Ixodes scapularis*. The disease usually begins with erythema chronicum migrans, an erythematous expanding annular skin lesion with central clearing, that occurs weeks to months after the tick bite. Joint involvement appears an average of 4 weeks after the onset of rash and usually persists for a few days to weeks. Most patients have recurrences with asymptomatic periods. A few patients have developed chronic arthritis, and most of these patients have been HLA-DRw2 positive. Other clinical manifestations include fatigue, fever, myalgias, nausea, vomiting, sore throat, lymphadenopathy, and central nervous system symptoms. Rheumatoid factor and antinuclear antibodies are negative, but cryoprecipitates containing IgM and thought to represent large circulating immune complexes have been identified.

VIRAL ARTHRITIS

Hepatitis B-associated Arthritis

A constellation of symptoms including arthralgias, arthritis, rash, and fever may constitute the presenting manifestations of hepatitis B infection. This serum sickness-like illness usually occurs in the preicteric phase of illness, lasting approximately 3 weeks and disappearing with the onset of clinical jaundice. The arthritis is an acute symmetric polyarthritis that may be migratory, and it involves most frequently the proximal interphalangeal and metacarpophalangeal joints of the hands. At times, acute rheumatoid arthritis is simulated. Laboratory test results are usually negative, with the exception of the presence of hepatitis B surface antigen in the serum, with decreased levels of complement and occasionally abnormal urinalysis if glomerulitis is present. Synovial fluid is mildly inflammatory and synovial fluid complement levels are decreased, suggesting that immune complexes may play a role in the pathogenesis of this syndrome.

Rubella Arthritis

Both natural rubella infection and rubella vaccination with live attenuated virus may be accompanied by arthritis. Joint involvement occurs primarily in adults and resembles that of viral hepatitis, with the small joints of the hands most frequently affected. Morning stiffness is often a prominent feature. The onset of rubella arthritis coincides with or follows development of the rash in naturally occurring infection and tends to occur an average of 2 weeks after live virus vaccination. In both cases, symptoms may last 1–2 months. Rheumatoid factor may become transiently positive. Serum hypocomplementemia has been reported, suggesting that immune complexes may play a role in the development of symptoms.

Other Viruses

Arthritis has been rarely reported in association with mumps, varicella, infectious mononucleosis, certain echoviruses, adenoviruses, arboviruses, and after smallpox vaccination.

The material in the section on *Gonococcal Arthritis* appears in similar form in Panush RS: Other rheumatic diseases with immunologic features, in Lockey RF (ed): *Allergy and Clinical Immunology*. Garden City, NY. Medical Examination Publishing Co, Inc, an Excerpta Medica company, © 1979, pp 273–274. Reprinted by permission.

BIBLIOGRAPHY

Bayer AS, Lucien BG: Fungal arthritis. *Semin Arthritis Rheum* 8:142, 1978.

Berney S, Goldstein M, Bishko, F: Clinical and diagnostic features of tuberculous arthritis.

Bayer AS, Lucien BG: Fungal arthritis. *Semin Arthritis Rheum* 8:200, 1978.
    Am J Med 53:36, 1972.

Brogadir SP, Schimmer BM, Myers AR: Spectrum of gonococcal arthritis-dermatitis syndrome. *Semin Arthritis Rheum* 8:177, 1979.

Goldenberg DL, Cohen AS: Acute infectious arthritis. *Am J Med* 60:369, 1976.

Hyer FH, Gottlieb NL: Rheumatic disorders associated with viral infection. *Semin Arthritis Rheum* 8:17, 1978.

Lang A, Peterson H: Osteomyelitis following puncture wounds of the foot in children. *J Trauma* 16:993, 1976.

Lisbona R, Rosenthall L: Observations on the sequential use of [99m]technetium phosphate complex and 67 gallium imaging in osteomyelitis, cellulitis, and septic arthritis. *Radiology* 123:123, 1977.

Newman JH: Review of septic arthritis throughout the antibiotic era. *Ann Rheum Dis* 35:198, 1976.

Tetzlaff TR, McCracken GH, Nelson JD: Oral antibiotic therapy for skeletal infections of children. *J Pediatr* 92:485–490.

22

Amyloidosis

Merrill D. Benson

Amyloidosis refers to a number of disease states characterized by the extracellular deposition of a homogeneous material having certain histologic traits. This material, which is composed mainly of fibrillar protein, may be deposited in any body organ and result in dysfunction of the organ by displacement of normal tissues. Amyloidosis may occur de novo (primary), in association with other diseases (secondary), or in predictable heredofamilial states. It may involve many organs (systemic) or be confined to one organ (localized). The most common forms of amyloidosis are primary with no associated disease and secondary with long-standing inflammatory disease such as tuberculosis, inflammatory arthritis, leprosy, or granulomatous colitis. Whatever the type of amyloid and composition of amyloid deposits, clinical disease is caused by the amount and strategic location of the deposits. The wide variation in organ involvement often makes amyloidosis an extremely difficult disease to diagnose.

PATHOLOGY

Morphology

Amyloid is found in body organs as amorphous extracellular deposits. In large amounts, it causes enlarged firm and friable organs. Virchow originally used the term *amyloid* because it stained with iodine and sulfuric acid in a manner similar to that of starch or cellulose. We now know that amyloid deposits are composed mainly of protein with varying amounts of carbohydrate. Histologically, amyloid is a homogeneous eosinophilic material on routine hematoxylin and eosin stain (H & E). It can be identified more specifically by staining tissue sections with crystal violet or Congo red.

In 1959, electron microscopy first showed that amyloid deposits had a substructure characterized by nonbranching fibrils measuring 75 to 100 Å in diameter. By x-ray defraction the conformation of amyloid fibril proteins is an antiparallel beta-pleated sheet. As opposed to the alpha helix of molecules such as collagen, the beta-pleated sheet structure has been identified in an increasing number of tissue proteins including, for example, the variable and constant domains of Ig molecules. This ordered structure gives amyloid its birefringence. Probably the best histologic definition of amyloid at this time includes three factors: (1) green birefringence on Congo red staining and polarization microscopy, (2) nonbranching fibrous appearance by electron microscopy, and (3) beta-pleated sheet configuration by x-ray defraction.

Chemistry

Although all amyloid deposits are histologically alike, chemical studies have recently shown that different types of amyloid have different compositions. In primary amyloidosis and in amyloidosis associated with malignant dysproteinemia, the major protein constituent is homologous to immunoglobulin light chain (Table 22.1). This protein may be an entire light chain (23,000 daltons) or only a fragment of a light chain with a molecular weight as low as 5,000. The majority of cases have only the variable segment of the light chain (VL) or a portion thereof. Patients with primary amyloidosis often have monoclonal Ig in their serum, which may appear in the urine when the nephrotic syndrome is present. For some unexplained reason, amyloid monoclonal Ig are more frequently lambda than kappa light chains. Several studies of individual cases of primary amyloidosis have shown that the serum monoclonal protein has the same amino acid primary structure as the protein isolated from amyloid deposits. This structure strongly suggests that the tissue protein is derived from the serum component or from a common source.

In secondary amyloidosis, the major protein constituent of the deposits has 76 amino acid residues in a single polypeptide chain with a molecular weight of approximately 8,400 (Table 22.1). Antiserum to this protein (AA) identifies an immunologically identical protein in the serum (SAA) that can be isolated from sera of patients with inflammatory diseases as a 12,000- to 14,000-molecular-weight protein. SAA appears to associate by noncovalent binding with other serum proteins and is, therefore, found in fractions of higher molecular weight. While SAA is found in normal serum in nanogram quantities, it acts as an acute phase reactant, increasing 300- to 500-fold during inflammation. Sustained high levels of serum SAA in those conditions that predispose to secondary amyloid suggest that serum SAA is the precursor of amyloid tissue protein AA.

Recent studies have shown that the amyloid found in medullary carcinoma of the thyroid contains a peptide with an amino acid sequence identical to that of a portion of the calcitonin molecule. The amyloid deposits in the Portuguese type of heredofamilial amyloidosis have a protein that cross-reacts with antiserum to prealbumin. Several cases of senile cardiac amyloid have been found to have a unique protein common to them all that is structurally related to prealbumin AA. These findings suggest that many uniquely different proteins may be deposited by similar mechanisms.

Table 22.1. Amyloid Fibril Protein N-terminal Sequences

Amyloid type	Protein Type	1 2 3 4 5 6 7 8 9 10
Primary	AL[a] Kappa I	Asp-Ile-Gln-Met-Thr-Gln-Ser-Pro-Ser-Ser-
Secondary	AA	Arg-Ser-Phe-Phe-Ser-Phe-Leu-Gly-Glu-Ala-

[a] AL, amyloid light chain.

IMMUNOLOGIC FACTORS

Patients with primary amyloidosis have few immunologic abnormalities other than the presence of serum monoclonal Ig. They have more of the features of a benign monoclonal gammopathy than of multiple myeloma—no increase in systemic infections, approximately 10%–15% mature marrow plasmacytes, and modest serum levels of polyclonal Ig. There have been reports of T-cell impairment as measured by lymphocyte stimulation with concanavalin A, but other measures of lymphocyte function are normal in primary amyloidosis. Similarly, few immunologic abnormalities have been noted in patients with secondary amyloidosis. Work with animal models of secondary amyloidosis, however, has shown T-cell impairment as measured by mitogen response and ability to reject skin grafts. An increase in B-lymphocyte function in the spleens of amyloidotic mice suggests a loss of suppressor cell function. The acute-phase nature of protein SAA suggests that this protein may be important in regulating the response to inflammatory or antigenic stimuli.

CLASSIFICATION

At our present level of understanding of amyloidosis, a usable classification along established lines can be made by adhering to a rigorous definition of terminology (Table 22.2). The term *primary* should be used for those cases of systemic amyloidosis that occurred de novo without an associated disease or family history of amyloidosis. Amyloidosis in patients with multiple myeloma, Waldenström's macroglobulinemia, or heavy chain disease can be referred to as *myeloma associated-* or *malignant dysproteinemia-associated amyloidosis*. Thus the term *secondary* refers only to those cases associated with chronic inflammatory diseases. At the present time, *heredofamilial amyloidosis* denotes those conditions seen in family

Table 22.2. Amyloid Classification

Clinical	*Chemical (major protein constituent)*
Primary	Immunoglobulin light chain (V_L)
Associated with malignant dysproteinemia Myeloma, Waldenström's, H-chain disease	Immunoglobulin light chain (V_L)
Secondary	AA
Heredofamilial	
Autosomal dominant	Several types related to prealbumin
Autosomal recessive (FMF)	AA
Localized	
Medullary carcinoma of thyroid	Peptide of calcitonin
Others (lichen amyloid, respiratory tract, urinary tract)	Unknown
Senile	
Cardiac	Related to prealbumin
Others (Alzheimer's plaques, diabetic islets of Langerhans)	Unknown

Table 22.3. Heredofamilial Amyloidoses

Neuropathy
  Lower limb (often with GI involvement, impotence, leg ulcers)
    Portuguese
    Japanese
    Swedish
  Upper limb (carpal tunnel syndrome, vitreous opacities)
    Swiss (Indiana)
    German (Maryland)
  Lower then upper limb with nephropathy
    Scot-English-Irish (Iowa)
Nephropathy
  Familial Mediterranean fever
  English—with urticaria and deafness
Cardiopathy
  Danish—progressive heart failure
  Persistent atrial standstill
Miscellaneous
  Medullary carcinoma of thyroid
  Lattice corneal dystrophy
  Cerebral hemorrhage

---

groups that are generally inherited as autosomal dominant traits with varying degrees of penetration. In the past, the amyloid associated with familial Mediterranean fever (FMF), which is inherited as an autosomal recessive trait, created a problem with classification. Chemical studies have now shown that the amyloid in FMF is of the AA protein type. This fact suggests that this type of amyloidosis is secondary to the chronic inflammatory condition (peritonitis, synovitis, pleuritis). Too little is known about the localized forms of amyloid, such as the deposits associated with medullary carcinoma of the thyroid, the deposits in the islets of Langerhans in diabetes mellitus, the cerebral plaques in Alzheimer's disease, or localized forms in the respiratory tract, to categorize these forms with certainty. At this time, we may include localized amyloid in the classification, realizing that this category may represent a collection of many disorders that can lead to fibrillar deposits. Recent reports of a unique protein common to amyloid deposits from the hearts of different patients suggest that senile cardiac amyloid may be a distinct entity.

Classification by organ system involvement may be of some value in the subclassification of heredofamilial disorders in which each family seems to have a consistent pattern and progression of organ involvement. A partial listing of heredofamilial amyloidoses by family origin and pattern of organ involvement is presented in Table 22.3.

CLINICAL PRESENTATION

Whatever the type of amyloidosis, the clinical presentation depends upon the pattern and degree of organ system involvement by amyloid deposits. A number of

well-recognized clinical syndromes can result from systemic amyloidosis and, while not specific for the disease, should raise the possibility of the diagnosis. These conditions include the nephrotic syndrome, congestive heart failure, malabsorption, and the carpal tunnel syndrome. Most of these syndromes may occur in each of the three major types of systemic amyloidosis (primary, secondary, heredofamilial). The carpal tunnel syndrome, however, has not been reported in secondary amyloidosis.

The most common presenting symptoms in systemic amyloidosis are fatigue, weight loss, peripheral edema, and shortness of breath. The most common findings on physical examination at presentation include hepatomegaly, edema, splenomegaly, macroglossia, purpura, and orthostatic hypotension. None of these findings is specific for any one type of amyloidosis. There are, however, certain patterns of organ system involvement that can be recognized in systemic amyloidosis. The classic description of primary amyloidosis with involvement of mesenchymal-derived tissue such as skeletal muscle, heart, and blood vessels usually is seen with some amount of proteinuria but not significant azotemia at the time of presentation. Death in this group is commonly from cardiovascular insufficiency with either cardiac arrhythmia, cerebral vascular accident, or prerenal azotemia being a major factor in the patient's demise. Another presentation of primary amyloidosis is with massive hepatomegaly, with or without large amounts of splenic amyloid. These patients may have varying amounts of proteinuria and often have significant azotemia at the time of death. Recently a group of patients with primary amyloidosis having either carpal tunnel syndrome or diffuse polyneuropathy has been identified who may go months to years before cardiac or renal deterioration occurs. Amyloid arthropathy, with large synovial deposits of amyloid, may occur in patients with primary or malignant dysproteinemic types of amyloidosis. Patients with neuropathy or arthropathy invariably have serum or urine monoclonal proteins, which are found in only approximately 50% of all primary amyloids. Muscle involvement may occur in any one of these types of appearance, although macroglossia occurs in only 10%–20% of patients with primary amyloidosis (Fig. 22.1).

While secondary amyloidosis often presents with proteinuria and renal impairment, hepatomegaly and serum enzyme changes may be the first abnormalities. Splenic amyloid deposition may lead to splenomegaly without clinical impairment unless ruptured by trauma. Diffuse cardiovascular involvement like that seen in primary amyloidosis may give the patient with secondary amyloidosis a poor prognosis. Clinical presentations of the autosomal dominant heredofamilial amyloidoses differ from one another but are often very specific for the particular familial form of the disease (Table 22.3).

LABORATORY FINDINGS

There are no specific laboratory findings for amyloidosis. Occasionally a selective deficiency of clotting factor X can be seen in primary amyloidosis, but this finding is not diagnostic. Abnormalities in laboratory test results really are a reflection of the organ system involvement by amyloid or accompanying disease. Patients with nephrotic syndrome may have depletion of serum proteins and very

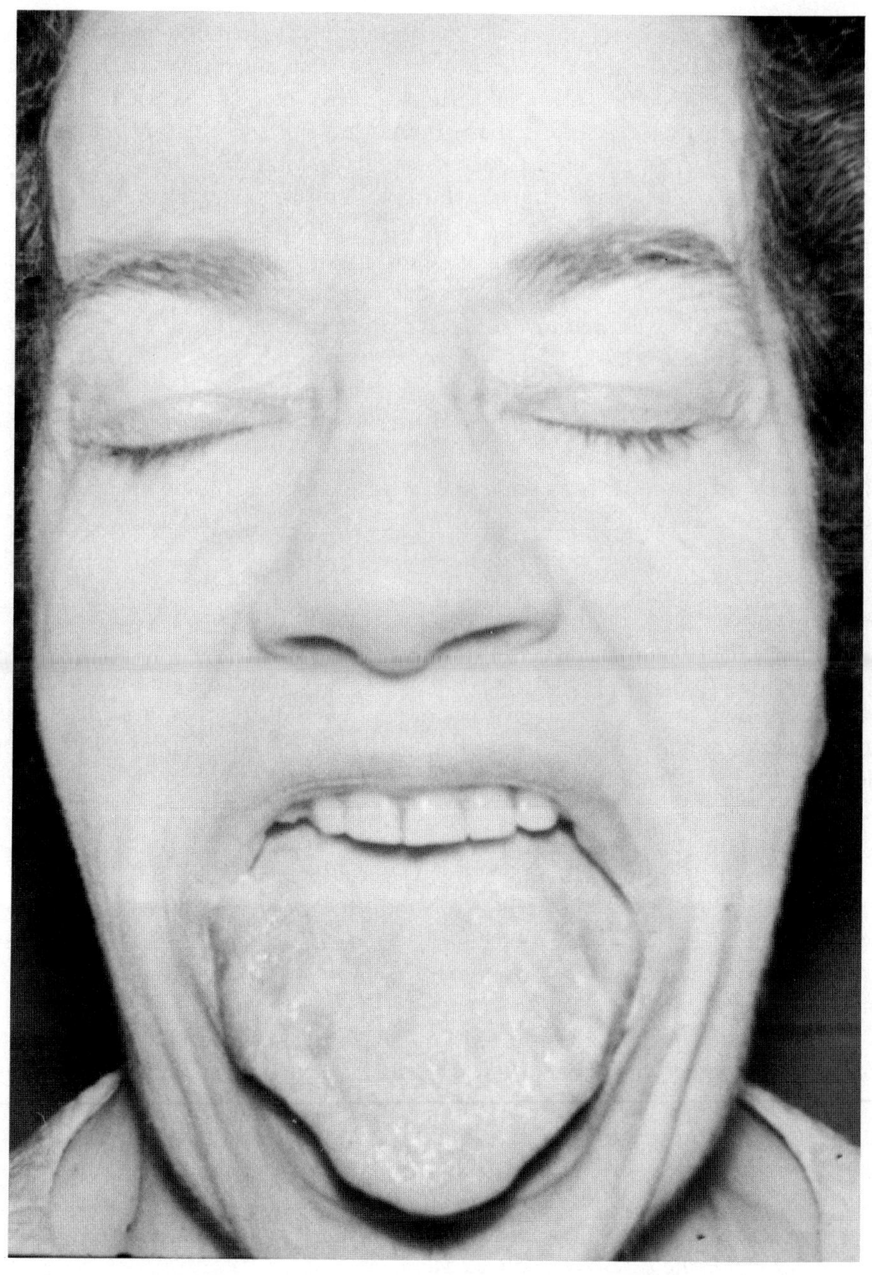

Figure 22.1. Macroglossia in a patient with primary amyloidosis. The size and firmness of the tongue cause indentations from the molars.

high serum cholesterol. Hepatic deposition very often elevates serum alkaline phosphatase. Bowel involvement often leads to abnormalities of absorption. An electrocardiogram often shows nonspecific conduction abnormalities and low voltage in the anterior precordial leads. Radionuclide scans of the liver and spleen may show organomegaly and a diffuse decrease in uptake. Chest x-rays may show large densities due to amyloid deposits in the lungs, and barium studies of the gastrointestinal tract may show a small bowel mucosal pattern of infiltrative disease. X-rays of the kidneys and intravenous pyelography may show large kidneys, but late in the course of the disease the kidneys are often small.

Approximately one-half of patients with primary amyloidosis will have monoclonal Ig spikes on serum or urine electrophoresis. This may be present as intact Ig or, less commonly, as free light chains in the serum or Bence Jones proteinuria. Lytic bone lesions can occur in primary amyloidosis and be indistinguishable on x-ray from those of multiple myeloma.

While most patients with secondary amyloidosis will have very high levels of SAA in the serum, this condition is probably a reflection of the underlying inflammatory disease and is not specific for amyloidosis. SAA may be elevated in primary amyloidosis but usually to a much lower level than in secondary disease. SAA has not been found to be elevated in patients with hereditary amyloidosis without concomitant inflammatory disease. SAA is elevated in FMF during the inflammatory attacks.

DIAGNOSIS

The diagnosis of amyloidosis depends mainly on the physician's ability to recognize the many syndromes caused by the different forms of amyloidosis coupled with a constant awareness of the disorder. The diagnosis of amyloidosis is frequently overlooked because the clinical findings can be explained on the basis of other diseases, and a definitive diagnosis can be made only by tissue biopsy. Certain findings in the history should increase the suspicion of amyloidosis—carpal tunnel syndrome, peripheral neuropathy, development of proteinuria, or heart failure. A history of chronic inflammatory disease, hepatosplenomegaly, or a family history of neuropathy or nephropathy should raise the suspicion of amyloidosis.

The physical examination often reveals multisystem involvement in systemic amyloidosis—hepatosplenomegaly, nephrotic syndrome, congestive heart failure with cardiomyopathy, or purpura. Deposition of amyloidosis in the posterior chamber of the eye (vitreous opacities) or a scalloped deformity of the pupil are essentially diagnostic of a hereditary type of amyloidosis.

Laboratory test results that suggest amyloidosis include monoclonal Ig (Fig. 4.1), abnormal liver enzyme test results, abnormal motility studies of the gastrointestinal tract, and impaired ability of the liver to conjugate bromosulfophthalein (BSP) or Cardio-Green (a sensitive function impaired very early in hepatic amyloidosis).

The diagnosis of amyloidosis really depends upon the demonstration of the typical deposits on tissue biopsy. It is considered safer to do a biopsy of an accessible site such as a rectal valve or gingiva, which can be observed for control of bleeding. Results of rectal biopsy will be positive in approximately 80% of pa-

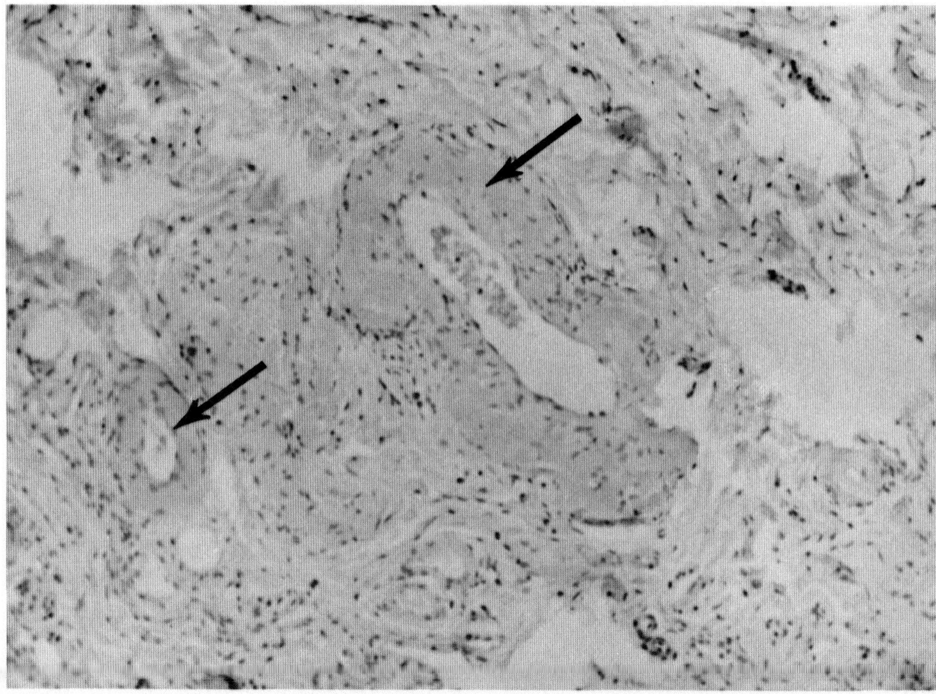

Figure 22.2. Rectal biopsy showing amyloid deposits throughout blood vessel walls. When viewed in a polarizing microscope, this Congo red-stained tissue will show green birefringence wherever amyloid is deposited.

tients with systemic amyloidosis regardless of the symptom complex of appearance (Fig. 22.2). Because amyloid is not always considered in patients with nephrotic syndrome or hepatomegaly, a considerable number of new cases are still diagnosed by kidney or liver biopsy. Once a biopsy is obtained, it is imperative to get appropriate stains. Often amyloid deposits go unrecognized on routine H & E sections. Congo red staining, which will give a characteristic green birefringence when the stained tissue is observed in the polarizing microscope, is felt to be the best means of detecting amyloid. Electron microscopy may be helpful in identifying deposits of amyloidosis but is often not readily available. If the result of a rectal biopsy is negative and the patient is still felt to be a strong candidate for having systemic amyloidosis, biopsy of an organ system that has definite clinical involvement is indicated. This procedure may involve sural nerve biopsy in a patient with peripheral neuropathy, kidney biopsy in a patient with nephrotic syndrome, or lung biopsy in a patient with pulmonary masses and cardiopulmonary dysfunction.

TREATMENT AND PROGNOSIS

There is no specific treatment for any type of amyloidosis. In localized forms of the disease, such as medullary carcinoma of the thyroid, resection will rid the patient of amyloid, but then the amyloid was of no great clinical significance in the first place. In secondary amyloidosis, it has long been felt that removal of an inflammatory stimulus such as chronic osteomyelitis may slow down or reverse the condition. There is little definite evidence of this process occurring in any predictable fashion. On the other hand, there have been well-documented cases of secondary amyloidosis occurring in patients with granulomatous colitis years after total colectomy with no further clinical evidence of active inflammatory disease. Although there have been scattered reports of effective results with immunosuppressive or cytotoxic drugs, no definite evidence is available to suggest that the progression of amyloid is affected by these drugs. Recently it has been found that colchicine will prevent the development of amyloid in the casein-treated mouse model of secondary amyloidosis. The use of colchicine in patients with FMF has now been reported to be associated with delay or prevention of the development of clinical renal involvement. No definite results on the use of colchicine in patients with either primary or secondary amyloidosis other than that with FMF have been reported. If the basis for the action of colchicine is to bind to cell microtubules and prevent degradation of precursor proteins to give fibril proteins, then it might be expected to have a similar effect in both primary and secondary amyloidosis.

The prognosis in systemic amyloidosis is probably better than thought in the past, when the diagnosis was often made at postmortem. With increasing awareness of this disease, the diagnosis has been made earlier in its course. Also, the development of many diagnostic techniques such as cardiac catheterization, gastrointestinal endoscopy, and radionuclide scanning has increased the chances of the physician stumbling onto the diagnosis. Patients with primary amyloidosis generally have a worse prognosis (median survival after diagnosis approximately 1.5 years) than patients with secondary amyloidosis. An associated malignant dysproteinemia (multiple myeloma or Waldenström's macroglobulinemia) portends the worst prognosis of all the systemic amyloidoses, with average survival after diagnosis being less than 6 months. In some patients with primary amyloidosis who appear with carpal tunnel syndrome, it is now obvious that the disease may be present for several years before significant systemic involvement, whereas patients who have congestive heart failure often die within 6 months. Secondary amyloidosis, if diagnosed early, may afford the patient a fairly good prognosis; well-documented survivals of greater than 10 years have been reported. The quality of life still depends upon the organ system involved and the means of treating the organ dysfunction. The newer diuretics have been very helpful in increasing a person's function in the presence of heart failure or nephrotic syndrome. Antibiotics may effectively treat gastrointestinal malabsorption when motility disturbances have caused bacterial overgrowth. Renal dialysis may afford several months of continued life for the patient with primary amyloidosis and actually add years to the life of a patient with secondary or hereditary amyloidosis. Renal transplantation has been tried in a modest number of patients. It would seem that secondary amyloidosis and particularly amyloidosis associated with FMF, in which renal involvement is the major manifestation of the disease, affords the best result for this form of therapy.

BIBLIOGRAPHY

Benditt EP, Eriksen N: Chemical classes of amyloid substance. *Am J Pathol* 65:231, 1971.

Brandt K, Cathcart ES, Cohen AS: A clinical analysis of the course and prognosis of forty-two patients with amyloidosis. *Am J Med* 44:955, 1968.

Cathcart ES, Ritchie RF, Cohen AS, et al: Immunoglobulins and amyloidosis. *Am J Med* 52:93, 1972.

Cohen AS: Amyloidosis. *N Engl J Med* 277:522, 574, 628, 1967.

Cohen AS, Benson MD: Amyloid neuropathy, in Dyck PJ, Thomas PK, Lambert EH (eds): *Peripheral Neuropathy*. Philadelphia, WB Saunders Co, Ltd 1975, p 1067.

Glenner GG, Terry W, Harada M, et al: Amyloid fibril proteins: Proof of homology with immunoglobulin light chains by sequence analyses. *Science* 172:1150, 1971.

Kyle RA, Bayrd ED: Amyloidosis: Review of 236 cases. *Medicine* 54:271, 1975.

Levin M, Franklin EC, Frangione B, et al: The amino acid sequence of a major non-immunoglobulin component of some amyloid fibrils. *J Clin Invest* 51:2773, 1972.

Levin M, Pras M, Franklin EC: Immunologic studies of the major nonimmunoglobulin protein of amyloid. I. Identification and partial characterization of a related serum component. *J Exp Med* 138:373, 1973.

Part 5

DEGENERATIVE AND METABOLIC DISEASES

mation involving the diaphyseal area and involving metacarpophalangeal, proximal interphalangeal, metatarsophalangeal and ankle joints, may develop in less than 1% of patients with Grave's disease. This syndrome is independent of the gland's secretory state and therapy; it is associated with increased levels of long-acting thyroid stimulator. Osteoporosis and a negative calcium and phosphorus balance can occur in patients with severe thyrotoxicosis. Syndromes similar to systemic lupus erythematosus (SLE) and rheumatoid arthritis (RA) have been reported secondary to treatment with some antithyroid drugs.

Parathyroid Hormone

Hyposecretion
Soft tissue calcifications have been reported in primary as well as in pseudohypoparathyroidism. A syndrome identical to osteitis fibrosa has been described in the latter patients, presumably because of end-organ unresponsiveness to parathyroid hormone and development of secondary hyperparathyroidism.

Hypersecretion
Hyperparathyroidism can present with skeletal and musculoskeletal symptoms in as many as 16% of patients. The classic lesion, osteitis fibrosa cystica, occurs more commonly in secondary hyperparathyroidism. It is best detected by radiographic evidence of subperiosteal resorption on the radial side of the middle phalanges. Bone cysts and brown tumors may develop as the disease progresses. An RA-like picture with sparing of proximal interphalangeal joints can also be seen. Gout occurs more frequently in these patients than in normal persons. Among patients with pseudogout, the prevalence of hyperparathyroidism ranges from 7% to 38%.

Growth Hormone

Hypersecretion
Carpal tunnel syndrome is seen in as many as 35% of patients with acromegaly and regresses with treatment. The typical changes of increased bone turnover and accretion are most prominent in the cranium, mandible, and phalangeal tufts. Overall, most of the skeleton is osteoporotic. Other changes include thickening of small and flat bones and a thickened heel pad. Hypertrophy of periarticular tissue also occurs and leads to premature osteoarthritis. Diffuse idiopathic skeletal hyperostosis (DISH) has been reported in some patients. An acromegalic myopathy, distinct from the arthropathy, has been described.

Insulin

Hyposecretion
Neuropathy (Charcot joint), especially of the midtarsal joint, occurs in 0.1% of diabetic patients, usually those with long-standing disease and peripheral neuropathy. These patients currently account for a majority of the new cases of neuroarthropathy. Osteolysis, primarily of the distal phalanges of the foot, occurs and can revert spontaneously. Chondrocalcinosis probably has no higher prevalence in diabetics, but symptomatic CPPD crystal-induced arthritis may. Peri-

arthritis, DISH, and early osteoarthritis have also been reported. There is no evidence of a primary association between gout and diabetes. Other rheumatic syndromes seen in diabetics include carpal tunnel neuropathy, Dupuytren's contracture, and reflex sympathetic dystrophy. Stiffness and decreased finger motion occur in juvenile diabetics. Diabetics may develop atrophy of the intrinsic muscles of the hand and median and ulnar neuropathy in the absence of an entrapment syndrome.

Adrenal Corticosteroids

Hyposecretion
When the disease is idiopathic (Addison's disease), antibodies to adrenal tissue and other endocrine cells are often found. During an adrenal crisis, flexion contractures of the abdominal and lower limb musculature may develop and are responsive to appropriate hormone and fluid replacement.

Hypersecretion (Primary, Secondary, or Exogenous)
Osteoporosis, mostly of the metacarpals, femoral neck, and spine, is common particularly in patients with RA, postmenopausal women, and nonexercising patients. Osteonecrosis of the proximal and distal femur, proximal humerus, and tibia is also seen. Definite evidence for the corticosteroids as etiologic agents for either condition is lacking. Proximal myopathy and elevated muscle enzyme levels can occur and will resolve with return of the plasma steroid level to normal (probably more common in exogenous hypercorticism). A pseudorheumatic syndrome can appear in patients on rapidly decreasing doses of exogenous steroids.

Progestational and Estrogenic Hormones

Hyposecretion
Postmenopausal osteoporosis appears in 25% of women at risk, although additional factors are also involved.

Hypersecretion (Pregnancy or Exogenous [i.e., birth control pills])
Significant titers of antinuclear antibodies have been reported in pregnancy and in patients on progestational agents. The true risk of developing SLE is unclear. Erythema nodosum and exacerbation of SLE have been reported. Partial remission of RA during pregnancy and worsening in the postpartum period can occur. Pregnancy is a recognized cause of carpal tunnel syndrome.

Rheumatic manifestations of endocrinopathies are summarized in Table 23.1.

RENAL DISEASE

The osteodystrophy of chronic renal failure develops as a result of abnormalities in calcium and phosphorus metabolism. Depending on whether parathyroid hormone secretion or vitamin D metabolism is most affected, the predominant lesion will be osteitis fibrosa cystica or osteomalacia. X-ray findings are more common than symptoms. Arthralgias, synovitis, septic arthritis, and myalgias are also de-

Table 23.1. Rheumatic Syndromes Associated with Endocrinopathies

Endocrinopathy	*Associated Rheumatic Syndrome*	*Prevalence*
Hypothyroidism	Carpal tunnel[a]	5%–10%
	Muscle cramps, pseudomyotonia[a]	?
	Proximal myopathy and high CPK[a]	?
	Joint effusions (> 50% contain crystals of calcium pyrophosphate)[a]	?
	Polyarthralgias[a]	?
	Hyperuricemia[a]	?
	Elevated erythrocyte sedimentation rate[a]	?
	Other autoimmune diseases in Hashimoto's	?
Hyperthyroidism	Proximal myopathy[a]	common
	Periarthritis[a]	5%–10%
	Acropathy of Graves' disease	0.1%–10%
	Osteoporosis[a]	?
Hypoparathyroidism	Soft tissue calcifications	?
Hyperparathyroidism	Musculoskeletal symptoms[a]	16%
	Osteitis fibrosa cystica[a]	?
	Gout	2%–3%
	Pseudogout	1%–10%
	Rheumatoid-like arthritis	?
Acromegaly	Carpal tunnel[a]	35%–50%
	Osteoporosis[a]	?
	Premature osteoarthritis	16%–62%
	Thickened heel pad	?
	Diffuse idiopathic skeletal hyperostosis	?
	Myopathy	?
Diabetes	Neuroarthropathy	0.1%
	Pseudogout	14%
	Premature osteoarthritis	?
	Osteolysis	?
	Diffuse idiopathic skeletal hyperostosis	13%–21%
	Carpal tunnel	?
	Periarthritis	11%
	Dupuytren's contracture	0.63%
	Reflex sympathetic dystrophy	?
	Atrophy of intrinsic hand muscles	?
	Joint contracture (in juvenile diabetes)	?
Addison's disease	Other autoimmune diseases when idiopathic	?
Cushing's syndrome	Osteoporosis[a]	?
	Osteonecrosis[a]	?
	Proximal myopathy and high CPK[a]	?
Postmenopause	Osteoporosis[a]	25%
Pregnancy	Carpal tunnel[a]	?

[a] Rheumatic syndrome resolves in parallel with the endocrinopathy.

scribed. Aseptic necrosis of bone may occur in patients on hemodialysis and in patients on high-dose steroid and immunosuppressive therapy secondary to renal transplant. The incidence has been reported as low as 1.4% and as high as 41%. Mechanisms may include fat embolization, osteoporosis, hemostatic abnormalities, vasculitis, infection, and secondary hyperparathyroidism. Surgical treatment has been recommended for early management and/or late joint reconstruction. Immune complexes have been demonstrated in a substantial proportion of patients with glomerulonephritis in whom they are thought to be pathogenic. The offending antigens have been identified in some instances.

Injury to the renal vessels, glomerular structures, and tubules are known complications of many rheumatic diseases—progressive systemic sclerosis (PSS), SLE, and Sjögren's syndrome. These complications are discussed in greater detail in the appropriate chapters.

HEPATIC AND GASTROINTESTINAL DISEASES

Hepatitis

Acute Hepatitis (B or non-B)

A prodromal syndrome resembling serum sickness and consisting of polyarthralgias and arthritis, urticaria, and skin eruptions can occur in 15%–20% of patients with acute hepatitis. The syndrome appears a few days or weeks before the onset of jaundice and resolves as icterus develops.

Hepatitis B Infection

Infection with hepatitis B virus can also produce several distinct syndromes in addition to various clinical forms of hepatitis. Polyarteritis nodosa may be ascribed to previous hepatitis B infection in as many as one-third of patients. Glomerulonephritis secondary to hepatitis B may account for 35% of children with the disease. Hepatitis B virus also may play an etiologic role in some cases of polymyalgia rheumatica and in some cases of essential cryoglobulinemia.

Chronic Liver Disease

Chronic Active Hepatitis

One-third of patients have Sjögren's syndrome, and a similar proportion have transient arthropathy involving small and large joints. Increased levels of autoantibodies and frequent association with other autoimmune conditions characterize these patients. Myopathy and neuropathy may also occur.

Primary Biliary Cirrhosis

Seventeen percent of patients with primary biliary cirrhosis were found to have PSS, many in association with Sjögren's syndrome (which has been reported in up to 70% of patients examined). Other autoimmune diseases (RA, Raynaud's phenomenon, and SLE) have also been reported. The presence of autoantibodies in serum helps confirm the diagnosis, and immune complexes and cryoproteins are found frequently.

Cryptogenic Cirrhosis

Sjögren's syndrome is found in almost 25% of patients with cryptogenic cirrhosis, while arthropathy is found in 3%.

Gastrointestinal Disease

Enteric Bypass Operations for Obesity

Polyarthralgias and arthritis are a known complication of this enteric bypass operation, occurring in 5%–25% of patients. The joint symptoms can develop within days to 2 years after the operation. Reversal of the procedure has led to complete resolution of the symptoms. Evidence suggests that the joint complications may be secondary to circulating immune complexes of antibody directed against gut bacterial antigens. Spondylitis and rheumatoid-like arthritis have been described much less frequently. Neuromyopathy can occur in up to 25% of patients postoperatively.

Inflammatory Bowel Disease

Ulcerative colitis and regional enteritis can both be associated with polyarthralgias, arthritis, and/or spondylitis. These associations, as well as arthritis after gastroenteritis with shigella, salmonella, and yersinia organisms, are covered in detail in Chapter 13.

Pancreatic Disease, Serositis, and Subcutaneous Nodules

Pancreatic diseases may be associated with subcutaneous nodules, arthritis, and inflammation of other serosal surfaces. The pancreatic disease is pancreatitis, cancer, or pseudocyst. Some patients have also been reported with peripheral blood eosinophilia, pleural effusion, and pericarditis. The presumed pathogenesis is liberation of pancreatic enzymes into the systemic circulation or through lymphatics with resultant fat necrosis. The findings in some patients of decreased cutaneous and in vitro lymphocyte reactivity (thought to be secondary to cancer); normal Ig and complement, depressed serum, pleural and pericardial CH50; and cutaneous vasculitis with pleural deposition of IgC and C3 have suggested the possible importance of immunologic mechanisms.

Rheumatic syndromes with gastrointestinal, hepatic, and pancreatic diseases are summarized in Table 23.2.

HEMATOLOGIC DISEASE

Hemarthrosis and Coagulopathy

The differential diagnosis of acute and subacute bleeding into the synovial space includes mechanical events, metabolic deficiencies, iatrogenic causes, hematologic defects in autoimmune diseases, and primary hematologic problems.

Acute mechanical trauma is a frequent cause of serosanguinous synovial effusions. While the trauma may be obvious in young persons, very mild trauma may produce a hemorrhagic effusion in the elderly. The presence of the serosanguinous products in the synovial space will often produce a tender, swollen, and warm joint. Vitamin deficiencies, particularly scurvy, may produce friable vasculature

Table 23.2. Rheumatic Syndromes Associated with Gastrointestinal, Hepatic, and Pancreatic Diseases

Gastroenteropathy	Associated Rheumatic Syndrome	Prevalence
Acute hepatitis B	Serum sickness[a]	15%–20%
Hepatitis B infection	Polyarteritis nodosa	?
	Glomerulonephritis	?
	Polymyalgia rheumatica	?
	Essential cryoglobulinemia	?
Chronic active hepatitis	Sjögren's syndrome	30%–40%
	Peripheral arthritis/arthralgias	30%–40%
	Other autoimmune diseases	?
Primary biliary cirrhosis	Scleroderma	15%–20%
Cryptogenic cirrhosis	Sjögren's syndrome	70%
	Peripheral arthritis/arthralgias	30%
Intestinal bypass surgery	Peripheral arthritis/arthralgias[b]	5%–25%
	Spondylitis	0.3%
	Neuromyopathy	Up to 25%
Ulcerative colitis	Peripheral arthritis/arthralgias[a]	10%–25%
	Spondylitis	2%–4%
	Osteoporosis/osteomalacia (?2° to steroid treatment)	3%
Regional enteritis	Peripheral arthritis/arthralgias[a]	10%–20%
	Spondylitis	4%
Whipple's disease	Peripheral arthritis/arthralgias	65%–90%
	Spondylitis	20%
	Granulomatous myositis	?
Yersinia enteritis	Erythema nodosum[a]	30%–40%
	Peripheral or central arthritis/arthralgias	30%–40%
Shigella or salmonella enteritis	Reiter's syndrome	1%–2%
Pancreatitis, pancreatic cancer, or pseudocyst	Serositis and subcutaneous nodules	?

[a] Rheumatic syndrome improves in parallel with underlying gastroenteropathy.
[b] Arthropathy resolves with reanastomoses of bypassed segment.

and predispose to hemarthrosis. A number of self-inflicted and iatrogenic agents may also contribute to a bloody synovial fluid. Coumadin overdose or coumadin inappropriately combined with antiplatelet drugs (e.g., acetylsalicylic acid) can cause a hemorrhagic synovial effusion. Underlying arthropathies predispose to bleeding in the patient with poorly controlled anticoagulation.

Recurrent monoarticular arthritis and hemarthrosis may be apparent manifestations of hemophilia A or B or pseudohemophilia (von Willebrand's disease). In patients with moderately reduced levels of factor VIII, recurrent hemarthrosis with mild trauma may be the only manifestation of the bleeding disorder. The knees, ankles, and elbows are the joints most commonly ($>85\%$) involved. Initial episodes are characterized by normal radiographic appearance of the affected joint. Evaluation includes a complete blood count, quantitative platelet count, prothrombin time (PT), and partial thromboplastin time (PTT). Bleeding time is normal in factor VIII and IX deficiencies. Specific assay for factor VIII or IX will confirm the diagnosis. Often the level of the factor will predict subsequent bleeding episodes for the patient. Prolonged bleeding time and abnormal platelet aggregation, in response to the antibiotic ristocetin, confirm the diagnosis of von Willebrand's disease. Therapy for the acute hemarthrosis consists of immobilization, elevation, and replacement of the deficient coagulation protein with cryoprecipitate. Arthrocentesis, for diagnostic or therapeutic purposes, may be performed after correction of the hemostatic defect. Recurrent hemorrhagic episodes lead to a proliferative synovitis with crepitation and limitation of movement on physical examination and radiographic osteoporosis in the epiphyses. Further hemarthroses cause subchondral cysts. However, the cartilaginous space may be preserved, and it is at this stage that the hemophilic arthropathy remains reversible. With subsequent hemarthroses, narrowing and destruction of the joint space become apparent with marked fibrous contracture, epiphyseal enlargement, and general disorganization of joint structure. Therapy of the subacute hemarthrosis without dramatic x-ray abnormalities includes 6–8 weeks of physical therapy, sufficient factor replacement three times weekly to raise the patient's plasma level to 20% or 30% of normal, and analgesia. Patients should avoid agents with antiplatelet activity (salicylates and other nonsteroidal anti-inflammatory drugs), and nontraumatic exercise is encouraged (bicycle riding or swimming). Synovectomies of the elbow and knee have been attempted for recurrent monoarticular hemarthrosis with proliferative synovitis. Careful coordination of the surgical and hemostatic laboratories is mandatory for a satisfactory result in hemophilia arthropathy. For more advanced disease, osteotomies are occasionally required for patients with significant flexion contracture especially of the knee. Total knee or total hip replacement has been successful in carefully selected patients.

Laboratory assessment of hemostatic deficiency may uncover abnormalities not apparent clinically. In SLE a prolonged PTT is noted in the absence of a hemorrhagic diathesis. The lupus anticoagulant appears to be an inhibitor that acts on the prothrombin activator complex. This entity is not unique to SLE and may occur with a number of diverse neoplastic, immunologic, and hematologic entities. The lupus anticoagulant is often associated with a positive Coombs' test in the SLE patient. The vast majority of the lupus anticoagulants in idiopathic SLE are discovered by an abnormal screening coagulation profile; bleeding disorders in the lupus patient are often a manifestation of uremia, thrombocytopenia, circulating anticoagulant, or a combination of these abnormalities. A peculiar and paradoxic observation in SLE is the association of thrombotic episodes with the presence of the lupus anticoagulant. The SLE patient with an isolated prolonged PTT will often tolerate biopsy, minor surgery, or major surgery without adverse effects in a carefully controlled environment.

Purpura and Platelet Abnormalities

Thrombotic episodes often accompany idiopathic thrombocythemia, thrombocythemia associated with myeloproliferative disorders, or thrombotic thrombocytopenic purpura (TTP). A significant number of persons with thrombotic thrombocytopenic purpura will manifest arthralgias and myalgias. Many diseases have been reported and associated with TTP. These have included infectious as well as rheumatic (SLE, Sjögren's syndrome, and polyarteritis nodosa) diseases. Rheumatic symptoms are uncommon manifestations of idiopathic thrombocytopenic purpura (ITP). The course of ITP varies with age of onset. Over 75% of children will recover in 4–6 weeks, with an extremely low mortality. The response is less predictable in adults, and corticosteroids are often required to achieve remission. Occasionally, splenectomy will be required in those persons unresponsive to steroids or incapacitated by steroid side effects. The thrombocytopenia of SLE also often responds to corticosteroids. The role of splenectomy is not well established in SLE.

Hemoglobinopathies

Arthropathy associated with hemoglobinopathies is most prevalent with homozygous S hemoglobin, with sporadic reports of SC and S-thalassemia-related arthropathies. Articular warmth and swelling are usually part of the overall picture of sickle cell crisis associated with fever, anemia, and abdominal pain. The arthropathy is usually migratory but may persist in the hands and feet; this sickle cell dactylitis, prominent in children, is often referred to as the *hand-foot syndrome*. Synovial fluid analysis has demonstrated noninflammatory effusions with white blood counts below 5,000/mm³ and mononuclear cell predominance.

HEAVY METAL AND LIPID STORAGE DISEASE

Hemochromatosis

Patients with hemochromatosis develop excessive iron stores. Over 50% of them have an arthropathy (most common among patients who first present after age 50), which is secondary to CPPD crystal deposition disease. It characteristically involves the second and third metacarpals and may also involve knees, wrists, hips and spine. A role for iron in producing the arthropathy has been postulated.

Copper Storage Disease (Wilson's Disease)

Patients with copper storage disease do not handle copper normally and develop abnormalities in the liver and basal ganglia and renal tubular defects secondary to excessive stores of the metal. Arthralgias are present in over 25% of patients and bone deformities (mostly asymptomatic) in 10%. Osteomalacia, osteoporosis, and rickets have been described and are probably secondary to the Fanconi syndrome present in these patients. Degenerative changes of the joint and periarticular structures and chondrocalcinosis have been reported. Patients treated with *d*-penicillamine can develop a lupus-like syndrome.

Lipid Storage Disease

The two most frequently noted presentations of adult Gaucher's disease are asymptomatic splenomegaly and recurrent articular complaints. Infiltration of the bone with the lipid-laden Gaucher cells increases the chance of vascular compromise,

Table23.3. Rheumatic Syndromes Associated with Pulmonary Manifestations

Systemic Rheumatic Disease (Frequency of Involvement)	Clinical/Radiographic Appearance	Associated Findings	Course/Management
Systemic lupus erythematosus (50%–70%)	Pleuritis[a] (± effusion), basilar atelectasis, diffuse interstitial disease, acute lupus pneumonitis	Exudative pleural effusions with low glucose and complement; intrinsic restrictive ventilatory defect	Superinfection must be excluded; most pleuropneumonic manifestations are steroid responsive
Rheumatoid arthritis (50%–70%)	Pleuritis[a] (± effusion), necrobiotic nodules, Caplan's syndrome, diffuse interstitial disease, pulmonary arteritis with pulmonary hypertension	Exudative pleural effusions with low glucose and complement; intrinsic restrictive ventilatory defect	Unpredictable response to therapy for articular problems
Progressive systemic sclerosis (70%–90%)	Basilar interstitial infiltrates,[a] aspiration pneumonitis, pulmonary hypertension, alveolar cell carcinoma	Intrinsic restrictive ventilatory defect, reduced diffusing capacity[a] often in the absence of radiographic features	Suspect aspiration; no proven therapy
Polydermatomyositis (10%)	Basilar interstitial infiltrates,[a] aspiration pneumonitis	Hypoventilation and intrinsic restrictive ventilatory defect	Hypoventilation and/or aspiration are ominous prognostic signs; respiratory deterioration can often be prevented by steroid treatment
Mixed connective tissue disease (40%–60%)	Interstitial infiltrates, pleuritis, aspiration pneumonitis	Reduced diffusing capacity, high-titer antibody to RNP	Appears steroid responsive
Sjögren's syndrome (10%–15%)	50%–60% of Sjögren's patients manifest stigmata of a systemic rheumatic disease; pleuritis,[a] interstitial infiltrates, occasional evolution to poorly differentiated lymphoma	May have small airway obstructive defects, fibrosing alveolitis	May be steroid responsive
Wegener's granulomatosis (90%–100%)	Sinus, pulmonary, and renal involvement; variable findings on chest x-ray	Necrotizing arteritis of upper and lower airway with granuloma; necrotizing glomerulitis	Cytoxan responsive

Allergic angiitis of Churg and Strauss (c. 25%)	CNS, pulmonary, sinus, dermal, and cardiac involvement; clinical asthma	Necrotizing angiitis with eosinophilia and granuloma formation; peripheral eosinophilia	? Steroid responsive
Polyarteritis nodosa (classic) (rare)	Visceral involvement, often sparing lungs; often involves muscle, testes, peripheral nerves	Necrotizing arteritis of medium-sized vessels; microaneurysms often demonstrable on visceral angiography	Steroids and/or immunosuppressives variably alter course
Pulmonary hemorrhage and glomerulonephritis (100%)	Hemoptysis and nephritis with diffuse alveolar hemorrhage	Circulating antibody to alveolar and glomerular basement membrane	Immunosuppression variably alters course
Relapsing polychondritis (55%–60%)	Auricular chondritis, nonerosive polyarthritis, tracheal chondritis, ocular inflammation	Biopsy of cartilage from ear, nose, or respiratory tract confirms diagnosis	? Steroid responsive
Behçet's disease (rare)	Oral and genital ulceration, iritis	Vasculitis and thrombosis of vessels may be noted on biopsy	Natural course and therapy are unclear
Sarcoidosis (90%)	Cough, dyspnea, polyarthritis, hilar adenopathy, interstitial pulmonary infiltrates	Noncaseating granulomata demonstrable in lymph node and pulmonary tissue	Course ameliorated with steroids
Lofgren's syndrome (rare)	Hilar adenopathy, erythema nodosum, painful nondeforming arthritis of ankles and knees	Pulmonary function studies usually normal	90% spontaneously resolve
Hypertrophic osteoarthropathy (common)	Proliferative periostitis in distal tibia, fibula, radius, and ulna; often associated with digital clubbing	Search for bronchogenic carcinoma	Symptoms improve with resection of malignancy

a More frequent manifestations.

traumatic damage, and impaired repair. Severe destructive changes resembling avascular necrosis may occur in the shoulder, hips, or knees. These articular manifestations begin in the third decade and may progress to severe degenerative changes by age 40 or 50. Characteristic radiographic features in the younger person include the "Erhlenmeyer flask deformity" of the distal femur. Radiographic features in the adult resemble those of severe and destructive degenerative changes. An elevated acid phosphatase level is a common feature of adult Gaucher's disease; however, a normal acid phosphatase value by no means excludes severe bony infiltration with the Gaucher's cells. Enzymatic replacement therapy appears theoretically feasible; however, conservative therapy with analgesics, physical therapy, and reconstructive surgery, when mandatory, constitute standard therapy at this time. Use of anti-inflammatory drugs with strong anti-platelet properties is discouraged in Gaucher's disease.

PULMONARY MANIFESTATIONS OF RHEUMATIC DISEASES

Several diseases that dramatically affect the lungs may have rheumatic manifestations—e.g., Goodpasture's syndrome, relapsing polychondritis, hypersensitivity pneumonitis, the hypereosinophilic syndromes, and the immunodeficiency diseases. Pulmonary complications of rheumatic diseases may be variable or stereotyped. Basilar interstitial fibrosis with intrinsic restrictive ventilatory defects are relatively common manifestations of RA, SLE, PSS, and mixed connective tissue disease. Apical interstitial fibrosis with fibronodular changes is a peculiar manifestation of ankylosing spondylitis.

The pulmonary manifestations of rheumatic disease may be subtle and detectable by pulmonary function testing long before clinical or radiographic disease appears (e.g., PSS). Other immunologic diseases may produce manifestations that vary significantly from day to day (e.g., hypereosinophilic syndromes and vasculitic syndromes); a precise radiographic description of these entities is therefore limited. The pulmonary associations of the various rheumatic syndromes are compared in Table 23.3.

OCULAR MANIFESTATIONS OF RHEUMATIC DISEASES

Ocular manifestations of connective tissue diseases are not always readily apparent. Pain, photophobia, foreign body sensation, subtle visual loss, and excess or decreased tearing are often overlooked. Certain ocular manifestations complicating rheumatic diseases may be iatrogenic (e.g., steroid-induced lenticular opacities) or may represent retinovascular complications of systemic vasculitis or severe systemic hypertension (e.g., SLE, polyarteritis, or PSS). Table 23.4 summarizes the ocular manifestations of rheumatic diseases.

INHERITED CONNECTIVE TISSUE DISEASES

The inherited connective tissue diseases may appear with a stereotyped musculoskeletal complaint. These complaints will, however, vary with the inherited defi-

Table 23.4. Ocular Manifestations of Rheumatic Diseases

Rheumatic Disease	Conjunctiva	Cornea/ Sclera	Uveal Tract	Retina	Periorbital Tissues
Arthritides					
Rheumatoid arthritis	+++	++			
Ankylosing spondylitis			+		
Reiter's and Psoriasis	++		++		
Juvenile pauciarticular chronic arthritis			+++		
Systemic rheumatic disease					
Systemic lupus erythematosus	+			+	
Sjögren's syndrome	+++	++			+
Polydermato-myositis			+		
Progressive systemic sclerosis				+^{a}	
Relapsing polychondritis	+		+		
Behçet's syndrome	+	+	+++	+	
Vasculitis					
Giant cell arteritis				+	
Wegener's granulomatosis				+	+
Polyarteritis nodosa				+^{a}	

[a] Hypertensive retinopathy (retina, uvea, cornea, sclera, lens).

ciency and in age of onset, extent, and type of disability. The salient features of the mucopolysaccharidoses are summarized and compared in Table 23.5. The main features of the collagen disorders are listed in Table 23.6.

MISCELLANEOUS RHEUMATIC DISEASES WITH IMMUNOLOGIC FEATURES

This section will review a number of entities with musculoskeletal manifestations and immunologic features. Most are diseases of unknown etiology and poorly understood pathogenesis that do not clearly fit into recognized categories of rheumatic diseases.

Table 23.5. Inherited Disorders of Connective Tissue: The Mucopolysaccharidoses (MPS)

Mucopolysaccharide (MPS) Designation	Onset/Course	Musculoskeletal Abnormalities	CV/Respiratory Abnormalities	HEENT Abnormalities	Urinary MPS
MPS I H Hurler syndrome	Clinically normal infant, severe deterioration by 18–24 months; 10-year survival rare	Loss of motion, short stature, thoracic cage deformity	Coronary pseudo-atheromata, thickened aortic and mitral valves, restrictive pulmonary defect	Coarse facies, corneal clouding, severe mental retardation	Dermatan sulfate Heparan sulfate
MPS I S Scheie syndrome	Progress to normal stature	Loss of motion, "claw hand," pes cavus, carpal tunnel syndrome	Aortic valve disease	Normal mental status, corneal clouding	Dermatan sulfate Heparan sulfate
MPS I H/S Hurler/Scheie	Early skeletal dysostosis, 20-year survival possible	Loss of motion, "claw hand," short stature	Valvular heart deformities, restrictive pulmonary defect	Coarse facies, mental retardation, corneal clouding	Dermatan sulfate Heparan sulfate
MPS II (severe) Hunter syndrome	Neurologic deterioration by 5 years, death at 10–13 years	Loss of motion, short stature, medial and ulnar nerve entrapment		Cornea clear, progressive deafness, coarse facies	Dermatan sulfate, Heparan sulfate
MPS II (mild) Hunter syndrome	Normal to minimal retardation, may survive to age 50–60	Loss of motion, short stature, nerve entrapment		Cornea clear, coarse facies	Dermatan sulfate, Heparan sulfate
MPS III A Sanfilippo syndrome A	Retardation and CNS deterioration apparent at 36–48 months	Moderately shortened stature and mild skeletal dysostosis	Mitral valve abnormalities	Cornea clear	Heparan sulfate
MPS III B Sanfilippo syndrome B	CNS deterioration noted at 6–8 years; may survive to third decade	Mild loss of motion, mild dysostosis	Valvular abnormalities	Cornea clear	Heparan sulfate

MPS IV Morquio syndrome	Growth abnormalities apparent at 24 months; may survive to sixth decade	Excessive joint motion, odontoid hypoplasia, short trunk	Severe restrictive pulmonary defect, aortic valve abnormality	Progressive deafness, mild corneal clouding	Keratan sulfate
MPS VI Maroteaux-Lamy	Growth retardation by 24–36 months; survival varies from 15–35 years	Mild to severe loss of motion, odontoid hypoplasia, short stature, nerve entrapment	Valvular abnormalities	Normal intelligence, corneal clouding	Dermatan sulfate
MPS VII Beta-glucuronidase deficiency	Variable	Variable, mild skeletal dysostosis		Coarse facies	Dermatan sulfate, Heparan sulfate

immune mechanisms, the cartilage lesions may result from either inherent abnormalities, biosynthetic defects, proteolysis of mucopolysaccharides, or vasculitis localized to tissues high in glycosaminoglycan content.

Immunodeficiency Diseases

Immunodeficiency diseases are discussed at length elsewhere in this volume (Chaps. 6–9). Interestingly, humoral immunodeficiencies are associated with systemic rheumatic diseases. Selective IgA deficiency is associated with adult and juvenile RA, SLE, vasculitis, Sjögren's syndrome, dermatomyositis, "lupoid" hepatitis, hemolytic anemia, thyroiditis, pernicious anemia, sarcoidosis, and inflammatory bowel disease. Cellular immunity in these patients is either normal or comparable to that seen in other patients with similar disorders. Impaired secretory immunity may possibly permit the invasion of foreign antigens, leading to the development of autoimmune diseases.

Rheumatoid-like arthritis occurs in up to one-third of hypogammaglobulinemic patients. Others develop SLE, PSS, or dermatomyositis. Studies of patients with hypogammaglobulinemia and RA identified C3, C3A, and properdin in synovium and synovial vessel walls and depressed synovial fluid C3. These observations suggest that the alternative complement system may mediate humoral immune events in these patients.

Pigmented Villonodular Synovitis

Pimented villonodular synovitis is an uncommon disease of young adults that affects the knee and, rarely, other joints and is characterized by sanguinous effusion. Unless roentgenograms or arthrography identify lobulated synovium with filling defects and joint destruction, diagnosis is made by biopsy. Histologic examination shows brownish discoloration, pedunculated hypertrophied villae containing connective tissue, pigmented giant cells, and round cells. Viral-like inclusions have implied a possible infectious cause. In another patient, Ig-containing synovial cells were identified and lymphocytes were unresponsive to phytohemagglutinin. This finding was interpreted as suggesting that immunologic events were associated with this illness.

Malignancies and Rheumatic Diseases

The occurrence of malignancies in patients with rheumatic diseases (not being treated with immunosuppressive drugs) has been described. Patients with SLE develop lymphoma, an illness like that in New Zealand black and white hybrid mice, leukemia, multiple myeloma, reticulum cell sarcoma, and others. Patients with RA may acquire plasma cell dyscrasias, heavy chain disease, and lymphoma. Patients with polydermatomyositis may have associated tumors. Patients with PSS have developed alveolar cell carcinomas. Additional tumors, usually reticuloendothelial, have been described in patients with RA or SLE who were using immunosuppressive drugs. Combinations of possible viral infection, chronic immunologic stimulation, and either generalized or selective abnormalities of cell-mediated immunity may lead to malignancy in some of these patients.

On the other hand, rheumatic symptoms may be a manifestation of underlying malignancy. Arthritis has occasionally been recognized as the predominant or apparent symptom of childhood leukemia, lymphoproliferative disorder, multiple myeloma, or reticulum cell sarcoma. Cutaneous vasculitis has been associated with lymphoproliferative disease, SLE with lymphoma, and RA and SLE with solid tumors.

Whipple's Disease

Whipple's disease is an uncommon disorder tending to affect white men in the fourth or fifth decade. It is characterized by systemic, gastrointestinal, and articular symptoms. Clinical features include constitutional symptoms (38%–55%), weight loss (95%–100%), diarrhea (72%–78%), abdominal pain (60%–72%), arthralgias/arthritis (65%–90%), adenopathy (52%–55%), splenomegaly (5%–18%), hyperpigmentation, malabsorption, peritonitis, pleuropericarditis, purpura, endocarditis, and neurologic abnormalities.

Laboratory findings are normocytic hypochromic anemia (90%), occasional leukocytosis, decreased vitamin B12 absorption, low folate concentrations, hypoalbuminemia, hypocalcemia, hypocholesterolemia, and steatorrhea (93%). Synovial fluids, when analyzed, showed 6,000–13,000 WBC/cu mm, good mucin clot, and 3.0–4.7 g/100 ml protein. Radiographic changes reveal coarsening of folds, dilatation, or edema of bowel. Joint films may show demineralization or narrowing and fusion of sacroiliac joints. Histologic changes, particularly in the small bowel, have been specific for Whipple's disease. Periodic acid–Schiff (PAS)-positive inclusions have been found within macrophages in most affected tissues, including synovium and mesothelial cells. These particles are thought to be partially digested bacterial components. Efforts to culture organisms or transmit disease to animals have not been uniformly successful. Based on a presumed bacterial etiology, Whipple's disease has been successfully treated with antibiotics.

Comprehensive immunologic studies of this disease have not been performed, but available data indicate abnormalities. Patients occasionally had reduced or elevated IgG, IgA, or IgM levels, often normalizing with treatment. Complement was normal. Skin test reactivity and in vitro lymphocyte responsiveness were reduced and did not consistently return to normal after treatment. Total lymphocyte counts were low before and normal after treatment.

Periodic Diseases

Certain rheumatic syndromes are uniquely characterized by episodic recurrences interspersed with asymptomatic intervals. Intermittent hydroarthrosis consists of recurrent effusions, usually of the knees. It affects more women than men, is of unknown etiology, often begins during adolescence, and occurs at 2- to 4-week intervals with painless effusions lasting 2 to 5 days. Laboratory studies are unremarkable. Evident radiologic changes do not occur. Pathologic changes vary from mild synovitis to changes described with RA. The course is variable and treatment palliative. Serum and synovial fluid complement levels have been normal, but a recent study found depressed serum CH50 and C1 inhibitor in some patients.

Palindromic rheumatism is characterized by recurrent episodes of inflammatory arthritis or tenosynovitis. Intervals, frequency of episodes, and sites of involvement vary. Attacks begin suddenly and generally resolve within 1 week. Transient subcutaneous nodules have been described. Laboratory studies show transient abnormalities consistent with acute inflammation. Roentgenographic findings are also unremarkable. Synovium shows inflammatory changes. The prognosis is good. More than half of patients have recurrent attacks without progression, 10% remit, and the remainder evolve into another recognizable rheumatic disease (RA, SLE, gout, etc.). Various antirheumatic therapies have been used. In one study, patients had increased anti-IgG levels, positive tests for rheumatoid factor, normal C1 esterase inhibitor, and cellular immunity to *Mycoplasma fermentans*—all abnormalities noted by the authors in patients with RA and interpreted as linking palindromic rheumatism with rheumatoid arthritis.

Familial Mediterranean fever is transmitted as an autosomal recessive trait with complete penetrance occurring predominantly in Sephardic Jews, Turks, Armenians, and Arabs. First attacks begin during the first 2 decades of life. They are characterized by acute periodic polyserositis—fever, peritonitis (95%–96%), pleuritis (40%–87%), pericarditis, or arthritis (37%–75%)—that resolves spontaneously over 3 to 7 days. Synovitis usually subsides without deformity. Other findings are rash, adenopathy, and myalgias. Roentgenographic changes are minimal. Acute-phase reactants are increased with attacks. Synovial fluids show 200–1,000,000 WBC/cu mm with a preponderance of neutrophils, good mucin clot, increased protein, and normal glucose. Histologic findings are low-grade acute or subacute inflammation. The duration and frequency of episodes are variable. Colchicine has proved effective in reducing recurrences. Amyloidosis occurs in about one-fourth of patients, usually eventuating in renal death. Some patients have reduced C1 inhibitor or CH50.

BIBLIOGRAPHY

Arkin CR, Masi AT: Relapsing polychondritis: Review of current status and case report. *Semin Arthritis Rheum* 5:41, 1975.

Arnold WD, Hilgartner MW: Hemophilic arthropathy. *J Bone Joint Surg* 59A:287, 1977.

Bland JH, Frymoyer JW, Newberg AH, et al: Rheumatic syndromes in endocrine disease. *Semin Arthritis Rheum* 9:23, 1979.

Byld WE, Matthews OP, Hunt RE: Left atrial myxoma presenting as a systemic vasculitis. *Arthritis Rheum* 23:240, 1980.

Calabro JJ: Cancer and arthritis. *Arthritis Rheum* 10:553, 1967.

Ehrlich GE: Intermittent and periodic rheumatic syndromes. *Bull Rheum Dis* 24:746, 1973–1974.

Golding PL, Smith M, Williams R: Multisystem involvement in chronic liver disease, studies on the incidence and pathogenesis. *Am J Med* 55:772, 1973.

Good RA, Rotstein J: Rheumatoid arthritis and agammaglobulinemia. *Bull Rheum Dis* 10:203, 1960.

Hamilton EBD: The arthritis of hyperparathyroidism, haemochromatosis and Wilson's disease. *Clin Rheum Dis* 1:109, 1975.

Hunninghake GW, Fauci AS: Pulmonary involvement in the collagen vascular diseases. *Am Rev Respir Dis* 119:471, 1979.

Ibels LS, Alfrey AC, Huffer WE, et al: Aseptic necrosis of bone following renal transplantation—experience in 194 transplant recipients and review of the literature. *Medicine* 57:25, 1978.

James DG, Neville E, Carstairs LS: Bone and joint sarcoidosis. *Semin Arthritis Rheum* 6:53, 1976.

Maizel H, Rubbin JM, Dobbins WO: Whipple's disease: A review of 19 patients from one hospital and a review of the literature since 1950. *Medicine* 49:175, 1970.

McCarty DJ, Silcox DC, Coe F, et al: Diseases associated with calcium pyrophosphate dihydrate crystal deposition—a controlled study. *Am J Med* 56:704, 1974.

Mills JA: A spectrum of organ systems that respond to cancer: The joints and connective tissue. *Ann NY Acad Sci* 230:443, 1974.

Pastan RS, Cohen AS: The rheumatologic manifestations of diabetes mellitus. *Med Clin North Am* 62:829, 1978.

Pennock CA: A review of simple laboratory methods used for the study of glycosaminoglycan excretion and the diagnosis of the mucopolysaccharidoses. *J Clin Pathol* 29: 111, 1976.

Tannenbaum H, Anderson LG, Schur PH: Association of polyarthritis, subcutaneous nodules and pancreatic disease. *J Rheumatol* 2:14, 1975.

Watson PG, Hayreh SS: Scleritis and episcleritis. *Br J Ophthal* 60:163, 1976.

Williams MH, Shelden PJHS, Torrigiani G, et al: Palindromic rheumatism: Clinical and immunological studies. *Ann Rheum Dis* 30:375, 1971.

24

Osteoarthritis and Other Degenerative Disorders

Gerald H. Stein

Arthur Mendelow

Osteoarthritis is a common disorder of the joints characterized by degeneration of the articular surfaces of single or multiple joints. It is also referred to as *degenerative joint disease* because of the slowly progressive deterioration of the joint cartilage. Further, it is also called *osteoarthrosis,* mainly by our British colleagues, because inflammation implied by the term *osteoarthritis* is a minimal contributor to the chronic disease process.

This chapter will review the clinical manifestations of the disorder and the current understanding of the etiology. However, discussion will be limited to osteoarthritis of the peripheral joints (see chaps. 29 and 30 for discussion of the arthritic involvement of the spine). Last, selected miscellaneous diseases of the joints will be briefly presented.

PREVALENCE

Autopsy studies indicate that 90% of all persons by age 60 have degenerative changes in the weight-bearing joints, but frequently this condition has been asymptomatic. Likewise, x-ray surveys of hands have shown a high rate of degenerative change that appears to be age related—starting at 4% of persons aged 18–24 years and increasing to 85% of those over 75 years. These studies suggest that at most 25% of those with demonstrable osteoarthritis have moderate or severe disease in terms of pain and disability. In other population surveys, men and women are equally affected by osteoarthritis when all ages are considered. Whereas osteoarthritis of the hands is more common in women, osteoarthritis of the hips is more common in men. Although clinical symptoms appear more prevalent in women, environmental and occupational factors have a greater impact on men. Race frequencies of osteoarthritis, with few exceptions, are not significant.

CLASSIFICATION

Osteoarthritis may be divided according to our understanding of the causes of the disorder. When these causes are unclear, as in most cases, the term *primary* or *idiopathic* osteoarthritis is best applied. When the causes are known, one refers to the arthritic process as *secondary* to the primary cause (see Table 24.1).

Osteoarthritis is most commonly a localized degenerative disorder of one or two large joints. However, a small percentage of patients have a more generalized variety involving the small as well as large joints (also called *Kellgren's syndrome*). More recently, a primary type of osteoarthritis in which inflammation appears to play a greater role has been defined as *erosive* or *inflammatory* osteoarthritis.

A secondary type of osteoarthritis encompasses those disorders in which an antecedent process has led to a secondary degeneration of the joint space. Injuries, accidents, and unusual stresses and strains are obvious direct causes of joint damage that can produce an osteoarthritic process. Harder to document are occcupational factors that may lead to joint damage by incongruity of articular surfaces or instability. An example seen in Florida is that of fruit sorters who spend their working hours continuously lifting oranges and grapefruit with their digits. In persons susceptible to what was thought to be a benign primary idiopathic pro-

Table 24.1. Classification of Osteoarthritis

Primary
  Idiopathic
  Generalized
Secondary
  Inflammatory
    Rheumatoid arthritis
    Septic—infectious
    Erosive
  Traumatic
  Metabolic
    Gout
    Calcium pyrophosphate deposition disease
    Hemochromatosis
    Ochronosis
    Paget's disease
    Acromegaly
    Wilson's disease
    Hyperparathyroidism
    Diabetes mellitus
  Congenital—genetic
    Neuropathic
    Others
      Osteonecrosis
      Hemophilia
      Tumors

cess, the stress of continuous squeezing of fingers produces an accelerated degenerative disease. For those persons with generalized inflammatory arthritis, like rheumatoid arthritis, a secondary degenerative process follows and may accelerate the joint damage, especially when the rheumatoid process is inadequately controlled. The accelerated inflammatory process, as in untreated septic arthritis, also produces an osteoarthritic condition.

Many metabolic causes can induce degenerative joint disease. These causes include the crystalline deposition disorders, such as gout (uric acid), pseudogout, (calcium pyrophosphate), and hemochromatosis. Hemochromatosis is characterized by iron storage problems most commonly involving the liver, skin, and terminally the heart and pancreas, and also may involve the joints, especially the metatarophalangeal joints. Paget's disease, one of pathologically increased turnover of bone, may cause an osteoarthritis due to joint incongruity.

Alkaptonuria, a condition associated with ochronosis, also produces degenerative arthritis. Although the degenerative process characteristically involves the spine with calcification of the intervertebral discs, the large peripheral joints, such as hips, knees, and shoulders, may become involved. Calcification of the menisci in the knees is not uncommon. Neuropathic disorders are thought to result from loss of proprioceptive or pain sensations, secondary to such diseases as syphilis and diabetes. Other degenerative processes are congenital ones, such as dysplasia of cartilage; osteonecrosis; genetic disorders, such as hemophilia with its concomitant bleeding into joints and its deleterious effects on cartilage; and the iatrogenic overuse of intra-articular adrenocorticosteroid therapy. These disorders will be discussed in greater detail toward the end of this chapter.

When clinically assessing a patient with osteoarthritis, one must be alert to some of these causes so that appropriate studies and subsequent forms of treatment may be initiated to impede these secondary degenerative processes.

SYMPTOMS

No matter which type of osteoarthritis is present, certain clinical features—pain, swelling, loss of function, deformity, and instability—are common to all.

Pain in the joint is the most troublesome symptom of osteoarthritis. Initially, the patient may have aching or nagging pain associated only with strenuous use of that extremity. Characteristically, the pain decreases or ends when the joint is not exercised and may be absent when the patient arises in the morning. Pain may increase in intensity during changes of weather, especially in cold, damp conditions. However, as the disease progresses, the pain may persist even during rest and may awaken patients from sleep.

The pain of osteoarthritis is exacerbated when muscles around the joints become involved. If the disease progresses, patients may complain of lost motion in a given joint with or without the pain complex. Generally, in osteoarthritis, morning stiffness lasts no more than a half an hour.

Patients often may have some of the nonspecific findings of osteoarthritis such as crepitation on moving the joint or x-ray changes of osteoarthritis with little or no manifestation of pain when the joint is examined or used.

SIGNS

In the examination of patients with osteoarthritis, the earliest detectable sign may be crepitation, which is a sensation of crackling or grating felt by the examiner as a joint is moved. This sensation results from alterations in the joint surface. Crepitus is more likely to be detected in the larger joints than in the smaller ones of the hands or feet. Palpating involved joints may reveal bony overgrowths, which are characteristically asymmetric. They occur at the edge of the articular cartilage and at the attachment of the joint capsule.

Sites of Involvement

One must differentiate between the osteoarthritis occurring in large weight-bearing joints (often in only one joint) and the osteoarthritis in multiple small joints, such as in the hands.

Hands

Idiopathic enlargement of the distal interphalangeal joints of the fingers is called *Heberden's nodes*. These nodules are cartilaginous and bony overgrowths at the joint margins. Similar processes occur in the proximal interphalangeal joints and are called *Bouchard's nodes*. This idiopathic type of small joint osteoarthritis is often associated with marked deformities, with medial deviation or instability, or both, of the distal or proximal phalanx. This process is frequently familial, with a higher prevalence in women. The specific genetic pattern has not yet been defined.

This degenerative process often begins gradually, with no symptoms, in the middle years. Many times, deformities will develop before any pain, and patients will complain of functional impairments. Relative sparing of the metacarpophalangeal joints is noted. Similarly, most wrist bones are spared in this process, but arthritis of the first carpometacarpal joint may cause a great deal of pain and discomfort and will interfere with common household tasks. Tenderness localized at the base of the first metacarpal bone may indicate damage of this joint.

A less common variant of osteoarthritis of the hands is the inflammatory form. This process characteristically affects middle-aged women, who appear with painfully enlarged distal or proximal, or both, interphalangeal joints of the hands. This disease may run a course of weeks or months or may cycle recurrently. Although the radiologic changes are characteristic of osteoarthritis, the additional finding of bony erosion in the para-articular area helps to distinguish this condition. The rheumatoid factor in these patients is characteristically negative, and they may have a mild elevation in the sedimentation rate.

Hip

Osteoarthritis often involves the hip joints and causes distressing pain and disability, at times bringing the patient to the clinician early in the course of the disease. This disorder assumes special significance for diagnostic purposes, since recently evolved surgical intervention offers impressive improvement for what previously was a bleak situation. At the hip joints the disease is often bilateral, and radiologic findings may correlate better with the clinical symptoms. Further, those patients with advanced x-ray findings tend to have the greatest amount of pain or disability. This condition appears, by radiologic examination, to be age related, and the incidence increases from 1% in those under 55 years to 10% in those over 85.

Osteoarthritis in adult life may be secondary to a preexisting primary process, such as osteochondritis, aseptic necrosis, or injury, in as many as 50% of patients with this problem.

Pain distribution in hip arthritis may vary widely from the low back to the gluteal areas or the thigh. One needs to recall that the pain may be referred to the knee joint; hence knee joint pain requires hip evaluation. Examination shows a decreased range of motion with tenderness. Ultimately, shortening of the extremity may occur.

Knees

The apparent problem in osteoarthritis of the knee is pain on walking or instability with deformity. The joints may be intermittently swollen because of an effusion, although synovitis with palpable synovium is generally minimal. Crepitation is also present. With disuse, quadriceps muscle atrophies; obesity may accelerate instability of the collateral ligaments, producing a valgus (leg turned laterally) or varus (leg turned inward) deformity.

Age-related degeneration of the menisci of the knee may lead to advancing destruction of the joint, with locking or giving way of the knee and localized tenderness.

Chondromalacia patellae may be thought of as a form of osteoarthritis that afflicts younger persons. In this disorder, there may be degeneration of the patellar cartilage as it articulates with the femur. Newer studies suggest that the condition may be a congenital malalignment of the patella on the femur, which leads to incongruities in the weight-bearing surfaces with pressure effects on the patello-femoral surfaces.

Feet

Osteoarthritis of the foot usually is manifested as bunion deformity (hallux valgus), which is subluxation of the great toe metatarsophalangeal joint with lateral deviation and instability of the great toe. Patients may complain that they have severe pain when walking. Less commonly, hammertoes, which may be secondary to inflammatory arthritis, mechanical problems (such as poorly fitted shoes), or heritable traits, cause a subluxation generally of all the metatarsal/phalangeal joints and result in thick callus formation along the plantar surface of the foot. The pain in this syndrome may be severely disabling when walking.

PROGNOSIS

The long-term outlook is generally variable and unpredictable. However, a few trends may be noted. The hip disease, once started, tends to progress inexorably to severe disability if untreated, whereas digital osteoarthritis will manifest advancing deformities with minimal restrictions in use. Nonetheless, patients need to be assured that the risk of significant disability and crippling of osteoarthritis is less than that of rheumatoid arthritis and that surgical treatment is more likely to be effective.

DIFFERENTIAL DIAGNOSIS

The apparent signs and symptoms of osteoarthritis can confuse the observer because many arthritic conditions have in common the pain and limitation of motion. Further, many causes of arthritis produce a secondary degenerative process, compounding the separation of the primary from the secondary causes. Table 24.2 shows the major differences between rheumatoid arthritis and osteoarthritis. The spondylarthritides, such as psoriatic arthritis and Reiter's syndrome, may be confused with osteoarthritis because both groups may involve the distal interphalangeal joints. The associated clinical aspects of the spondylarthritides usually allow one to clarify the diagnosis. Infection (septic arthritis) is important, since failure to recognize this cause will indeed lead to a destroyed joint. Last, the presence of an effusion may suggest gout or pseudogout which have a different course and treatment; these can be rapidly excluded by a careful analysis of the synovial fluid (see Chap. 3).

Table 24.2. Clinical Features of Osteoarthritis and Rheumatoid Arthritis

Features	Osteoarthritis	Rheumatoid Arthritis
Age	Elderly	Variable
Sex ratio	Equivalent	Female predominant
Onset	Gradual	Variable
Pain	With use	With use and rest
Morning stiffness	Brief	Prolonged
Hands	Bony overgrowth, Herberden's and Bouchard's nodes	Ulnar drift Swan-neck deformities Boutonniere deformities
Hips	End stage: nonspecific degeneration	End stage: protrusion of acetabulum
Knees	Asymmetric degeneration of each joint, varus deformity	Symmetric joint compartment involvement, valgus deformity
Feet	Bunion: mortise ankle joint	Bunion: metatarsal and phalangeal subluxation with calluses, subtalar ankle involvement
Swelling of joints	May be absent	Always present
Deformities	Variable	Specific
Sedimentation rate	Normal	Elevated
Rheumatoid factor	Negative	Positive
Synovial fluid	Noninflammatory	Inflammatory
X-rays	Loss of cartilage, bony sclerosis, and osteophytes	Osteoporosis, erosions, cartilage loss

LABORATORY AND X-RAY FINDINGS

Laboratory tests are not helpful in diagnosing osteoarthritis except as they relate to the exclusion of secondary causes of this disorder. The complete blood count, routine blood chemistry, and erythrocyte sedimentation rate are normal. Similarly, synovial fluid examination, which should be done in the initial evaluation of all patients who have significant effusion in accessible joints, is helpful because this examination can exclude important pertinent secondary causes. The synovial fluid in osteoarthritis is a noninflammatory type with good viscosity and mucin clot and low white cell counts (generally less than 5,000/mm^3). The presence or absence of fibrils in the synovial fluid is of little diagnostic significance.

The characteristic x-ray appearances are more fully described in Chapter 4 and include narrowing of the joint, reactive subchondral bony sclerosis, marginal osteophyte formation, bone cysts, and loose bodies. Deformity with subluxation and instability occurs in more advanced situations.

MANAGEMENT

No curative treatment exists for established osteoarthritis. Successful intervention is designed to allow the patient to be more comfortable and to prevent or retard progression of the disease. Treatment can best be considered by three aspects: (1) a basic program applicable to virtually all patients with chronic arthritis, (2) use of anti-inflammatory and analgesic medication, and (3) the judicious timing and application of surgery (Table 24.3).

Basic Program

Although adequate rest combined with appropriate exercise is accepted as essential in managing any patient with a chronic arthritis, there is no scientific way

Table 24.3. Management of Osteoarthritis

Conservative
Rest
Avoidance of trauma or abnormal use of affected joints
Weight reduction for lower extremity involvement in obese patients
Physical therapy
Orthopedic appliances
Vocational and family alterations
Medical
Anti-inflammatory agents
Aspirin
Nonsteroidal anti-inflammatory agents
Analgesic agents
Intra-articular corticosteroids
Surgical
Osteotomy
Joint replacement

to gauge the degree of rest or activity for a specific person with a given arthritic problem. General guidelines imply that the painful joint needs to be rested after it has been put through an adequate range-of-motion program together with muscle-strengthening exercises on a regular daily basis. In some cases, patients are unaware that they are overstressing the affected joint, and simple counseling about everyday use of the involved site can be extremely helpful. It is impossible to specify the number of minutes of rest for a diseased joint or the number of repetitions in an exercise regimen. Persons who are stoic or deny the degree of discomfort may inadvertently damage the joints by excessive use. Consequently, all patients who have advanced signs or symptoms of osteoarthritis should avoid stressful use of the affected joint.

Weight reduction is deemed appropriate for obese patients with lower extremity involvement. Although experimental and clinical evidence of obesity as a specific factor in the induction or aggravation of degenerative arthritis is not firmly established, most clinicians believe it prudent to reduce to an ideal weight in all cases.

A clear understanding of the specific employment tasks of a patient may uncover stressful physical factors that can readily be improved. However, if insurmountable problems seem apparent, consultations with vocational counselors are frequently of help.

Similarly, the family situation may improve or worsen the pain and disability of an osteoarthritic patient. Inappropriate attention may reinforce pain behaviors and lead to further disability out of proportion to the evident damage in the joint. The guidelines for specific family therapy are beyond the scope of this chapter, but the clinician should look for family problems that could be contributing to the disability of the patient.

Recent studies have indicated that the major continuing crisis facing patients with unremitting arthritis is the loss of income because of inability to work. It is sometimes successful to combine community resources of various allied health professionals with the team approach of physicians and surgeons working in consort to assist in the patient's management. These general supportive measures, as well as other environmental manipulations to accommodate the disabilities, offer the best chance for helping these patients cope with their day-to-day problems.

Of obvious value is the judicious use of canes, crutches, hand-gripping appliances, braces, and other aids, to assist or stabilize damaged joints mechanically.

Medications

In considering drug treatment in osteoarthritis, one should not rely on medication alone for its palliative effects. The basic program discussed in the previous section may obviate the need for drugs, which decreases the expense of treatment and virtually eliminates the side effects of medication. Most of the medications used in treating patients with osteoarthritis have evolved empirically, that is, through studies to evaluate the effectiveness of the drug in reducing pain and stiffness. The disease process, however, remains basically unaltered by such therapeutic interventions; hence no one drug or group of drugs has proved to be consistently beneficial in retarding the pathologic changes of osteoarthritis. Medications can be considered palliative in the management of arthritis.

Aspirin

Acetylsalicylic acid, aspirin, is a basic form of drug therapy for patients with primary osteoarthritis. One uses this medication in a fashion similar to that used for rheumatoid arthritis, aiming for a blood value at the lower end of the therapeutic range, that is, $\sim$ 15–20 mg salicylate per 100 ml serum. This value is generally achieved by beginning with 650 mg of aspirin four times a day in divided doses, generally at mealtimes and in the evening with a snack. Since aspirin requires 4–6 days to obtain a plateau of blood levels, alterations in doses should not be made until after the first week of the initial dose. Thereafter, the dose can be increased or decreased, depending on the balance between lack of therapeutic effect and troublesome side effects. Patients should be warned about gastrointestinal complaints and tinnitus. Hence, in the absence of a therapeutic effect, one may increase the dose weekly by 650 mg/day, generally not to exceed 5,120 mg/day (equivalent to 16 5-grain aspirin tablets). Those persons who suffer the troublesome gastrointestinal side effects of aspirin may be unable to achieve a successful therapeutic response and should supplement their aspirin regimen with full therapeutic doses of antacids or use one of the buffered aspirin preparations.

More recently, salicylic acid compounds with the acetyl moiety substituted by chlorine or magnesium or both have demonstrated efficacy in the management of chronic arthritic disorders and at the same time have lessened gastrointestinal blood loss and dyspeptic symptoms.

The theoretic considerations for using aspirin are based on both its anti-inflammatory and its analgesic properties, as will be described more fully later in this chapter. The inflammatory components of osteoarthritis are minimal in the pathophysiologic mechanisms initiating the disorder and in the gross pathologic specimens seen at the time of surgery. Hence, the anti-inflammatory suppression by aspirin may not be its principal mode of alleviating pain in such persons.

Nonsteroidal Anti-Inflammatory Agents

The basis for using nonsteroidal anti-inflammatory agents is similar to that for using aspirin, namely, their anti-inflammatory and analgesic properties. Although there is some divergence of opinion, most rheumatologists in U.S. medical centers still believe that aspirin continues to be the basic starting agent because of similar efficacy and significantly lower cost. Nonetheless, there is a class of patients, not readily identifiable, that does not appear to respond to aspirin but may respond to a nonsteroidal anti-inflammatory agent. Side effects from aspirin also may preclude its continuation in these patients, and they become candidates for treatment with nonsteroidal anti-inflammatory agents.

It is difficult to know which anti-inflammatory agents other than aspirin to start with, especially since no adequate comparative study exists to allow one to make a rational choice. Clinicians probably have the greatest cumulative experience with indomethacin because it is one of the earliest and safest agents introduced by studies reporting efficacy in osteoarthritis. Nonetheless, well-designed studies showed no advantage of indomethacin over adequate doses of aspirin. Indomethacin remains ulcerogenic but has a low incidence of associated blood dyscrasias. Phenylbutazone (Butazolidin) is probably as efficacious as indomethacin in the management of osteoarthritis, but it is rarely used by rheuma-

Table 24.4. Medications Used in the Treatment of Osteoarthritis

Name		Usually Effective Dosage	Principal Side Effects	Half-life
Generic	*Proprietary*			
Anti-inflammatory agents				
Acetylsalicylic acid	Many others	0.65–1.3 g qid	GI irritation, bleeding, anemia, tinnitus	4.7 hr, but increases in proportion to serum salicylate level
Choline salicylate	Arthropan	0.87–1.75 g qid	GI irritation, salicylism in large doses	—
Choline magnesium trisalicylate	Trilisate	1 g bid	Nausea, dyspepsia, heartburn	Almost 12 hr
Nonsteroidal anti-inflammatory agents				
Fenoprofen Calcium	Nalfon	300–900 mg qid 1,600 mg/day	GI irritation, bleeding, pruritis, constipation, tinnitus, blurred vision,	3 hr
Ibuprofen	Motrin	400–600 mg tid 900–1,200 mg/day	GI irritation, bleeding, blurred vision, possible liver toxicity	2 hr
Indomethacin	Indocin	25–50 mg tid 50–75 mg/day	GI irritation, headache, dizziness—psychic disturbances	6–8 hr
Sulindac	Clinoril	150 mg bid	GI irritation, bleeding, blurred vision, headache, dizziness, and rash	16 hr (active sulfide metabolite)
Analgesic agents				
Propoxyphene	Darvon	65 g qid	Dizziness, nausea, vomiting	—
Acetaminophen	Tylenol, others	650 mg qid	Rare hypersensitivity	—
Intra-articular steroids				
Methylprednisolone	Depo-Medrol	20–40 mg with lidocaine	Local: increasing pain and rare infection	—
Triamcinolone hexacetonide	Aristospan	10–40 mg with lidocaine	Local: increasing pain and rare infection	—

Table 24.5. Comparison of Other Therapeutic Agents with Aspirin in Treatment of Osteoarthritis

Agent	Comparison with Aspirin	Comments
Acetylsalicylic acid	—	Tinnitus defines limit of tolerance; least expensive
Choline salicylate	More rapidly absorbed, decreased GI toxicity	In liquid form, may be mixed with fruit juice
Choline magnesium trisalicylate	Milder side effects, longer acting	—
Fenoprofen calcium	Aspirin increases excretion of fenoprofen, fewer GI complaints	Food decreases absorption; give ½ hr before or 2 hr after meals; get periodic renal function tests
Ibuprofen	Aspirin reduces ibuprofen blood levels; fewer GI complaints with ibuprofen	—
Indomethacin	—	Interferes with probenecid (Benemid)
Sulindac	—	Inhibitor of platelet function
Propoxyphene	—	May cause seizure in chronic abusers
Acetaminophen	—	May cause hepatotoxicity
Methylprednisolone	—	May cause increased joint destruction
Triamcinolone hexacetonide	—	May cause increased joint destruction

tologists in most arthritis centers because it has a high incidence of side effects with chronic use. Much interest has been shown in the recently released nonsteroidal anti-inflammatory agents. Some of these drugs have been specifically studied in patients with osteoarthritis; others have not. Nonetheless, these drugs all have the same advantages and disadvantages in the degenerative disorders. Tables 24.4 and 24.5 as well as Table 10.6 describe these agents.

Corticosteroids

The use of systemic corticosteroids is discouraged in the management of localized or generalized osteoarthritis. The risks of side effects from chronic administration far exceed the potential benefits in these minimally inflammatory degenerative disorders. Nonetheless, there is a distinct role for intra-articular injections of corticosteroids when administered judiciously. It is generally recommended that the maximum number of intra-articular injections per joint per years be three to four to avoid the deleterious effects of excessive use of corticosteroids on joint structure. Tables 24.4 and 24.5 list various aspects of their use.

Analgesic Agents

Standard analgesic agents often are as effective as the anti-inflammatory agents in alleviating the pain of osteoarthritis. The drug of first consideration is acetaminophen. This agent suppresses pain reasonably well and has minimal accompanying side effects. The usual regimen is 640 mg in divided doses three or four times a day at the maximum. Patients with underlying liver disorders are susceptible to hepatic toxicity. Propoxyphene (Darvon) may be slightly more potent than acetaminophen on a per tablet basis (acetaminophen, 640 mg versus propoxyphene hydrochloride, 65 mg), but conclusions on comparative degrees of analgesia are far from complete. The hazards of propoxyphene abuse include habituation and seizure disorder from abrupt discontinuation when excessive amounts have been taken. An occasional patient may require codeine for control of pain.

Surgery

The progression of osteoarthritis produces mechanical changes in the joint surfaces that no medication available currently or in the near future could reverse. Hence, it is exceedingly important to consider advanced degenerative arthritis as a disorder to be managed surgically. Surgery may be performed for several reasons: to maintain or increase joint mobility or stability, or both; to relieve pain; or to correct deformities.

The different types of surgery are as follows. (1) Osteotomy is a realignment of the bones near the articular nondegenerative cartilage surface of the joint to allow contact between uninvolved surfaces. This procedure permits transmission of forces through normal cartilage rather than through the diseased cartilage. (2) Arthroplasty is a resurfacing of the joint cartilage, generally with prosthetic devices such as a metallic cup (an older operation) or, more recently, by the use of low-friction arthroplasty, which is a total joint replacement. (3) Arthrodesis means fusion of the joint, a decision not lightly taken except in severe cases. (4) Finally, flail joint is resection of the articular bones of the joint. Although use of that joint is limited, the patient is free of pain.

The most beneficial reconstructive surgical procedure is total joint replacement of the hip or knees, but a skilled surgeon may be able to improve the status of any joint damaged by osteoarthritis. The clinician should freely consult qualified surgeons so that a cooperative plan can be selectively applied to optimize restoration of patients to their fullest functional capabilities.

Research Aspects of Patient Management

Many frontiers currently are being explored for the treatment of osteoarthritis. Two major areas are the development of more potent medical measures and newer surgical devices and techniques. Regarding the former, investigators are actively seeking inhibitors of cartilage destruction in the hope that such chemicals could be administered orally or injected into joints to inhibit or nullify the effects of destructive enzymes. Newer surgical investigations include the experimental application of Bioglass, a silicon polymeric coating that permits a more perfect union of the foreign metallic substance with surrounding bone. This substance is an improvement because methylmethacrylate cement currently used in total joint replacement causes necrosis of the surrounding bone. Last, selective applications of electric current are being studied to stimulate bone and cartilage regeneration.

Articular Bone Transplantation

Attempts at transplantation of cartilage from one person to another have not been successful (in this country). Allogeneic grafting has a high rate of failure in spite of the appropriate use of immunosuppressive agents. It has been recently demonstrated that chondrocytes contain major histocompatibility antigens as well as their own unique surface antigens. The role these histocompatibility antigens play in graft acceptance and rejection is poorly understood; nonetheless, hope remains that transplantation may be effective, since it is known that the matrix offers an effective barrier to the destructive immune responses.

BASIC ASPECTS OF JOINTS

Normal Articular Cartilage

Cartilage is a specialized tissue that has the main purpose of acting as a bearing surface for movable joints. The cartilage covering the ends of diarthrodial joints is specialized connective tissue that permits joint motion because of its anatomic, biochemical, and physical characteristics.

The major weight of cartilage is made of the extracellular connective tissue called *matrix*. Interspersed in the matrix are the cellular component chondrocytes. Significantly absent are vascular, neural, and lymphatic channels. Nutrients must therefore pass through a diffusion process to nourish the chondrocytes; more specifically, substances must diffuse across the synovial membrane into synovial fluid and then across the matrix of articular cartilage to reach the chondrocyte cell membrane. The lower one-third of articular cartilage receives nutrition by diffusion from the underlying bone.

We are beginning to understand the role of the chondrocyte in maintaining normal cartilage. The cell density is low compared with other body tissues. Although the histologic appearance suggests that these cells are inactive, recent studies have disclosed that the cells are indeed metabolically active. Nonetheless, the number of cells and mitotic figures clearly diminish in animals and humans from some time shortly after birth, through puberty, and into adulthood.

Similarly, the matrix, previously thought to be relatively inert, has now been shown to be in a state of metabolic activity; its biochemistry is being analyzed in detail. Water, existing in a hyperhydrated form, makes up 60% of the cartilage weight. The remaining organic component consists of about equal parts of collagen and proteoglycans. This collagen is distinctly different in structure from that of bone and skin, with characteristic changes in biochemical chains.

Whereas the collagen imparts toughness to the cartilage, the proteoglycans are important in maintaining the high water content and the functional resiliency for surface motion. The proteoglycan macromolecules, referred to as *protein-polysaccharides* in earlier reports, have now been shown to be composed of specific glycosaminoglycan subunits linked in a specific fashion to form the aggregated proteoglycan unit. The principal glycosaminoglycan in adults is chondroitin 6-sulfate. Chondroitin 4-sulfate is present in higher concentrations in immature animals but greatly diminishes in adulthood. Conversely, keratan sulfate, present in small amounts in immature cartilage of humans, increases in concentration in tissue of adults. Further, these macromolecules contain an increased negative charge, which helps to maintain the stiffness property of the tissue as well as being important in its water aggregation.

Metabolism of Cartilage

Chondrocytes actively synthesize component portions of proteoglycans and collagen, assemble them intracellularly, and extrude them into the surrounding matrix. Further, current data suggest that an internal remodeling system acts in normal cartilage in a twofold manner: (1) to degrade the aged portion of cellular matrix and then (2) to synthesize or reconstruct the replaced components. For this remodeling to occur, the chondrocytes synthesize lysozymes necessary for the normal turnover of the proteoglycan components.

Last, normal mature adult chondrocytes are capable of cell division when stressed under certain types of physiochemical or physiologic stimuli.

Biochemical Changes in Osteoarthritis Cartilage

One of the initial biochemical changes of cartilage in osteoarthritis is the early depletion of glycosaminoglycan components. Specific alterations have been described as the osteoarthritic process advances. Further, the total collagen content of osteoarthritic cartilage does not appear to vary from that of normal tissue; nonetheless, the type of collagen synthesized by the osteoarthritic chondrocytes is not that of articular cartilage but rather that of skin and bone. Also, the diametric and spatial arrangements of these collagen fibers are likewise altered from the normal in osteoarthritis. These changes apparently increase the functional capability of the proteoglycans to contain water.

When the chondrocytes in early osteoarthritis were carefully examined, the rate of proteoglycan synthesis in osteoarthritic cartilage was markedly increased as compared with normal. Protein synthesis is increased in mildly osteoarthritic cartilage. However, in cartilage with moderate to advanced disease, the ability to synthesize matrix component falls off markedly.

Another area of intense investigation of osteoarthritic cartilage focuses on the role of proteolytic enzymes in the degenerative process. Catheptic enzymes, which are lysosomal in origin, and acid phosphatase appear to increase in human osteoarthritic cartilage in direct proportion to the severity of the degradation process. These proteolytic enzymes apparently provide the mechanism to effect the destruction of the proteoglycan. It has only recently been demonstrated that collagenase is activated in severe osteoarthritic human cartilage and participates in the destruction of collagens and the total loss of cartilage substance (see Table 24.6).

Osteoarthritis may be viewed as a series of biochemical and metabolic reactions of articular cartilage to chronic unspecified stresses. This process results in an initial cellular and synthetic reparative reaction and a subsequently decreased rate of proteoglycan synthesis as the severity of the disease increases. Further, although the rate of matrix synthesis is increased, the resultant products are abnormal and hence may contribute to the degradation process.

Table 24.6. Biochemical Alterations in Osteoarthritic Articular Cartilage

---

Collagen: Changes in structure, chemistry, and rate of synthesis

Water: Increase in total content of water-binding capacity

Chondrocytes: Increase in number and rate of cell proliferation until severe disease reverses this process

Proteoglycans: Initial increase in synthesis with mild disease, decrease with progressive destruction of the cartilage

Glycosaminoglycans: Alteration in subunits with moderate disease

Lysosomal enzymes: Increase in concentration with severity of the process

---

PATHOLOGY OF OSTEOARTHRITIS

The pathologic changes of osteoarthritis may be best considered in terms of the three joint structures—the articular cartilage, the bone, and the surrounding soft tissues. The osteoarthritic process is a focal and local one with a multiplicity of patterns that vary widely and depend on the underlying abnormalities, the duration of the disease, and the clinical appearance. There is early softening of the cartilage with disruption of the superficial layers, which produces either flaking on the surface or splits called *fibrillations* in the deeper layers. Abrasion of the fibrillated cartilage occurs with progressive disease and results in exposure of the underlying bony cortex in the process referred to as denudation (see Table 24.7).

As deterioration of the cartilage progresses, the supporting bone may undergo several reactions. Most characteristic is the formation of marginal osteophytes produced by ossification secondary to vascularization of heaped-up cartilage; these bony spurs may protrude into the joint space or develop within the capsular and ligamentous attachments at the joint margins. The osteophyte consists of newly formed bone that merges with the subchondral bone. Often its surface contains a reparative type of cartilage that becomes continuous with the adjacent synovial lining. When the denuded surface of cartilage exposes bone, the surface develops a smoothed, rubbed appearance referred to as *eburnation*. On x-ray examination of such a joint, the eburnated surface frequently appears sclerotic—that is, there is an increase in subchondral bone density, reflecting an abortive

Table 24.7. Gross Pathologic Features of Osteoarthritis

Degenerative changes
    Loss of cartilage
    Juxta-articular bone cysts

Reparative changes
    Subchondral bone sclerosis
    Marginal osteophyte formation

Inflammatory changes
    Synovitis
    Joint effusion

---

reparative attempt. Further, the bone may undergo a cystic degenerative change; these cysts form below the surface of the cartilage. The trabeculae disappear and are replaced by mucoid or fibrous tissue. The surrounding areas are often encircled by a rim of active new bone. These cysts are thought to be formed from pressure transmitted from the joint directly to the bone in the absence of the supporting cartilage. These degenerative cysts are often difficult to differentiate from those caused by rheumatoid arthritis or gout.

Role of Inflammation in Osteoarthritis

Although osteoarthritis is not primarily an inflammatory disorder, small foci of inflammatory cells are often present in surgically removed specimens. The synovial thickening may be so gross as to simulate that of rheumatoid arthritis. Indeed, there exists the syndrome of inflammatory or erosive osteoarthritis in which a distinct inflammatory component is present in the synovium without the associated well-known features of rheumatoid arthritis. This syndrome has led some students in the field to speculate that osteoarthritis may indeed be secondary to inflammation. More specifically, if the inflammation is brief, as is frequently the case with trauma, or if repetitious or of low grade, as with joint overuse, the osteoarthritic process may be slow to develop; and hence the features of inflammation may be minor. In rheumatoid arthritis, the profound degree and duration of inflammation clearly result in early osteoarthritis. More recently, collagen has been demonstrated to be antigenic and to stimulate humoral antibodies and cell-mediated immunity against proteoglycan components in chondrocytes. These antibodies and immunity have been detected in degenerative arthritis as well as other conditions. Cartilage is an ideal entrapment medium for the slow release of antigens or proteolytic enzymes. Thus, there may be a possible role for inflammation in the pathogenesis of osteoarthritis.

Effects of Aging

Osteoarthritis has generally been thought to be a widespread senescence of cartilage, with the degenerative changes in major joints of the body increasing concomitantly with age. It is now believed that localized nonspecific osteophyte lesions are indeed associated with age but are of limited progression. Although found in older persons, these osteophytes are not associated with clinical symptoms and hence do not cause the syndrome of osteoarthritis. Consequently, one should consider osteoarthritis an articular disease of cartilage that is distinct from the aging process of cartilage.

Genetic and Metabolic Factors

The study of Heberden's nodes affords the opportunity to consider the interplay of genetic and metabolic factors in osteoarthritis. Pathologically, these lesions are similar if not identical to those of osteoarthritis in the weight-bearing joints. Although mechanical explanations have been offered, there is a remarkable prevalence of the lesions in women and in certain families. Some studies suggest that a single dominant gene might determine the occurrence. Further, because Heberden's nodes often evolve around the time of menopause, hormonal factors, although poorly defined, may be involved in this disorder.

Mechanics of Joints

In spite of newer findings concerning the role of metabolic, biochemical, enzymatic, hereditary, inflammatory, and anatomic disturbances occurring in osteoarthritis, the question of the cause of these changes still remains. Hence, it is important to consider mechanical factors in this process. Synovial fluid, which may increase in the osteoarthritic process and cause a joint effusion, performs its normal lubricant function. Cartilage has compressibility and elasticity, features that create a lubricating film that keeps the articular surfaces from touching. Hence, with even minimal amounts of fluid, it is impossible for rubbing to cause degeneration of cartilage. However, cartilage can be made to degenerate mechanically by simulating the compression forces of everyday life. In such settings without added synovial fluid, cartilage may wear out very quickly. Cartilage seems to act as a bearing surface and a redistributor of load, rather than as a shock absorber alone. Nonetheless, this absorption of shock needs to occur for the safety of the joint. The shock-absorber function is maintained by the supporting muscles and the subchondral bone. Although subchondral sclerotic bone was originally thought to be a reaction to the degenerative process, more recent studies have suggested that the bone stiffening occurs at the beginning of the degenerative disorder. This idea suggests that small, repetitive "shock loading" has deleterious effects not only on the cartilage but also on the underlying subchondral bone. More specifically, small microfractures of the trabeculae may be one of the earliest lesions in this sequence.

Pathophysiology of Osteoarthritis

Poorly defined physical stresses probably cause injury to the chondrocytes. The release of the lysozymes would then cause matrix-proteoglycan degeneration. Subsequently, there is local chondrocyte stimulation in an abortive attempt at repair, with increased production of the proteoglycan collagen components early in the course of the disease. Nonetheless, this repair process is ineffective, and because of the initial injury to the cartilage, further loss of elasticity and the lubricating properties of the cartilage leads to its erosion. The cycle of cartilage degeneration may continue permanently at variable rates of joint damage (see Table 24.8).

OTHER JOINT DISEASES

Neuropathic Joint Disease

Neuropathic joint disease represents the most advanced and severe form of chronic degenerative arthropathy. Although the peripheral joints are most characteristically involved, the spine may not be spared in this process. The hallmark of this destructive process is the alteration in the normal proprioceptive sensory innervation of the joints. There is almost always a readily identifiable cause of

Table 24.8. Pathophysiology of Osteoarthritis

Initiating Factors	*Degenerative Processes*	*Abortive Reparative Processes*

Intrinsic
  Age
  Gender
  Heredity
  Obesity
  Inflammation
Extrinsic
  Mechanical factors
  Trauma
	Exposure to destructive enzymes
	Breakdown of proteoglycans and collagen
	Cartilage erosion
		Chondrocyte proliferation
		Increased proteoglycan synthesis
		Reactive bone formation
		  Bony spurs
		  Bony sclerosis

this neurologic deficiency. The most common etiologic disorders include alcoholic neuropathy, diabetic neuropathy, syphilitic tabes dorsalis, syringomyelia, and calcium pyrophosphate deposition diseases. Several other neurologic disorders may be associated with this syndrome, including tertiary syphilis, paraplegia, pernicious anemia, and nerve damage. More recently, the disease has been associated with calcium pyrophosphate deposition disorder and has possibly occurred from too vigorous and frequent intra-articular injections of corticosteroids (cortisone arthropathy). Indomethacin analgesic arthropathy has been recently reported.

Patients often come to the clinician with advanced monoarticular osteoarthritis, exhibiting gross deformity of the joint in a setting of remarkably little pain; rarely, pain may be present. At times, the diagnosis is suspected after x-ray films of the affected joint show marked erosions, sclerosis, and spurs.

In diabetic patients, this destructive process is generally monoarticular and is found primarily in the small joints of the mid-foot, but the ankle joints and knees may be similarly involved. Because of the lack of pain, an occasional patient will have protrusion of bone through the skin with accompanying osteomyelitis and an unbelievable lack of complaints.

The management of these disorders is generally supportive—that is, immobilizing and restricting weight bearing of the affected joint. Frequently, these relatively simple measures cause the disorder to improve significantly. Surgical attempts to control the process through joint fusion (arthrodesis) are not uniformly effective.

Hence, close collaboration with an orthopedic surgeon is essential in managing these patients. It should, of course, be stated that the underlying neurologic disorder is generally not amenable to any form of treatment, and improvement by altering the course of the underlying disease is generally not to be expected.

Osteonecrosis

Osteonecrosis has been referred to by such names as *aseptic* or *avascular* necrosis of bone. This disorder is characterized clinically by pain in the involved joints that is generally monoarticular but sometimes bilateral and polyarticular. When there is a clear history of injury to the joint, such as a fracture, the cause is generally ascribed to that event. These traumatically caused osteonecrotic joints are seen commonly by orthopedic surgeons. About half of the cases, however, are not due to evident injury. A primary necrotic disorder may then be considered.

The joint most commonly involved is the femoral head; but the femoral condyle, humeral head, wrist bones (such as the lunate), and almost any other bone may be involved.

In the nontraumatic cases, the diagnosis can be made only from a high index of suspicion in the appropriate clinical setting of joint pain and characteristic x-ray changes. The x-ray changes depend on the stage of evolution of the disorder. More specifically, when x-ray examinations are performed early in the course of the disease, there may be no discernible changes. Early x-ray changes include the crescent-shaped separation of the subchondral areas from the trabecular bone, caused by an abortive healing attempt by granulation tissue, producing the radiolucency; structural deficits in the dome of a joint, with areas of partial collapse; and ultimately, total collapse of the head of the joint. Last, as changes progress, end-stage osteoarthritis is evident. All of these x-ray changes are indeed late in the course of the disease, since the earliest radiologic appearance reflects the reparative and degenerative processes rather than initial bone death.

The nontraumatic causes of osteonecrosis are most commonly associated with alcoholism or corticosteroid use. In alcoholics with osteonecrosis, the accompanying problems include hyperlipidemia, hyperuricemia, pancreatitis, and overuse of steroids. In patients treated with corticosteroids, associated problems include hyperuricemia, systemic lupus erythematosus, rheumatoid arthritis, and alcoholism. Osteonecrosis is prevalent in patients receiving high-dose steroid treatment for renal transplants. Less commonly, osteonecrosis may occur in patients with sickle cell disorders, Gaucher's disease, liver disorders, caisson disease, polycythemia, diabetes, obesity, and lipid disorders.

In trying to explain a single common mechanism for osteonecrosis in such a large variety of diseases, many investigators believe that alterations in body lipids in conjunction with vascular compromise of end arteries are the final pathways leading to the bone necrosis. However, results of animal studies show clearly that although the interaction of steroids and lipids with compromised vasculature can cause the disorder, this is not uniformly the case; hence, these results suggest that other mechanisms, heretofore unidentifiable, may be operating.

The importance of early diagnosis cannot be overemphasized because the only treatment, surgery, depends on the stage of progress of the disorder. When a disease is in the earliest stage, as determined by minimal x-ray findings, specialized allograft procedures sometimes succeed. In a later stage of disease, with collapse of the articular surfaces of the joint, the entire joint may be replaced.

Osteochondritis

Osteochondritis dissecans is a disease of unknown cause, affecting mostly youngsters and adolescents and characterized by separation of a devitalized fragment of subchondral bone. At times, progression of the disease results in "loose" bodies with an accompanying increase in pain and locking. Although an injury may precipitate the osteochondritis, in many cases the exact cause is unknown.

Patients characteristically appear with mild discomfort that is increased by use. Initial x-rays are often negative, but with advancing disease, there is a bony sequestrum in a sharply defined cavity. The most common sites are the knees, hips, and shoulders, but other joints may also be sites of this disorder. It usually occurs in joints with convex surfaces, thus substantiating the theory of end artery obstruction from whatever cause.

Epiphyseal osteochondritis refers to necrosis of the entire epiphysis and is usually a localized disorder of childhood. Although injury may be an etiologic factor, vascular insufficiency is thought to be a more prominent one. When the disease is localized in the hip joint (Legg-Calve-Perthes disease), the younger child usually has a limp and pain referred to the knee.

The condition should be diagnosed as early as possible, because it can be conservatively managed by not permitting the joints to bear weight for an extended period, which will prevent the later sequela. Surgical extrication of loose fragments may occasionally be necessary.

Tumors of the Joint Area

Although tumors of articular structures are uncommon, they do occur, and improper diagnosis may cause inappropriate delays in treatment. The hallmark for suspicion is the bloody aspirate of joint fluid when nontumorous conditions (e.g., recent injury, traumatic tap, or even inflammatory arthritis), have been ruled out. Unexplained radiologic findings should encourage consultation with an orthopedic surgeon.

Pigmented villonodular synovitis refers to benign tumorous overgrowth of the linings of the synovium, bursa, or tendons and is often associated with bleeding into the joint or tendon. The patient, generally a man, appears with symptoms like those in types of inflammatory arthritis—pain and swelling (intermittent, recurring, or persistent) mostly in the knee, but sometimes in other major joints. The aspirate from a hemorrhagic joint is noninflammatory. Multiple loose bodies may be seen on x-ray.

Although the cause of pigmented villonodular synovitis is unclear (i.e., inflammatory components may be the basis of the disorder), the appropriate treatment clearly is surgical. The general principle of exploring any joint with undiagnosed monoarticular arthritis holds true in general and for this disorder specifically.

Synovial chondromatosis refers to the benign focal metastatic growth of normal-appearing cartilage in the synovium. When this cartilage becomes calcified, the condition may be called *synovial osteochondromatosis*. This cartilage will break off and form loose bodies. The knee is often the site of involvement in young or middle-aged men. Although the crepitation may lead the clinician to suspect osteoarthritis, the radiologic picture generally confirms the diagnosis of synovial chondromatosis by disclosing several small rounded opacities within the confines of the joint cavity. The treatment is a surgical synovectomy.

Benign tumors of the joint include those characteristically found in connective tissues—for example, hemangiomas, lipomas, and fibromas.

Primary malignant tumors of the joint area are rare and include synovial sarcomas and synovial chondrosarcomas. Synovial sarcomas are highly malignant and occur mostly in adolescents or young adults, with a higher prevalence in

men. Joints in the lower extremities are more frequently involved than those in the upper extremities. Pain is usually not a feature because these tumors often originate in the para-articular tissues. They are generally suspected when there is an overgrowth of soft tissue in the vicinity of the joints. Obviously, biopsy is necessary to establish the diagnosis, but it should be done only in technically competent centers because partial resection may lead to rapid spread of the cancer. The tumor metastasizes very early, often through regional lymph nodes. Surgery is the preferred treatment, although an occasional patient may respond to chemotherapy or irradiation. The 5-year survival rate is approximately 30%.

Metastatic malignancies to the joints may be found in careful inspection of the synovium in postmortem specimens, but very rarely does the metastasis appear with clinical problems. Besides solid tumors, hematologic malignancies, such as leukemias, may infiltrate the synovium, and the patient may have an unexplained monoarticular noninflammatory arthritis. Here again, the biopsy of any unexplained synovial reaction is strongly recommended.

BIBLIOGRAPHY

American Academy of Orthopaedic Surgeons: *Symposium on Osteoarthritis.* (Meeting Chicago, Ill, Oct 1974.) St Louis, CV Mosby Co, 1976.

Howell DS, Moskowitz RW (eds): Symposium on osteoarthritis. *Arthritis Rheum* 20 (Suppl):S96, 1977.

Jones JP Jr (ed): Symposium: Osteonecrosis. *Clin Orthop* 130:2, 1978.

Lee P, Rooney PJ, Sturrock RD, et al: The etiology and pathogenesis of osteoarthritis: A review. *Semin Arthritis Rheum* 3:189, 1974.

Marmor L: Surgery in osteoarthritis. *Semin Arthritis Rheum* 2:117, 1972.

Moskowitz RW: Cartilage and osteoarthritis: Current concepts. *J Rheumatol* 4:329, 1977.

Peyron J: Epidemiologic and etiologic approach of osteoarthritis. *Semin Arthritis Rheum* 8:288, 1979.

Radin EL: The physiology and degeneration of joints. *Semin Arthritis Rheum* 2:245, 1972.

25

Crystal-induced Arthritis

Robert G. Gray

Roy D. Altman

Certain crystalline substances, when released into the joint space, may elicit an inflammatory response. Crystals known to cause acute synovitis in humans include (1) monosodium urate monohydrate (MSU) (in gout), (2) calcium pyrophosphate dihydrate (CPPD) (in pseudogout), and (3) microcrystalline corticosteroid esters (in postinjection flare-ups).

Properties common to MSU, CPPD, and corticosteroid crystals include sparing solubility in water, size (0.5–20 μm), and the capacity to be readily phagocytosed by polymorphonuclear and mononuclear leukocytes. Hydroxyapatite crystals have been identified in synovial effusions, but their relationship to arthritis has not been clearly defined.

CRYSTAL IDENTIFICATION

A diagnosis of acute gouty arthritis requires the identification of intracellular MSU crystals in synovial fluid. One places a drop of the fluid on a clean glass slide which is mounted with a coverslip. In general, the morphologic characteristics of MSU crystals are readily appreciated on this type of wet mount microscopy: a needle shape, length roughly up to twice the diameter of a polymorphonuclear leukocyte, and refractility. Urate phagocytosis often makes it appear that the crystal is "spearing" the engulfing white blood cell (Fig. 25.1). In questionable cases, compensated polarized microscopy confirms the strongly negative birefringent nature of MSU crystals. Two polarizing lenses are aligned to prevent unrefracted light from reaching the eye; an intervening red filter (compensator) changes the black background to a reddish blue. If the microscope stage is rotated so that the crystals are parallel to the slow phase of light vibration, MSU crystals appear deep yellow. CPPD crystals are rhombic or rod-shaped and usually shorter (3–15 μm) than MSU crystals (Fig. 25.2). They exhibit weakly positive birefringence and thus appear faintly blue when parallel urate crystals are deep yellow; if the microscope stage is rotated 90 degrees, the crystal colors are reversed. Definitive identification of MSU crystals by uricase digestion or of

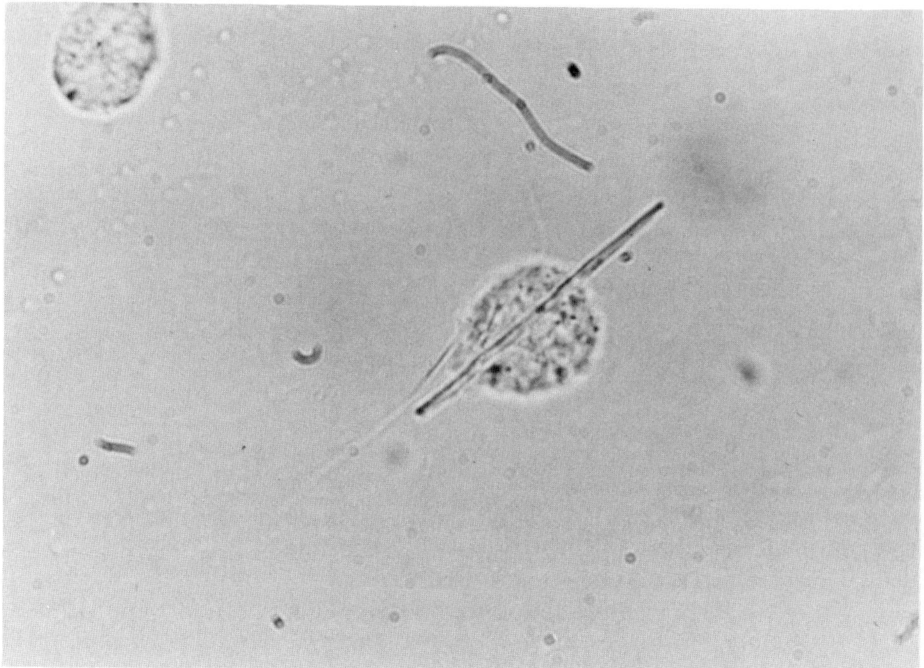

Figure 25.1. Note the large toothpick-shaped crystal partially engulfed by a polymorphonuclear leukocyte. The lack of a double density about the portion of the crystal engulfed by the cell indicates a loss of the phagosomal membrane. Note the thin fibrin strand on the left of the cell and various debris that should not be confused with crystals.

either MSU or CPPD crystals by x-ray diffraction is neither readily available nor clinically necessary.

Occasionally, other crystalline and birefringent material may be confused with gout or pseudogout crystals. Corticosteroid ester crystals may be seen in synovial fluid a month or longer after intra-articular injection. Betamethasone crystals can be indistinguishable from urate, appearing needle-shaped and showing negative birefringence. Triamcinolone hexacetonide crystals usually are wider and longer than MSU and may exhibit negative or positive birefringence. Other corticosteroid preparations produce branching and amorphous patterns. Cholesterol crystals have no proven phlogistic properties and are observed most often in long-standing rheumatoid arthritis effusions. They assume a large rectangular plate-like configuration with a notched edge and display positive birefringence; rarely, long, needle-shaped forms have been described. Calcium oxalate, used as an anticoagulant in some complete blood count tubes, often appears as a pyramid-shaped crystal. One should use caution so as not to confuse crystals with cellular inclusions, thin fibrin strands, scratches on the slide, or other debris.

PATHOGENESIS OF THE ACUTE GOUTY ATTACK

The acute gouty attack is triggered by the discharge of MSU crystals from the synovial membrane into the joint space and, possibly, also by the de novo pre-

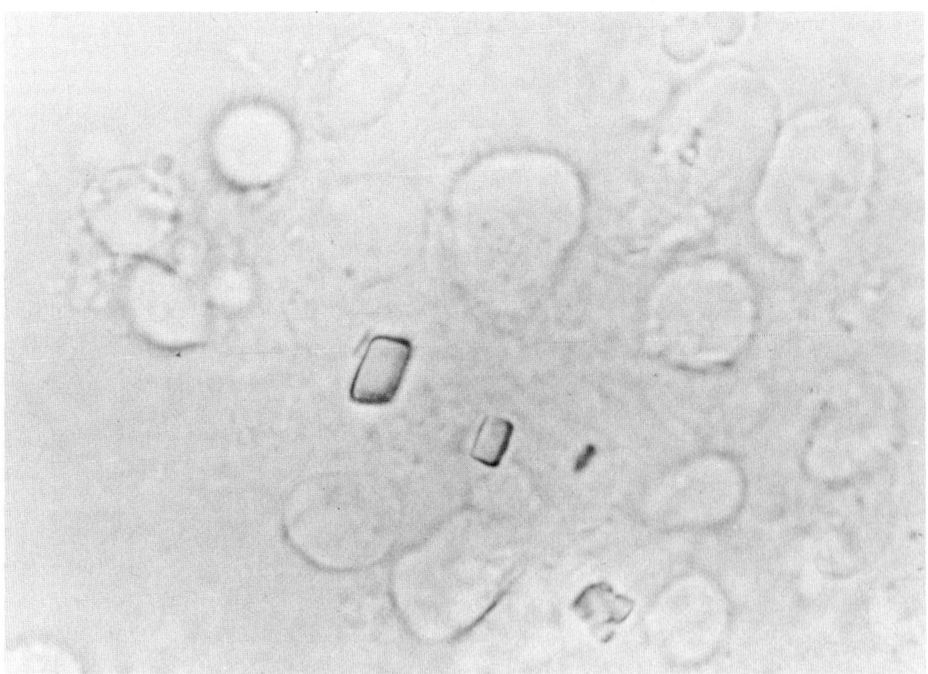

Figure 25.2. Note the rhomboid-shaped crystals lying in the debris of ruptured polymorphonuclear leukocytes.

cipitation of synovial fluid urate. Prolonged hyperuricemia permits the deposition of urate in subsynovial tissue but is not essential to the genesis of acute gout. The majority of hyperuricemic persons never develop gout, and acute gouty synovitis may begin at a time when serum uric acid is normal. More importantly, an acute rise or fall of serum urate appears to predispose to the extrusion of MSU from the synovium.

Several local factors (Table 25.1) seem to contribute to the onset of acute gout. Joint trauma may dislodge subsynovial microtophi. Intact proteoglycans enhance urate solubility; increased proteoglycan turnover, suggested by elevated serum uronic acid levels in gouty patients, may diminish urate solubility. Also, the diffusion of synovial fluid urate molecules is one-half that of water. It was proposed that equilibration is attained between plasma and synovial fluid urate levels during the day. However, during nocturnal recumbency, the resorption of water from small, traumatic effusions in dependent joints (e.g., the first meta-

Table 25.1. Proposed Local Triggers of Acute Gout

Joint trauma and dislodgement of subsynovial urate deposits

Increased proteoglycan turnover resulting in decreased urate solubility

Selective nocturnal water resorption from traumatic, dependent joint effusions, increasing urate concentration

Lower temperature of acral joints, favoring decreased urate solubility

---

tarsophalangeal joint) increases the synovial fluid urate concentration and the propensity to acute gout. The lower temperature of acral joints further favors reduced urate solubility.

The two essential ingredients of acute gout are the presence of MSU crystals and polymorphonuclear leukocytes. Smaller urate crystals (< 0.05 μm) and soluble, noncrystalline urate exert no significant inflammatory effects. Animals rendered severely leukopenic fail to develop gout after the intraarticular instillation of MSU crystals. The recent report of typical acute gout with intrasynovial MSU crystals but no leukocytic response is unexplained, but it suggests that the primary inflammatory process resides in the synovial membrane rather than the contiguous joint space.

Urate crystals are avidly phagocytosed by synovial fluid polymorphonuclear cells and, to a lesser extent, by mononuclear leukocytes and synovial lining cells (Fig. 25.1). MSU crystals extruded into the synovial cavity are coated with protein adsorbed from serum; at least a portion of the protein coat appears to be immunoglobulin (Ig) G, oriented for functional contact with the Fc receptors of ambient leukocytes (Fig. 25.3). This interaction between urate-bound IgG and leukocytic receptors enhances phagocytosis and may also promote the noncytolytic release of lysosomal enzymes. White blood cell ingestion of MSU crystals causes the release of a nondialyzable 8,500-dalton glycopeptide with strong chemo-

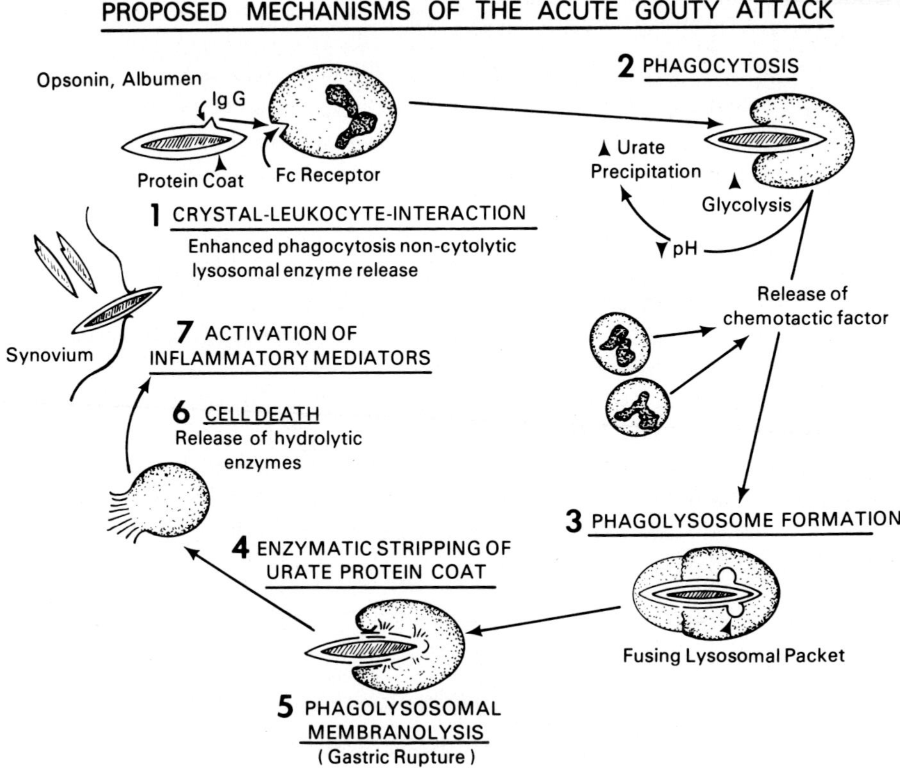

Figure 25.3. Possible pathogenesis of crystal-induced inflammation.

tactic properties. The arrival of more inflammatory cells through chemotaxis and random locomotion accelerates crystal phagocytosis and accounts for the brisk synovial fluid leukocytosis observed during a gouty attack (1,000 > 100,000/cu mm; more than 75% polymorphonuclear cells). The enhanced glycolytic activity of phagocytosing leukocytes may reduce local pH and predisposes to further urate precipitation.

The ingested crystal is surrounded by a leukocytic cell membrane (phagosome) that ultimately fuses with intracytoplasmic lysosomal packets (phagolysosome). After enzymatic stripping of the crystal protein coat, hydrogen bonding mediates lysis and rupture of the phagolysosomal membrane. Release of hydrolytic enzymes rapidly produces cell death. The consequent discharge of cellular and enzymatic products into the synovial space promotes the inflammatory process.

Hageman factor is activated by urate and, in turn, is capable of triggering a cascade of inflammatory mediators that dilate capillaries, enhance leukocytic margination and diapedesis, promote chemotaxis, and activate the kallikrein-kinin system. However, acute gout may be produced in animals lacking Hageman factor, and at least one of the kinins (bradykinin) seems nonessential to gouty synovitis. The role of the complement pathways and prostaglandins is presently being investigated.

The number of observed synovial fluid MSU crystals appears to correlate poorly with the intensity of the gouty attack. Occasionally, very few crystals are identified, probably reflecting extensive prior digestion by myeloperoxidases. Infrequently, the initial synovial fluid crystal search is unrevealing, yet numerous urate crystals are seen in an aliquot of joint fluid aspirated shortly thereafter. Sequestration or clumping of crystals in synovial recesses may be partly responsible. Synovial fluid MSU crystals may be seen in asymptomatic joints of gouty patients during intercritical periods. However, the crystals generally are scanty in number and predominantly extracellular; the minimal crystal phagocytosis observed is mostly by mononuclear, rather than polymorphonuclear, leukocytes.

The seemingly self-perpetuating, self-augmenting acute gouty attack gradually subsides spontaneously. The role of inactivators of chemotaxis and inflammation currently is poorly understood (Fig. 25.3).

PATHOGENESIS OF ACUTE PSEUDOGOUT

CPPD crystals, responsible for acute pseudogout, are derived primarily from deposits in articular cartilage and menisci. Deposits may be found in connective tissue elsewhere (synovium, tendons, bursae, ligaments, dura mater) but not in other types of tissue or viscera. Thus, it appears that primary alterations in connective tissue matrix or metabolism permit local CPPD crystal accumulation. In cartilage, CPPD seems to appear first along midzone collagen fibers and aggregates in the proteoglycan mold surrounding chondrocytes.

Several mechanisms have been proposed to explain the periodic "autoinjection" of CPPD crystals from cartilage into the joint space. A drop in serum ionized calcium markedly reduces CPPD crystal solubility in vitro and seems likely to free crystals from their proteoglycan mold and permit "crystal shedding" into the synovial cavity. Indeed, acute pseudogout attacks correlate clinically with falling serum calcium levels in the postoperative state and during various acute medical illnesses. Trauma may disrupt the cartilage architecture via subchondral bone microfractures and thus release CPPD crystals. Hydrolytic and proteolytic enzymes engendered in the joint as a result of various arthritides (septic arthritis, acute gout, osteoarthritis) may degrade the cartilage matrix ("enzymatic strip mining") that retains CPPD crystals. Recently, acute pseudogout has been reported after hormonal replacement therapy of hypothyroidism; restoration of a euthyroid state may somehow loosen the cartilaginous mold in which CPPD crystals are embedded. Synovial fluid pyrophosphate levels exceed plasma values in patients with both CPPD deposition disease and other forms of arthritis. It is unclear if such changes promote crystal deposition.

Upon access to the joint, CPPD crystals appear to initiate a sequence of events similar to those observed in acute gout (Fig. 25.3). However, the phagocytosis-inducing, chemotactic, and phagolysosomal membranolytic effects of the CPPD crystals are less intense than those of MSU. The ensuing synovitis procedures an inflammatory joint fluid with characteristics similar to those of gouty effusions. Occasionally, synovial fluid leukocyte counts are only minimally elevated despite obvious clinical synovitis.

Why most attacks of pseudogout subside spontaneously while in others a chronic low-grade inflammatory arthritis develops is uncertain. Synovial membrane uptake of CPPD crystals, in part, may help attenuate the acute joint inflammation.

MICROCRYSTALLINE CORTICOSTEROID-INDUCED SYNOVITIS

Intra-articular corticosteroid ester injections are used extensively in the palliation of inflammatory synovitides. In 2%–5% of cases, local injection is followed 4–12 hours later by an acute, self-limited synovitis. Joint pain and swelling generally are mild and resolve rapidly within 12–48 hours. However, intense synovitis with joint fluid leukocyte counts of > 100,000/cu mm, large effusions, and fever may occur. Polymorphonuclear leukocytic phagocytosis of steroid crystals is readily evident and supports a true crystal-induced synovitis. Reaspiration of the joint serves to abort the attack and permits exclusion of iatrogenic septic arthritis when the flare-up is inordinately intense or prolonged. Traumatic technique appears to increase the risk of steroid flare-up.

APATITE CRYSTAL ARTHRITIS

Calcium hydroxyapatite may be deposited in various soft and para-articular structures. This process accounts for calcific tendonitis and bursitis, the calcific periarthritis of dialysis patients, fluffy synovial calcification associated with hypercalcemic states, and the calcinosis of scleroderma and polymyositis.

Recently, apatite crystals, too small (< 0.5 μm) to be visualized by conventional light microscopy, have been identified by electron microscopy within synovial fluid leukocytes of osteoarthritic effusions. The intra-articular injection of apatite crystals produces an acute arthritis in dog knees. It has been proposed that synovial deposits of these crystals may account for some exacerbations of osteoarthritis and other cases of acute, nonspecific synovitis in humans.

BIBLIOGRAPHY

Bennett RM, Lehr JR, McCarty DJ: Crystal shedding and acute pseudogout. *Arthritis Rheum* 19:93, 1976.

Denko CW: A phlogistic function of prostaglandin E_1 in urate crystal inflammation. *J Rheumatol* 1:222, 1974.

Denko CW: A phlogistic function of PGE_1 in calcium pyrophosphate dihydrate crystal-induced inflammation. *J Rheumatol* 2:251, 1975.

Giclas PC, Ginsberg MG, Cooper NR: Immunoglobulin G independent activation of the classical complement pathway by monosodium urate crystals. *J Clin Invest* 63:759, 1979.

Ginsberg MH, Kozin F, O'Malley M, et al: Release of platelet constituents by monosodium urate crystals. *J Clin Invest* 60:999, 1977.

Halverson PB, McCarty DJ: Identification of hydroxyapatite crystals in synovial fluid. *Arthritis Rheum* 22:389, 1979.

Hasselbacher P: C3 activation by monosodium urate monohydrate and other crystalline material. *Arthritis Rheum* 22:571, 1979.

Holmes EW, Blondet P: Urate binding to serum albumin. *Arthritis Rheum* 22:737, 1979.

Kahn CB, Hollander JL, Schumacher HR: Corticosteroid crystals in synovial fluid. *JAMA* 211:807, 1970.

Kellermeyer RW: Hageman factor and acute gouty arthritis. *Arthritis Rheum* 11:452, 1968.

Kozin F, Ginsberg MH, Skosey JL: Polymorphonuclear leukocyte responses to monosodium urate crystals: Modification by absorbed serum proteins. *J Rheumatol* 6:519, 1979.

McCarty DJ: Mechanisms of the crystal deposition diseases—gout and pseudogout. *Ann Intern Med* 78:767, 1973.

Melmon KL, Webster ME, Goldfinger SE, et al: The presence of a kinin in inflammatory synovial effusion from arthritides of varying etiologies. *Arthritis Rheum* 10:13, 1967.

Perricone E, Brandt KD: Enhancement of urate solubility by connective tissue. I. Effect of proteoglycan aggregates and buffer cation. *Arthritis Rheum* 21:453, 1978.

Spilberg I: Urate crystal arthritis in animals lacking Hageman factor. *Arthritis Rheum* 17:143, 1974.

Spilberg I: Current concepts of the mechanism of acute inflammation in gouty arthritis. *Arthritis Rheum* 18:129, 1975.

Spilberg I, Gallacher A, Mehta JM, et al: Urate crystal-induced chemotactic factor. Isolation and partial characterization. *J Clin Invest* 58:815, 1976.

26

Gout and Hyperuricemia

Roy D. Altman

Gout is a disease that has been known since the time of Hippocrates. The term is based on the Latin *gutta* or drop, reflecting the theory that a bad humor had "dropped" into a weak joint. The disease is a complication of usually prolonged hyperuricemia, whereby monosodium urate monohydrate crystals form in the synovial cavity, synovium, or periarticular bone and soft tissues as well as occasionally in the kidneys. Until the twentieth century, the term *gout* was applied to many subacute or chronic arthritides. At present, it applies most often to a moderately severe acute intermittent arthritis.

URIC ACID METABOLISM

Humans lack the enzyme uricase and are therefore able to accumulate uric acid. Uric acid is produced in the body from the catabolism of purines as part of the de novo synthesis of nucleic acids. A lesser source of uric acid is from dietary purine-containing foods. Uric acid, in the form of monosodium urate, is soluble at body pH. It comprises about 1.2 g in the normal human. Approximately 60% is replaced daily, with 60% of that amount excreted in the urine (average urine excretion 420 ± 80 SD mg/24 hr on a purine-free diet). About one-third of the uric acid produced is excreted into the gastrointestinal tract and is promptly degraded by intestinal bacteria. The scheme for purine biosynthesis has been carefully elaborated and is summarized diagramatically in Figure 26.1.

CLASSIFICATION

Primary Gout

Primary gout refers to hyperuricemia due to endogenous defects in metabolism. The majority of patients with primary gout have no definable defect. The most common definable defect (80%) is due to hypoexcretion of uric acid by the kidneys. This condition tends to be familial, and hyperuricemia may be affected by dietary alterations or indiscretions. Less common forms are the heritable forms of pathologic overproduction of uric acid, apparently related to enzymatic defects

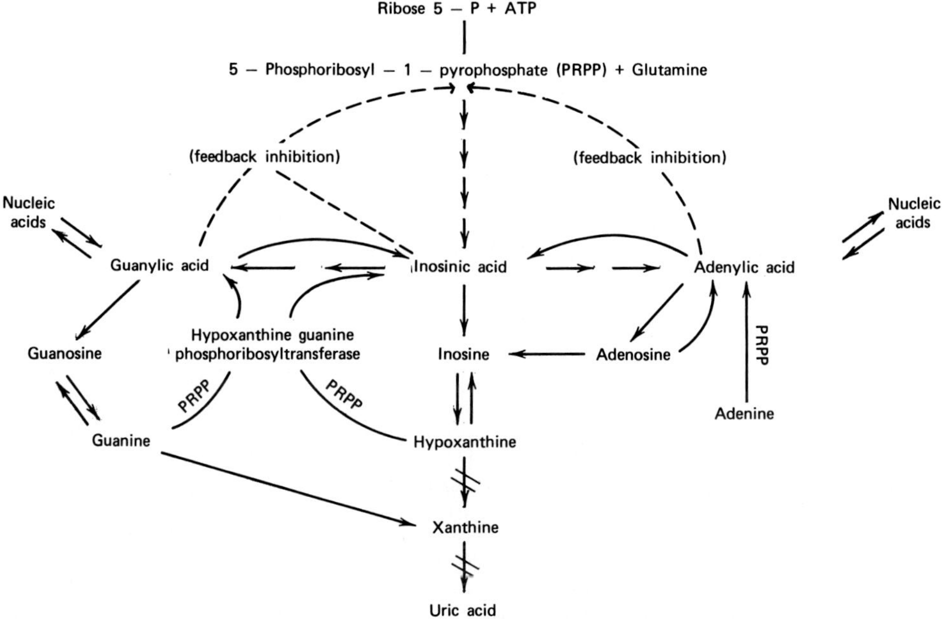

Figure 26.1. Diagrammatic summary of major steps of purine biosynthesis.

in purine biosynthesis. The enzymatic defects have been defined in rare subgroups of this disorder—Lesch-Nyhan, glycogen storage diseases, and others. Incomplete enzyme defects have also been defined.

Secondary Gout

Secondary gout is commonly associated with many underlying disorders in which uric acid overproduction results from nucleic acid turnover. These disorders are primarily related to blood dyscrasias (polycythemia vera, secondary polycythemia, leukemia) and other neoplastic diseases (multiple myeloma, Hodgkin's disease). However, gout can be caused by chronic renal disease of various etiologies and chronic lead poisoning (saturnine gout) (see also Table 4.2).

GOUTY ARTHRITIS

Acute Gout

There is a strong male predominance in gout (> 80%). The first attack may occur at any age but is most common between the ages of 40 and 50. The younger the person, the more likely a definable defect (i.e., enzymatic, secondary, metabolic).

The acute attack most often has its onset in the early morning hours. The joint becomes acutely painful, with all the cardinal signs of inflammation (heat, redness, pain, swelling, and loss of function). The periarticular tissues become edematous, giving the appearance of a cellulitis with a red, sometimes violaceous center. The onset of gout may take several hours to reach a peak. The pain is severe enough to be aggravated by touching the joint to the bedsheet. The attack may be accompanied by a tachycardia, fever, chills, and leukocytosis.

The acute attack of gout may be precipitated by dietary indiscretion, fasting, any event that may be associated with sharp changes in serum uric acid, a postoperative period of bed rest, earlier trauma to the involved joint, or treatment with allopurinol, or it may have no known precipitating event. Most attacks of gout resolve in 7–10 days if untreated; occasional attacks will last considerably longer. Upon the resolution of the attack, there may be desquamation of the skin over the involved joint and usually full return of the joint to its normal status. Occasionally, patients will have minor periarticular pains that do not evolve into full-blown gouty attacks. Frequently these minor pains are a prodrome of the attack, and patients can predict their own course.

The most frequently involved joint in the acute attack is the bunion joint or first metatarsal-phalangeal joint (podagra). The second most common area is the fifth tarsal-metatarsal joint. The next most common are the ankle, knee, olecranon bursae, wrists, fingers, and elbows. Gout is particularly uncommon in the spine, temporomandibular joints, hips, and shoulders. Occasional attacks may be polyarticular.

Intercritical Gout

It is important to note that the intervals between gouty attacks are asymptomatic. Chronic inflammation is strongly suggestive of another diagnosis. The intervals between the first several attacks of gout are frequently months or years. These attacks become closer in time. Attacks are also more severe as the patient ages.

Chronic Gout

Initially, attacks of gout are most often monoarticular. With time, attacks may become oligoarticular or even polyarticular. In general terms, the more joints involved, the more protracted the acute attack and the more difficult it is to treat. The more frequent and severe attacks are often associated with tophaceous gout.

If hyperuricemia is untreated for 8–10 years, tophaceous deposits will develop in about 50% of patients. They develop most often in synovium, bursae, tendons, or bone. The most common areas are the olecranon bursa, juxta-articular interphalangeal joint of the first toe, or other pressure points such as the Achilles tendon, pretibial bursa, or knuckles (Figs. 26.2, 26.3). The pinnae of the ear are an infrequent site for tophi.* Tophi are frequently almost rock hard, in contrast to the firm but less hard feel of rheumatoid arthritis nodules. Histologically, the tophus is a mass of monosodium urate crystals surrounded by inflammatory cells including foreign body giant cells. Tophi may be subcutaneous and are rarely intracutaneous. When exposed in the skin, they appear white. Tophi may drain through fistulous tracts in the skin or lead to overt ulcers. These chronically draining lesions, surprisingly, are rarely infected. Tophi are frequently not

---

* A microscope glass slide pressed against a protrusion from the pinna can differentiate the tophus (white) from cartilage (same color as the surrounding tissue) from a sebaceous cyst (yellow).

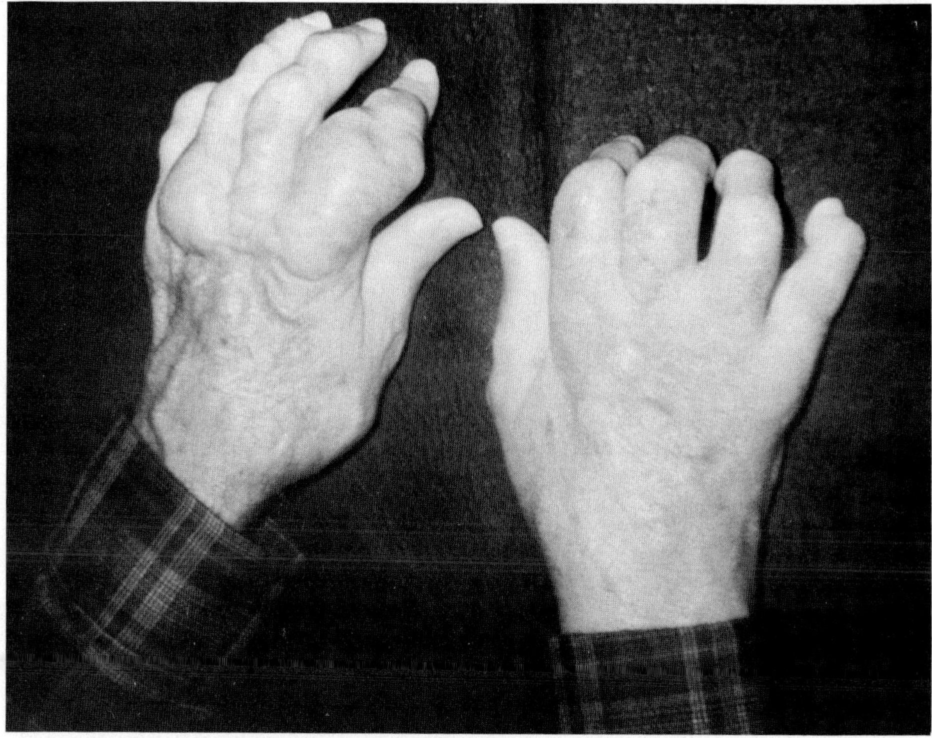

Figure 26.2. Note the massive tophaceous deposits on the left hand of this 56-year-old watchmaker. Surgical excision of tophi and reconstruction of tendinous insertions of the right hand have improved function to a modest degree.

overtly inflamed, but when deposited in or near joints, they may cause erosion of cartilage with bony destruction leading to a deforming arthritis known as *chronic gouty arthritis*. This deformity may be incorrectly diagnosed as rheumatoid arthritis. When biopsy is done of a suspected tophaceous deposit, the tissue should be fixed in 95% alcohol, as the crystals dissolve in water-based fixatives, such as formalin.

Destruction of cartilage may lead to secondary osteoarthritis and possibly chondrocalcinosis. Rarer locations of tophaceous deposits include the spine (gibbus formation), myocardium (conduction defects), vocal cords, carpal tunnel, and aorta.

SECONDARY HYPERURICEMIA AND GOUT

Numerous medications can be responsible for induction of hyperuricemia. The most common is any diuretic, particularly thiazide diuretics. The hyperuricemia of diuretics is probably caused by increased urate reabsorption at the proximal tubule. The second most common drug implicated in hyperuricemia is aspirin at doses of less than 2 g daily. Those low doses inhibit tubular secretion of urate (larger doses inhibit reabsorption and are uricosuric). Several antituberculous

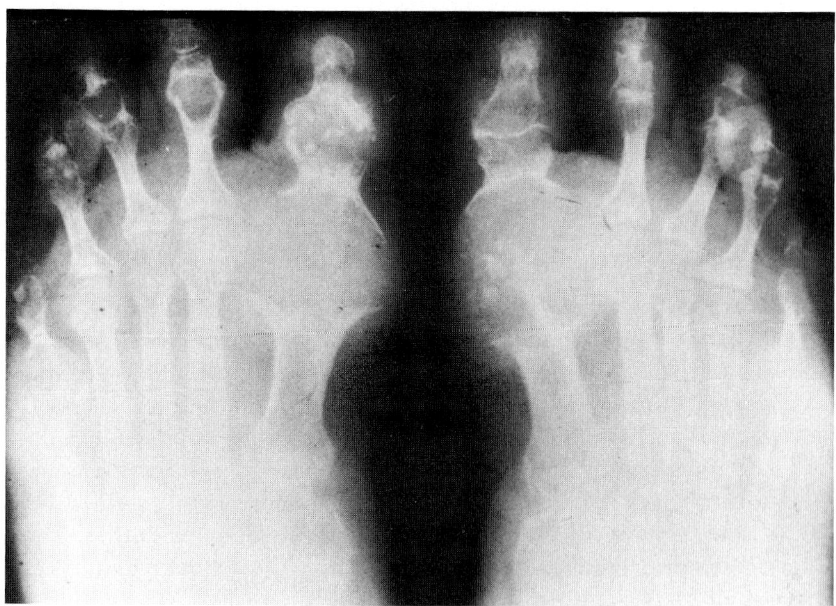

Figure 26.3. Note the massive replacement of bone by tophaceous deposits with total destruction of several joints, particularly the first metatarsophalangeal joints.

medications can cause hyperuricemia, most notably ethambutal. Alcoholism can be related to hypouricemia but is more often related to hyperuricemia by lactic acidosis (lactic acid interferes with tubular secretion of urate). Although hyperuricemia due to drugs is common, the relation of drug-induced hyperuricemia to gout is not as clear. It is probable that other factors, such as a genetic predisposition, must be present for the precipitation of crystals and acute gouty arthritis.

Hyperuricemia and gout may be due to metabolic abnormalities or associated diseases. Lactic acid production is increased and can cause hyperuricemia in starvation, diabetes mellitus, and excessive exercise. Reduced renal clearance of urate has been associated with sickle cell disease, hyperparathyroidism, hypoparathyroidism, and hyperthyroidism.

Other disease states that may be associated with hyperuricemia include sarcoidosis, beryllium disease, psoriasis, Down's syndrome, infectious mononucleosis, hypertension, hyperlipidemia, and obesity (Table 4.2).

The acute arthritis of secondary gout is identical to that of primary gout. When the hyperuricemia is related to myeloproliferative disorders, it is often marked, attacks are frequent and severe, and tophi may develop rapidly. Sex incidence is almost equal, and uric acid stone formation is common. The hyperuricemia is often due to nucleoprotein breakdown of highly metabolic cells. This breakdown may be precipitated or aggravated by chemotherapy or radiation therapy.

In chronic renal disease, the hyperuricemia is related to poor excretion of urate. Attacks of gout may not be as severe, perhaps due to the chronic illness itself or to solubility factors in the serum.

ENZYME DEFECT DISEASES

The most excessive overproduction of uric acid is associated with the Lesch-Nyhan syndrome, a sex-linked disorder of boys. This condition is characterized by hyperuricemia, compulsive self-mutilation in spite of conscious efforts by the child to prevent them, mental and growth retardation, hyperuricosuria, uric acid calculi, spasticity, and choreo-athetosis. There is a deficiency of hypoxanthine-guanine phosphoribosyl transferase (HGPRTase) (Fig. 26.1). The nearly total absence of this enzyme leads to increased purine production and hyperuricemia.

HGPRTase is the enzyme possible for conversion of guanine to guanosine monophosphate and of hypoxanthine to inosine monophosphate. Absence of this enzyme causes the failure of the body to reuse hypoxanthine; absence also augments de novo purine synthesis. Also, the coenzyme phosphoribosyl pyrophosphate synthetase (PRPPase) increases in intracellular concentration, also augmenting de novo purine synthesis. There are less complete deficiencies of this enzyme in numerous genetic forms. Increased enzyme activity of PRPPase exists in at least three genetic variants, leading to increased de novo purine biosynthesis.

Recently, deficiencies of three enzymes involved in the degradation of purines were reported in patients with immunodeficiency diseases. These enzymes were adenosine deaminase in children with severe combined immunodeficiency disease; ecto-purine-5′-nucleotidase in patients with X-linked agammaglobulinemia, and purine nucleoside phosphorylase in subjects with T-cell dysfunction.

RENAL DISEASE

There are four components for handling uric acid in the kidney: (1) filtration through the glomerulus, (2) reabsorption in the proximal tubule of 98%–100% of that filtered, (3) secretion of a variable percentage back into the distal region of the proximal tubular lumen, and (4) postsecretory reabsorption at the last portion of the proximal tubule and/or distal tubule. This process finally results in the passage of about 12% of the filtered load of uric acid into the urine. Early in chronic renal failure of various etiologies, there is increased uric acid clearance relative to creatinine. Hyperuricemia results, with progressive renal failure.

Gouty Nephropathy

Gouty nephropathy is an often loosely used term that should apply to the presence of uric acid crystals in the renal parenchyma. This deposition is of unknown physiologic and clinical significance. Renal biopsy is usually not helpful, as the crystals rarely form in the cortex but rather in the papillae, pyramids, and medullary interstitium of the kidney, where the concentration of uric acid is greatest. Deposition of crystals may stimulate foreign body reactions. It is felt that crystal deposition in the kidneys may be associated with the inability to concentrate the urine and eventually with proteinuria, pyuria, and hematuria; perhaps these problems are related to uric acid calculi. Subsequently, chronic renal insufficiency and hypertension may develop. There is increasing evidence that long-standing hyperuricemia per se is not related to progressive renal insufficiency.

Nephrolithiasis

Nephrolithiasis is a more established complication of hyperuricosuria. Hyperuricosuria is most often related to hyperuricemia. The frequently acid pH of urine decreases uric acid solubility and tends to favor precipitation of these radiolucent stones. Alkalinization of the urine will prevent most uric acid calculi. However, many stones in these patients are composed of mixed uric acid and oxalate; perhaps the uric acid or monosodium urate crystal forms a nidus that allows radiopaque stone formation. Some patients with hyperuricosuria simply form oxalate stones with no detectable urate.

The most severe form of uric acid stone formation is that associated with myelo- or lymphoproliferative diseases in which hyperuricemia is marked and further accentuated by chemotherapy. In these patients, acute renal failure can be considered to be due to uric acid if the urine urate:creatinine ratio is greater that 1.0 (persons over the age of 10 (Chap. 4).

ROENTGENOGRAMS

X-rays of the involved joints most often show soft tissue swelling unless tophaceous material has been deposited about the joints.

The most typical finding of tophi are well-defined punched-out areas of subchondral bone erosion most often of phalanges or at the ulna styloid. These deposits can extend to involve the major portion of the shaft of bone. There may be outward displacement of the cortex, with a tumor-like appearance of the eroded joint. There may be calcification within this tumorous enlargement, and chondrocalcinosis may occur. Recurrent attacks of arthritis with intrasynovial tophus may be associated with periarticular osteopenia.

DIAGNOSIS

The sine qua non for the diagnosis of gout is demonstration by arthrocentesis of negative birerefringent, toothpick-shaped, needle-like crystals of monosodium urate. These crystals may be intra- or extracellular, range in size from 1 to 5 μm in synovial fluid, and be somewhat larger in tophi. The typical appearance of these crystals "skewering" or ingested by a mononuclear leukocyte will allow the diagnosis in the absence of a polarizing light microscope.

The diagnosis may otherwise be suspected in the presence of a typical history of intermittent acute arthritis attacks that have a predominance for the lower extremity, particularly the bunion joint (see above). In these patients, there should be demonstrable hyperuricemia. Another aid to the diagnosis is a therapeutic response to colchicine.

THERAPY

Therapy for gout should be divided into two phases: (1) treatment of the acute attack and (2) prevention of recurrent attacks. The latter phase should include an approach to (a) prophylaxis for prevention of attacks and (b) control of uric acid metabolism by inducing uricosuria or inhibition of uric acid production.

Acute Attack

Traditionally, the acute attack has been treated with colchicine at 0.5 or 0.6 mg per hour for 8 hours or two tablets every 2 hours for four doses orally until the patient improves and/or toxicity develops. Dramatic but incomplete improvement can be expected within 6 hours in most patients. This is an excellent means of treating the patient with suspected gout in which the response to colchicine is one of the diagnostic criteria. In the patient whose diagnosis has been established, any of the nonsteroidal anti-inflammatory drugs (NSAID) will provide more dramatic relief with potentially fewer side effects. In patients in whom hypertension or cardiac failure is not a problem, the most potent medication might be phenylbutazone or oxyphenbutazone. This medication can be administered as 600 mg in 12 hours as a single dose or in divided doses. In patients in whom heart failure or hypertension is a problem, indomethacin may be administered as 200 mg in the first 24 hours in divided doses. In patients with active peptic ulcer disease or nothing per os, intravenous colchicine is still useful; the dose is 1–2 mg intravenously every 4 hours, and there are fewer gastrointestinal side effects than by oral use. Occasional patients will be refractory to the initial course of therapy and will require 2–5 days of NSAIDs. In these patients ACTH at 40 units intramuscularly or oral corticosteroids may be useful.

It should be pointed out that arthrocentesis may have a dual role in the acute attack. Not only can the diagnosis be established, but removal of crystals and inflammatory cells may be of benefit. However, considerable benefit can be achieved by injection of crystalline corticosteroid derivatives such as prednisolone tertiary butyl acetate, methylprednisolone acetate, or triamcinolone acetonide or hexacetonide.

Prophylaxis

Prophylaxis for recurrent attacks has been adequately achieved in most patients by the use of colchicine in doses of 0.5 or 0.6 mg daily. Persons may require up to four tablets daily for control. Colchicine is indeed the safest prophylactic medication available. On rare occasions, massive doses have been used in suicide attempts.

Control of Uric Acid Metabolism

Control of uric acid metabolism may be necessary under special circumstances (Table 26.1).

Uricosuria

Uricosuria can be obtained in the patient who is a hypoexcretor. Urate resorption can be blocked in the renal tubule by probenecid, sulfinpyrazone, and high doses of aspirin. The congener of sulfinpyrazone, phenylbutazone, is also urico-

Table 26.1. Hyperuricemia: Indications for Therapy

Frequent, uncontrolled attacks of gout
Tophaceous gout
Uric acid or combined uric acid/oxalate stones
Chronic renal disease
Lymphoproliferative or myeloproliferative diseases with/without therapy
Overproduction of uric acid (excretion of >800 mg/24 hr with a purine-free diet)
Hyperuricemia in excess of 3 mg/100 ml over the normal upper range

suric but is not generally prescribed for long-term use. Alkalinization of the urine to a pH of greater than 6 is required with this therapy. These agents are most helpful when the serum uric acid elevation is 2 mg/100 ml or less. Probenecid is initially used as 500 mg daily and gradually increased to 2 g daily; long-term safety is established with this agent. Sulfinpyrazone is used initially at 80 mg daily, with gradual increases to 400 mg if needed.

Uric Acid Production

Uric acid production can often be inhibited in hypoexcretors by reduction of purine foods in the diet. However, in most patients, diet control alone is not adequate. Allopurinol is metabolized to oxipurinol by xanthine oxidase in about 3 hours. Oxipurinol has a prolonged half-life and, as with allopurinol, inhibits the enzyme xanthine oxidase; this inhibition lowers the intracellular concentration of PRPPase. A single daily dose of 100–300 mg of allopurinol is usually adequate to bring serum uric acid into the normal range. This is a potent agent usually with minor toxicity related to gastrointestinal symptoms. However, in the indiscriminant use of this agent there is potential danger of granulomatous hepatitis with hepatic necrosis, exfoliative dermatitis or toxic epidermal necrolysis, agranulocytosis, and hypersensitivity vasculitis. Care should be used when administering purine antagonists such as azathioprine and 6-mercaptopurine; doses reduced to 20%–30% should be employed when allopurinol is used. There are increased dermatologic reactions when using allopurinol and ampicillin in combination. Use of allopurinol has been associated with precipitating acute attacks of gout; colchicine should be maintained for at least the first 6 weeks of allopurinol therapy and perhaps indefinitely.

Treatment of asymptomatic hyperuricemia should be performed only when there is great risk of some complication, such as gout or stone formation.

Additional therapeutic measures that may be of value in tophaceous gout include orthopedic excision of tophi and arthroplasty, particularly when impaired function or drainage is present.

BIBLIOGRAPHY

Bluestone R, Waisman J, Klinenberg JR: The gouty kidney. *Semin Arthritis Rheum* 7:97, 1977.

Boss GR, Seegmiller JE: Hyperuricemia and gout. *N Engl J Med* 300:1459, 1979.

Hadler NM, Franck WA, Bress NM, et al: Acute polyarticular gout. *Am J Med* 56:715, 1974.

Hall AP, Barry PE, Dawber TR, et al: Epidemiology of gout and hyperuricemia: A long-term population study. *Am J Med* 42:27, 1967.

Holmes EW, Kelley WN, Wyngaarden JB: Control of purine biosynthesis in normal and pathologic states. *Bull Rheum Dis* 26:848, 1975–1976.

Kelley WN: Pathophysiology of purine metabolism in man. *Enzyme* 18:161, 1974.

Kelley WN: Current therapy of gout and hyperuricemia. *Hosp Pract* 11:69, 1976.

Lesch M, Nyhan WL: A familial disorder of uric acid metabolism and central nervous system function. *Am J Med* 36:561, 1964.

Seegmiller JE: Human aberrations of purine metabolism and their significance for rheumatology. *Ann Rheum Dis* 39:103, 1980.

Simkin PA: Management of gout. *Ann Intern Med* 90:812, 1979.

Talbott JH, Yii T: *Gout and Uric Acid Metabolism*. Stratton Intercontinental Medical Book Corp, 1976.

Wallace SL: The treatment of gout. *Arthritis Rheum* 15:317, 1972.

Wallace SL, Robinson H, Masi AT, et al: Preliminary criteria for the classification of the acute arthritis of primary gout. *Arthritis Rheum* 20:895, 1977.

27

Chondrocalcinosis and Pseudogout

Robert G. Gray

Roy D. Altman

A form of ectopic calcification in the articular and para-articular structures is called *calcium pyrophosphate dihydrate crystal deposition disease (CPPD)*. CPPD generally occurs sporadically, although familial aggregation has been described. Sporadic CPPD rarely is manifest under the age of 50 years, exhibits no clear sex preference, and may be associated with various metabolic and endocrinopathic disorders in a minority of patients (Table 27.1).

Chondrocalcinosis is relatively common in the aged. Radiologic surveys of knee joints have detected meniscal calcification in 7%–28% of elderly populations. Only a minority of persons with chondrocalcinosis appear to develop the symptomatic arthropathy termed *pseudogout*. Diagnostic criteria for pseudogout are (1) the presence of calcium pyrophosphate dihydrate crystals, (2a) monoclinic and triclinic crystals with weakly positive birefringence by compensated polarized light microscopy, (2b) the radiographic presence of typical calcifications, (3a) acute arthritis, and (3b) chronic arthritis. A definite diagnosis is accepted when criterion 1 or 2a plus 2b is fulfilled. A probable diagnosis is entertained when either criterion 2a or 2b is met. Possible disease should be considered when either criterion 3a or 3b is appreciated.

CLINICAL FEATURES

The clinical spectrum of CPPD extends from a noninflammatory degenerative arthropathy simulating osteoarthritis to an inflammatory polyarticular disease that resembles rheumatoid arthritis. Five clinical patterns of CPPD have been characterized by McCarty (Table 27.2).

Acute pseudogout is a mono- or oligoarticular crystal-induced synovitis of sudden onset. This condition occurs in nearly 25% of all patients with CPPD. The acute attack is self-limited, with spontaneous resolution within days to weeks. Diagnosis requires identification in synovial fluid of intracellular positively birefringent rhomboid-shaped crystals. The radiologic finding of chondrocalcinosis

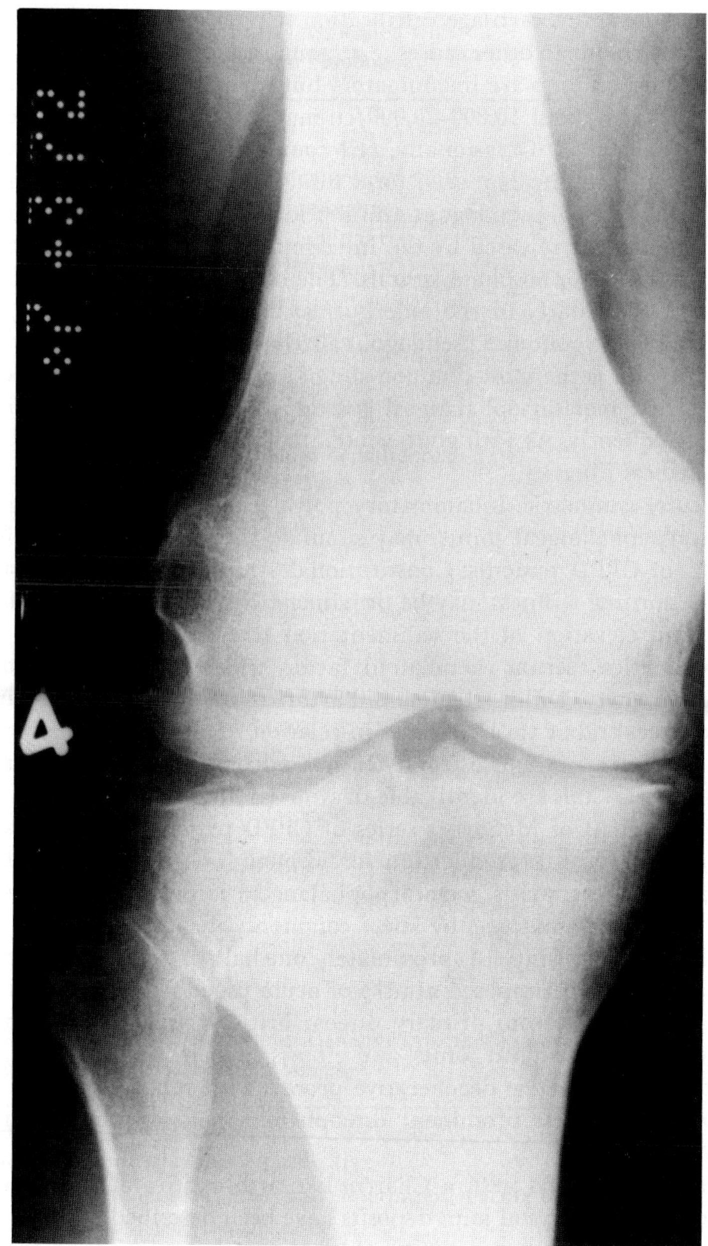

Figure 27.1. Note both meniscal calcification of the knee in the lateral and medial compartments and cartilaginous calcification at the lateral surface of the medial femoral condyle.

pubis, shoulder labra, and the annulus fibrosis of intervertebral discs). Hyaline cartilage calcification appears as a linear deposit paralleling the joint line. Capsular, bursal, and tendinous calcification is frequent and often appears more fluffy and amorphous than cartilage deposits. Occasionally, acute pseudogout is demonstrated in joints lacking chondrocalcinosis. In such cases, cartilage deposits of calcium pyrophosphate may be insufficiently dense to be radiologically visible or may be masked by extensive degenerative changes with joint space (cartilage) loss.

Subchondral cysts, often large, and erosive changes resembling the destructive process of rheumatoid arthritis may be seen. Osteophyte formation is common but usually less than one might anticipate on the basis of cartilage loss. Hook-like osteophytes of the metacarpophalangeal joints appear to be characteristic. An unusual erosive change of the anterior femur, associated with patellofemoral compartment osteoarthritis, has been reported.

A radiologic screening for CPPD should include anteroposterior views of the knees and pelvis and a posteroanterior view of the wrists.

PATHOGENESIS

The pathogenesis of CPPD is detailed, in part, in Chapter 25. Although the pathogenesis of the disease is not known, some insights are possible. Crystal deposition may well be the final common pathway of many metabolic disturbances (as for urate). The crystals themselves do provoke synovitis when injected intra-articularly. Tentative reports of increased synovial fluid pyrophosphate and decreased alkaline phosphate suggest that impaired pyrophosphatase activity may be important in crystal accumulation and deposition. Rupture of preformed crystalline deposits into the joint space probably results in phagocytosis, lysosomal enzyme release, and subsequent inflammation. Crystal deposition in cartilage leads to chondrocyte death and degenerative changes.

TREATMENT

The acute attack of pseudogout responds readily to thorough joint aspiration and the instillation of microcrystalline corticosteroid preparation. Colchicine (orally and intravenously) reportedly has produced a rapid response in some patients. Polyarticular pseudogout and CPPD characterized by subacute or chronic inflammatory or degenerative arthritis may be managed by a variety of non-steroidal anti-inflammatory agents (salicylates, phenylbutaone, indomethacin, ibuprofen, and others).

Treatment or control of associated disorders does not seem to prevent the recurrence of acute attacks.

The material in the *Pathogenesis* section appears in similar form in Panush RS: Other rheumatic diseases with immunologic features, in Lockey RF (ed): *Allergy and Clinical Immunology.* Garden City, NY, Medical Examination Publishing Co, Inc, an Excerpta Medica company, © 1979, pp 277–278. Reprinted by permission.

BIBLIOGRAPHY

Genant H: Roentgenographic aspects of calcium pyrophosphate dihydrate crystal deposition disease (pseudogout), *Arthritis Rheum* 19:307, 1976.

Gerster JC, Vischer TL, Boussina I, et al: Joint destruction and chondrocalcinosis in patients with generalized osteoarthrosis. *Br Med J* 4:684, 1975.

Glass JS, Grahame R: Chondrocalcinosis after parathyroidectomy. *Ann Rheum Dis* 35: 521, 1976.

Hamilton EBD: Diseases associated with CPPD deposition disease. *Arthritis Rheum* 19: 353, 1976.

Hamilton EBD, Richards AJ: Destructive arthropathy in chondrocalcinosis articularis. *Ann Rheum Dis* 33:196, 1974.

Jacobelli S, McCarty DJ, Silcox DC, et al: Calcium pyrophosphate dihydrate crystal deposition in neuropathic joints: Four cases of polyarticular involvement. *Ann Intern Med* 79:340, 1973.

Martel W, Champion CK, Thompson GR, et al: A roentgenographically distinctive arthropathy in some patients with pseudogout syndrome. *Am J Roentgenol Rad Ther Nucl Med* 109:587, 1970.

McCarty DJ: Diagnostic mimicry in arthritis—patterns of joint involvement associated with calcium pyrophosphate dihydrate crystal deposits. *Bull Rheum Dis* 25:804, 1975.

McCarty DJ: Calcium pyrophosphate dihydrate crystal deposition disease—clinical aspects. *Clin Rheum Dis* 3.01, 1977.

McCarty DJ, Gatter RA: Pseudogout syndrome (articular chondrocalcinosis). *Bull Rheum Dis* 14:331, 1964.

McCarty DJ, Hogan JM, Gatter RA, et al: Studies on pathological calcifications in human cartilage. I. Prevalence and types of crystal deposits in the menisci of two hundred fifteen cadavera. *J Bone Joint Surg* 48A:309, 1966.

McCarty DJ, Silcox DC, Coe F, et al: Diseases associated with calcium pyrophosphate dihydrate crystal deposition: A controlled study. *Am J Med* 56:704, 1974.

O'Duffy JD: Clinical studies of acute pseudogout attacks: Comments on prevalence, predispositions, and treatment. *Arthritis Rheum* 19:349, 1976.

Utsinger PD, Zvaifler, NJ, Resnick, D: Calcium pyrophosphate dihydrate deposition disease without chondrocalcinosis. *J Rheumatol* 2:258, 1975.

28

Paget's and Metabolic Diseases of Bone

Roy D. Altman

PAGET'S DISEASE

Paget's disease is a chronic abnormality of the adult skeleton in which localized areas of hyperactive bone are replaced by a softened and enlarged osseous structure; involved bones have a tendency toward bowing, fracture, and malignant degeneration. Sir James Paget gave the first clear clinical and pathologic description of the disease in 1877.

Incidence

Paget's disease is particularly common in Great Britain, Western Europe (except Scandinavia), Australia, and New Zealand. In Great Britain the incidence appears to be about 3% of the adult population. The disease occurs in men 1.5 times as often as in women. It is detected above the age of 50 in over 80% of cases and rarely below the age of 30. It is most common in Caucasians, with only occasional reported cases in blacks, Orientals, and natives of India. The etiology is unknown. There is some familial tendency, but no genetic pattern has yet been defined.

Pathology and Pathophysiology

Histologically, involved bone demonstrates an increase in the active bone surface and in the number of bone surface cells (osteoclasts and osteoblasts). There is considerable variation in the size of the osteoclasts, which often contain several nuclei. Osteoclastic nuclei contain inclusions suggesting a viral etiology. The normal lamellar pattern is replaced by a coarse woven pattern (mosaic). An elevation of bone collagen destruction and synthesis is reflected in high values of urine hydroxyproline peptide excretion. Increased bone formation surface is registered by an elevation in serum alkaline phosphatase and isocitrate dehydrogenase activity. The most common sites of predilection are (in decreasing order of frequency) the pelvis and sacrum, femur, tibia, skull, lumbar and dorsal vertebrae, and clavicle, with a slight preponderance of lesions on the right side of the body; however, virtually any bone in the body may become diseased.

Afflicted long bones become structurally weakened, with a tendency to deformity and fracture. Complete fracture or microfractures (infarctions) of long bones and compression fractures of vertebrae at Paget's disease sites are common. Rapid bone replacement leads to enlargement of the existing bone, which may precipitate compression neuropathy. Juxtaposition of Paget's disease to an articulation may lead to degenerative joint disease. Extensive bone remodeling is associated with a local increased bony blood flow; a resultant high-output cardiac state with or without cardiac failure may ensue. Sarcomatous degeneration occurs in less than 1% of pagetic lesions but is 40 times the frequency of a nonpagetic population. These tumors are usually osteogenic sarcomas encompassing varying histologic types.

Clinical Features

Most of the disease is asymptomatic. Often the early diagnosis is made accidentally by elevated serum alkaline phosphatase or by a roentgenologic examination for other purposes. Initial knowledge of the disease may occur when the patient appears with a fracture through a Paget's disease site, the most common serious complication of the disease.

When symptoms occur, their onset is insidious and clinical manifestations may often be realized only after 20–30 years of disease. They include general stiffness and fatigability, deformity, pain, headaches, dizziness, tinnitus, decrease of auditory and visual acuity, increased hat size, and excessive heat over a long bone or clavicle. Pain in Paget's bones is aching, deep, occasionally severe, reminiscent of osteomalacic bone pain, and may be accentuated at night. Often pain arises from compression neuropathy or associated secondary arthritis. In the presence of osteoarthritis, one must be wary of attributing pain to juxta-articular Paget's disease.

Signs of the disease may be bitemporal skull enlargement with frontal "bossing," dilated scalp veins, nerve deafness or otosclerosis in one or both ears with or without vestibular signs, angioid streaks of the optical fundus, a short kyphotic trunk with simian appearance and hobbling gait, anterolateral bow of the femur or tibia, warmth, or periostial tenderness. The intensity of symptoms and signs is highly variable (Fig. 28.1).

Roentgenologic Manifestations and Bone Scans

The initial radiologic lesion is a radiolucent zone of bone resorption that follows the histologic pattern. This "lytic" zone is replaced by a coarse, heavy, abnormal-appearing trabecular pattern, frequently heavily calcified and accompanied by enlargement of the external contours of the bone (Fig. 28.2).

Areas of early, active, and symptomatic Paget's disease may be detected by bone scans before a change appears in the roentgenographic pattern. The bone scan is useful in delineating the extent of Paget's disease.

Diagnosis

In its advanced stages, this disease should be readily distinguishable from other disorders. The serum alkaline phosphatase is elevated in active Paget's disease

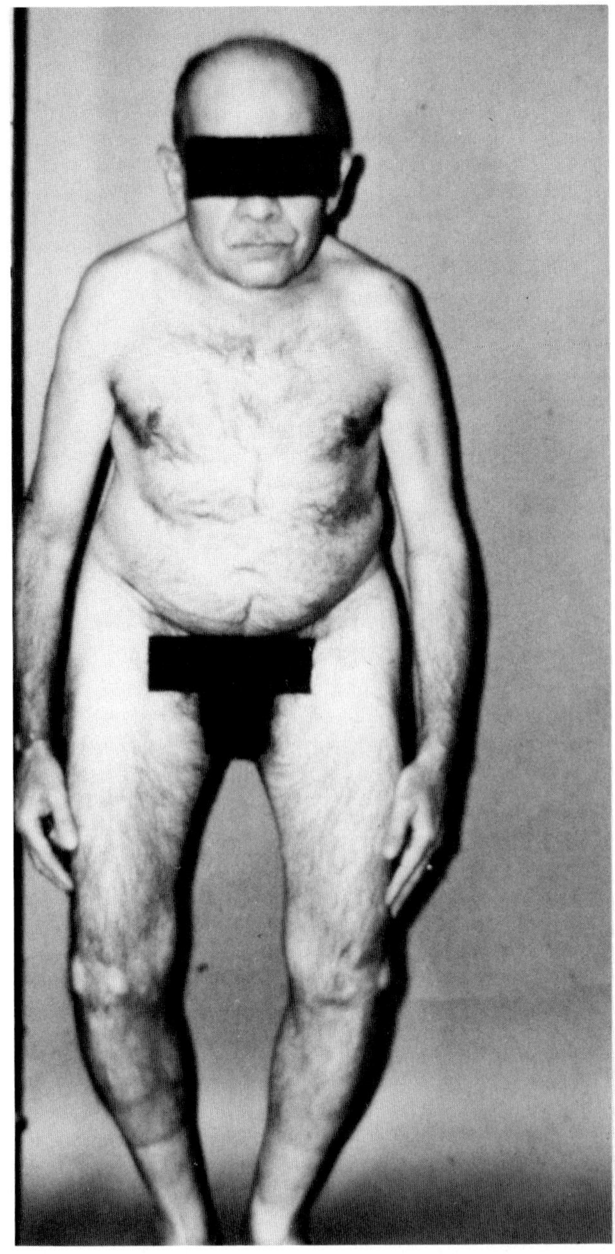

Figure 28.1. A subject with severe Paget's disease of bone demonstrating physical findings of a shortened stature with simian posture, frontal bossing, enlarged right clavicle, and anterior and lateral bowing of thighs and legs.

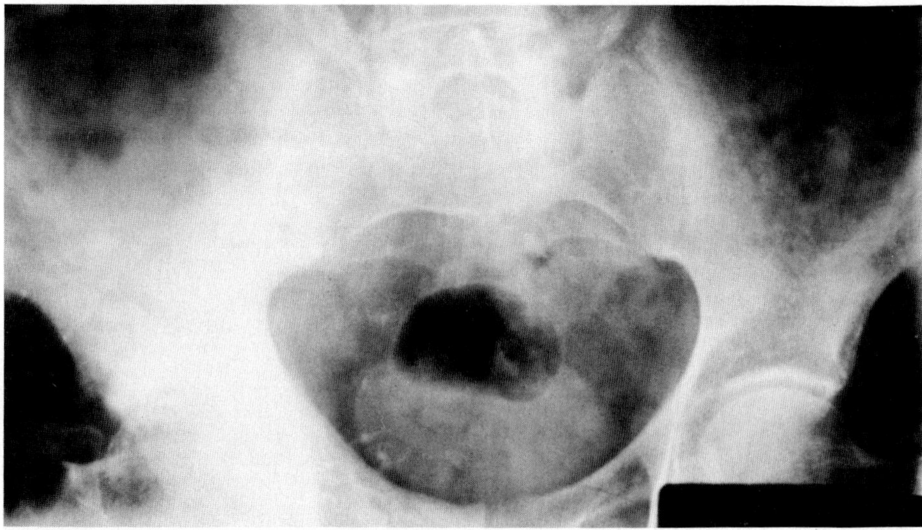

Figure 28.2. Pelvis x-ray of a subject with extensive involvement of the entire pelvis and both femora. The disorganized coarse trabecular pattern is characteristic of this disease. Note the thickened ileopectineal line. There is loss of the radiologic joint space of the right hip.

unless the condition is limited. Serum and urine calcium determinations are normal unless immobilization has accelerated calcium absorption from bone. When serum acid phosphatase is slightly to moderately elevated, Paget's disease must be differentiated from metastatic prostatic carcinoma. Extreme elevation of serum acid phosphatase is distinctly uncommon in Paget's disease. Prostatic carcinoma does not involve the iliopectineal line radiographically.

Only an occasional patient will need bone biopsy to differentiate Paget's disease from other bone disease, unless there is progressive severe pain and/or a radiologic suggestion of malignant degeneration or coexistent malignant disease.

For the workup of increased serum alkaline phosphatase on routine examination, at present there is no method that consistently differentiates serum alkaline phosphatase related to bone anabolism from other sources, for example, the liver. Inasmuch as leucine aminopeptidase is handled similarly to alkaline phosphatase in the liver, when elevated, it suggests the hepatic origin of the alkaline phosphatase. When serum alkaline phosphatase is from bone, the bone scan will help define the site of origin. An x-ray is then needed to define further the bony abnormality.

Therapy

Most often the disease is localized, asymptomatic, and requires no treatment. Therapy is often aimed at the correction of a specific complication such as a neural compression.

Salicylates or nonsteroidal anti-inflammatory agents may reduce the pain of osteoarthritis. Synthetic salmon calcitonin is administered subcutaneously and has demonstrated reduction of bone turnover in Paget's disease. Initially, it inhibits osteoclasts and stimulates osteoblasts. It may be useful in retarding the advancing "osteolytic wedge." After prolonged use, the osteoblasts are also inhibited, but prolonged therapy has demonstrated some return of a more normal histologic picture. Several patients have demonstrated bradyphylaxis after 1–2 years of therapy. Some of these patients have demonstrated antibodies to the calcitonin. Synthetic salmon calcitonin is usually administered as 50–100 mrc subcutanteously daily or up to once weekly adjusted to the response. Disodium etidronate (a salt) is a pyrophosphate analogue that has demonstrated a reduction in the indices of bone turnover in Paget's disease. It reduces osteoclastic activity and tends to return bone to a more normal histologic picture. The initial course is 5 mg/kg/day po for 6 months. Mithramycin is a potent antibiotic causing a reduction of osteoclasts (cytotoxic). It is administered intravenously at 15–25 mg/kg/day for 10 days. Common side effects are nausea and vomiting. Potential hematologic, hepatic, and renal toxicity should limit its use to disabled or severely affected persons. There is evidence that mithramycin, calcitonin, and disodium etidronate reduce the high-output cardiac state toward normal. Patients treated with mithramycin or disodium etidronate may have complete or near-complete remission of their disease for years after the initial therapy.

OSTEOPOROSIS

Osteoporosis is characterized by a bone that has become lighter with loss of calcium and matrix. Osteoporosis is the most common metabolic bone disorder in clinical practice, involving as many as 25% of 70-year-old women.

Bone mass is anabolic before the age of 20, related to growth and a balance between resorption and deposition of new bone. Bone mass becomes maximum at ages 20–35. After the age of 35, a slight imbalance between resorption and deposition of bone leads to decreasing increments of bone each year. It has been noted that men have a greater total bone mass than women and that blacks have a greater total bone mass than whites. Removal of gonads appears to hasten this imbalance. Central bones (vertebrae) lose a greater percentage of bone mass than do more peripheral (long) bones. Numerous other factors may hasten this imbalance, for example, starvation; malignancy; hyperthyroidism; acromegaly; Cushing's syndrome (idiopathic or iatrogenic); immobilization due to splints, casts, or paralysis; diabetes mellitus; chronic heparin therapy; and chronic disabling illnesses such as rheumatoid arthritis. Postmenopausal women comprise 80% of persons with this affliction.

Histologically, the bone is porous, with large vascular channels separated by thinned and sparse trabeculae. There is an increase in resorptive surface and numerous lytic osteocytes with calcification of their lacunea.

Most commonly, patients report pain related to spinal compression fractures, but they may incur long bone fractures, particularly of the femoral neck. Of note is that increasing osteoporosis relates to fractures more distal to the femoral head.

Postmenopausal patients are usually stooped over with a "dowager's hump," flared pelvis, short stature, and thin body build. Roentgenography reveals osteopenia, but this osteoporosis cannot be differentiated from other losses of body calcium such as by osteomalacia or multiple myeloma. Vertebrae may lose their height, particularly in the center of the vertebra, giving a "codfish" biconcave indentation in the vertebrae by the intervertebral disc.

There is no presently known effective medication for this condition. Perhaps newer vitamin D derivatives and diphosphonate salts will prove of benefit in the future. Presently, in the immediate postmenopausal state, female hormone replacement may have benefit. No benefit has been detected if this treatment is begun more than 10 years after menopause. These agents have the added risk of increasing uterine carcinomas and might best be used in patients who have had a prior hysterectomy.

Calcium salts have demonstrated the least risk and possibly the greatest benefit. The addition of vitamin D (D_2) has no proven benefit but is in regular use on teleologic grounds. The use of fluoride is controversial. The role of 1,25dihydrocholecalciferol ($1,25OHD_3$) or 25hydroxycholecalciferol ($25OHD_3$) in the routine patient is uncertain at this time. Careful use of $1,25OHD_3$ or $25OHD_3$ is limited to hemodialysis patients.

General measures should not be overlooked. Pain relief is important. Activities are to be encouraged, as bed rest aggravates the osteoporosis. Analgesics, splinting, and exercise are encouraged. Diet has not been shown to alter the course of this disease.

OSTEOMALACIA

Osteomalacia is characterized by inadequate calcification of bone matrix (osteoid), causing weakening and structural alteration of bone. The disease is related to inadequate calcium or vitamin D due to dietary or metabolic causes.

Although osteomalacia (adults) or rickets (children) has many etiologies, the most common causes in the United States are related to chronic renal failure and malabsorption syndromes. Occasionally osteomalacia is seen in undernourished subjects (drug addiction, malignancy), related to specific congenital defects (renal tubular vitamin D-resistant rickets, Fanconi's syndrome), or growth that exceeds dietary calcium (pregnancy, hyperthyroidism).

Pathophysiologically, osteoblastic activity synthesizes adequate osteoid matrix, but the calcification process is disrupted. The resulting trabeculae are normal except for widened seams with uncalcified osteoid. Numerous osteoblasts are present. The resultant bone is softened, demonstrating stress fractures (Looser zones, microfractures) of long bones. The serum alkaline phosphatase is elevated. Serum calcium is most often normal but may be reduced. Serum phosphorus is most often low.

Spine and long bone pain with tenderness is aggravated by activities often leading to a waddling type of gait. Chvostek's or Trousseau's signs may predict reduced serum calcium. Spinal compression fractures may lead to radicular pain. Pathologic fractures, particularly of the femoral neck, may occur. Growing bones may demonstrate poorly mineralized epiphyseal plates, particularly long bones.

The diagnosis may be suspected by the radiographic findings of osteopenia with an elevated serum alkaline phosphatase, normal serum calcium, and reduced serum phosphorus. However, many patients have combined metabolic bone diseases, and a bone biopsy may be needed to determine the defects. Processing of undecalcified bone biopsy specimens greatly aids this differentiation.

Therapy includes vitamin D, 50,000 units daily, and a calcium salt, up to 30 g daily, until healing is noted on the x-ray, and the serum alkaline phosphatase returns toward normal. One should follow urine and serum calcium and alter the dose of vitamin D2 and calcium if elevations occur, in order to prevent iatrogenic nephrolithiasis and hyperparathyroidism.

HYPERPARATHYROIDISM

Hyperparathyroidism, a metabolic bone disease of parathormone (PTH) excess, is characterized by accelerated diffuse bone destruction resulting in large bone cysts and giant cell tumors—Von Recklinghausen's disease.

Chief cell adenomas of one or more of the parathyroid glands or hyperplasia related to carcinoma comprise the primary forms. Most secondary forms are related to chronic renal disease, osteomalacia, and hyperthyroidism.

Pathologically, bone matrix reveals bone cysts, increased resorptive surface, and "brown tumors" composed of masses of osteoid cells.

Laboratory findings are characterized by an elevated serum calcium, depressed serum inorganic phosphate, and normal or mildly increased alkaline phosphatase.

Many patients with increased PTH are asymptomatic, which may be related to the high calcium-phosphorus diet in the United States. When symptoms occur, they include anorexia, epigastric distress, nausea, vomiting, weakness, constipation, change in mental status with possible psychosis and coma, renal lithiasis, and possible progressive renal failure.

In patients with a low calcium-phosphorus diet, diffuse extremity pain with bone tenderness may often be mistaken for arthritis or neuritis. Chronic disease may lead to deposition of calcium in unusual places such as cartilage, inducing chondrocalcinosis and possibly pseudogout. Kyphosis, bending of long bones, loss of teeth, and pigeon breast deformity may be found in physical examination.

X-rays demonstrate the brown tumors, often in the jaw, metacarpals, metatarsals, and ends of long bones. Osteopenia on x-ray may relate to codfish deformities of vertebrae, subperiosteal bone resorption, "ground glass" texture of the skull, jagged resorption of the distal digital tufts, nephrolithiasis, and resorption of the lamina dura about the teeth.

Hyperparathyroidism must be differentiated from other causes of hypercalcemia such as metastatic bone disease. On some occasions, particularly in the presence of chronic renal disease, the serum calcium is normal. A bone biopsy may be necessary to differentiate hyperparathyroidism from osteomalacia. Although methods are variable, more laboratories are providing reliable serum parathormone values. This information simplifies an often difficult task of diagnosis. No present method consistently localizes the parathyroid gland containing the tumor.

Removal of the parathyroid tumor leads to rapid repair of bone; this process requires aggressive replacement of calcium with a vitamin D supplement. A magnesium supplement may be necessary to prevent tetany. Perhaps in the near future, oral suppressive therapy of PTH will replace surgery in many cases.

BIBLIOGRAPHY

Barry HC: *Paget's Disease of Bone*. Edinburgh, E and S Livingston, 1969.

Frame B, Parfitt AM: Osteomalacia: Current concepts. *Ann Intern Med* 89:966, 1978.

Gallagher JC, Riggs BL: Current topics in nutrition: Nutrition and bone disease. *N Engl J Med* 248:193, 1978.

Haddad JG: Caldwell JG: Calcitonin resistance: Clinical and immunologic studies in subjects with Paget's disease of bone treated with porcine and salmon calcitonins. *J Clin Invest* 51:3133, 1972.

Hahn TJ, Hahn BH: Osteopenia in patients with rheumatic diseases: Principles of diagnosis and therapy. *Semin Arthritis Rheum* 6:165, 1976.

Kairi MRA, Altman RD, DeRosa GP, et al: Sodium etidronate in the treatment of Paget's disease of bone. *Ann Intern Med* 87:656, 1977.

Lutwak L, Singer FR, Urist MR: Current concepts of bone metabolism. *Ann Intern Med* 80:630, 1974.

Nagant de Deuxchaisnes C, Krane SM: Paget's disease of bone: Clinical and metabolic observations. *Medicine* 43:233, 1964.

Paget J: On a form of chronic inflammation of bones (osteitis deformans). *Med Chir Trans* 60:37, 1877.

Ryan WG, Schwartz TB, Northrop G: Treatment of Paget's disease with mithramycin: Further experiences. *Semin Drug Treat* 2:57, 1972.

Part 6

NONARTICULAR RHEUMATISM

29

Regional Musculoskeletal Syndromes: The Neck and Upper Extremities

Bernard F. Germain

Painful musculoskeletal syndromes are a leading cause of office consultation. These disorders are commonly encountered in the practice of family physicians, internists, rheumatologists, and orthopedists. They are a source of potential misdiagnosis and mistreatment. A number of common musculoskeletal pain syndromes involve the neck and upper extremities. A thorough history and a careful examination combined with a basic knowledge of anatomy permit an accurate diagnosis.

THE CERVICAL SPINE

Cervical Disc Disease

The most common condition causing a painful neck is cervical disc disease or cervical spondylosis. In this disease there are degenerative changes of the intervertebral discs of the cervical spine. This degeneration usually occurs at C4–5 and C5–6. The patient complains of posterior neck pain, sometimes radiating up the back of the head. Extension of the neck (looking upward) or lateral movement often exacerbates the pain. The patient may hear or feel a grinding noise in the posterior neck; the discomfort may be constant or intermittent. Radicular pain occurs if the protruded disc material presses on a nerve root; this pain may radiate to the shoulder or down the arm.

Cervical disc-derived pain may also be referred to the interscapular area. Cervical disc disease should always be considered in a patient with upper back pain, particularly between the scapulae. Physical examination reveals limitation and pain with motion of the cervical spine. Frequently the patient's pain can be reproduced by a particular movement of the cervical spine; this process is very helpful diagnostically. The cervical spine should be gently extended, flexed, rotated to the left and right, and then laterally flexed both to the right and to the left.

Limited or painful motion will be evident if cervical disc disease is present. Testing of muscle strength, sensory intactness, and reflexes will indicate the extent of neurologic involvement. Most patients with painful disc disease will not have a neurologic deficit.

Radiologic examination of the cervical spine is important only to rule out other causes of neck pain and to satisfy the curiosity of the physician and patient. The severity of x-ray evidence of disc disease correlates poorly with the clinical picture. Typically, there is loss of disc space height, sclerosis of the contiguous vertebrae, and osteophyte formation (Figs. 5.13 and 29.1). These conditions are particularly evident on the lateral film. Oblique films demonstrate osteophyte encroachment on intervertebral neural foramina (Fig. 29.2).

Treatment is for the most part conservative. Nonsteroidal anti-inflammatory drugs are helpful—aspirin, indomethacin, ibuprofen, fenoprofen, naproxen, tol-

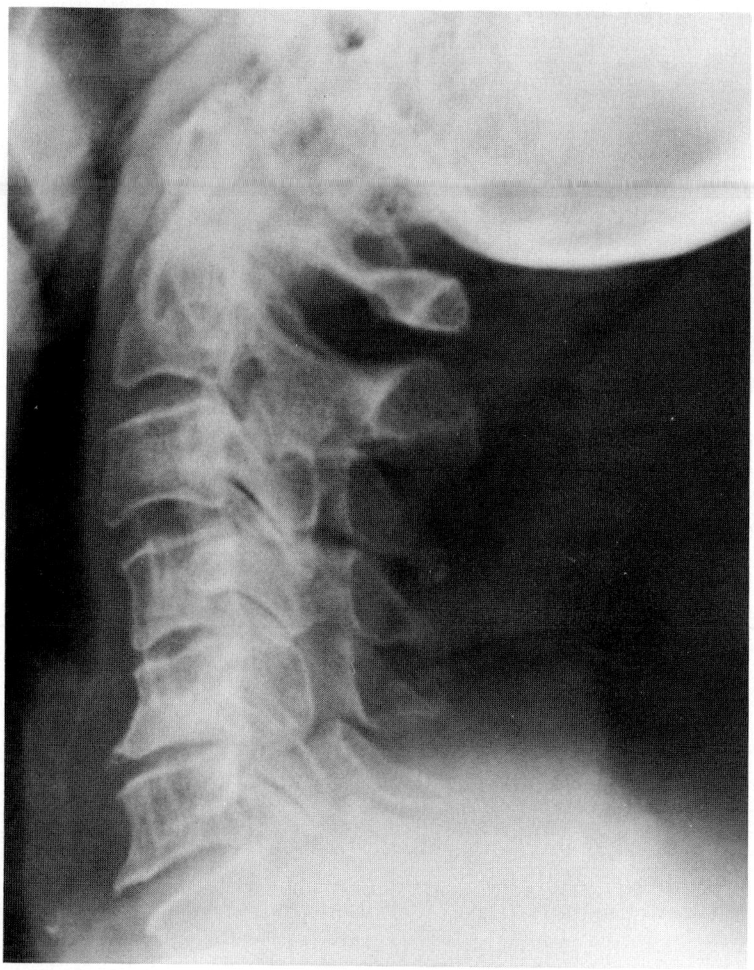

Figure 29.1. Cervical disc disease; note narrowing of the intervertebral discs at C4–5, C5–6, and C6–7. Both anterior and posterior osteophytes are present.

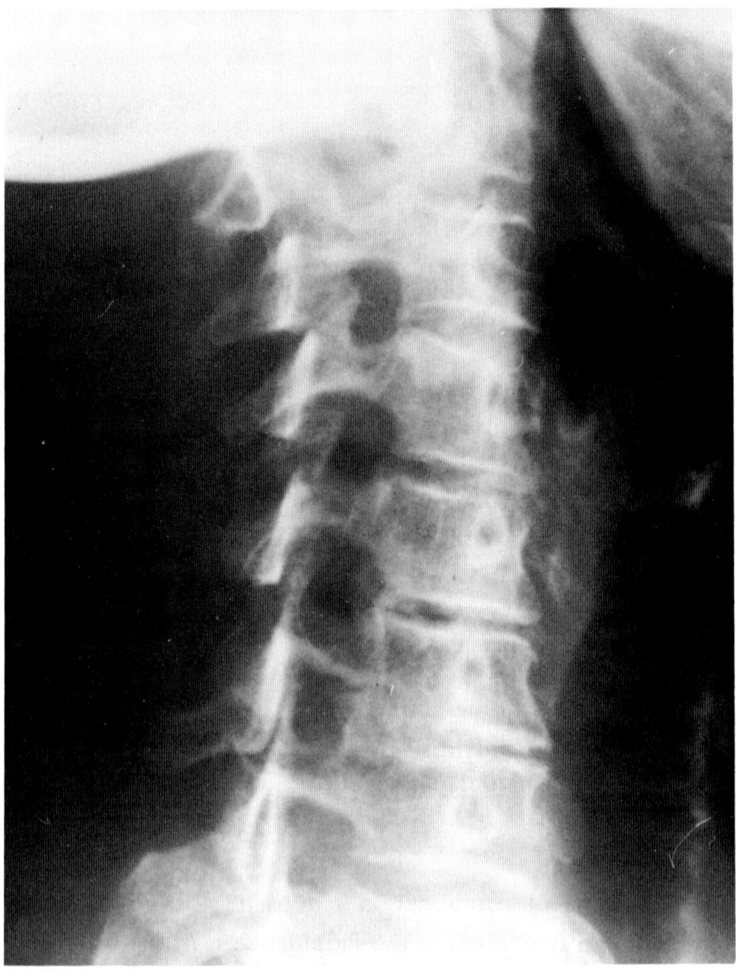

Figure 29.2. Cervical disc disease; oblique view demonstrating osteophytes encroaching on the intervertebral foramina.

metin, and sulindac. Analgesics such as propoxyphene and acetaminophen are also useful. The application of wet heat may relieve muscle spasm and pain, and isometric exercises are often beneficial. Posture is of great importance; the patient should avoid hypertension and prolonged flexion of the neck. Television viewing provides a daily period of poor posture, as may certain work habits. The patient should sleep supine, arms by the side, with either no pillow or a thin pillow under the neck. A soft cervical collar worn for a short period (1 week) helps to remind the patient to keep the neck in a neutral position. Home traction using 6–8 lb of weight twice daily for 15–20 minutes can be effective when employed on a regular basis. Surgical intervention is rarely necessary but should be considered if radicular symptoms do not respond to good medical management. A progressive neurologic deficit would hasten the surgical approach.

If osteophytes occur posteriorly and impinge on the spinal column, cervical

wrist drop and may mimic a ruptured extensor tendon, as commonly occurs in the rheumatoid hand. Differentiation includes numbness in the first dorsal webb space and an inability to extend the interphalangeal joint of the thumb when the radial nerve is involved.

BIBLIOGRAPHY

Bland JH, Merrit JA, Boushey DR: The painful shoulder. *Semin Arthritis Rheum* 7:21–47, 1977.

Cailliet R: *Neck and Arm Pain*. Philadelphia, FA Davis Co, 1964.

Cailliet R: *Shoulder Pain*. Philadelphia, FA Davis Co, 1966.

Cailliet R: *Hand Pain and Impairment*. Philadelphia, FA Davis Co, 1971.

Germain BF (ed): *Osteoarthritis and Musculoskeletal Pain Syndromes*. Garden City, NY, Medical Examination Publishing Co (in preparation).

Kopell HP, Thompson WAL: *Peripheral Nerve Entrapment Neuropathies*. Baltimore, Williams & Wilkins Co, 1963.

Marmor L: Surgery of osteoarthritis. *Semin Arthritis Rheum* 2:117–156, 1972.

30

Regional Musculoskeletal Syndromes: The Back and Lower Extremities

Selden Longley

Regional musculoskeletal syndromes may be manifestations of purely local phenomena or of systemic disease. Not only rheumatic but also vascular, neurologic, or metabolic problems may appear as regional pain syndromes. Recognition and accurate diagnosis of these conditions are challenging, satisfying, and necessary for appropriate treatment of systemic or local disease.

This section will address first the hip and thigh, then the knee and calf, and last the ankle and foot. The low back will be addressed indirectly as pain reflected in the lower extremity. Emphasis will be placed on distinguishing historic features and physical maneuvers. Radiographs and special ancillary tests will be discussed last and their role in differential diagnosis emphasized.

HIP AND THIGH

Hip problems should be considered by sequential assessment of the systems that may affect the area; muscular, vascular, bone, and neurologic.

Muscular Diseases

Polymyositis

Hip girdle musculature is commonly a source of disability with both polymyositis and polymyalgia rheumatica. A patient with polymyositis is typically a 45-year-old woman with symmetric proximal muscle weakness. Both hip and shoulder girdle musculature are affected. The patient has difficulty in both rising from a chair and abducting the shoulder to brush her hair or teeth. Inflammatory muscle disease is confirmed by the elevation of muscle enzymes—creatine phosphokinase (CPK), serum glutamic oxaloacetic transaminase (SGOT), and lactic dehydrogenase (LDH)—and abnormalities on electromyogram and muscle biopsy (Chap. 4).

Table 30.1. Muscular Diseases Affecting the Hip Girdle/Lower Extremity

Major Categories	Type of Inheritance	Clinical Onset	Initial Symptoms
Myositis			
Polymyositis/ dermatomyositis (P/DM)	—	Fifth decade	Proximal muscle weakness, 25% experience myalgias, often with a reddish skin eruption on face and upper trunk
P/DM	—	Third–fourth decades	Similar to above, with features of SLE and PSS
P/DM	—	Seventh decade	Similar to above; may be associated with malignancy
Polymyalgia rheumatica	—	Seventh decade	Severe myalgia without weakness
Neuromuscular junction disease			
Myasthenia gravis	—	Second decade in women, fourth–sixth decades in men	Ptosis, difficulty in swallowing or speaking, often weakness in leg or arm muscles, especially after activity
Eaton-Lambert syndrome (carminomatous neuromyopathy)	—	Fifth–seventh decades	Spares cranial muscles; otherwise resembles myasthenia gravis
Muscular dystrophy			
pseudohypertrophic (Duchenne)	Sex-linked recessive	Early childhood	Swayback, a waddling gait, difficulty in rising from the floor and climbing stairs, pelvic girdle muscle weakness
Pseudohypertrophic (Becker)	Sex-linked recessive	Second–third decades	Similar to Duchenne, but milder
Fascioscapulo humeral	autosomal dominant	Childhood young adult	Facial muscle weakness (sparing EOMs), shoulder girdle weakness, often asymmetrical
Limb girdle (includes juvenile dystrophy of ERB)	Autosomal recessive	Any time from first to third decades of life	Usually weakness of the proximal muscles of both the pelvic and shoulder girdles
Muscular dystrophy of late onset	Not known; affects both sexes	Fourth or fifth decade of life	Weakness of the proximal muscles of the pelvic girdle
Myotonia			
myotonic dystrophy (Steinert's disease)	Autosomal dominant	Young adulthood, occasionally as early as puberty	Weakening of hand and forearm muscles, with myotonic stiffness and inability to relax handgrip; eye and tongue muscles often affected

Progression	Muscle Enzyme Elevation	Electromyogram	Muscle Biopsy
Variable, may be mild and chronic, severe and chronic or rapidly fatal; steroid responsive	Yes	Myopathic	Inflammatory
Similar to P/DM; steroid responsive	Yes	Myopathic	Inflammatory
Often steroid responsive	Yes	Myopathic	Inflammatory
Exquisitely steroid sensitive; high association with giant cell arteritis	No	Normal	Normal
Variable, 20% may spontaneously remit	No	Characteristic; may be normal in 40% of cases	Normal
Variable, high association with oat cell carcinoma	No	Characteristic changes; normal EMG excludes diagnosis	Normal
Rapid, ultimately involving all the voluntary muscles; death usually occurs within 10–15 years of clinical onset	Yes	Nonspecifically abnormal	Dystrophic changes
50% survive to age 40	Yes	Nonspecifically abnormal	
Variable, may plateau, some patients severely disabled	Mild	"Myopathic"	"dystrophic" changes, may show inflammatory changes
Variable; some patients live to old age	Yes		May be diagnostic in advanced cases
Variable	Variable	Nonspecifically abnormal	
Variable, but reaches a stage of severe disability 15–20 years after onset; patients rarely attain a normal life span	No	Excellent screening test, "myotonic"	

Polymyalgia Rheumatica

While pain in a muscle is a feature of only 25% of cases of polymyositis, it is the primary complaint of patients with polymyalgia rheumatica (PMR). The patient with PMR is over age 60 and bitterly complains of hip and shoulder girdle pain. The pain is symmetric and not associated with activity. There is neither weakness nor inflammation of muscle. The absence of muscle damage and the presence of an elevated erythrocyte sedimentation rate, with the typical history, are sufficient to confirm the diagnosis of PMR (Chap. 18).

Muscular Dystrophy

Muscular dystrophy may be difficult to distinguish from polymyositis. Weakness is insidious in onset, and pain is not common. The important historic feature is the family history of muscle disease. The CPK may be elevated, and the electromyogram may resemble polymyositis. However, the results of muscle biopsies do not show prominent inflammation. On rare occasions, it is not possible to distinguish polymyositis from muscular dystrophy, and a trial of steroids may be undertaken. Polymyositis usually responds to steroids, whereas muscular dystrophy rarely improves. The salient features of the myopathies are compared in Table 30.1.

Fibrositis

Fibrositis affects persons of middle age with chronic and recurrent pain that is often accentuated by rest and relieved by modest activity. The thigh and lumbar area are frequently involved, as is the shoulder girdle musculature. The diagnosis should be reserved for those persons with no evidence of muscle weakness or damage and with (1) exquisite point tenderness, (2) circumscribed painful hardening in muscle, and (3) reproduction of the pain by palpation of the trigger point. Mechanical impairment is unusual, and the pain is relieved by infiltration with local anesthetic. Pain may recur during emotional stress or sleep deprivation. In spite of the excellent mechanical prognosis, the patient with fibrositis requires a great deal of support and reassurance.

Trauma

Acute muscle strain or trauma is usually asymmetric. Tenderness to palpation is prominent but often poorly localized. Weakness is not a feature. Elevation of CPK may reflect even minimal muscle trauma. Careful search for a precipitating event, the asymmetry of the lesion, and the absence of weakness will help to exclude inflammatory and dystrophic muscle disease.

Vascular Diseases

Atherosclerosis/Arterial Insufficiency

Vascular insufficiency often appears with pain in the lower extremity. The Leriche syndrome is manifested by an aching pain increasing in severity with walking or climbing steps. The pain is appreciated in the buttocks, hip, or thigh and gradually subsides several minutes after exercise. Confusion with articular disease of the hip is understandable, as radiographic evidence of degenerative joint disease is often detectable in the older person with vascular insufficiency of the terminal aorta. The arterial pulses are feeble in the lower extremities and bruits are auscultated over the abdominal aorta, the iliac, or the femoral vessels. Requiring the patient to stoop, lift, or passively moving the hip through its full range of flexion, abduction, and external rotation does not reproduce the pain; the true nature of intermittent claudication will be established by repetitive exercises such as walking or climbing steps.

Aseptic Necrosis

A number of diverse entities may compromise the vascular supply to the bone. Interruption of the blood supply will produce ischemia and ultimate cellular necrosis. Repair is accomplished by revascularization, reossification, and resorption of dead bone. Ischemic necrosis of bone has been variably classified as *avascular, aseptic,* or *ischemic* necrosis. The proximal femur and femoral head are particularly susceptible areas. A variety of entities may cause this condition— fracture or dislocation, infiltrative disease of bone (Gaucher's disease, histiocytosis X), hemoglobinopathies (SS and SC), polycythemia rubra vera, hyperviscosity syndromes, nitrogen emboli (decompression sickness), chronic alcohol abuse, chronic pancreatitis, chronic steroid therapy, and/or systemic lupus erythematosus or rheumatoid arthritis. Clinical manifestations of avascular necrosis of the femoral head are remarkably similar irrespective of the associated disease. The onset of the pain is slow and usually monoarticular. It is worse with activity and weight bearing. Early in the course of the illness, radiographs may not be dramatically abnormal. The earliest radiographic features are best appreciated with an AP view of the pelvis combined with frog-leg lateral views of the hips, as illustrated in Figure 5.20*a* and *b*. Failure to revascularize the femoral head leads ultimately to its fragmentation and collapse, with resultant severe degenerative joint disease. Therapy is conservative and consists of weight reduction and limitation of weight bearing and correction, when possible, of the precipitating entity.

Bone Disease

Severe pain with motion and weight bearing associated with transient osteoporosis of the hip has been variously recorded as *transient osteoporosis of the hip, regional migratory osteoporosis, and migratory osteolysis.* The patients are usually middle-aged men without a history of antecedent trauma. Early radiographs (AP pelvis with lateral hip) may be minimally abnormal and the radioisotope uptake increased on bone scan. The disorder is self-limited, and conservative treatment with nonweight bearing for several months is usually sufficient. The disorder may equally affect the knee or foot, and although it resembles Sudek's atrophy, the precise etiology is not understood. Prognosis for a full recovery is excellent, and it is questionable whether any therapy beyond the limitation of weight bearing is justified. A comparison of vascular and vascular-related phenomena is found in Table 30.2.

Neurologic Conditions

Herniated Nucleus Pulposus

Pain or disability in the lower extremity that is dramatically affected by one's position should arouse suspicion of entrapment or impingement of neurologic

Table 30.2. Vascular and Related Phenomena

Condition	Symptoms	Physical Examination	Ancillary Studies
Vascular insufficiency			
Terminal aorta (Leriche syndrome)	Hip claudication	Bruits, decreased pulses	Arteriography; bone x-rays often show degenerative changes
Femoral vessels	Calf claudication	Decreased pulses	Arteriography
Small vessels	Paresthesias	Delayed capillary filling Loss of dermal appendages	
Embolic phenomena	Abrupt asymmetric pain	Abdominal or femoral bruits Abnormal cardiac exam	Arteriography
Vasculitis	Rarely appears as local phenomenon	Purpura, muscle weakness, neurologic deficits	Biopsy of affected vessels
Thrombophlebitis (compare with ruptured Baker's cyst)	Edema and pain in affected extremity	Minimal pain in thigh and pelvis, positive Homans' in calf (also positive Homans')	Ultrasonography (± venogram)
Avascular necrosis	Insidious hip, knee, or ankle pain	Decreased range of motion; no obvious synovitis	Plane radiographs of affected area
Transient painful osteoporosis	Subacute hip, knee, ankle, or forefoot pain	Decreased range of motion, edema, and erythema over involved foot	Early bone scans show increased uptake

structure. Herniated nucleus pulposus (HNP) or *slipped disc* is characterized by pain of recent onset in the active 30- to 40-year-old person. Sharp, radiating pain exacerbated by stooping, bending forward, lifting, or walking is typical. Exacerbation of the pain may be noted with coughing, sneezing, or defecation. Relief of pain is usually accomplished by bed rest, most commonly with the patient maintaining the hips in the flexed position. The most frequent level of involvement includes first the L5–S1, then the L4–5, and then the combination of L5–S1 and L4–5. The characteristic physical findings (for lesions affecting these disc spaces) are summarized in Table 30.3. Initial plane films of the pelvis and lumbar spine may be normal; myelography may be required to establish the diagnosis. The initial therapy for HNP is conservative and consists of bed rest, anti-inflammatory, and analgesic therapy. Modification of work or recreational habits and use of a corset may accelerate recovery. Severe and incapacitating pain may re-

Table 30.3. Neurologic Conditions Affecting the Lower Extremity

Condition	History	Examination			
		Reflex	Motor	Sensory	Ancillary Study
Herniated nucleus pulposus	S1 (L5–S1): third–fourth decade; abrupt onset, sharp unilateral radiating pain to lower leg	Depressed ankle jerk	Weakness and atrophy of calf	Deficit in lateral border and sole of foot and toes	Myelogram
	L5 (L4–5); same as S1	No deficit	Weakness—toe extensors	Deficit in lateral leg, mediodorsal aspect of foot	Myelogram
	L4 (L3–4); same as S1 and L5	Depressed knee jerk	Weakness—knee extensors	Deficit along shin	Myelogram
Spinal stenosis	Posterior laminar compression, sixth–seventh decade; gradual onset of backache	Rare	Rare	Rare	Myelogram or myelogram + CAT[a]
	Lateral apophyseal root compression, sixth–seventh decade; gradual onset, proximal claudication pain		Several roots involved; findings represent a combination of individual compressed roots		Myelogram or myelogram + CAT[a]
Meralgia paresthetica	Lateral femoral cutaneous nerve, third–fifth decade; burning over anterolateral thigh	No deficit	No change	Normal early, decreased late	Plane x-ray normal
Peroneal nerve	External compression of peroneal nerve at fibular neck or compression in posterior fossa	No deficit	Weakness of dorsiflexion of foot, extension of great toe, eversion of foot	Lower lateral aspect of leg dorsum of foot	Distal slowing only of nervs conduction velocity
Tarsal tunnel syndrome	Posterior tibial nerve entrapped beneath flexor retinaculum; burning pain over sole of foot, worse at night	No deficit; positive Tinnel's sign	Weakness of intrinsic foot musculature; difficult to detect	Deficit over sole of foot, late	Slowing of distal sensory nerve conduction

[a] Computerized axial tomography.

473

quire prolonged bed rest. Immobilization and traction are not universally indicated and should be reserved for cases refractory to conservative therapy. Failure to respond to medical management raises the possibility of surgical intervention.

Other neurologic entities may be confused with HNP. These conditions include neurofibromata, neurolemmoma, and ependymoma, which may involve nerve roots in the lumbar spine. Pain from these entities may resemble that of HNP and require clarification by myelography or myelography combined with computerized axial tomography.

Spinal Stenosis

Narrowing of the bony spinal canal is termed *spinal stenosis*. This condition may occur laterally (apophyseal), compressing emerging nerve roots, or in the midline (produced by laminae), compressing the cauda equina. The pain is often of many months' duration and is typically experienced by patients over age 50. Cauda equinal compression may produce backache only; lateral compression may produce radicular pain. Unlike the radicular pain of disc compression, the pain of lateral spinal stenosis is exacerbated by walking and is localized proximally in the thigh. Unlike claudication, the pain does not promptly resolve with rest. Straight leg raising is rarely restricted. Plane radiographs, and occasionally myelograms, may fail to establish the diagnosis if restriction is limited to the lateral recesses. Myelography combined with computerized axial tomography has been suggested to establish the diagnosis in such cases. Conservative therapy consists of bed rest and anti-inflammatory therapy. As the osteophytic encroachment on the spinal canal may involve several adjacent vertebrae, surgical intervention may be an extensive procedure. The role of surgical intervention for spinal stenosis is not well established at this time.

Meralgic Pain

Meralgia paresthetica is the result of entrapment of the lateral femoral cutaneous nerve beneath the inguinal ligament near the anterior superior iliac spine. Pregnancy, a pendulous abdomen, or a tight belt or corset may precipitate symptoms. Since the nerve is entirely sensory, the patient will complain of paresthesias, burning, and ultimately sensory deficits over the anterolateral thigh. Rest and removal of the offending belt or corset usually provide relief; surgical decompression is rarely required.

Bursitis

Irritation and inflammation of the bursae in the hip area may superficially mimic articular pain. As a general rule, periarticular inflammation, that is, tendinitis/bursitis, will produce discretely localized tenderness. In addition, pain may be reproduced by putting the articular structure through only one of its several ranges of motion. In contrast, pain due to synovitis in the hip usually produces pain throughout all the normal ranges of motion.

Trochanteric Bursitis

The pain of trochanteric bursitis is aggravated, in the standing position, by external rotation of the extremity; flexion and extension of the affected extremity are not painful. The pain may be referred down the lateral aspect of the calf and is characteristically exacerbated when the patient lies on the affected side. Tenderness to palpation is usually localized to a 2-cm circular area over the greater trochanter. The history of antecedent trauma is obtainable in the minority of cases. Infiltration of the area with a local anesthetic and sustained-release steroids produces prompt relief.

Ischial Bursitis

Weaver's bottom refers to inflammation of the bursa overlying the ischial tuberosity. The bursa is under the gluteus maximus muscle while standing; when sitting, the bursa is not protected by the gluteus musculature. The pain in the buttock is therefore exacerbated by sitting, and flexion of the hip is often painful. The painful hip with flexion may force the patient to shorten the stride and produce a shuffling gait. Identification and palpation of the painful area are facilitated with the patient on the side with the hips flexed. As in trochanteric bursitis, the radiographs are usually normal in ischial bursitis. A combination of anti-inflammatory therapy, local infiltration with steroids, and several days' rest may be required to alleviate the symptoms of ischial bursitis. The mechanical and traumatic phenomena affecting the lower extremity are compared in Table 30.4.

Systemic Conditions

Many patients will experience anxiety when the clinician is not promptly able to establish a diagnosis after consideration of the entities described above. Additional confusion of the picture by emotional overtones is a frequent problem. A purely psychogenically induced back or hip pain, however, is unusual. If the diagnosis is not clear after a symptomatic evaluation of the muscular, vascular, neurologic, periarticular, and articular structures, one must consider systemic problems with local manifestation of systemic or visceral disease. In this unusual situation, the history will establish that viscerogenic pain is not aggravated by activity or relieved by rest. Physical examination will confirm a painless full range of motion in the periarticular and articular structures; the examiner will then continue the evaluation with a pelvic and rectal exam. In the absence of a local genitourinary or gastrointestinal explanation, one must consider metabolic and infiltrative bone disease. Such diverse entities as osteomalacia, osteoporosis, hyperparathyroidism, Paget's disease of bone, myeloma, and metastatic malignancies should be included in the differential diagnosis.

Only when one has failed to establish a diagnosis and must consider these diverse problems should one resort to profile laboratory screens and survey radiographs. When confronted with a patient who has pain with no readily explicable cause, our initial evaluation includes a complete blood count with a differential count and sedimentation rate, urinalysis, and serum creatinine, calcium, phosphorous, serum protein electrophoresis, acid and alkaline phosphatase, and lipoprotein electrophoresis and thyroid function studies. Survey radiographs include the affected painful area plus an AP pelvis and a PA and lateral chest film. A normal screen of this type will exclude most of the previously mentioned diverse systemic problems that may appear with pelvic or hip pain. With such normal

Table 30.4. Mechanical Problems

Condition	Symptoms	Physical Examination	Ancillary Study
Bursitis			
"Weaver's bottom"	Pain on sitting	Focal tenderness over ischial tuberosity, normal range of motion in hip	plane radiographs of affected area
Trochanteric bursitis	Pain with external rotation of limb	Focal tenderness over greater trochanter, normal range of motion in hip	plane radiographs of affected area
"Housemaid's knee"	Pain over prepatellar bursa on extension of knee	Focal prepatellar swelling, normal range of motion in knee	plane radiographs of affected area
Anserine bursitis	Pain on climbing steps	Pain under insertion of sartorius, medial aspect of knee, normal range of motion in knee	plane radiographs of affected area
"Pump bumps"	Pain with dorsi-plantar flexion of foot	Focal pain under Achilles tendon	plane radiographs of affected area
(compare with Achilles tendinitis)	(similar)	(tendon is tender) (normal range of motion in ankle for both)	
"Policeman's heels"	Pain with ambulation	Pain with pressure on calcaneal bursa, normal range of motion in ankle	plane radiographs of affected area
Trauma			
Knee	Acute pain, swelling, limitation of motion	Focal instability early, general loss of motion late	Arthrocentesis serosanguinous fluid with rare WBC
Ankle	Acute pain, swelling, limitation of motion	Focal instability early, generalized edema and limitation of motion late	"Stress x-ray"
Anterior compartment	Pain over anterior compartment (antero-lateral calf)	Crepitance, erythema over peroneal musculature	plane radiographs of affected area

tests, we reassure the patient and do not hesitate to offer a reevaluation in 2–4 months, should the condition deteriorate or change in any fashion.

KNEE AND CALF PAIN AND DISABILITY

Muscular

Posterior Compartment Injuries

Acute pain of the calf musculature is a common sequel of trauma. *Tennis leg* refers to partial rupture of one of the calf muscles, often the plantaris or a belly of the gastrocnemius. The history includes a "snap" with a sudden burning pain in the calf during vigorous muscular contraction. This condition is not unique to tennis but may follow any explosive start-and-stop motions. The physical exam discloses tenderness to palpation extending along the calf muscle to the popliteal space and blood pooling about the ankle, visible in fascial planes. The pain is exacerbated by dorsiflexion of the foot. Conservative treatment consists of rest and immobilization of the ankle for several weeks.

Anterior Compartment Injuries

The *anterior tibial compartment syndrome* describes edema and inflammation in the anterior compartment. The history includes a repetitive dorsiplantar motion of the ankle (running), and the patient describes exquisite pain over one or both anterior compartments lateral to the proximal two-thirds of the tibia. Crepitance and erythema may be appreciated over the anterior compartment with dorsiflexion of the foot. Edematous muscle, in this confined space, may further compromise the vascular supply to muscle and the deep peroneal nerve. Therapy consists of rest, anti-inflammatory therapy, and often fasciotomy to relieve pressure. Pain in the anterior compartment may occur with minimal swelling and without the dire consequences of the frank anterior compartment syndrome; *shin splints* probably belong in this latter category.

Popliteal Cyst

Acute unilateral painful swelling in the gastrocnemius area may occur in a setting of chronic or recurring effusions in the synovial compartment of the adjacent knee. The synovial effusion may have been the result of either internal derangement of the knee or inflammatory synovitis. The acute swelling often appears in the absence of unusually vigorous exercise or trauma. Warmth is appreciated over the painful area, the calf is greater in circumference than its neighbor, and there is pain with dorsiflexion of the foot. Radiopaque dye injected into the synovial space of the knee will appear in the Baker's cyst in the popliteal space and distally adjacent to the gastrocnemius musculature. Rest and treatment of the synovial inflammation with intra-articular steroids often obviate the need for surgery. Deep vein thrombois also appears with a painful, warm, swollen calf that is made more painful with dorsiflexion of the foot (Homans' sign). The differential between deep vein thrombosis and dissecting Baker's cyst can be difficult. We hesitate to undertake venography with its well-known potential to initiate deep vein thrombosis. Detection of patent deep veins and venous flow with ultrasonography has been useful in the hands of experienced persons. In the painful swollen calf with no detectable deep venous flow via ultrasonography and no obvious distension of the popliteal space, we have assumed a diagnosis of deep vein thrombosis and treated it accordingly.

Vascular Diseases

Atherosclerosis

Arterial compromise or inflammation may cause pain in the lower extremity. Atheromatous vascular disease may produce the typical intermittent claudication described for the Leriche syndrome. More dramatic may be the sequel of atheromatous emboli. A large embolus with obvious perfusion defects presents no diagnostic difficulty. Showers of small emboli may be more subtle and induce calf muscle inflammation with mechanical obliteration of the vascular supply or with inflammatory changes. Cholesterol crystals may activate the complement cascade, induce vascular inflammation, and secondarily produce muscle inflammation. The calf is tender to palpation with either mode of vascular compromise. The CPK may be elevated, and inflammatory cellular infiltrates are noted on biopsy.

Vasculitis

Generalized inflammation in medium-sized arteries (polyarteritis nodosa, PAN) may affect the musculature of the calf, producing acute pain, or the peripheral nerves, producing mononeuritis multiplex. Symptoms of PAN are rarely localized to one extremity and usually reflect multisystem disease (Chap. 18). Biopsy of the involved muscle or nerve will show the typical panarteritis. We have stressed the pain and disability of calf musculature due primarily to a vascular phenomenon; the corollary is that isolated distal muscle pain and disability are not common features of primary myopathic illness, that is, polymyositis or polymyalgia rheumatica.

Bone Diseases

Transient painful osteoporosis or migratory osteolysis may affect the knee, like the hip. Avascular necrosis of the distal femur may also be a source of pain and disability in the knee. For both of these illnesses, the precipitating features, associated phenomena, management, and prognosis are similar to those for the same entities in the hip.

Neurologic Conditions

Neurologic deficits in the lower extremity may represent the referred pain of more proximal phenomena (e.g., HNP) or local phenomena.

Entrapment Neuropathies

Both the posterior tibial and peroneal nerves may be compromised near the knee. The posterior tibial nerve may be entrapped by a mass lesion in the popliteal fossa, the most common being a Baker's cyst. Entrapment occurs more commonly at the medial aspect of the ankle, involving the plantar nerve and the terminal branches of the posterior tibial nerve. The physical findings and the differentiation of proximal versus distal injury to the posterior tibial nerve will be discussed nerve may be trapped by the same phenomena that compromise the posterior tibial nerve; however, it is more often subject to external trauma as it courses near the fibular neck. The peroneal nerve may be involved more often than the posterior tibial with the various vasculitis syndromes. Compression of the peroneal nerve against the fibular neck occurs in the obtunded patient with the leg resting against a bedrail or other unforgiving surface. It may also occur in the trauma patient with a swollen extremity and an unusually tight cast. The compromised peroneal nerve produces weakness and dorsiflexion of the foot, extension of the great toe, and eversion of the foot; inversion is usually strong, differentiating peroneal nerve injury from L5 root compression. Sensation is diminished over the lateral aspect of the lower leg and the dorsum of the foot. Remembrance of the precipitating factors of peroneal nerve injury and avoidance of such factors are encouraged. Functional recovery, even with a release procedure, cannot be guaranteed.

The peroneal nerve may be trapped by the same phenomena that compromise the posterior tibial nerve under "Foot and Ankle Conditions." Within the popliteal fossa, the peroneal

Mechanical Injuries

Internal Knee Derangements

Periarticular structures are particularly subject to trauma at the knee. The inherent unstable configuration of the knee places tremendous requirements on the supporting structures. We will emphasize only the general principles of investigation of knee injuries.

Precision in diagnosis of knee injury is best obtained within minutes of the injury; the isolated instability of a medial collateral ligament tear may be appreciated only in the first 30 minutes after the insult. A precise history is useful in evaluating the knee injury. The soccer player or football player struck from the rear or from the side is subject to medial collateral ligament tear, medial meniscus tear, and cruciate tear. Tenderness over the medial collateral ligament implies damage to that ligament but obviously does not exclude damage to menisci or cruciates. Instability is best assessed by examining the unaffected knee first to establish the normal range of motion and laxity. Comparison with the injured knee may then reveal subtle increases of motion due to tearing of the collateral ligament or cruciate. Examination of synovial fluid is helpful; grossly hemorrhagic fluid is unlikely in an isolated meniscus or collateral ligament tear and suggests a cruciate tear or fracture. Hemorrhagic fluid with fat globules suggests a fracture. Arthrography may be required to establish the nature of an internal derangement. Severe pain over the lateral aspect of the knee near the fibular head is commonly encountered in runners. Unusually tight lateral collateral and fibular collateral ligaments contribute to the pain; many runners have been able to avoid such injuries with expansion of their stretching exercises.

Patellar Injuries

Injuries to the patella are a common source of impairment in extension. Lateral dislocation of the patella may occur in the setting of a shallow lateral femoral condyle, shallow patellar groove, marked genu valgum, or laxity of the extensor mechanism. Women are more commonly affected than men. Symptoms include a tendency for the knee to buckle, accompanied by pain and occasionally mild effusion. Therapy has included changing the line of quadriceps pull, strengthening the quadriceps pull, and restoring the depth of the femoral sulcus. Recurrent patellar dislocation plays a role in development of *chondromalacia patellae*. This term denotes the painful conditions arising from cartilaginous abnormalities of the posterior aspect of the patella. Patients are young persons who complain of retropatellar pain exacerbated by climbing stairs or rising from a chair; stiffness and crepitance may be noted after prolonged sitting. Pain and crepitance are elicited by downward pressure on the patella during a forced quadriceps contraction. Effusions are rare; both plane radiographs and arthrograms are normal except in advanced cases. Conservative therapy of nonweight bearing, physical therapy to prevent quadriceps atrophy, and anti-inflammatory drugs are beneficial. Indications for surgical intervention are not universally agreed upon for either patellar dislocation or chondromalacia patellae.

Bursitis

Prepatellar Bursitis

The descriptive term *housemaid's knee* emphasizes the role of kneeling and pressure in the initiation of prepatellar bursitis. Warmth, erythema, and swelling in the prepatellar bursa are common; there is no loss of motion. Rest and local infiltration with steroids will produce prompt relief. Recurrences are common even if undue pressure in the prepatellar area is avoided. Recalcitrant cases may require long-leg splinting to protect the bursa from the trauma of flexion-extension motion in the knee. Infrapatellar bursitis usually occurs from overactivity with undue friction against the upper tibia. Tenderness is elicited by pressure behind the infrapatellar tendon and from passive forced flexion and active extension of the knee. Conservative therapy consists of aspiration and immobilization.

Anserine bursitis

Anserine bursitis is due to inflammation of the bursa under the insertion of the sartorius muscle on the medial aspect of the proximal tibia. Pain is typically elicited when climbing stairs. As in the previously discussed bursitis syndromes, there is no loss of motion or instability in the joint, and conservative therapy is sufficient.

In our discussion of pain and disability of the knee and calf, we have deemphasized the role of ancillary studies. Plane radiographs of the knee are normal in the vast majority of the previously described entities, and only rarely, for example, in arthrogragraphy for Baker's cyst dissection, will additional studies be necessary. The history should suggest the diagnosis, and a knowledgeable physical examination will provide confirmation.

FOOT AND ANKLE CONDITIONS

Vascular Disease

The distal lower extremity, foot and ankle, is commonly affected by vascular insufficiency and may exhibit the same intermittent claudication as the calf. Inflammation in small blood vessels may involve the ankle and foot. Manifestations include purpura, small ulcers, and occasionally a "stocking glove" dysesthesia from damage to superficial nerves. The differential diagnosis for small vessel inflammation is the same in the foot and ankle as in other areas of the body.

Bone Disease

Avascular necrosis may affect the ankle but much less commonly than the hip or knee. Transient painful osteoporosis or migratory osteolysis may involve the foot, like the hip, and enjoys the same favorable prognosis.

Neurologic Conditions

Neurologic defects in the ankle and foot may be local or reflect more proximal damage. The local phenomena will be discussed. The reader is referred to Table 30.2 for differentiation of local from proximal problems.

Entrapment Neuropathies

The posterial tibial nerve may be damaged in the foot and ankle, producing two separate syndromes. The first is the tarsal tunnel syndrome—entrapment of the posterior tibial nerve within the fibro-osseous canal beneath the flexor retinaculum in the medial side of the ankle. The patient complains of burning pain and dysesthesia over the toes and the entire sole of the foot. As in carpal tunnel syndrome, the pain may be worse at night, and a positive Tinnel's sign is present in the vast majority of cases. Motor findings are particularly difficult to assess in the foot. Sensory nerve conduction may be useful in documenting delayed conduction. As in carpal tunnel syndrome, surgical intervention with a release procedure may provide relief.

The second entrapment syndrome involving branches of the posterior tibial nerve is plantar nerve compression. This condition reflects entrapment of the terminal branches of the posterior tibial nerve as they course around the medial edge of the foot. The complaints, findings, and conduction studies are often similar to those of the tarsal tunnel syndrome. Occasionally, diagnosis may be made only after a negative exploration of the tarsal tunnel and extension of the same surgical procedure to the terminal portion of the nerve.

Morton's neuroma refers to an interdigital neuroma. This condition is a fusiform enlargement in a digital nerve, commonly located between or distal to the heads of the third and fourth metatarsal bones. It is usually unilateral and produces pain that is sharp or burning, occurring initially with activity and later also at rest. The typical feature of the history is the release of pain obtained when the shoe is removed and the foot is massaged. Sharply localized tenderness is characteristic. Occasionally, soft tissue swelling may be noted in the area of the pain. The location of the tenderness between or distal to the metatarsal heads allows differentiation from abnormalities in the metatarsophalangeal joint. Occasionally, altered sensation may be found over the lateral aspect of the third toe and the medial aspect of the fourth toe. Successful therapy involves supporting the transverse arch of the foot in a suitable broad shoe. Local infiltration with steroid therapy may often provide transient relief. However, surgical excision of the neuroma may ultimately be required.

Mechanical Injuries

Trauma plays a prominent role in irritation, inflammation, and disruption of the periarticular structures of the ankle and foot.

Ankle Sprains

Ankle sprain is a very common cause of pain in the ankle. Forceful inversion of the plantar-flexed ankle causes undue stress on the lateral collateral ligaments. Similar force with eversion produces stress on the medial collateral ligament. Excessive force usually occurs during athletic events or when running or walking over uneven ground. The physical examination of the injured ankle is most precise immediately after the injury. With increasing time, swelling and ecchymoses obscure the physical findings, and the patient's recollection of details becomes vague. The diagnosis of sprain implies the rupture of some of the fibers of the supporting ligament but also implies that the continuity of the ligament remains intact. This diagnosis therefore excludes complete rupture of the ligament, avulsion of the ligament, dislocation, or fracture.

Inversion injury, with lateral collateral ligament damage, is more common than eversion injury. The physical examination will confirm tenderness to palpation immediately distal to the lateral malleolus. Plantar or dorsiflexion is not limited. Inversion is limited and painful; one should not be able to invert the ankle beyond its normal range of motion. With a partial ligamentous tear, the talus remains in the appropriate position and no gap can be palpated between the talus and the lateral malleolus. Complete tearing often allows excessive inversion, and a sulcus may be palpated between the talus and the lateral malleolus. Protective spasm may mask unusual laxity, and the value of a radiographic examination of the acutely injured ankle cannot be overemphasized. Plane films should be obtained with the ankle in the neutral position and repeated with the examiner attempting to stress the ankle in the direction of the precipitating injury. Malalignment may then be detected as the ankle, injured in inversion, is further inverted by the examiner; comparison with the uninjured ankle on the opposite side will establish a normal range of motion for the joint. The radiographic approach will thus identify complete tearing with excessive joint laxity, as well as avulsion of the distal fibula or significant dislocation. The treatment of inversion injuries is conservative and consists of immobilization, elevation, and cooling in the first 48 hours. Any suggestion of excessive instability on physical examination or radiographic evaluation merits a prompt orthopedic evaluation.

Eversion injury may often cause bony damage as well as spraining or tearing of the medial collateral ligament. The medial collateral ligament is so sturdy that severe force will often cause fracture or evulsion of the tibia before a significant ligament tear. The physical findings are similar to those of inversion sprain; however, the tenderness to palpation will be appreciated immediately distal to the medial malleolus. The radiographic approach is also similar. Because of the greater propensity for bony damage and disruption of normal joint architecture, we encourage an orthopedic evaluation as quickly as possible after significant eversion injury. An additional source of instability with damage to the medial ligament subsequent to eversion is injury to the tibiofibular ligament. A tear in this ligament permits the ankle to widen and further produces an unstable ankle joint. The radiographic evaluation of a tibiofibular tear will demonstrate a widened joint space between the distal tibia and fibula. The pathognomonic sign of tibiofibular tear is widening of the joint space between the medial border of the talus and the medial malleolus. This sign may occasionally be missed on the routine anteroposterior view of the ankle. An oblique view, when compared with the unaffected ankle, will often reveal the separation. The cursory examination of the acutely injured ankle often leads to an underestimation of the extent of damage. It cannot be overemphasized that one must have a high index of suspicion of significant tearing or dislocation and must be aware of the appropriate radiographic techniques. The prompt evaluation by an orthopedist is to be encouraged in all but the most insignificant injuries to the ankle.

It is noteworthy that the enthesopathy of Reiter's disease may also appear with an asymmetric arthritis and periarticular inflammation of the foot and ankle.

Bursitis/Tendinitis

Achilles Tendinitis and Bursitis

Injury to the Achilles tendon may occur after violent exercise such as sprinting or jumping in volleyball or basketball. There may be a partial tear at the musculotendinous junction or avulsion at the attachment of the calcaneus. Erythema and pain may be apparent with acute injury. However, with chronic injury and irritation, edema around the tendon is often prominent. Pain is particularly pronounced with passive but vigorous dorsiflexion of the foot. Therapy consists of rest and immobilization with the foot in plantar flexion. Surgical intervention is usually required for extensive or complete tears.

Irritation of the bursa underlying the Achilles tendon may be precipitated by the same injury that initiates Achilles tendinitis. The bursa may also be irritated by particularly tight-fitting shoes and has led to the descriptive term *pump bumps*. Conservative therapy is indicated for Achilles bursitis, as for Achilles tendinitis.

Calcaneal Bursitis

Policeman's heel stresses the role of pressure in prolonged ambulation in the production of calcaneal bursitis. The tenderness is immediately below the calcaneus. Pressure produces exquisite pain. Reduction in weight bearing may be all that is required to relieve the irritation of calcaneal bursitis. Should this remedy fail, injection as has previously been described for the bursitis syndrome seems appropriate. Irritation of the periosteal structures at the calcaneus is often associated with Reiter's disease and may, if prolonged, initiate typical radiographic features of the heel spur.

Plantar Fasciitis

Plantar fasciitis is a common occurrence in Reiter's disease and is also a feature of occupations that entail excessive walking. Pain and tenderness beneath the anterior portion of the heel radiating to the sole are usually the apparent complaints. Examination reveals a point of deep tenderness at the anterior medial aspect of the calcaneus at the point of attachment of the plantar fascia. Treatment is usually directed to alleviating the pressure of weight bearing. Raising the heel one-quarter inch removes the tension placed on the calcaneus by the Achilles tendon and releases the tension placed on the fascia by plantar flexion of the forefoot. As in the previously described tendinitis/bursitis syndromes, local infiltration with steroids and local analgesics often provides dramatic relief. Unfortunately, recurrence is common unless the aggravating stimuli are removed or modified.

Successful evaluation of the foot and ankle, as with the knee and hip, relies predominantly on the history and physical examination. As with the hip and knee, we have stressed recognition of the phenomena, the initial conservative therapy where appropriate, and the need for modification of the precipitating activity.

BIBLIOGRAPHY

Cailliet R: *Foot and Ankle Pain*. Philadelphia, FA Davis Co, 1968.

Cailliet R: *Knee Pain and Disability*. Philadelphia, FA Davis Co, 1973.

Cailliet R: *Soft Tissue Pain and Disability*. Philadelphia, FA Davis Co, 1977.

Fessel WJ: Muscle diseases in rheumatology. *Semin Arthritis Rheum* 3:127, 1973.

Hunder GG, Kelly PJ: Roentgenologic transient osteoporosis of the hip. *Ann Intern Med* 68:539, 1968.

Kopell HP, Thompson WAL: *Peripheral Entrapment Neuropathies*. Baltimore, Williams & Wilkins Co, 1963.

MacNab I: *Backache*. Baltimore, Williams & Wilkins Co, 1977.

Marcus ND, Enneking WF, Massam RA: The silent hip in idiopathic aseptic necrosis. *J Bone Joint Surg* 55A:1351, 1973.

Polley HG, Hunder GG: *Physical Examination of the Joints*. Philadelphia, WB Saunders Co, Ltd 1978.

Rowland LP, Layser RB: Muscular dystrophies, atrophies and related diseases, in Baker AB (ed): *Clinical Neurology*. Hagerstown, Md, Harper & Row Publishers Inc, 1977.

Index